CLINICAL PRIMER OF RHEUMATOLOGY

CLINICAL PRIMER OF RHEUMATOLOGY

Editors

WILLIAM J. KOOPMAN, M.D.
Professor and Chairman
Department of Medicine
University of Alabama at Birmingham
Birmingham, Alabama

DENNIS W. BOULWARE, M.D.
Professor
Department of Medicine
University of Alabama at Birmingham
Birmingham, Alabama

GUSTAVO R. HEUDEBERT, M.D.
Associate Professor
Department of Medicine and School of Public Health
University of Alabama at Birmingham
Birmingham, Alabama

LIPPINCOTT WILLIAMS & WILKINS
A **Wolters Kluwer** Company
Philadelphia • Baltimore • New York • London
Buenos Aires • Hong Kong • Sydney • Tokyo

Acquisitions Editor: Rich Winters
Developmental Editor: Brigitte P. Wilke
Production Editor: Jonathan Geffner
Manufacturing Manager: Benjamin Rivera
Cover Designer: Christine Jenny
Compositor: Lippincott Williams & Wilkins Desktop Division
Printer: Maple Press

Library of Congress Cataloging-in-Publication Data
Clinical primer of rheumatology / by William J. Koopman, Dennis W. Boulware,
Gustavo R. Heudebert.
    p. ; cm.
  Includes bibliographical references and index.
  ISBN 0-683-30648-0
  1. Rheumatism. 2. Rheumatology. I. Koopman, William J. II. Boulware, Dennis W.
III. Heudebert, Gustavo R.
  [DNLM: 1. Rheumatic Diseases. 2. Arthritis, Infectious. 3. Complex Regional Pain
Syndromes. WE 544 C6409 2003]
RC927.C535 2003
616.7'23—dc21

                  2002034037

Where would we be without our beloved wives, Lillianne Koopman, Diane Boulware, and Carmen Heudebert, and our families? For their endless love, support, patience, understanding, and tolerance of our absences as we developed this book and our careers, this book is dedicated to all of them.

CONTENTS

CONTRIBUTING AUTHORS

Graciela S. Alarcón, M.D., M.P.H. Jane Knight Lowe Chair, Professor, Department of Medicine, Division of Rheumatology, The University of Alabama at Birmingham, Birmingham, Alabama

Roy D. Altman, M.D. Professor, Department of Medicine, University of Miami; Clinical Director, Geriatrics Research, Education and Clinical Center, Miami Veterans Affairs Medical Center, Miami, Florida

Frank C. Arnett, Jr., M.D. Professor and Chairman, Department of Internal Medicine, University of Texas School at Houston; Chief, Department of Internal Medicine, Memorial Hermann Hospital, Houston, Texas

J. D. Bartleson, M.D. Associate Professor, Department of Neurology, Mayo Medical School; Consultant, Department of Neurology, St. Mary's Hospital, Rochester, Minnesota

Michael A. Becker, M.D. Professor, Department of Medicine, University of Chicago Prtizker Medical School; Attending Physician, Department of Medicine, University of Chicago Hospitals, Chicago, Illinois

Robert M. Bennett, M.D. Professor, Department of Medicine, Oregon Health and Science University, Portland, Oregon

Joseph J. Biundo, M.D. Medical Director, Department of Physical Medicine and Rehabilitation, Kenner Regional Medical Center, Kenner, Louisiana

Dennis W. Boulware, M.D. Professor, Department of Medicine, Division of Rheumatology, The University of Alabama at Birmingham, Birmingham, Alabama

Stephanie Ann Call, M.D., M.S.P.H. Assistant Professor, Department of Medicine, University of Louisville, Louisville, Kentucky

W. Winn Chatham, M.D. Associate Professor, Department of Medicine, Division of Rheumatology, The University of Alabama at Birmingham; Clinical Director, University of Alabama at Birmingham Arthritis and Musculoskeletal Center, Birmingham, Alabama

Marta L. Cuellar, M.D. Associate Professor, Department of Medicine, Tulane Health Sciences Center, New Orleans, Louisiana

Martha R. Curry, M.S., R.N., C.P.N.P. Instructor, Department of Pediatrics, Division of Rheumatology, Baylor College of Medicine; Pediatric Nurse Practitioner, Division of Pediatric Rheumatology, Texas Children's Hospital, Houston, Texas

John J. Cush, M.D. Chief, Rheumatology and Clinical Immunology, Department of Internal Medicine, Presbyterian Hospital of Dallas, Dallas, Texas

Filip De Keyser, M.D. Department of Rheumatology, University Hospital, Ghent, Belgium

M. Franklin Dolwick, D.M.D., Ph.D. Chairman, Department of Oral and Maxillofacial Surgery, University of Florida College of Dentistry; Chairman, Department of Hospital Dentistry, Shands at the University of Florida, Gainesville, Florida

N. Lawrence Edwards, M.D. Professor and Program Director, Department of Medicine, University of Florida; Clinical Chief, Department of Rheumatology, Shands Hospital at the University of Florida, Gainesville, Florida

Luis R. Espinoza, M.D. Professor and Chief, Department of Medicine, Section of Rheumatology, Louisiana State University Health Sciences Center, New Orleans, Louisiana

Allan Gibofsky, M.D., J.D. Professor, Departments of Medicine and Public Health, Weill Medical College of Cornell University; Attending Rheumatologist, Department of Rheumatology, Hospital for Special Surgery, New York, New York

James T. Halla, M.D. Abilene, Texas

Joe G. Hardin, M.D. Professor, Department of Internal Medicine, Division of Rheumatology, University of South Alabama College of Medicine; Attending Physician, Department of Internal Medicine, University of South Alabama Hospitals, Mobile, Alabama

Gustavo R. Heudebert, M.D. Associate Professor, Department of Medicine and School of Public Health; Director, Internal Medicine Residency Training Program, The University of Alabama at Birmingham, Birmingham, Alabama

Kenneth A. Jaffe, M.D.   American Sports Medicine Institute; Alabama Sports Medicine and Orthopedic Center, Birmingham, Alabama

Bruce A. Julian, M.D.   Professor, Department of Medicine, Division of Nephrology, The University of Alabama at Birmingham; Active Staff, Department of Medicine, University of Alabama Hospital, Birmingham, Alabama

Arthur Kavanaugh, M.D.   Professor; Department of Medicine; Division of Rheumatology, Allergy, and Immunology; University of California at San Diego, San Diego, California

Janet M. Kim, M.D.   Assistant Professor, Department of Medicine, University of California, San Diego School of Medicine, La Jolla, California

Ramesh Kumar, M.D.   Fellow, Department of Medicine, Division of Clinical Immunology and Rheumatology, University of Alabama at Birmingham Medical School, Birmingham, Alabama

Peter E. Lipsky, M.D.   Scientific Director, National Institute of Arthritis and Musculoskeletal and Skin Diseases, National Institutes of Health, Bethesda, Maryland

Michael D. Lockshin, M.D.   Professor, Departments of Medicine and Obstetrics–Gynecology, Joan and Sanford Weill Medical College of Cornell University; Director, Barbara Volcker Center for Women and Rheumatic Disease, Co-Director, Mary Kirkland Center for Lupus Research, Hospital for Special Surgery, New York, New York

Carlos J. Lozada, M.D.   Associate Professor, Department of Medicine, Director, Rheumatology Training Program, Division of Rheumatology and Immunology, University of Miami School of Medicine; Attending Physician, Department of Medicine, Director, Rheumatology Outpatient and Consultation Services, Jackson Memorial Hospital, Miami, Florida

Maren Lawson Mahowald, M.D.   Professor, Department of Internal Medicine, University of Minnesota; Rheumatology Section Chief, Department of Internal Medicine, Minneapolis VA Medical Center, Minneapolis, Minnesota

Thomas A. Medsger, Jr., M.D.   Professor, Department of Medicine, University of Pittsburgh School of Medicine; Division of Rheumatology and Clinical Immunology, University of Pittsburgh Medical Center, Pittsburgh, Pennsylvania

Herman Mielants, M.D.   Professor, Department of Rheumatology, University Hospital, Ghent, Belgium

Frederick W. Miller, M.D., Ph.D.   Chief, Environmental Autoimmunity Group, Office of Clinical Research, National Institute of Environmental Health Sciences, National Institutes of Health, Bethesda, Maryland

Gerald F. Moore, M.D.   Professor, Department of Internal Medicine, Section of Rheumatology and Immunology, University of Nebraska Medical Center, Omaha, Nebraska

Sarah L. Morgan, M.D., R.D.   Professor of Nutrition Sciences and Medicine, Department of Nutrition Sciences, The University of Alabama at Birmingham; Medical Director, University of Alabama at Birmingham Osteoporosis Prevention and Treatment Clinic, The Kirklin Clinic, Birmingham, Alabama

Barry L. Myones, M.D.   Associate Professor, Departments of Pediatrics and Immunology, Baylor College of Medicine; Director of Research, Pediatric Rheumatology Center, Texas Children's Hospital, Houston, Texas

Kenneth K. Nakano, M.D., M.P.H., S.M.   Neurologist, Department of Neurology, Straub Beretania Clinic, Honolulu, Hawaii

James R. O'Dell, M.D.   Professor and Vice Chairman, Department of Internal Medicine; Chief, Section of Rheumatology and Immunology, University of Nebraska Medical Center, Omaha, Nebraska

Maria D. Perez, M.D.   Associate Professor, Department of Pediatrics, Baylor College of Medicine; Texas Children's Hospital, Houston, Texas

Michelle Petri, M.D., M.P.H.   Professor, Department of Rheumatology, Johns Hopkins Hospital, Baltimore, Maryland

Perry J. Rush, M.D.   Assistant Professor, Department of Medicine, University of Toronto; Staff Physician, Department of Medicine, St. John's Rehabilitation Hospital, North York, Ontario, Canada

Kenneth G. Saag, M.D., M.Sc.   Associate Professor, Department of Medicine, Division of Clinical Immunology and Rheumatology, The University of Alabama at Birmingham, Birmingham, Alabama

Kenneth E. Sack, M.D.   Professor of Clinical Medicine, Director of Clinical Programs in Rheumatology, Department of Medicine, University of California at San Francisco, San Francisco, California

Randy R. Sibbitt, M.D.   Director, Neuroradiology, Department of Radiology, St. Peter's Hospital, Helena, Montana

Wilmer L. Sibbitt, Jr., M.D.   Professor of Rheumatology and Neurology, Department of Internal Medicine, University of New Mexico Health Sciences Center, Albuquerque, New Mexico

Eric M. Veys, M.D. Department of Rheumatology, University Hospital, Ghent, Belgium

Robert W. Warren, M.D., Ph.D., M.P.H. Associate Professor, Department of Pediatrics, Baylor College of Medicine; Chief, Department of Rheumatology, Texas Children's Hospital, Houston, Texas

Andrew P. Wilking, M.D. Associate Professor, Department of Pediatrics, Baylor College of Medicine; Active Staff, Department of Pediatrics, Texas Children's Hospital, Houston, Texas

Yusuf Yazici, M.D. Clinical Assistant Professor, Department of Medicine, State University of New York; Attending Physician, Department of Rheumatology, Long Island College Hospital, Brooklyn, New York

PREFACE

The impetus for *Clinical Primer of Rheumatology* was the recent trends in clinical medicine that created a need for such a book. Extraordinary scientific advances in the treatment of rheumatic diseases recently have been made. These new discoveries have generated an enthusiasm for the treatment of rheumatic diseases, the like of which has not been seen since the discovery of cortisone. The prevalence of arthritis and associated conditions continues to increase, making it a part of every clinician's practice. Finally, the increased pace of clinical medicine demands that clinicians have practical clinical information readily available at their fingertips, and in a format that is easily digestible and ready for clinical use. With these trends in mind, *Clinical Primer of Rheumatology* was planned to meet the clinician's needs and was based on a similar blueprint used for another successful textbook, *Arthritis and Allied Conditions: A Textbook of Rheumatology*.

To meet the needs of the busy clinician, the chapters are arranged in a manner that facilitates accessing information easily and quickly. Early chapters address patient problems that present themselves as a complaint and may be the result of a sports-related consequence or an occupational consequence. Patients are usually seen in the initial visit with a regional problem—low back pain, painful feet, or knee pain. These chapters are written in a manner intended to guide the clinician to a specific diagnosis quickly and efficiently.

Most of the chapters are arranged by diagnosis and are clustered by the pathologic mechanism—such as autoimmune-mediated diseases, degenerative diseases, arthritides resulting from metabolic causes, and infectious arthropathies. These chapters will lead the reader through the relevant epidemiology, pertinent pathology, clinical evaluation, therapy, and prevention.

The final section addresses special therapeutic considerations, including the use and monitoring of medication commonly used in rheumatology cases, and techniques of arthrocentesis and injection therapy.

We deeply appreciate the time and efforts of the many authors who have contributed toward this new textbook and shared their knowledge, skills, and clinical judgment for the benefit of all of our patients.

William J. Koopman, M.D.
Dennis W. Boulware, M.D.
Gustavo R. Heudebert, M.D.
Birmingham, Alabama

ACKNOWLEDGMENTS

Our deepest appreciation is extended to Brigitte P. Wilke, Developmental Editor, for her excellent nurturing and guidance through this first edition and also to Richard Winters and Danette Knopp, Acquisitions Editors, for their patience, encouragement, and advice. Ms. Wilke, Mr. Winters, and Ms. Knopp—all of Lippincott Williams & Wilkins—kept us on track through the difficult trials and tribulations of a first edition. We are also indebted to our colleagues in the Divisions of Clinical Immunology and Rheumatology, and General Internal Medicine for their authorship, support, and encouragement throughout the years. We would also like to recognize the many contributors to *Clinical Primer of Rheumatology* and *Arthritis and Allied Conditions: A Textbook of Rheumatology* for their generous contribution of time and effort toward this book.

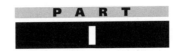

PART

I

INTRODUCTION TO THE RHEUMATIC DISEASES

EVALUATION OF PATIENTS WITH RHEUMATIC DISORDERS

GUSTAVO R. HEUDEBERT

Patients with rheumatic conditions present to physicians with a myriad of complaints. Signs and symptoms can be localized and specific for a certain diagnosis; however, on many occasions symptoms can be ill defined and physical findings subtle. For example, fatigue might be the dominant feature of seemingly disparate conditions such as systemic lupus erythematosus (SLE) and fibromyalgia. Conversely, monoarticular arthritis, although circumscribed, could still generate a lengthy list of differential diagnoses shaped by the age, gender, and underlying comorbid conditions of the patient. In other words, it is unlikely that one particular sign or symptom will have enough discriminatory quality to diagnose a disease with certainty.

Rheumatic diseases lend themselves well to a systematic approach of diagnosis based on demographics (i.e., young female with malar rash and diffuse articular pain should evoke the diagnosis of SLE), pattern of joint involvement (i.e., painful first metacarpal of acute onset should evoke the diagnosis of gout), pattern of muscle involvement (i.e., insidious painless weakness of muscles of the forearm should evoke the diagnosis of inclusion body myositis), or pattern of involvement of different organs (i.e., sinusitis and glomerulonephritis should evoke the diagnosis of Wegener granulomatosis).

This chapter is organized in sections, each of which attempts to capture patterns of presentation of rheumatic diseases based on patient demographics and nature of joint involvement. We recognize that in only a few instances does a pattern fit one disease perfectly; however, we hope to present a framework that will allow clinicians to recognize disease patterns leading to the formulation of a relatively narrow differential diagnosis while using time and resources efficiently.

APPROACH TO THE PATIENT WITH ARTICULAR COMPLAINTS

An important first step in patients presenting with complaints related to the joints is to determine if the problem is articular, periarticular, or nonarticular. Careful examination of periarticular ligamentous structures, pain at the site of tendon insertion (i.e., enthesitis), or pain around the joint itself (periarthritis) is important to determine the likely etiology of the patient's "articular" complaint.

Demographics

Age, gender, and ethnicity alone, or more commonly, in combination, can provide useful clues for patients presenting with signs or symptoms consistent with a rheumatic disease. We will consider each of these demographic characteristics separately and then finish the section with examples illustrating several useful combinations of age, gender, and/or ethnicity.

Age

We discuss only adult patients, with the exception of a few disorders in which the clinical condition might be a continuum between pediatric and young adults. We divide this section based on etiologic causes.

The infectious etiology of arthritis varies based on age, absence or presence of a disease process affecting a native joint, and presence of a prosthetic device. A combination of these risk factors is very helpful in trying to determine the best choice of empirical antibiotic coverage.

Gonococcal arthritis is diagnosed almost exclusively in sexually active individuals less than 40 years of age. It can present as monoarthritis, polyarthritis, or more commonly, oligoarthritis. *Neisseria gonorrhoeae* organisms can infect joints in the absence of underlying synovial damage (i.e., rheumatoid arthritis, crystal induced).

Patients more than 40 years of age are more likely to be immunosuppressed [e.g., diabetes mellitus, acquired immunodeficiency syndrome (AIDS), chemotherapy] or to have underlying rheumatic disease affecting their joints; similarly, this population is most likely to have been subjected to either an arthroplasty or joint replacement procedure. These affected joints are more vulnerable to synovial invasion, especially in the presence of bacteremia. In order of frequency the organisms more likely to be found in septic joints in this age group are: *Staphylococcus aureus, Staphylococcus epidermidis, Streptococci* spp., and Gram-negative enteric organisms (*Escherichia coli, Proteus mirabilis, Pseudomonas aeruginosa*).

Many of the inflammatory arthropathies exhibit age-related patterns. Rheumatoid arthritis (RA) presents characteristically in the fourth and fifth decades of life; SLE affects predominantly women during their reproductive years. Systemic sclerosis is more commonly diagnosed in the third and fourth decades of life. The seronegative spondyloarthropathies (Reiter syndrome, ankylosing spondylitis, psoriatic arthritis, reactive arthritis) are more commonly seen in young adulthood.

Systemic vasculitis exhibits a wide range of age distribution, although most affected individuals are diagnosed between the fourth and sixth decades of life. Some notable examples are worth mentioning: Henoch–Schönlein purpura is seen mostly in pediatric patients, with some patients being diagnosed in their twenties; diagnosis after 50 years of age is highly unusual. Takayasu arteritis (pulseless disease) is diagnosed almost exclusively in young females. Giant cell arteritis is a disease seen more commonly in elderly individuals. Polymyalgia rheumatica is seldom seen in individuals less than 50 years of age.

Crystal-induced arthropathies (gout and pseudogout) are seen over a wide a range of ages, although pseudogout has a stronger predilection for individuals in the fifth or sixth decade of life. Gout diagnosed in the twenties should alert the clinician to the possibility of lead exposure (saturnine gout), increased endogenous production of uric acid (i.e., a lymproliferative disorder), or an inherent defect of production or excretion of uric acid.

Osteoarthritis (OA) is characteristically diagnosed in the sixth and seventh decades of life. OA can be diagnosed at a younger age in patients with a history of significant trauma of a specific joint (i.e., elite athletes) or in the familial form of the disease.

Gender

It has long been recognized that a number of rheumatic diseases exhibit a strong gender predilection; best known to clinicians is the well-established relationship between SLE and young women.

In addition to SLE, a number of rheumatic conditions exhibit strong gender preponderance. For example, of the seronegative spondyloarthropathies, Reiter syndrome and ankylosing spondylitis are more likely to occur in males. Psoriatic arthritis affects both genders evenly.

Most of the inflammatory arthropathies exhibit a strong female preponderance. Rheumatoid arthritis is seen more frequently in women, although this gender difference tends to diminish with increasing age. The female-to-male ratio is particularly impressive in systemic sclerosis, peaking at 15:1 in the third and fourth decades of life. Sjögren syndrome is another disorder in which women are more commonly affected than men.

Of the crystal-induced disorders, gout has a male preponderance, whereas pseudogout affects both males and females similarly. Most of the systemic vasculitides exhibit a very small male preponderance, with the exception of Takayasu arteritis and giant cell arteritis, which are much more common in females.

Ethnicity

A few rheumatic disorders have a clear ethnic predilection. The HLA-27-positive seronegative spondyloarthropathies (Reiter syndrome and ankylosing spondylitis) are much more common in whites. On the other hand, at least in the United States, sarcoidosis is more common in young blacks. In a young black patient with ankle arthralgias sarcoidosis should be considered in the differential diagnosis.

Systemic sclerosis is slightly more common in young black females; rheumatoid arthritis affects all ethnic groups equally. Of patients with vasculitis, those with giant cell arteritis are predominantly whites, and patients with Takayasu arteritis tend to be women of Asian descent.

For reasons that are not well understood OA is more common among whites than among any other ethnic group even after controlling for well-known risk factors such as obesity.

In certain instances ethnicity is more related to prognosis than diagnosis. The best example is SLE, where black patients have a generally worse prognosis than whites in the United States. Although less well established, this relationship might also be true in patients with systemic sclerosis.

Finally, a number of rheumatic conditions have strong geographic predilection. Behçet disease is more common in the Mediterranean basin, especially among Turkish people. Familial Mediterranean fever is seen much more commonly in individuals from the Middle East.

Summary

Although a significant number of rheumatic disorders are more commonly seen in young females, important age, gender, and ethnic differences characterized an important number of these disorders. Table 1.1 presents a matrix con-

TABLE 1.1. RELATIONSHIP BETWEEN DIFFERENT COMBINATIONS OF DEMOGRAPHIC CHARACTERISTICS AND DIAGNOSIS IN PATIENTS WITH ARTICULAR COMPLAINTS

	Female	Male	AA	Whites
Age ≤40	Takayasu arteritis, SLE, SS	Reiter syndrome, AS	Sarcoidosis	Reiter syndrome, AS
Age ≥50	RA, OA, GCA	Gout, pseudogout		OA, GCA

AS, ankylosing spondylitis; GCA, giant cell arteritis; OA, osteoarthritis; RA, rheumatoid arthritis; SLE, systemic lupus erythematosus; SS, systemic sclerosis.

taining several rheumatic diseases with a unique combination of demographic characteristics.

Pattern of Joint Involvement

One of the most important aspects of the interview and the physical examination of the patient with joint complaints is to determine the symmetry of joint involvement (symmetric versus asymmetric), the number of joints affected (mono-, oligo- or pauci-, poly-), the location of joints (axial versus peripheral), presence of inflammation (arthralgias versus arthritis), anatomic involvement [i.e., proximal (PIP) versus distal interphalangeal (DIP)], and the evolution of joint involvement (additive versus migratory). A classical description of a pattern of joint involvement is best exemplified by that of patients with RA: a *symmetric* (both hands and/or feet), *peripheral* (hands and/or feet), *additive* (goes from hands to feet with hands still being affected), and *polyarthritic* (inflammatory changes in greater than three joints) condition affecting predominantly the metacarpophalangeal (MCP) and PIP joints.

Presence of Inflammation

One of the most important aspects in the evaluation of patients with joint complaints is to determine the presence of inflammatory changes. The history is helpful, as patients can accurately describe if a joint has been or is currently warm, red, and swollen. The physical examination is very helpful in confirming or refuting the complaints of the patient. Another important aspect in the history of present illness is determining the presence of morning stiffness. The duration of morning stiffness is very helpful; characteristically, patients with RA and other inflammatory arthropathies experience this symptom more than 1 hour after awakening, whereas OA patients usually feel loosening of their joints before 1 hour has elapsed.

Bacterial causes of infectious arthritis are likely to present with obvious inflammatory changes; the most common clinical pattern is that of an acute monoarthritis. Inflammatory changes might not be present in patients on steroids or those with severe neutropenia. Another special case of infectious arthritis without or with minimal inflammation is that of bacterial infections in prosthetic devices. Fungal and mycobacterial infections can present with little or no inflammatory changes. Viral infections present clinically more like arthralgias than arthritis; parvovirus B19 infections usually present as a very acute and disabling polyarthralgia.

Rheumatoid arthritis almost universally presents with inflammatory changes in the affected joints. The symptoms are present for several weeks and the physical examination usually confirms the history obtained by the patient. Patients with "burnout" rheumatoid joints present with severe deformities associated with little or no appreciable inflammatory changes. Presence of prolonged morning stiffness is frequently elicited. Conversely, the clinical picture of patients that ultimately carry the diagnosis of OA is dominated by pain with little or no inflammatory changes; over time patients with advance OA exhibit deforming changes of the affected joints. The main difference between advanced RA and OA with deformities resides in the joints being affected (i.e., large joints in OA like the knee versus small joints in RA like MCP or PIP). The presence of a new inflamed-appearing joint in a patient with OA should alert the clinician to the possibility of an infectious or crystal-induced etiology.

Patients with connective-tissue diseases can present with either arthralgias or arthritis. Characteristically, the joint involvement in SLE tends to be more of a polyarthralgia than a polyarthritis. Patients with systemic sclerosis present with diffuse arthralgias; the changes observed in the digits (sausage-like changes) are due to infiltration of the skin and not to that of the synovial space.

Patients with seronegative spondyloarthropathies can manifest joint involvement in various ways: those with psoriatic arthritis can have a symmetric polyarthritis indistinguishable from that in patients with RA; the most severe form of psoriatic arthritis produces a classic destruction of the distal phalanx known as *arthritis mutilans*. A careful joint examination in patients with Reiter often reveals pain at the site of insertion of tendons (enthesitis), the classic site of involvement of the insertion of the Achilles tendon in the calcaneous bone. Patients with ankylosing spondylitis usually present with little or no evidence of a peripheral arthritis; these individuals have predominant involvement of the axial skeleton. Individuals with inflammatory bowel disease can present with either oligoarthritis or, more commonly, oligoarthralgias.

Crystal deposition disease is usually present with a history and physical examination consistent with an inflammatory process. Gout tends to be an acute monoarthritis affecting, in order of frequency, the first metatarsal joint (podagra), the knee (gonagra), or the wrist (chinagra). Occasionally, gout can mimic RA with polyarticular involvement. Usually, patients with this condition have manifestations of tophaceous gout elsewhere. Pseudogout can mimic gout in terms of acuteness and degree of inflammation. The joints most commonly affected in pseudogout are the knee, shoulder, and wrist.

Patients with systemic vasculitis commonly complain of diffuse, symmetric arthralgias. Of patients with a diagnosis of vasculitis, those with Henoch–Schönlein purpura and cryoglobulinemia are more likely to have prominent arthralgias. For example, patients with chronic hepatitis C infection can produce mixed cryoglobulins, resulting in a clinical triad of purpura, arthralgias, and proteinuria.

Joint Involvement

The number of joints involved, evolution of joint involvement, site of involvement, and symmetry are important features in the history and physical examination of patients with joint complaints.

Monoarticular involvement is defined as one joint being affected; polyarticular involvement is defined as more than three joints being involved; oligo- or pauciarticular involvement is defined as two or three joints being affected. In general terms, monoarticular involvement is characteristic of bacterial infections, trauma, and crystal-induced disease. Patients with seronegative spondyloarthropathies and juvenile RA usually exhibit oligoarticular involvement. Adult-onset RA is characterized by polyarthritis; polyarthritis is also frequently seen in SLE and systemic sclerosis.

Additive articular involvement refers to consecutive joints being affected over time with involvement of the first joint still present at the onset of symptoms in the second joint; this additive pattern is characteristic of RA and Reiter syndrome. Migratory articular involvement refers to consecutive involvement of joints with resolution of articular involvement in the first joint when the second joint becomes symptomatic. Examples of this pattern are gonococcal arthritis and viral arthritis.

Joints in the skeleton are broadly divided as peripheral and axial. The spine, sacroiliac, sternoclavicular, acromioclavicular, shoulder, and hip joints are considered part of the axial skeleton. The remaining joints of both the upper and lower extremities are considered part of the peripheral skeleton. Diseases that typically involve the axial skeleton include the seronegative spondyloarthropathies and osteonecrosis; peripheral involvement is characteristic of RA and many of the connective-tissue diseases. Within each of these two skeleton areas, distinct joints can help in the differential diagnosis. For example, in the hand, involvement of the MCP and PIP joints is characteristic of RA, whereas involvement of the DIP joints is seen more commonly in psoriatic arthritis and OA. The combination of an enthesitis (i.e., Achilles tendonitis, plantar fasciitis) with sacroiliitis should raise the suspicion of Reiter syndrome.

A final aspect of the pattern of joint involvement refers to the symmetry of the joints affected. Monoarticular and oligoarticular diseases are by definition asymmetric; most of the spondyloarthropathies, infections, OA, crystal-induced processes are asymmetric. Important exceptions are the symmetry of the DIP joints seen in psoriatic arthritis, and occasional cases of polyarticular gout and OA. Of the polyarticular entities, RA and the connective-tissue diseases are more likely to present in a symmetric fashion.

Summary

Table 1.2 presents a matrix of combinations of pattern involvement. Together with the information contained in Table 1.1, it allows for the recognition of the most likely rheumatic disease affecting the patient.

Miscellaneous

Occasionally, patients present with unusual patterns of articular involvement that might be highly characteristic of certain clinical entities. We would like to highlight these unusual presentations to heighten the awareness of these conditions. Patients with hemochromatosis can present with pain across the MCP joints with sparing of the DIP and PIP joints. Furthermore, there are little inflammatory changes appreciable in these joints. Individuals affected with OA can visit your office with complaints of isolated first carpometacarpal area pain and subluxation. Patients with SLE can occasionally exhibit deforming but nonerosive articular changes known as Jaccoud arthritis. A symmetric additive polyarthritis affecting the ankles and knees associated with erythema nodosum should suggest sarcoidosis. The association of these two symptoms with bilateral hilar adenopathy is known as Lofgren syndrome and suggests a good long-term prognosis for patients with sarcoidosis. Painless bilateral ankle joint deformity in a patient with long-standing diabetes mellitus should alert the clinician to the possibility of neuropathic joint damage due to loss of proprioception (Charcot arthropathy). Long-standing diabetics can also present with diffuse thickening of the digits that has a major resemblance to scleroderma. A symmetric polyarthritis with widening of the joint space and puffiness of the fingertips should suggest the diagnosis of acromegaly arthropathy. Occasionally, patients with hypertrophic arthropathy come to the attention of the physician with complaints of knee and ankle pain. The presence of

TABLE 1.2. RELATIONSHIP BETWEEN DIFFERENT COMBINATIONS OF PATTERNS OF JOINT INVOLVEMENT AND DIAGNOSIS IN PATIENTS WITH ARTICULAR COMPLAINTS

	Axial	Peripheral	Additive	Migratory	Symmetric	Asymmetric
Mono-	OA	Gout, OA, pseudogout				
Oligo-	Reiter syndrome, AS		Rheumatic fever, gonococci	Gonococci, viral		Reiter syndrome, AS
Poly-		SLE, RA, SS, psoriatic	RA, rheumatic fever	Gonococci, viral	SLE, RA, SS, psoriatic	Reiter syndrome, AS

AS, ankylosing spondylitis; OA, osteoarthritis; RA, rheumatoid arthritis; SLE, systemic lupus erythematosus; SS, systemic sclerosis.

clubbing and deformity of visible joints (i.e., ankles, wrist) should alert the clinician to the possibility of this paraneoplastic syndrome. The most likely related malignancy is bronchogenic carcinoma.

APPROACH TO PATIENTS WITH MUSCLE DISORDERS

The patient with myopathy may present to the physician with one of three complaints: (a) a clinical picture dominated by painless weakness that is either diffuse (i.e., polymyositis) or localized (i.e., distal as seen in inclusion body myositis); (b) a clinical picture dominated by painful weakness (i.e., polymyalgia rheumatica); (c) a clinical picture dominated by pain without associated weakness that can be generalized (i.e., influenza, systemic infections) or localized (i.e., fibromyalgia). As in patients with articular complaints, the combination of demographic factors and patterns of muscle involvement is helpful in generating a list of potential diagnoses.

Demographics

Certain demographic characteristics can be linked to specific inflammatory muscle disorders. For example, polymyalgia rheumatica is seen almost exclusively in individuals more than 50 years of age; there is no gender predilection. However, this disease is more common in whites. Inclusion body myositis is characteristically seen in elderly men. Polymyositis/dermatomyositis (PM/DM) occurs more commonly in females. Blacks are more likely to be affected. In polymyositis/dermatomyositis the age of presentation varies with the type of PM/DM syndrome: Patients with adult polymyositis and adult dermatomyositis are usually diagnosed in the fifth decade of life. A similar age distribution is seen in patients with polymyositis as part of an overlap syndrome. Patients with paraneoplastic PM present at around 60 years of age.

Age is an important criterion for differentiation between inflammatory and noninflammatory myopathies. Most patients with glycogen storage and lipid storage diseases (noninflammatory) present either in childhood or in early adulthood. Although patients with connective-tissue disease, who are usually in their second or third decade of life, can present with a prominent myopathy, most patients with a primary inflammatory myopathy present later in life.

Pattern of Muscle Involvement

Distinguishing muscle weakness of a neuropathic versus myopathic etiology can be very difficult. Among patients with a neuropathic etiology, those with upper motor neuron disease are easier to differentiate because of asymmetric weakness (i.e., hemiparesis) and presence of associated physical examination findings, including hyperreflexia, positive Babinski sign, and ultimately spasticity. Patients with lower motor neuron disease might be more challenging to differentiate from patients with a primary myopathic process. The following clinical characteristics might prove useful: (a) patients with lower motor neuron disease are more likely to manifest distal muscle weakness, which is unusual in patients with a primary myopathic process; (b) patients with lower motor neuron disease often have fasciculation of the muscle(s) affected, hyporeflexia, and ultimately decreased muscle tone. The most challenging to differentiate are disorders affecting the neuromuscular junction, as they share clinical characteristics (i.e., proximal distribution) and physical examination findings (i.e., normal reflexes, no Babinski sign, normal muscle tone) similar to those elicited in patients with a primary myopathic process. Not uncommonly, clinicians resort to electromyographic studies (EMG/NCV) and even muscle biopsies to distinguish between these two groups of patients.

The pattern of muscle involvement can be helpful in generating a differential diagnosis in patients with weakness. Among the inflammatory myopathies, proximal muscle weakness of insidious onset is more characteristic of polymyositis. Individuals with inclusion body myositis tend to have both proximal and distal muscle weakness. Otherwise, most of the metabolic myopathies (i.e., hypokalemia, hypercalcemia) and the myopathies associated with endocrine disorders (i.e., thyroid disorders, hypercalcemia) are usually proximal. It is worth remembering that patients with periodic hypokalemic paralysis can present with profound generalized weakness of rather acute onset. A search for hyperthyroidism is warranted in such patients, especially if they are of Asian descent.

Individuals presenting with regional pain and/or weakness need to be approached in a different manner. Patients with clear regional muscle pain should be carefully questioned for a history of trauma. Occasionally, infections might be responsible for the regional nature of the pain. Pyomyositis, a relatively unusual disorder outside of the tropics, should be suspected in patients with known human immunodeficiency virus that present with fever and localized muscle pain. On occasion these patients might also have associated weakness. The presence of gluteal muscle weakness and atrophy among diabetics should alert the clinician to the possibility of diabetic amyotrophy. Diabetics with long-standing, poorly controlled diabetes can present with localized pain and weakness due to diabetes myonecrosis. Much more common, however, is the patient with fibromyalgia who presents to the clinician with complaints of profound generalized fatigue and diffuse muscle pains. Differentiating fatigue from weakness can be challenging. In these patients documentation of normal muscle strength and tone is of great importance. Elicitation of painful trigger points (see chapter 20) might help the clinician to make this diagnosis.

TABLE 1.3. DEMOGRAPHIC AND CLINICAL CHARACTERISTICS OF PATIENTS PRESENTING WITH MUSCULAR COMPLAINTS

	Male	Female	Proximal	Distal
Age >50	Inclusion body myositis	PM/DM	PM/DM, endocrine	Inclusion body myositis
Age >50		CTD	Endocrine, CTD	LMN (?)

CTD, connective-tissue disorder; DM, dermatomyositis; LMN, lower motor neuron disease; PM, polymyositis.

Summary

Table 1.3 presents a matrix with a different combination of demographic and muscle involvement patterns that might give a clue to the diagnosis of patients with muscle disorders.

SUGGESED READING

Bellamy N, Buchanan WW. Clinical evaluation in the rheumatic diseases. In: Koopman WJ, ed. *Arthritis and allied conditions: a textbook of rheumatology*, 14th ed. Baltimore: Lippincott Willliams & Wilkins, 2001.

Felson DT. Epidemioloy of the rheumatic diseases. In: Koopman WJ, ed. *Arthritis and allied conditions: a textbook of rheumatology*, 14th ed. Baltimore: Lippincott Wlliams & Wilkins, 2001.

Gordon DA, Hastings DE. Clinical features of rheumatoid arthritis: early, progressive and late disease. In: Klippel JH, Dieppe PA, eds. *Practical rheumatology*. London: Time Mirror International Publishers Limited, 1995.

Helliwell PS, Wright V. Clinical features of psoriatic arthritis. In: Klippel JH, Dieppe PA, eds. *Practical rheuumatology*. London: Time Mirror International Publishers Limited, 1995.

Hoffman BI. The musculoskeletal system. In: Mangione S, ed. *Physical diagnosis secrets*. Philadelphia: Hanley & Belfus, Inc., 2000.

Ingram Jr, RH, Braunwald E. Dyspnea and pulmonary edema. In Braunwald E, Fauci AS, Kasper DL, eds. *Harrison's principles of internal medicine*. 15th ed. *Vol. 1*. McGraw-Hill, 2001.

Khan MA. Clinical features of ankylosing spondylitis. In: Klippel JH, Dieppe PA, eds. *Practical rheuumatology*. London: Time Mirror International Publishers Limited, 1995.

Liang MH, Sturrock RD. Evaluation of musculoskeletal symptoms. In: Klippel JH, Dieppe PA, eds. *Practical rheuumatology*. London: Time Mirror International Publishers Limited, 1995.

Mangione S. The extremities. In: Mangione S, ed. *Physical diagnosis secrets*. Philadelpia: Hanley & Belfus, Inc., 2000.

McCarty DJ. Differential diagnosis of arthritis: analysis of signs and symptoms. In: Koopman WJ, ed. *Arthritis and allied conditions: a textbook of rheumatology*, 14th ed. Baltimore: Lippincott Williams & Wilkins, 2001.

Olney RK, Aminoff MJ. Weakness, myalgias, disorders of movement, and imbalance. In: Braunwald E, Fauci AS, Kasper DL, eds. *Harrison's principles of internal medicine*, 15th ed. vol. 1. McGraw-Hill, 2001.

Sapira JD. The musculoskeletal system. In: *The art and science of bedside diagnosis*. Baltimore and Munich: Urban & Schwarzenberg, 1990.

Sapira JD. The extremities. In: *The art and science of bedside diagnosis*. Baltimore and Munich: Urban & Schwarzenberg, 1990.

Schumacher Jr H, ed. *Primer on the rheumatic diseases*, 12th ed. Atlanta, GA: Arthritis Foundation; 2001.

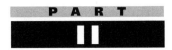

PART

II

SPORT-RELATED, OCCUPATIONAL, AND OTHER REGIONAL PAIN SYNDROMES

CERVICAL SPINE PAIN

JOE G. HARDIN
JAMES T. HALLA

Neck pain is a common problem in the general population, whether or not a well-defined rheumatic disorder exists. It occurs at some time in one-third or more of the population (1). Typically, the pain is perceived not only in the neck itself, but also in other regions, such as the back of the head, shoulder girdle, arm, and anterior chest. Pain originating from neck structures might be perceived exclusively in extracervical areas. In patients with unequivocal cervical trauma, cervical degenerative disc and joint disease, or inflammatory arthropathies, the origin of the pain in the neck might be easy to establish, at least by inference. In individuals with pain but with none of these conditions, the cause is often impossible to establish with certainty. Fortunately, many of these pain syndromes are transient. The neck is a complex anatomic structure with many components that lend themselves poorly to diagnostic investigation.

It can be assumed that pain derived from the cervical spine originates in one or more of a limited number of structures: joints (either synovial or cartilaginous), ligaments, neural tissue (especially nerve roots), muscles, and tendons. Disease in one structure (e.g., a joint) often leads to symptoms in another (e.g., a nerve). Available diagnostic modalities can identify joints or neural tissue as a probable source of pain with relative ease; however, some of these techniques have been shown to be overly sensitive. Recognition of pathology in muscle or ligament is much more difficult, which accounts for the difficulty in precise identification of the origin of cervical pain in individuals with no underlying rheumatic disorders.

The functional anatomy of the cervical spine and structures related to it will first be addressed, followed by a review of cervical spine syndromes commonly encountered in otherwise normal individuals, syndromes associated with trauma, syndromes associated with degenerative disc and joint disease, syndromes resulting from inflammatory arthropathies, and finally a summary of conservative approaches to chronic neck pain in a primary-care setting.

FUNCTIONAL ANATOMY

Emphasis is on the spine, its articulations, and their relationship to neural structures. Individual cervical vertebrae and their components are illustrated in Fig. 2.1. The atlas (C1) (Fig. 2.1A) is a ring of bone modified by articular facets anterolaterally. The superior facets articulate with the skull, forming relatively stable joints that permit only flexion–extension. The inferior facets articulate with their counterparts on the axis (C2) (Fig. 2.1B). A third C1–C2 articulation also plays an important role in the motion between these two vertebrae. This is the joint formed between the odontoid process of C2 and the anterior chamber of C1—the atlantoodontoid articulation. This joint is stabilized by the transverse ligament of C1 behind the odontoid and by ligaments between the odontoid and the occiput. The head and C1 move as a unit on C2 during cervical flexion. This motion stresses the stability of the atlantoodontoid articulation and tends to force the odontoid posteriorly into the area occupied by the spinal canal. The three C1–C2 articulations contribute about 50% of the rotational motion of the cervical spine, and all three are synovial-lined joints.

Below the axis the remaining five cervical vertebrae (Fig. 2.1C) are relatively constant; their articulations account for the remaining motions permitted by the cervical spine. Anteriorly, the vertebral body articulates with its counterpart via the cartilaginous intervertebral disc. During youth the disc is typical of others elsewhere in the spine with a dense outer annulus fibrosus and a central nucleus pulposus. Laterally, near the intervertebral neural foramina, the vertebral bodies are modified by superior uncinate processes (neurocentral lips) that articulate with a region of the vertebral bodies above them, forming the so-called joints of Luschka. The adult cervical disc loses its nucleus pulposus, and clefts develop at the site of the uncinate processes. With increasing age these clefts dissect medially, bisecting the disc but not forming a true synovial joint (2,3). According to this observation Luschka joints are mythic (2,3).

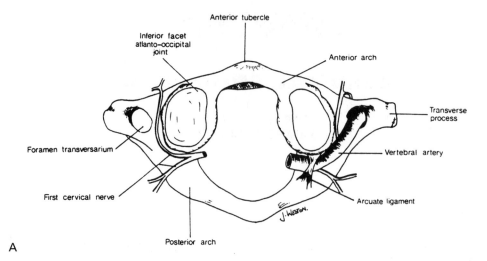

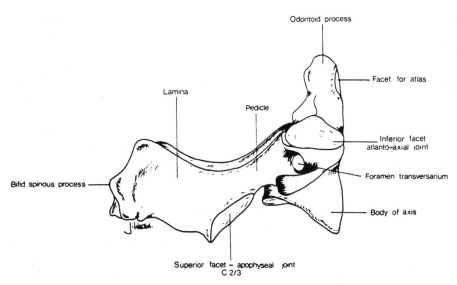

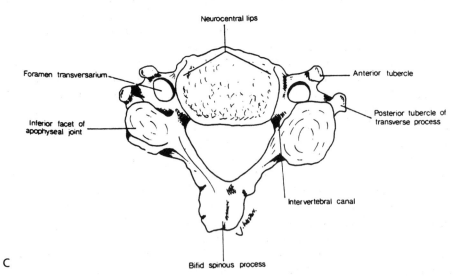

FIGURE 2.1. Atlas, axis, and typical lower cervical vertebra: **A:** Atlas, superior aspect. **B:** Axis, lateral view. **C:** Typical cervical vertebra, superior view. (From Jeffreys E. *Disorders of the cervical spine.* London: Butterworth, 1980:3, with permission.)

The posterior elements of C2 and the lower five cervical vertebrae form the neural arch surrounding the spinal canal laterally and posteriorly. Laterally, the narrow pedicles provide for the oval intervertebral neural foramina (Fig. 2.2), and the transverse processes, extending anterolaterally from the pedicles, form shelves or gutters for the exiting nerves. Except for that of C7 each transverse process, including those of C1 and C2, is perforated by a foramen for the vertebral artery (foramen transversum). The intervertebral neural foramina are best viewed obliquely in the anterolateral plane. Posterior to the pedicle the neural arch flares inferiorly and superiorly to form the articular facets that lie considerably posterior to the articular facets of C1 and C2. The articulating surfaces of the facets face each other at an angle of about 45 degrees. The facet (apophyseal) joints are true synovial joints. The posterior elements (lamina) of the neural arch complete the spinal canal.

Motions permitted by the cervical articulations vary with age, sex, and the observer measuring them. Average ranges are as follows: flexion–extension, 106 degrees; lateral flexion or bending, 178 degrees; and rotation, 131 degrees. Ranges in all directions decrease significantly with increasing age (4,5).

The first cervical nerve exits superior to C1 and posterior to the articular facet, and the second cervical nerve exits similarly superior and posterior to the superior articular facet of C2. All other cervical nerves pass anterolaterally through their respective gutters and posterior to the vertebral artery. After exiting the spinal canal the posterior and anterior nerve roots join within their dural sleeve in the gutter to form the cervical nerve, with the posterior root lying superior to the anterior root. Their position in the foramina and the uncinate processes serves to protect the roots from protrusion or herniation of disc material.

Important ligaments add support to the cervical spine below the C1–C2 articulations. The anterior longitudinal ligament is bound to the front of the vertebral bodies, its fibers blending loosely with the annulus fibrosus as it crosses the disc spaces. The reverse is true for the posterior longitudinal ligament, which is loosely bound to the posterior aspects of the vertebral bodies but more firmly attached to the discs. The posterior longitudinal ligament is much thicker in the cervical area than in the thoracolumbar regions. The lamina or posterior aspects of the neural arch are bound to their inferior and superior counterparts by the tough elastic ligamenta flava, which extend anteriorly to blend in with the capsules of the facet joints.

A large muscle mass occupies the posterolateral cervical area. For the most part these muscles are attached to the spine and to the skull, especially the occiput. In concert with the sternomastoid and the anterior neck muscles, they move the head and neck, support and stabilize the head and neck, and balance the head on the spine.

GENERAL APPROACHES TO CERVICAL SYMPTOMS

Most symptoms perceived in the neck are transient and of uncertain cause. Many probably qualify as myofascial (6). Symptoms are typically rapid in onset, are associated with limited or painful mobility of the neck and shoulder girdle, and seldom last longer than a week. The neurologic examination is normal; other physical findings are nonspecific, and diagnostic imaging is not helpful. This syndrome is often referred to by patients as a "crick." What appears to be persistent myofascial pain (in the presence or absence of an accompanying fibromyalgia syndrome) may also be a

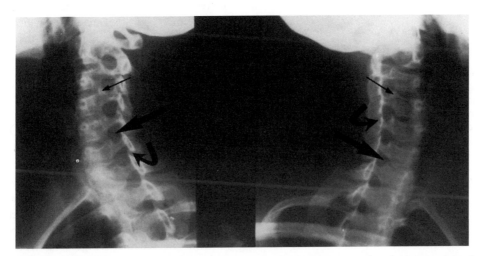

FIGURE 2.2. Right and left oblique views of the cervical spine demonstrating the intervertebral neural foramina (*large arrows*). Sites of the uncinate processes are indicated by *small arrows* and the facet joints are indicated by *curved arrows*. (From Hardin JG Jr, Halla JT. Cervical spine syndromes. In: Koopman WJ, ed. *Arthritis and allied conditions: a textbook of rheumatology,* 14th ed. Philadelphia: Lippincott Williams & Wilkins, 2001:2009–2018, with permission.)

common cause of chronic symptoms in the neck region (7). Appropriate cervical contour pillows may be useful in alleviating this more persistent myofascial pain.

Symptoms persisting beyond 1 or 2 weeks or associated with certain other manifestations must be taken more seriously. Other features suggesting a potentially serious or diagnosable cause include pain in other parts of the body, neurologic symptoms, abnormal neurologic findings, fever, and palpable or audible cervical crepitus. Polymyalgia rheumatica, fibromyalgia, and some of the inflammatory arthropathies might begin or predominate in the cervical region, as outlined in Table 2.1 (8). Symptoms or signs in other areas of the body might suggest one of these conditions. Cervical injuries might also trigger or precipitate a fibromyalgia syndrome. In a survey of patients with recent neck or lower-extremity injuries, fibromyalgia was 13 times more frequent in those with the neck injury (9).

When the diagnosis is not apparent and the symptoms persist or seem potentially serious, further diagnostic efforts are indicated, as listed in Table 2.2. The history and physi-

TABLE 2.1. DISORDERS THAT MAY PRESENT WITH SYMPTOMS IN THE NECK REGION

Rheumatic diseases
  Fibromyalgia
  Polymyalgia rheumatica
  Rheumatoid arthritis
  Juvenile rheumatoid arthritis
  Ankylosing spondylitis
  Peripheral spondyloarthropathies
  Crystal deposition diseases
  Degenerative disc and joint diseases
  Diffuse idiopathic skeletal hyperostosis
Trauma
  Fractures–dislocations
  Soft-tissue injuries
Regional cervical disorders
  Myofascial pain
  Osteomyelitis
  Septic discitis
  Septic arthritis
  Congenital and acquired torticollis syndromes
  Other congenital disorders of the cervical spine
  Cervical lymphadenitis
  Hyoid bone syndrome
  Neck–tongue syndrome
  Longus colli muscle tendinitis
  Facet joint synovial cyst
  Thyroiditis
  Thoracic outlet syndrome
Bone diseases
  Paget disease
  Osteomalacia
  Osteoporosis
  Metastatic tumor
Neuromuscular disorders
  Meningitis
  Cerebral palsy and other spastic conditions
  Paralysis of cervical muscles from any cause

TABLE 2.2. USEFUL DIAGNOSTIC MANEUVERS IN PATIENTS WITH SYMPTOMS IN THE NECK REGION

History
  Duration
  Trauma
  Pain or similar symptoms elsewhere
  Pain related to head–neck motion or position
  Referral pattern and nature of referred pain
  Neurologic symptoms
Physical examination
  Abnormal head position
  Neck motion and pain on motion
  Spine tenderness
  Tender or trigger points in neck area
  Motor or sensory deficits or reflex abnormalities, especially in the arms
Diagnostic imaging
  Routine radiographs (with oblique views)
  Radioisotope scanning
  Conventional tomography
  Computed tomography
  Magnetic resonance imaging
  Myelography
Electrodiagnostic studies
  Nerve conduction studies
  Electromyography

cal examination maneuvers are routine but very important. Cervical spine radiographs—anteroposterior, lateral, right and left oblique, and flexion and extension views in the lateral projection—are usually indicated. The facets between C1 and C2 are generally visualized by a view taken through the open mouth. Conventional tomography can be helpful if a bony defect or spinal derangement is suspected but not well defined by routine radiography or radioisotopic scintigraphy. Electrodiagnostic studies might confirm or better define a suspected neurologic deficit. Computed tomography (CT), magnetic resonance imaging (MRI), and myelography are used to define the source of a neurologic sign or symptom. Neural compression syndromes may be best defined by MRI (10,11); however, care must be taken not to overinterpret normal and age-related changes (12).

NECK PAIN ASSOCIATED WITH TRAUMA

Fractures and dislocations of the cervical spine must be excluded in symptomatic patients with a recent history of cervical trauma; however, blunt trauma elsewhere does not necessarily require cervical spine evaluation (13). A number of terms are used interchangeably to refer to the typical soft-tissue injury syndrome, including *whiplash,* cervical *sprain* or *strain,* and *posttraumatic cervical syndrome.* Although industrial or sports injuries might cause the problem, in the United States, most such injuries result from automobile collisions from the rear, most often with the victim using a seat belt (14). Medicolegal considerations can complicate and confound the clinical picture. The typical injury occurs as the head is first flexed and then forcibly hyperextended beyond its normal range of motion. Presumably, the affected tissues include muscles, tendons, joints, ligaments, and perhaps nerve roots. The pathogenesis of the injury is not well understood. Usually, the pain begins within hours of the accident and predominates in the neck and medial aspects of the shoulder girdle. Headaches are common, and posttraumatic audiologic and vestibular dysfunction have been reported (15). Cervical radiographs can show loss of lordosis secondary to cervical muscle spasm; however, the significance of this finding may have been overinterpreted (16).

In one series the syndrome had resolved in 52% of patients at 8 weeks and in 87% of patients at 5 months (17), but the natural history continues to be highly variable. In recent reviews, psychologic and medicolegal factors appear to have the major influence on the course and severity of the problem (18,19). The cervical zygapophyseal joints have long been implicated as a source of persisting pain after cervical flexion extension injuries, and provocation and blocking maneuvers have been used to support this notion (20). A recent controlled study failed to demonstrate any benefits of intraarticular corticosteroid injections in the implicated zygapophyseal joints in subjects with chronic whiplash pain (21). Collars, traction, other physical therapies, and analgesic agents can help symptomatically, though they do not seem to affect the course of the syndrome. A conservative approach is generally recommended (22,23).

DEGENERATIVE DISC AND JOINT DISEASES (INCLUDING DIFFUSE IDIOPATHIC SKELETAL HYPEROSTOSIS)

Although diffuse idiopathic skeletal hyperostosis (DISH) is usually readily identifiable from plain radiographs and typically produces few neck symptoms, degenerative disease of the spinal articulations can result in a confusing array of symptoms that are often difficult to explain. Table 2.3 summarizes confounding observations that can account for this difficulty. Despite these difficulties, diagnoses continue to be made, and the conditions often are treated successfully. In few cases, however, is the precise pathogenesis clearly understood. Four syndromes will be addressed: presumed herniation of the nucleus pulposus (HNP), presumed osteophytic neural and vascular encroachment, facet joint osteoarthritis, and DISH.

Herniation of the Nucleus Pulposus

Disc ruptures, protrusions, and extrusions are used synonymously with *herniation of the nucleus pulposus.* Much of the literature concerning cervical disc disease fails to distinguish between HNP and osteophytic encroachment on neural structures, apparently because the two often appear to occur together. A distinctive clinical syndrome might be apparent, however. The HNP syndrome occurs at a younger age than the osteophytic one and affects men more often than women. Protrusion tends to occur acutely on one side and at one level (most often C6–C7), dorsolaterally (apparently compressing intrameningeal nerve roots), or intraforami-

TABLE 2.3. FEATURES ASSOCIATED WITH DEGENERATIVE CERVICAL SPINE DISEASE THAT LEND DIFFICULTY TO PRECISE DIAGNOSES

Symptoms may arise from the facet joints or anulus fibrosus.
Radiographic abnormalities are almost universal in the elderly population, most of whom are asymptomatic.
Diagnostic imaging abnormalities may correlate poorly with symptoms.
Distribution of diagnostic imaging abnormalities may correlate poorly with location of symptoms.
Neurologic physical findings are most often absent.
With age the ligamenta flava become inelastic and may buckle into the spinal canal, causing symptoms.
With age the posterior longitudinal ligament may further thicken, encroaching on the spinal canal and causing symptoms.
Even lesions that appear to encroach on neural structures (by diagnostic imaging) may not cause symptoms.
By 40 years of age the nucleus pulposus appears to be no longer present in the cervical discs (suggesting that it cannot herniate) (3,24).
The posterior longitudinal ligament and the uncinate processes provide formidable barriers to disc herniation (3,24).
The lower cervical nerve roots appear to exit below the disc level, apparently protecting them from herniation in any event (3,24).
The anterior nerve roots appear to be too low in the intervertebral foramina to be vulnerable to osteophytic encroachment (3,24).

nally (apparently compressing the exiting nerve roots). Most often there is no history of trauma sufficient to account for the event. Symptoms often begin with neck pain that progresses to involve the scapular area, anterior chest, or arm, depending on which root is affected. Hyperextension of the neck or deviation of the head toward the side of the HNP can aggravate the pain. Neurologic findings and other signs are often present, depending on the site of the lesion (24–26).

The diagnosis may be supported by electromyography and confirmed by myelography, MRI, or CT. The procedure of choice is a matter of opinion, but most current experience favors MRI (27). Therapy is also a matter of opinion. Progressive neurologic deficits, signs of myelopathy, and intractable pain usually indicate surgery, however. Conservative therapy consists of intermittent or continuous cervical traction, bed rest, analgesics, and cervical collars for comfort (28).

Osteophytic Disease (Spondylosis)

Anterior osteophytes arising at the disc margins might imply more posterior disease but of themselves are typically asymptomatic. The uncinate processes enlarge with age, so that what appear to be osteophytes in that area radiographically might not be, but foraminal bony encroachment from that region is seen commonly, as is similar encroachment from facet joint osteophytes posteriorly. Only the facet osteophytes are in a position to impinge on a nerve root, and only the posterior root is vulnerable (3,23). Posterior osteophytes from the vertebral bodies at the disc margins are common and can be sufficiently large to compress the spinal cord, though they too are most often asymptomatic. In general, the lower cervical spine, especially C5–C6, is most prominently involved. Three overlapping syndromes can result from spondylitic osteophytic neural or vascular encroachment: nerve root compression (radiculopathy),

spinal cord compression (myelopathy), and vertebral artery compression.

It might not be possible, even at surgery, to distinguish clearly between a radiculopathy due to an HNP and one due to osteophytic encroachment, and the reported clinical syndromes resulting from these events are similar, except as already mentioned. HNP tends to occur in younger patients, affecting a single root. Approaches to diagnosis and therapy are also similar (29). A less dramatic and more ill-defined syndrome is more common than the classic one usually reported in textbooks. Older patients commonly experience neck, shoulder area, and arm pain, often aggravated by neck motion, and sometimes associated with intermittent paresthesias. Sometimes tests listed in Table 2.4 are positive but neurologic deficits are absent. Plain cervical radiographs document neural foraminal osteophytic encroachment, often at several levels. More expensive diagnostic studies are seldom indicated. Symptoms tend to respond to conservative therapy, perhaps improving with time alone. Intermittent cervical traction is frequently helpful, and may be dramatically so. It is seldom possible to clearly document an association between a given osteophytic encroachment and the symptoms.

Bland and Boushey suggest that spondylitic myelopathy is more common than radiculopathy (2). The syndrome is seen more often in older men and is typically gradual in onset. Leg symptoms predominate and spasticity is common. Radicular symptoms frequently accompany the myelopathy. A congenitally narrow spinal canal and posterior longitudinal ligament thickening or ossification may contribute to the compression. Myelography or MRI confirms the diagnosis, and surgical therapy is often indicated (30–33).

Many symptoms can result from osteophytic compression of the vertebral artery, especially in the upper cervical region. These include autonomic symptoms, transient ischemic attacks, dizziness, vertigo, and headaches; symp-

TABLE 2.4. CLINICAL TESTS FOR CERVICAL NERVE ROOT COMPRESSION

Test	Technique
Neck compression test	With the patient sitting, the examiner laterally flexes, slightly rotates, and then compresses the patient's head with a force of about 7 kg. Positive result is pain or paresthesias in distribution of affected root.
Axial manual traction test	With the patient supine, the examiner applies manual traction to the neck with a force of 10 to 15 kg. Positive result is relief of radicular symptoms.
Shoulder abduction test	With the patient sitting, the arm is actively abducted above the head. Positive result is relief of radicular symptoms.

Based on the results of myelography or magnetic resonance imaging, these tests are highly specific, but together have a sensitivity only in the range of 50% (25).

toms are often related to cervical motion. The association of cervical spondylosis with headache has been questioned, however (34). The diagnosis of vertebral artery compression is usually made by angiography, and the treatment often involves surgical decompression.

Facet Joint Osteoarthritis

It is widely assumed, but difficult to prove, that neck discomfort in the older population is related to the radiographic findings of facet joint osteoarthritis (facet joint OA). In one follow-up study of 205 patients, such an association could not be documented (35). A few patients with cervical OA have symptoms arising primarily from the C1–C2 facet joints, however. Patients with this syndrome tend to be older women complaining primarily of occipital pain. Crepitus in the upper cervical spine, occipital tender points, and a rotational head tilt deformity are common. These patients usually respond to conservative therapy, but surgical fusion is occasionally indicated for intractable pain (36).

Diffuse Idiopathic Skeletal Hyperostosis

The anterior longitudinal ligament of the cervical spine is commonly ossified in patients with diffuse idiopathic skeletal hyperostosis (DISH), and sometimes the ossification is luxuriant (Fig. 2.3). Although most often asymptomatic, extensive ossification can be associated with limited neck mobility, anterior cervical masses, and dysphagia from esophageal

compression (37). DISH has also been associated with ossification of the posterior longitudinal ligament, sometimes resulting in myelopathy with quadriplegia (38).

INFLAMMATORY ARTHROPATHIES

Neck syndromes are common in the inflammatory arthropathies (Table 2.1), especially rheumatoid arthritis (RA).

Rheumatoid Arthritis

Neck pain occurs in half of the patients with RA, but half of these symptomatic patients have normal cervical spine radiographs. Abnormalities of the rheumatoid cervical spine and its supporting structures occur in three patterns: (a) atlantoaxial (C1–C2) complex involvement with subluxation anteriorly or posteriorly with or without odontoid erosion; (b) C1–C2 lateral facet joint and/or atlantooccipital joint involvement with lateral or rotatory subluxations; and (c) subaxial involvement with subluxation and/or spondylodiscitis (39).

More than one pattern might be seen in any individual patient, and each pattern might be associated with a distinctive clinical profile. For example, involvement of the C1–C2 lateral facet joints, either unilaterally or bilaterally, is characterized by pain that parallels the degree of radiographic involvement, by restricted neck motion, and by a nonreducible rotational head tilt to the side of collapse and paralleling the degree of lateral mass collapse (Fig. 2.4).

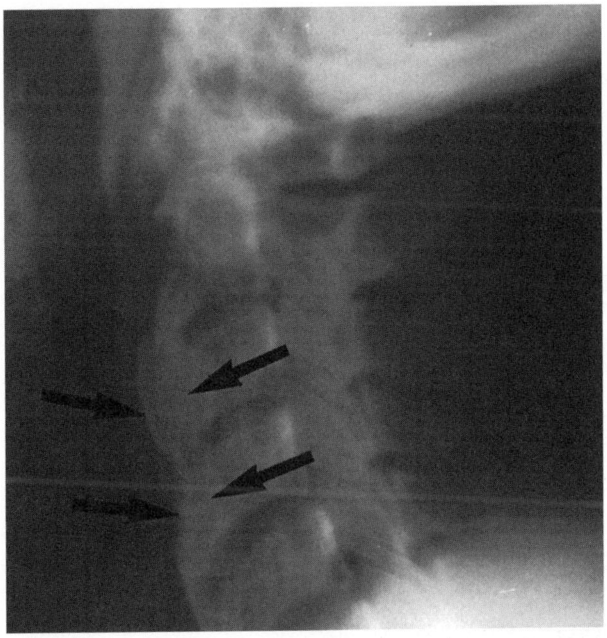

FIGURE 2.3. Cervical diffuse idiopathic skeletal hyperostosis (DISH). *Arrows* indicate the extent of the anterior longitudinal ligament ossification. (From Hardin JG Jr, Halla JT. Cervical spine syndromes. In: Koopman WJ, ed. *Arthritis and allied conditions: a textbook of rheumatology,* 14th ed. Philadelphia: Lippincott Williams & Wilkins, 2001:2009–2018, with permission.)

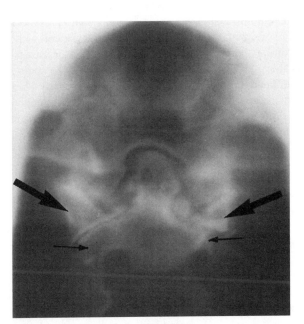

FIGURE 2.4. Conventional anteroposterior tomography of C1–C2 in a patient with severe rheumatoid arthritis. *Large arrows* indicate C1 lateral mass collapse and *small arrows* indicate C2 lateral mass collapse. (From Hardin JG Jr, Halla JT. Cervical spine syndromes. In: Koopman WJ, ed. *Arthritis and allied conditions: a textbook of rheumatology,* 14th ed. Philadelphia: Lippincott Williams & Wilkins, 2001:2009–2018, with permission.)

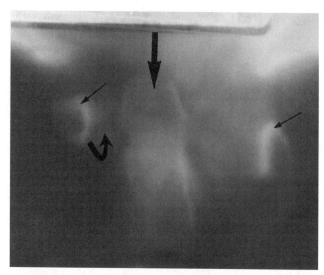

FIGURE 2.5. Conventional lateral tomography of C1–C2 area in a patient with severe rheumatoid arthritis. *Small arrows* indicate C1 and *large arrow* indicates the odontoid process. The spinal canal is to the left (*curved arrow*). This patient had severe C1–C2 anterior subluxation with no symptoms! (From Hardin JG Jr, Halla JT. Cervical spine syndromes. In: Koopman WJ, ed. *Arthritis and allied conditions: a textbook of rheumatology*, 14th ed. Philadelphia: Lippincott Williams & Wilkins, 2001:2009–2018, with permission.)

Neurologic symptoms are uncommon unless cranial settling is present (40,41).

Neck symptoms resulting from anteroposterior subluxations at the C1–C2 complex are less distinctive (Fig. 2.5). Anterior C1–C2 subluxation is the most frequent radiographic abnormality. The correlation between the degree of subluxation demonstrated radiographically and symptoms, especially neurologic symptoms, is poor (42). However, patients with the following abnormalities are at the greatest risk for irreversible paralysis: (a) atlantoaxial subluxation and a posterior atlantoodontoid interval of ≤14 mm; (b) atlantoaxial subluxation and at least 5 mm of cephalad migration of the odontoid tip due to cranial settling; and (c) subaxial subluxation and a sagittal diameter of the spinal canal of ≤14 mm (43).

Subaxial involvement includes vertebral endplate erosions, disc space narrowing without osteophytes, spondylodiscitis, and subluxation. Subluxation, either at single or multiple levels, is not uncommon, but rarely causes symptoms unless accompanied by discitis (39).

Treatment of neck pain in patients with RA should be guided by the radiographic pattern and by the nature of symptoms. Sometimes no therapy is necessary and conservative measures, including physical therapy and drugs, suffice. If pain is intractable, surgical fusion (occiput to C2 or C3) might give dramatic pain relief; this is especially true if the pain is due to C1–C2 lateral facet joint disease (40,41,44,45).

Juvenile Rheumatoid Arthritis

Cervical spine involvement occurs in up to 50% of patients with juvenile rheumatoid arthritis (JRA) and is most prominently associated with polyarticular disease, a positive rheumatoid factor, or both. Manifestations include loss of cervical lordosis; apophyseal joint erosions and ankylosis, especially in the upper cervical spine; failure of vertebral body growth; C1–C2 anterior subluxation; and lateral facet joint disease with nonreducible rotational head tilt (46–48).

Neck pain can be either the presenting feature or a later manifestation of adult-onset Still disease. Because the childhood and adult forms of Still disease are similar in presentation and course, radiographic similarities are not unexpected. Unlike the childhood form, the adult disease tends to involve both the upper and lower cervical segments (49).

Ankylosing Spondylitis

Neck pain in ankylosing spondylitis (AS) is common. As many as 5% to 10% of patients present with neck pain in the absence of back pain (50). Neck pain usually correlates with radiographic changes but can occur in their absence. Conversely, radiographic abnormalities without neck pain are sometimes seen. Cervical spine involvement usually accompanies disease in the thoracolumbar spine, though women may have a higher frequency of isolated cervical spine disease (51).

Involvement of the C1–C2 complex occurs uncommonly; subluxation, usually anterior, and odontoid erosions are its usual manifestations (52). However, in one series, 22 of 103 ankylosing spondylitis patients had anterior subluxations, and they progressed over a 2-year period in about one-third, five of whom required cervical fusion (53). The C1–C2 lateral facet joints might be the commonest source of severe neck pain in ankylosing spondylitis (47).

Cervical spine fracture, usually with minor trauma, is another cause of neck pain in patients with ankylosing spondylitis and is easily overlooked. These patients tend to be older men (mean age, 55 years) with advanced disease (average duration, 25 years). Neurologic deficits are common and mortality is as high as 35% (54).

Spondylodiscitis is another source of neck pain in patients with AS. This radiographic finding occurs in 1% to 28% of patients, usually during the first 10 years of disease. The more destructive the lesion, the more likely there is to be widespread spinal ankylosis (55). Infectious spondylitis must be excluded.

Ossification of the posterior longitudinal ligament of the cervical spine occurs commonly in ankylosing spondylitis and other spondyloarthropathies. It generally correlates with disease severity, and may cause or contribute to myelopathy (56).

Reiter Syndrome

Cervical spine involvement in Reiter syndrome is uncommon; fewer than 6% of patients demonstrate radiographic abnormalities. Manifestations include C1–C2 subluxations; C1–C2 lateral facet joint disease, including nonreducible rotational head tilt, atlantooccipital joint involvement, anterior longitudinal ligamentous ossification, and spondylitis (57,58). All of these can be a source of neck pain.

Psoriatic Arthritis

Involvement of the cervical spine in psoriatic arthritis occurs in two patterns: a pattern similar to rheumatoid arthritis and a pattern similar to ankylosing spondylitis (59). Neck pain is common and neurologic complications occur, especially in those patients with a rheumatoid arthritis–like pattern (60). The duration of psoriatic arthritis and the number of peripheral joints involved appear to be the major factors in determining cervical spine involvement (61).

Crystallopathies

As a group, the crystallopathies rarely affect the cervical spine. Gout can produce neck symptoms in a variety of ways, however, including intradural deposition of urate, discitis, and subluxations (62). In a group of 85 patients with calcium pyrophosphate deposition disease, 10 had neck symptoms (63). Radiographic abnormalities included disc space loss with vertebral sclerosis and osteophyte formation, facet joint abnormalities, and crystal deposition in synovial and ligamentous structures, including the ligamenta flava.

Crystal deposition, usually in the form of hydroxyapatite, can also occur in periarticular locations in the spine. Calcification within the longus colli muscle and tendon can be responsible for acute neck and occipital pain with or without dysphagia (64). Hydroxyapatite crystal deposition has also been reported in the infraoccipital region, interspinous bursae, and ligamenta flava, and has been associated with neck pain and neurologic manifestations (65).

SUMMARY OF CONSERVATIVE APPROACHES TO CHRONIC NECK PAIN IN A PRIMARY CARE SETTING

A large number of patients with chronic pain in the vicinity of the cervical spine will not be candidates for surgical or aggressive drug therapy. These patients will not have neurologic signs or symptoms, serious anatomic derangements of the cervical spine, or active systemic inflammatory disease. Most will probably have a trauma history ("chronic whiplash") or degenerative disc or joint disease as the suspected cause of their chronic pain. Standard initial therapies typically consist of simple analgesics and/or drugs sold as skeletal muscle relaxants; soft cervical collars, perhaps with cervical contour pillows at night; physical therapy maneuvers, such as traction, massage, and heat; and manipulation. Chiropractic manipulation often results in patient satisfac-

tion but lacks a scientific basis (66,67). In osteopathic treatment or physical therapy, manipulation and mobilization are almost as controversial but may have somewhat more of a scientific basis in terms of controlled clinical trials (67–69).

In the absence of satisfactory scientific data (controlled clinical trials), a stepwise approach might be appropriate. A contour pillow or soft collar for use at night with simple analgesics and a "muscle relaxant" such as cyclobenzaprine (perhaps only at night) could be the initial approach. Ideally, the simple analgesic would be acetaminophen or low doses of a nonsteroidal antiinflammatory drug. (Maximum or antiinflammatory doses are not indicated.) The next step might be home traction. Over-the-door devices with water bag weights are simple to use and inexpensive. A few pounds for 5 to 10 minutes can be gradually increased to 16 pounds for 30 minutes twice a day. If home traction fails to benefit the patient, referral to a physical therapist would allow for more aggressive manipulation with simultaneous use of other symptomatic therapies such as massage, heat, and ultrasound. If a course of physical therapy fails to benefit the patient, referral to a specialist in pain management is a reasonable alternative. Various anesthetic maneuvers can result in lasting pain relief, and many specialists in pain management are knowledgeable about nonnarcotic agents, such as gabapentin (Neurontin) that might be useful in controlling chronic pain. Chronic use of sustained-release narcotics will remain controversial in a benign chronic pain situation, but the practice is becoming more accepted, especially if all else fails.

REFERENCES

1. Bovin G, Schrader H, Sand T. Neck pain in the general population. *Spine* 1994;19:1307–1309.
2. Bland JG, Boushey DR. Anatomy and physiology of the cervical spine. *Semin Arthritis Rheum* 1990;20:1–20.
3. Bland JH. Basic anatomy. In: Bland JH, ed. *Disorders of the cervical spine*, 2nd ed. Philadelphia: WB Saunders, 1994:41–70.
4. O'Driscoll SL, Tomenson J. The cervical spine. In: Wright V, ed. *Clinics in rheumatic diseases*. Philadelphia: WB Saunders, 1982:617–630.
5. Kuhlman KA. Cervical range of motion in the elderly. *Arch Phys Med Rehabil* 1993;74:1071–1079.
6. Rachlin ES. History and physical examination for regional myofascial pain syndrome. In: Rachlin ES, ed. *Myofascial pain and fibromyalgia*. St. Louis: Mosby, 1994:159–172.
7. Smythe HA. The C6–7 syndrome: clinical features and treatment response. *J Rheumatol* 1994;21:1520–1526.
8. Bland JH. Differential diagnosis and specific treatment. In: Bland JH, ed. *Disorders of the cervical spine*. Philadelphia: WB Saunders, 1994:223–270.
9. Buskila D, Neumann L, Vaisberg G, et al. Increased rates of fibromyalgia following cervical spine injury. *Arthritis Rheum* 1997;40:446–452.
10. Kuroki T, Kumano K, Hirabayashi S. Usefulness of MRI in the preoperative diagnosis of cervical disk herniation. *Arch Orthop Trauma Surg* 1993;112:180–184.
11. Goto S, Mochizuki M, Watanabe T, et al. Long-term follow-up

study of anterior surgery for cervical spondylotic myelopathy with special reference to the magnetic resonance imaging findings in 52 cases. *Clin Orthop Rel Res* 1993;291:142–153.

12. Lehto IJ, Tertti MO, Komu ME, et al. Age-related MRI changes at 0.1 T in cervical discs in asymptomatic subjects. *Neuroradiology* 1994;36:49–53.

13. Roth BJ, Martin RR, Foley K, et al. Roentgenographic evaluation of the cervical spine. *Arch Surg* 1994;129:643–645.

14. Bauer W. Neck pain. In: Weisel SW, Feffer HL, Rothman RH, eds. *Neck pain.* Charlottesville, VA: Michie Company, 1986: 1–17.

15. Hildingsson C, Wenngren BI, Toolanen G. Eye motility dysfunction after soft-tissue injury of the cervical spine. *Acta Orthop Scand* 1993;64:129–132.

16. Helliwell PS, Evans PF, Wright V. The straight cervical spine: does it indicate muscle spasm? *J Bone Joint Surg* 1994;76B: 103–106.

17. Pennie BH, Agambar LJ. Whiplash injuries. *J Bone Joint Surg* 1990;72B:277–279.

18. Ferrari R, Russell AS. The whiplash syndrome: common sense revisited. *J Rheumatol* 1997;24:618–623.

19. Radanov BP. Common whiplash-research findings revisited. *J Rheumatol* 1997;24:623–625.

20. Bogduk N, Aprill C. On the nature of neck pain, discography and cervical zygapophysial joint blocks. *Pain* 1993;54:213–217.

21. Barnsley L, Lord SM, Wallis BJ, et al. Lack of effect of intraarticular corticosteroids for chronic pain in the cervical zygapophyseal joints. *N Engl J Med* 1994;330:1047–1050.

22. Carette S. Whiplash injury and chronic neck pain. *N Engl J Med* 1994;330:1083–1084.

23. Bogduk N, Lord SM. Cervical spine disorders. *Curr Opin Rheumatol* 1998;10:110–115.

24. Bland JH. New anatomy and physiology with clinical and historical implications. In: Bland JH, ed. *Disorders of the cervical spine,* 2nd ed. Philadelphia: WB Saunders, 1994:71–91.

25. Viikari-Juntura E, Porras M, Laasonen EM. Validity of clinical tests in the diagnosis of root compression in cervical disc disease. *Spine* 1989;14:253–257.

26. Dubuisson A, Lenelle J, Stevenaert A. Soft cervical disc herniation: a retrospective study of 100 cases. *Acta Neurochir* 1993;125: 115–119.

27. Van de Kelft E, Van Vyve M. Diagnostic imaging algorithm for cervical soft disc herniation. *J Neurol Neurosurg Psychiatry* 1994;57:724–728.

28. Maigne JY, Deligne L. Computed tomographic follow-up study of 21 cases of nonoperatively treated cervical intervertebral soft disc herniation. *Spine* 1994;19:189–191.

29. Yu YL, Woo E, Huang CY. Cervical spondylotic myelopathy and radiculopathy. *Acta Neurol Scand* 1987;75:367–373.

30. Bernhardt M, Hynes RA, Blume HW, et al. Current contents review: cervical spondylotic myelopathy. *J Bone Joint Surg* 1993;75A:119–128.

31. Sadasivan KK, Reed RP, Albright JA. The natural history of cervical spondylotic myelopathy. *Yale J Biol Med* 1993;66:235–242.

32. Law MD Jr, Bernhardt M, White AA. Cervical spondylotic myelopathy: a review of surgical indications and decision making. *Yale J Biol Med* 1993;66:165–177.

33. Houser OW, Onofrio BM, Miller GM, et al. Cervical spondylotic stenosis and myelopathy: evaluation with computed tomographic myelography. *Mayo Clin Proc* 1994;69:557–563.

34. Appenzeller O. The autonomic nervous system in cervical spine disorders. In: Bland JH, ed. *Disorders of the cervical spine.* Philadelphia: WB Saunders, 1994:313–327.

35. Gore DR. Sepic SB, Gardner GM, et al. Neck pain: a long-term follow-up of 205 patients. *Spine* 1987;12:1–5.

36. Halla JT, Hardin JG. Atlantoaxial (C1–C2) facet joint osteoarthritis: a distinctive clinical syndrome. *Arthritis Rheum* 1987;30:577–582.

37. Kritzer RO, Rose JE. Diffuse idiopathic skeletal hyperostosis presenting with thoracic outlet syndrome and dysphagia. *Neurosurgery* 1988;22:1072–1074.

38. Pouchot J, Watts CS, Esdaile JM, et al. Sudden quadriplegia complicating ossification of the posterior longitudinal ligament and diffuse idiopathic skeletal hyperostosis. *Arthritis Rheum* 1987;30:1069–1072.

39. Halla JT, Hardin JG, Vitek J, et al. Involvement of the cervical spine in rheumatoid arthritis. *Arthritis Rheum* 1989;32:652–659.

40. Halla JT, Fallahi S, Hardin JG. Non-reducible rotational head tilt and lateral mass collapse: a prospective study of frequency, radiographic findings, and clinical features in patients with rheumatoid arthritis. *Arthritis Rheum* 1982;25:1316–1324.

41. Halla JT, Hardin JG. The spectrum of atlantoaxial (C1–C2) facet joint involvement in rheumatoid arthritis. *Arthritis Rheum* 1990;33:325–329.

42. Weissman B, Aliabadi P, Weinfeld M, et al: Prognostic features of atlantoaxial subluxation in rheumatoid arthritis patients. *Radiology* 1982;144:745–751.

43. Boden SC, Dodge LD, Bohlman HH, et al. Rheumatoid arthritis of the cervical spine. *J Bone Joint Surg* 1993;75A:1282–1297.

44. Oostveen JCM, van de Laar MAFJ, Geelen JAG, et al. Successful conservative treatment of rheumatoid subaxial subluxation resulting in improvement of myelopathy, reduction of subluxation, and stabilization of the cervical spine. A report of two cases. *Ann Rheum Dis* 1999;58:126–129.

45. Rawlins BA, Girardi FP, Boachie-Adjei O. Rheumatoid arthritis of the cervical spine. *Rheum Dis Clin North Am* 1998;24:55–65.

46. Ansell B, Kent P. Radiological changes in juvenile chronic polyarthritis. *Skeletal Radiol* 1977;1:129–144.

47. Halla JT, Fallahi S, Hardin JG. Non-reducible rotational head tilt and atlantoaxial lateral mass collapse. *Arch Intern Med* 1983;143: 471–474.

48. Uziel Y, Rathaus V, Pomeranz A, et al. Torticollis as the sole initial presenting sign of systemic onset juvenile rheumatoid arthritis. *J Rheumatol* 1998;25:166–168.

49. Elkon K, Hughes G, Bywaters E, et al. Adult onset Still's disease: twenty-five-year follow-up and further studies of patients with active disease. *Arthritis Rheum* 1982;25:647–654.

50. Hochberg M, Borenstein D, Arnett F. The absence of back pain in classic ankylosing spondylitis. *Johns Hopkins Med J* 1978;143: 181–183.

51. Wiesner K, Bryan B. Clinical and radiographic abnormalities in ankylosing spondylitis: a comparison of men and women. *Radiology* 1976;119:293–297.

52. Sorin S, Askari A, Moskowitz R. Atlantoaxial subluxation as a complication of early ankylosing spondylitis. *Arthritis Rheum* 1979;22:273–276.

53. Ramos-Remus C, Gomez-Vargas A, Hernandez-Chavez A, et al. Two year follow-up of anterior and vertical atlantoaxial subluxation in ankylosing spondylitis. *J Rheumatol* 1997;24:507–510.

54. Murray G, Persellin R. Cervical fracture complicating ankylosing spondylitis. *Am J Med* 1981;70:1033–1041.

55. Dihlmann W. Current radiodiagnostic concept of ankylosing spondylitis. *Skeletal Radiol* 1979;4:179–188.

56. Ramos-Remus C, Russell AS, Gomez-Vargas A, et al. Ossification of the posterior longitudinal ligament in three geographically and genetically different populations of ankylosing spondylitis and other spondyloarthropathies. *Ann Rheum Dis* 1998;57:429–433.

57. Melsom R, Benjamin J, Barnes C. Spontaneous atlantoaxial subluxation: an unusual presenting manifestation of Reiter's syndrome. *Ann Rheum Dis* 1989;48:170–172.

58. Halla JT, Bliznak J, Hardin JG. Involvement of the craniocervi-

cal junction in Reiter's syndrome. *J Rheumatol* 1988;15: 1722–1725.

59. Blau R, Kaufman R. Erosive and subluxing cervical spine disease in patients with psoriatic arthritis. *J Rheumatol* 1987;14:111–117.

60. Fam A, Cruickshank B. Subaxial cervical subluxation and cord compression in psoriatic spondylitis. *Arthritis Rheum* 1982;25:101–106.

61. Jenkinson T, Armas J, Evison G, et al. The cervical spine in psoriatic arthritis: a clinical and radiological study. *Br J Rheumatol* 1994;33:255–259.

62. Resnick D, Niwayama G. Gouty arthritis. In: *Diagnosis of bone and joint disorders,* 2nd ed. Philadelphia: WB Saunders, 1988: 1618–1671.

63. Haselwood D, Wiesner K. Clinical, radiographic and pathologic abnormalities in calcium pyrophophate dihydrate deposition disease: pseudogout. *Radiology* 1977;122:1–15.

64. Resnick D, Niwayama G. Calcium hydroxyapatite crystal deposition disease. In: *Diagnosis of bone and joint disorders,* 2nd ed. Philadelphia: WB Saunders, 1988;1733–1764.

65. Nakajima K, Miyaoka M, Sumie H, et al. Cervical radiculomyelopathy due to calcification of the ligamenta flava. *Surg Neurol* 1984;21:479–488.

66. Hadler NM. Complementary and alternative therapies for rheumatic diseases II. Chiropractic. *Rheum Dis Clin North Am* 2000;(26):97–102.

67. Justus J, Fiechtner MD, Raymond R, Brodeur MC. Complementary and alternative therapies for rheumatic diseases. Manual and manipulation techniques for rheumatic disease. *Rheum Dis Clin North Am* 2000;26:83–96.

68. Aker PD, Gross AR, Goldsmith CH, et al. Conservative management of mechanical neck pain: systematic overview and meta-analysis. *BMJ* 1996;313:1291–1296.

69. Hurwitz EL, Aker PD, Adams AH, et al. Manipulation and mobilization of the cervical spine: a systematic review of the literature. *Spine* 1996, 21:1746–1759.

70. Jeffreys E. *Disorders of the cervical spine.* London: Butterworth, 1980.

LOW BACK PAIN
AND LUMBAR STENOSIS

J. D. BARTLESON

ACUTE, RECURRENT, AND CHRONIC LOW BACK PAIN IN ADULTS

Epidemiology

Low back problems are extremely common and affect virtually every person at some point during their life. In the United States the yearly prevalence of back pain has been reported to be 15% to 20%, and 50% of working-age individuals admit to back pain each year (1–3). Prevalence increases in early adulthood and reaches a peak between the ages of 35 and 55 and then declines somewhat thereafter (less so for women). There is little difference in the prevalence of back pain between men and women, but men are twice as likely as women to undergo surgery for a herniated lumbar disc. In one U.S. study, blacks had a slightly lower lifetime prevalence of back pain than whites and "nonblack, nonwhite" individuals had an even lower risk. Higher levels of education are associated with a somewhat lower prevalence of back pain. Heavy physical work, lifting, bending, and twisting are associated with an increased risk of occupational low back pain (1). In general, there is no correlation between back pain and body habitus except that increased height is a risk factor for lumbar disc herniation (1).

The impact on society of acute and chronic back pain is substantial. For those under the age of 45, low back problems are the most common cause of disability (1–3). About 1% of the U.S. population is chronically disabled because of back pain and another 1% is temporarily disabled at any one time. About 2% of the U.S. workforce sustains compensable back injuries each year. Lower back problems are the second most common reason for physician visits and the third most common reason for surgery in the United States. Hospitalization for medical treatment of low back pain has declined in recent decades, whereas the number of low back operations has increased (1). There is marked variation between countries and between regions within the United States in the use of diagnostic tests and surgery for patients with back pain

(1,3). Back pain represents about 25% of all lost workdays in the United States and accounts for a similar percentage of Workers' Compensation claims (1). Estimates of the total annual societal cost of back pain in the United States range from $38 billion to more than $50 billion (1). Low back pain can be divided broadly into acute pain (less than 3 months' duration) and chronic (more than 3 months' duration). Many patients experience recurrent episodes of acute low back pain (LBP). While chronic low back problems represent less than 5% of the total group with lower back complaints, they account for up to 60% of the societal costs for this condition (3).

Pathophysiology and Pathogenesis

LBP is not a single disorder and is usually not due to simple mechanical problems. LBP can be caused by multiple pathophysiologic mechanisms affecting the region of the lower spine and adjacent structures. Occasionally, low back pain represents the local manifestation of a systemic illness. Table 3.1 shows the major sources of LBP and referred lower limb pain suggestive of sciatica, which is defined as pain extending from the low back into the lower extremity in the distribution of the sciatic nerve. Although all pain is either carried by or brought to awareness by nerves, most pain is not caused by nerve compression or injury. Most causes of LBP are spondylogenic (from the structures of the spine and their attachments). Most patients with true sciatica have lumbosacral nerve root impingement by a protruded or extruded lumbar disc. A protruded disc is still contiguous with the bulk of the nucleus pulposus, whereas an extruded disc refers to a piece that has broken off from and is no longer attached to the main disc. Some authors believe that inflammation of the impinged nerve root is necessary for referred pain (sciatica). Clinicians should be aware that even with extensive evaluation, only about 15% of patients with LBP can be given a definitive diagnosis (3).

TABLE 3.1. MAJOR SOURCES OF LOW BACK AND REFERRED LOWER LIMB PAIN

Spondylogenic (from the spine)
 Bones
 Muscles
 Ligaments
 Joints
 Discs
Neurogenic
 Central nervous system
 Nerve roots
 Peripheral nerves
 Meninges
Viscerogenic
 Pancreas
 Kidneys
 Bowel
 Uterus
 Ovaries
 Bladder
 Prostate
Vascular
 Abdominal aortic aneurysm
 Atherosclerotic peripheral vascular disease
Psychogenic
 With an additional source of pain
 Rarely, without an additional source

Data from McCulloch JA, Transfeldt E. In: *Macnab's backache*, 3rd ed. Baltimore: Williams & Wilkins, 1997.

Clinical Features: Symptoms and Signs

Up to 90% of patients with acute low back problems recover within 1 month with very conservative treatment (2,3). Because the causes of LBP are manifold, our diagnostic studies are imprecise, and the natural history for most patients is benign, clinicians are only able to determine a definite diagnosis in a minority of patients with acute low back pain. Given these facts, the clinician's task is to determine if there is a potentially serious spine condition (such as tumor, infection, fracture, or cauda equina compression), or lower limb symptoms due to nerve root pathology (true sciatica) versus nonspecific back symptoms that are likely to improve on their own.

The clinician's job has been greatly aided in recent years by the development of evidence-based clinical practice guidelines for evaluation and treatment of low back problems (2–4).

General information about patients and their back pain should be elicited. Their age and gender, current symptoms, how the symptoms began, how the symptoms limit the patient, the duration of symptoms, the results of previous testing and treatment, and the temporal trend should be determined (Table 3.2).

Evaluation of psychologic and socioeconomic factors may also be helpful, especially for patients with recurrent flares or chronic LBP. Substance abuse, anxiety, depression, job dissatisfaction, family problems, and stress can con-

TABLE 3.2. DEMOGRAPHICS AND GENERAL QUESTIONS

Age and gender
What are your symptoms?
 Do you have pain, numbness, weakness, stiffness?
 Located primarily in back, lower limb, or both?
 Constant or intermittent?
 Improving or worsening?
How do your symptoms limit you?
 How long can you sit, stand, walk?
 How much can you lift?
How and when did your symptoms begin?
 Was there an injury, and if so, please describe.
Have you had similar episodes in the past?
Have you had previous testing and/or treatment?
What do you hope we can accomplish during this visit?

Modified from Bigos S, Bowyer O, Braen G, et al. *Acute low back problems in adults: clinical practice guideline*, Quick Reference Guide Number 14. Rockville, MD: U.S. Department of Health and Human Services, Public Health Service, Agency for Health Care Policy and Research, AHCPR Pub. No. 95-0643. December 1994.

tribute to prolonged symptoms and disability. The evidence-based guidelines strongly recommend that certain "red flag" inquiries be conducted to help exclude tumor, infection, fracture, or major neurologic compromise such as a cauda equina syndrome (CES). Table 3.3 lists the worrisome questions and neurologic findings and the corresponding potentially serious conditions.

TABLE 3.3. RED FLAGS FOR POTENTIALLY SERIOUS CONDITIONS

Possible fracture	Major trauma such as motor vehicle accident or fall from height
	Minor trauma or lifting a weight in an older or potentially osteoporotic patient
Possible tumor or infection	Age >50 or <20
	History of cancer
	Recent fever or chills or unexplained weight loss
	Recent bacterial infection, intravenous drug abuse, or immunosuppression
	Pain that worsens when supine or wakes patient from sleep at night
Possible cauda equina syndrome	History or examination evidence of perianal/perineal sensory loss
	Recent onset of bladder or bowel dysfunction or unexpected weakness of anal sphincter on examination
	History of severe or progressive lower limb neurologic deficit
	Major motor weakness in lower limb on examination

Modified from Bigos S, Bowyer O, Braen G, et al. *Acute low back problems in adults: clinical practice guideline*, Quick Reference Guide Number 14. Rockville, MD: U.S. Department of Health and Human Services, Public Health Service, Agency for Health Care Policy and Research, AHCPR Pub. No. 95-0643. December 1994.

Physical and neurologic examination of the patient will be directed by the patient's history and should include general observation of the patient, a regional back examination, neurologic screening, and testing for lumbosacral nerve root irritation. Many of the physical findings require patient cooperation and input, although a few, such as deep tendon reflexes and muscle atrophy, do not. For the patient with acute LBP of 6 to 12 weeks' duration or less, the evidence-based guidelines suggest that the following basic examination be performed: inspection of the lumbar region with palpation for spinal tenderness (with or without assessment of spinal range of motion) and screening tests for neurologic involvement (Table 3.4). Vertebral point tenderness may be suggestive of but not specific for spinal fracture or infection. Marked limitation of range of motion may suggest spinal infection, ankylosing spondylitis, or simply muscle spasm. The neurologic screening tests include assessing lower limb muscle strength; measuring the circumference of the leg (defined as the lower limb between the knee and ankle) and thigh (defined as the lower limb from hip to knee) and looking for a difference of 2 cm or more between the two sides; testing the knee and ankle reflexes; checking for Babinski signs; testing sensation in the medial, dorsal, and lateral aspects of the foot and perianally if there is any question of CES; and performing tests for L5 and/or S1 nerve root irritation using the straight-leg raising (SLR) test (Fig. 3.1).

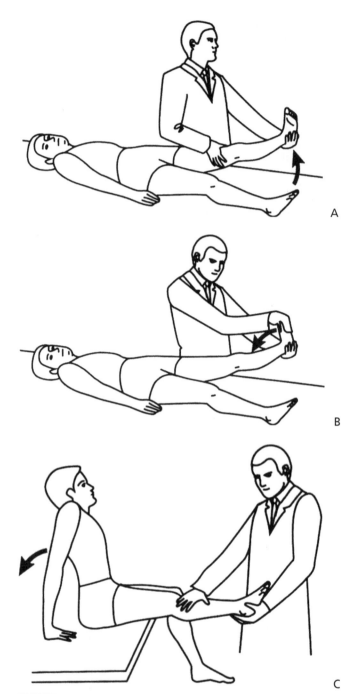

FIGURE 3.1. Straight-leg raising (SLR) test. **A:** With the patient supine, raise one lower limb while keeping the knee fully extended. Ask the patient to report when and where he or she experiences pain as the leg is raised. Estimate the degree of leg elevation. Symmetric hamstring tightness should be ignored. SLR is positive if sciatic nerve distribution pain occurs at elevations of 70 degrees or less. **B:** Accentuation of the patient's pain with foot dorsiflexion suggests nerve root impingement. **C:** With the patient sitting and the hips flexed at 90 degrees, extend one knee. This stretches the lumbosacral nerve roots about the same as moderate supine SLR. (Modified from Bigos S, Bowyer O, Braen G, et al. *Acute low back problems in adults: clinical practice guideline*, Quick Reference Guide Number 14. Rockville, MD: U.S. Department of Health and Human Services, Public Health Service, Agency for Health Care Policy and Research, AHCPR Pub. No. 95-0643. December 1994.)

TABLE 3.4. SCREENING EXAMINATION FOR ACUTE AND RECURRENT LOW BACK PAIN

Spine	Inspection
	Vertebral tenderness
	Range of motion (optional)
Neurologic screening	
Muscle strength testing—L4	Quadriceps strength—ascend step with one limb
Muscle strength testing—L5	Walk on heels, dorsiflexion of great toe and foot
Muscle strength testing—S1	Walk on toes, rise on toes of one foot alone, plantar flexion of great toe
Atrophy—L4	Thigh
Atrophy—L5	Leg
Atrophy—S1	Leg
Reflexes—L4	Knee
Reflexes—L5	None
Reflexes—S1	Ankle
Sensory loss—L4	Medial leg
Sensory loss—L5	Lateral leg, dorsum foot
Sensory loss—S1	Posterior leg, lateral foot
Straight-leg raising—L4	±
Straight-leg raising—L5	+
Straight-leg raising—S1	+

The most commonly encountered acute back and limb pain syndromes will be described briefly. Pain of spinal origin can be broadly divided into that arising from the musculoskeletal components alone and that arising as a direct result of compression or irritation of the spinal nerve roots. The most common presentation is acute pain confined to the lower back region with or without a history of bending, lifting, or making a mismove. Most of these patients are presumed to have a musculoligamentous "strain," but some probably have a disturbance of the facet joints or a ruptured intervertebral disc without nerve root impingement. In general, these patients do very well with conservative therapy but can experience recurrences over time.

Less common but more worrisome are patients with pain that includes the back and lower limb, where there is a likelihood of nerve root impingement or irritation. Some feel that pain that does not extend below the knee is less likely to be neurogenic than pain that extends below the knee. Obviously, the presence of neurologic symptoms and especially signs increases the likelihood of neurogenic pain. In adults, the spinal cord ends at about the level of the L1 vertebral body. The nerve roots of the cauda equina descend within the lumbar spinal canal and paired nerve roots exit at each interspinal level. The exiting nerve roots migrate laterally and exit beneath the pedicle of the vertebral body with the same number as the nerve root (L4 nerve root exits beneath the pedicle of the L4 vertebral body). Because the pedicle is above the interspinal disc, a ruptured disc characteristically impinges on the nerve root that is migrating laterally to exit beneath the pedicle of the next lower vertebral segment. For this reason, in the lumbar region a lumbar disc rupture characteristically affects the nerve root that is one higher in number (and lower in the spinal canal). Therefore the L4 disc typically impinges on the L5 nerve root, and the L5 disc impinges on the S1 nerve root.

More than 90% of disc herniations occur at L4–L5 (and potentially cause L5 radiculopathy) and L5–S1 (and potentially cause S1 radiculopathy). Disc herniations less commonly occur at L3–L4 (which can cause L4 radiculopathy) and L2–L3 (which can cause L3 radiculopathy). Of course, large disc herniations can compress more than one nerve root on one side and, if they are large enough, can cause nerve root compression bilaterally and thus result in CES. Low back pain with radiculopathy is usually, but not always, caused by disc herniations and/or bony nerve root impingement. Intraspinal masses such as synovial cysts and benign and malignant tumors can also cause a radicular pain syndrome.

There are some common characteristics of lumbar disc herniation syndromes. These include subacute or acute onset; pain that is more apt to be aching than sharp; aggravation with sitting; positive cough, sneeze, and/or strain effect on the limb pain; and night waking from pain. In addition to neurologic symptoms and findings, there may be tenderness of the sciatic nerve in the sciatic notch or in the popliteal fossa.

SLR is positive if it elicits pain along the course of the sciatic nerve, especially leg pain, at elevations of 70 degrees or less. Provocation of LBP alone does not suggest nerve root impingement. SLR is positive for L5 and S1 nerve root impingement but not usually for L4 nerve root impingement and not at all for L2 or L3 nerve root impingement. This occurs because the L5 and S1 much more than the L4 nerve roots contribute to the sciatic nerve and thus the impinged nerve roots are irritated when the sciatic nerve is stretched via the SLR maneuver. Pain in the lower limb, more than in the buttock, and much more than in the lower back, is positive in the SLR test. Crossed SLR in which pain in the affected lower extremity is brought out by SLR of the asymptomatic limb is said to be highly suggestive of nerve root compression. Reverse SLR in which the knee is passively flexed maximally while the patient is prone is positive if this maneuver brings out the patient's limb pain more likely than if it aggravates the back pain in patients with L2, L3, or L4 nerve root impingement, because these three roots contribute to the femoral nerve and are stretched by this test. Hip and/or knee pathology can limit the utility of reverse SLR testing. If there is a tilt of the lumbar spine laterally when the patient is standing or if the patient "corkscrews" or bends to the side while attempting to flex forward and/or return to an upright posture, disc herniation with nerve root impingement is thought to be more likely. Be aware that an occasional patient will report improvement in radicular pain coincident with worsening disc-induced nerve root compression. In this situation the patient or examiner will note significant progression of the neurologic deficits. Table 3.5 shows the neurologic changes in L2, L3, L4, L5, and S1 nerve root injuries.

Recognition of the uncommon CES is imperative. The patient can have prodromal unilateral symptoms and then develop bilateral lower limb symptoms that can be asymmetric. Bilateral pain with or without weakness is then accompanied by perianal and perineal numbness and tingling and difficulty with bladder more often than bowel control. Patients note an inability to void, decreased force of the urinary stream, inability to sense bladder fullness, and incomplete emptying, indicating involvement of the sacral nerve roots. SLR may be absent but perianal sensation and sacral reflexes (anal wink and bulbocavernosus) may be lost along with the lower limb deep tendon reflexes. Rectal examination should be performed if CES is suspected and will show anal sphincter weakness when the patient is asked to squeeze the examiner's finger. The condition is usually caused by massive midline disc herniation most frequently at L4–L5, but other intraspinal mass lesions can cause the same syndrome. CES is a neurosurgical emergency. If CES is suspected, additional investigation is mandatory.

TABLE 3.5. LUMBOSACRAL NERVE ROOT IMPINGEMENT SYNDROMES

	L2	L3	L4	L5	S1
Pain	Anterior thigh	Anterior thigh	Anterolateral thigh, anteromedial leg	Lateral thigh and leg	Posterior thigh and leg
Motor weakness	Hip flexion	Hip flexion, knee extension, thigh adduction	Knee extension, foot dorsiflexion	Ankle and great toe dorsiflexion	Foot and great toe plantar flexion
Sensory loss	Lateral thigh	Anterior and medial thigh	Medial leg	Lateral leg, dorsum foot	Posterior leg, lateral foot
Reflex depression	None	Knee, adductor	Knee	None	Ankle
Atrophy	± Thigh	Thigh	± Thigh	± Leg	Leg
SLR test	–	–	±	+	+
RSLR test	+	+	+	–	–

RSLR, reverse straight-leg raising; SLR, straight-leg raising.

Acute Versus Chronic Low Back Pain

Most authors and algorithms differentiate between acute [less than 6 weeks (4) or less than 12 weeks in duration (2,3)] and chronic LBP. Most "serious" and surgical causes of back pain present as acute syndromes. One exception is lumbar spinal stenosis (LSS), which is described separately later in this chapter. Of course, there is no sharp cutoff between acute and chronic with respect to symptoms or underlying etiologies. Patients with "serious" causes can present with acute symptoms superimposed upon chronic complaints. Most patients with chronic LBP with or without lower-extremity pain have an underlying musculoskeletal cause for their discomfort and, with the exception of LSS, do not have an underlying surgically treatable cause. Patients with chronic LBP can be difficult to evaluate because of lingering uncertainty about the true cause of their symptoms. Treatment of patients with chronic LBP is frustrating because of the resistance of their symptoms to therapy and complicating psychologic and disability/workers' compensation factors (5).

Evaluation of the Patient with Acute Low Back Pain

Excellent, evidenced-based clinical practice guidelines are available for the evaluation and management of patients with acute and chronic LBP (2–4,6). Acute LBP will be defined as occurring in patients with new or recurrent symptoms of less than 6 to 12 weeks' duration. Although some algorithms define sciatica as pain in the lower extremity below the knee (3,4), patients with upper lumbar radiculopathies can experience pain limited to the thigh, and a true definition of sciatica refers to pain radiating into the lower extremity without differentiating between pain that affects the thigh versus leg. Therefore the quoted algorithms have been modified such that sciatica is defined as pain in the lower extremity below the buttock affecting the thigh or leg (or both).

The initial evaluation of acute or recurrent LBP with or without lower limb discomfort follows directly from the history and physical findings outlined earlier and is shown in Fig. 3.2. If there are no red flags from the history and no significant findings on neurologic examination, diagnostic testing is not clinically helpful in the first 4 weeks of symptoms. Appropriate evaluation is conducted for symptoms of possible spine fracture [plain films, then possibly bone scan and/or computed tomographic (CT) scan], cancer or infection (blood count, sedimentation rate, other blood tests, urinalysis, then plain x-ray, bone scan, and possibly magnetic resonance imaging), and for rapidly progressive neurologic symptoms, including CES [magnetic resonance imaging (MRI) or myelography with CT scanning and consultation with a neurologist and/or spine surgeon]. Oblique projections rarely add helpful information, double the patient's radiation exposure, and are not recommended. Some plain x-ray findings are of doubtful clinical relevance because they are commonly found and often unrelated to acute back pain. These findings include narrowing of a single disc space, spondylolysis (a defect in pars interarticularis of the vertebral body arch), partial lumbarization of the sacrum or sacralization of a vertebral body, Schmorl node (herniation of a disc upward or downward into a vertebral body), spina bifida occulta, disc calcification, and mild thoracolumbar scoliosis.

For patients without red flags and without neurologic signs, conservative treatment is recommended for the first 1 to 2 months (see later). When the patient is seen in follow-up, the clinician again looks for red flags and/or signs of neurologic involvement. If none are found, continued conservative management is recommended, but if red flags or deficits emerge, investigation should be considered. Although more than 90% of patients will completely recover within 12 weeks of the onset of symptoms, up to 10% of patients may have continuing symptoms. Of the patients with symptoms that persist for more than 2 to 3 months after onset, about 90% will have LBP alone and 10% will have LBP with lower limb discomfort. For patients with pain that persists for more than

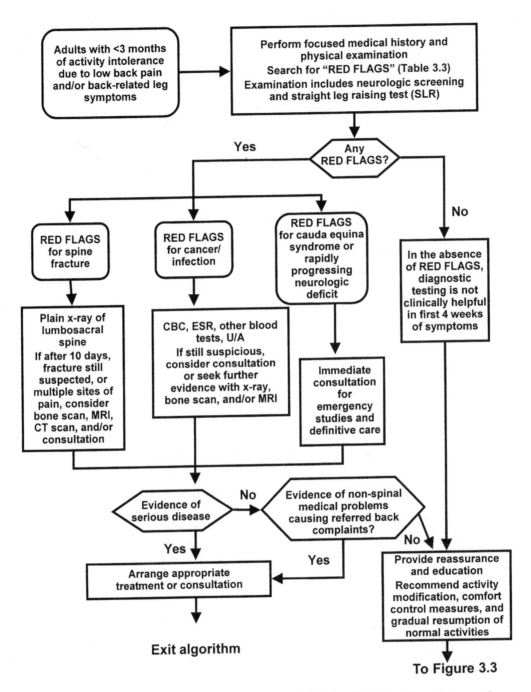

FIGURE 3.2. Initial evaluation of acute low back pain (LBP). (Modified from Bigos S, Bowyer O, Braen G, et al. *Acute low back problems in adults: clinical practice guideline*, Quick Reference Guide Number 14. Rockville, MD: U.S. Department of Health and Human Services, Public Health Service, Agency for Health Care Policy and Research, AHCPR Pub. No. 95-0643. December 1994.)

4 to 6 weeks without improvement, additional investigation should be considered (Fig. 3.3). For patients with LBP alone, plain anteroposterior and lateral x-rays of the lumbar spine may be sufficient, but additional tests such as blood count, sedimentation rate, prostate-specific antigen, serum protein electrophoresis, MRI, and bone scan can be conducted for specific, suspected conditions. For patients with persisting

low back and lower limb pain, MRI of the lumbar spine can be considered to look for evidence of nerve root impingement and/or inflammation. For patients who are extremely claustrophobic or have a pacemaker, magnetic prosthetic heart valve, wire in the spinal canal, metallic foreign body in a critical location, or ferromagnetic intracranial aneurysm clip, plain CT scan or myelography with CT scanning can be

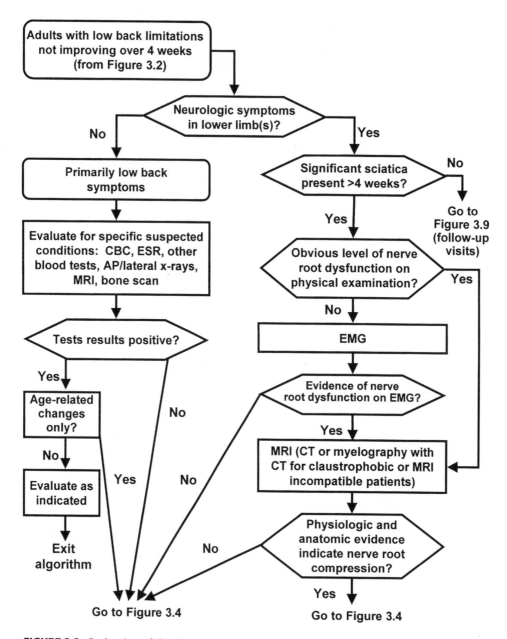

FIGURE 3.3. Evaluation of the slow-to-recover patient. (Modified from Bigos S, Bowyer O, Braen G, et al. *Acute low back problems in adults: clinical practice guideline,* Quick Reference Guide Number 14. Rockville, MD: U.S. Department of Health and Human Services, Public Health Service, Agency for Health Care Policy and Research, AHCPR Pub. No. 95-0643. December 1994.)

used. Myelography with CT scanning is preferred over plain CT, especially for possible surgical candidates because of superior imaging of the nerve roots. In this setting, electromyography (EMG) with nerve conduction velocity testing could also be considered. EMG changes may not be evident for 3 to 4 weeks after nerve injury. Interpretation of EMG depends upon the expertise of the electromyographer, and old, chronic changes in the distribution of a lumbosacral nerve root can be confused with acute abnormalities. EMG can help determine if there is nerve root involvement, which

level(s) is involved, and whether the nerve injury is old, active, or improving.

If the patient's symptoms and signs persist despite conservative treatment, instruction in a back exercise program should be considered. The primary care physician may elect to refer the patient for consultation with a nonsurgical back specialist (physical medicine and rehabilitation, neurology, or rheumatology) or to a back surgeon if the patient has indications for and is willing to accept surgical intervention (Fig. 3.4). To consider surgery,

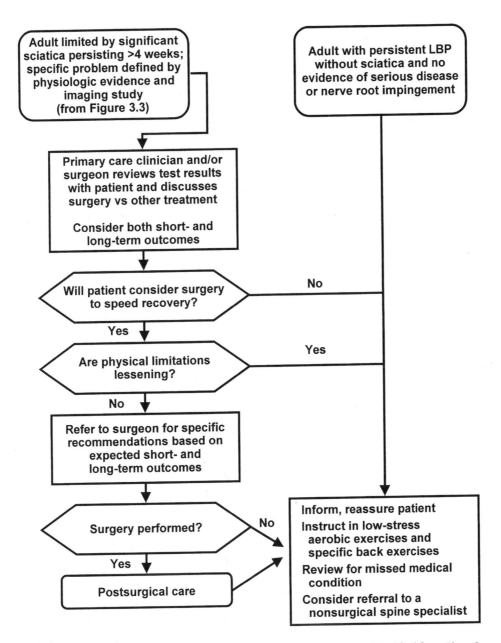

FIGURE 3.4. Additional considerations for patients with persistent pain. (Modified from Bigos S, Bowyer O, Braen G, et al. *Acute low back problems in adults: clinical practice guideline*, Quick Reference Guide Number 14. Rockville, MD: U.S. Department of Health and Human Services, Public Health Service, Agency for Health Care Policy and Research, AHCPR Pub. No. 95-0643. December 1994.)

Agency for Health Care Policy and Research (AHCPR) criteria call for all three of the following to be present: sciatica that is both severe and disabling, symptoms of sciatica that persist without improvement for more than 4 weeks or with extreme progression, and very strong physiologic evidence of dysfunction of a specific nerve root with intervertebral disc herniation confirmed at the corresponding level and side by findings on an imaging study (2).

Chronic Low Back Pain with or Without Lower Limb Pain

Recurrent episodes of acute symptoms separated by essentially pain-free intervals are approached as though the patient has acute symptoms. More than 90% of patients with acute symptoms will clear or improve substantially within 4 to 6 weeks of symptom onset. Of the 10% or less of patients who have chronic symptoms lasting more than

6 to 12 weeks, about 90% have LBP alone and about 10% have LBP with sciatica.

For purposes of evaluation, patients with chronic pain can be divided into those with LBP alone and those with low back and lower limb pain.

The patient with chronic symptoms should undergo a thorough evaluation (or reevaluation if the patient is receiving ongoing care from a single provider) similar to that outlined earlier. Testing of the patient with chronic pain will depend on the duration of the pain, whether the pain is worsening, the results of prior testing, and the provider's clinical suspicions. There are few evidence-based guidelines for the evaluation of patients with chronic back pain. If not previously obtained, plain x-rays of the lumbar spine should be ordered; anteroposterior and lateral views will suffice in most patients. If there is any evidence of instability, oblique and flexion–extension films can be obtained to look for spondylolysis and spondylolisthesis (slippage of one vertebral body forward or backward on the vertebra below). Similarly, screening blood and urine tests (blood count, sedimentation rate, other blood tests, and urinalysis) should be considered. Especially for patients with sciatica, more precise imaging of the lumbosacral spine and EMG should be considered. As noted earlier, EMG can show evidence of previous nerve root injury that does not correlate with current symptoms. MRI is the preferred, more precise imaging test because it clearly shows the soft tissues and nervous structures as well as the bones, at least to some extent. Patients and their families are aware of the availability of powerful imaging studies such as MRI and may request that such a test be performed. A normal MRI study can be persuasively reassuring, but incidental findings abound. When MRI is performed in volunteers without signs or symptoms of back problems, about one-third show one or more herniated intervertebral discs. Myelography with CT scanning is an alternative for patients with low back and lower limb pain if MRI cannot be performed because of claustrophobia, pacemaker or intraspinal wires, metal prosthetic heart valves, metallic foreign bodies in critical locations, or ferromagnetic intracranial aneurysm clips. Plain CT scanning of the lumbar spine can be helpful for patients with suspected bony lesions. Nuclear medicine bone scans can be helpful for patients with LBP alone or LBP with sciatica if spine tumor, infection, or occult fracture is suspected.

The patient with chronic low back and/or lower limb pain is challenging, and primary care physicians should consider referral to a medical nonsurgical back specialist (physical medicine and rehabilitation, neurology, or rheumatology) or to a conservative surgical back specialist (neurosurgeon or orthopedic surgeon) for help with evaluation and management.

All authors (1–3,5–7) describe the psychosocial factors that can promote chronic pain and disability. These include disability and workers' compensation issues, problems at work and at home, primary psychiatric disorders, and difficulty coping with pain that might be considered physiologic or normal for aging. The ICSI guideline suggests use of the *Diagnostic and Statistical Manual of Mental Disorders,* 4th ed. (DSM-IV), screening checklist for depression (Table 3.6), a pain drawing that the patient completes looking for evidence of nonanatomic and/or exaggerated pain reporting (Fig. 3.5), and Waddell's signs for nonorganic pathology and pain magnification (Table 3.7) (4). Of course, patients with underlying organic disease can also have psychosocial problems. Although addressing psychosocial factors is difficult, their recognition can help explain the chronicity of symptoms.

Differential Diagnosis of Acute and Chronic Low Back Pain

The differential diagnoses of acute and chronic LBP with and without lower limb radiation are somewhat different and are shown in Tables 3.8 and 3.9 (7). Images of selected diagnoses are shown in Figs. 3.6, 3.7, and 3.8.

TABLE 3.6. DSM-IV SCREENING CHECKLIST FOR DEPRESSION

1. Depressed mood.
2. Markedly diminished interest or pleasure in all or almost all activities.
3. Significant (>5% body weight) weight loss or gain or decrease or increase in appetite.
4. Insomnia or hypersomnia.
5. Psychomotor agitation or retardation.
6. Fatigue or loss of energy.
7. Feeling of worthlessness or inappropriate guilt.
8. Diminished concentration or indecisiveness.
9. Recurrent thoughts of death or suicide.

For a diagnosis of a major depressive episode, at least five of the symptoms listed above must be present nearly every day for at least two weeks and represent a change from previous functioning. At least one of the symptoms must be either #1, depressed mood, or #2, loss of interest or pleasure.
From *Diagnostic and Statistical Manual of Mental Disorders,* 4th ed. Washington, DC: American Psychiatric Association, 1994:327, with permission.

Name_____   Date_____

Where is your pain now?

Mark the areas on your body where you feel the sensations described below, using the appropriate symbols. Mark the areas of radiation, including all affected areas.
Please mark an (X) (X within a circle) on the area where the pain is now worst.

Aching	Numbness	Pins and needles	Burning	Stabbing
zzz	===	OOO	XXX	///

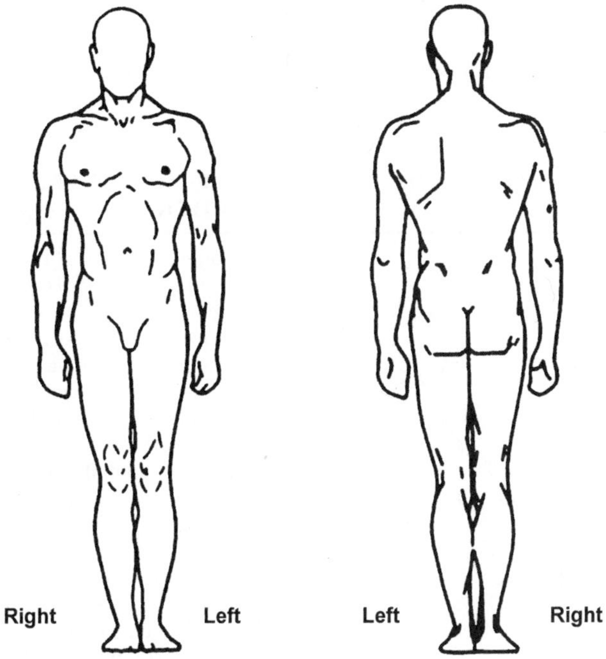

Right   Left   Left   Right

How bad is your pain?

On a scale of 1 to 10, circle your pain

At its very worst	No pain	1 2 3 4 5 6 7 8 9 10
At its best	No pain	1 2 3 4 5 6 7 8 9 10
Now		1 2 3 4 5 6 7 8 9 10

Overall, is your pain generally (circle one): Improving   Same   Worsening

FIGURE 3.5. Pain drawing. (Modified from Institute for Clinical Systems Improvement Health Care Guideline. Adult low back pain, May 2001. Used with permission.)

TABLE 3.7. WADDELL'S NONORGANIC PHYSICAL SIGNS IN LOW BACK PAIN

Tenderness: Tender to superficial pinch in the lumbar area or deep tenderness in a wide, nonanatomic distribution
Simulation of an organic test: Low back pain caused by axial loading (pressure on top of the head) or rotation of the hips/pelvis and shoulder in the same plane while the patient is standing
Distraction: A positive finding (e.g., straight-leg raising when supine) is not present when the patient is distracted or tested in a different way (e.g., straight-leg raising when seated)
Regional disturbances: Weakness or sensory loss that follows a regional, nonanatomic distribution
Overreaction: Dramatic verbalization, facial expression, muscle tension, tremor, and collapse— "an academy award performance"

If three or more of the tests listed above are positive, there is a high probability of nonorganic disease.
Modified from Waddell G, McCulloch JA, Kummel E, et al. Nonorganic physical signs in low-back pain. *Spine* 1980;5:117–125.

TABLE 3.8. DIFFERENTIAL DIAGNOSIS OF LOW BACK PAIN

Musculoskeletal
   Herniated nucleus pulposus
   Facet joint arthritis
   Spondylolisthesis
   Muscle origin
   Trauma, including compression fracture
Referred from abdomen or pelvis
   Abdominal aortic aneurysm
   Peptic ulcer
   Genitourinary (infection, stone, tumor, endometriosis)
   Pancreatitis
   Diverticulitis
Infection
   Disc
   Epidural
   Bone
Tumor
   Primary bone
   Metastatic
   Intraspinal (neural)
Rheumatologic
   Ankylosing spondylitis
   Polymyalgia rheumatica
   Other inflammatory arthritides
Metabolic and bone diseases
   Osteoporosis
   Paget disease
   Fluorosis

TABLE 3.9. DIFFERENTIAL DIAGNOSIS OF SCIATICA

Neurogenic at level of conus medullaris, cauda equina, or exiting nerve roots
   Tumor
      Primary (e.g., neurofibroma, ependymoma)
      Metastatic to bone or epidural space
      Meningeal involvement by cancer or lymphoma
   Herniated nucleus pulposus
   Stenosis of canal or lateral recess
   Sterile inflammatory arachnoiditis
   Synovial cyst
   Infection
      Disc space
      Epidural space
      Ganglionitis (herpes zoster)
Neurogenic outside the spine
   Lumbosacral plexus
      Tumor
      Idiopathic inflammatory
   Sciatic neuropathy
      Compression
      Tumor
   Diabetic polyradiculoneuropathy
   Peripheral neuropathy
Nonneurogenic
   Orthopedic (e.g., arthritis of hip or knee; effects of trauma)
   Peripheral vascular disease
      Arterial
      Venous
   Bone disease
      Tumors
      Osteoporosis
   Genitourinary

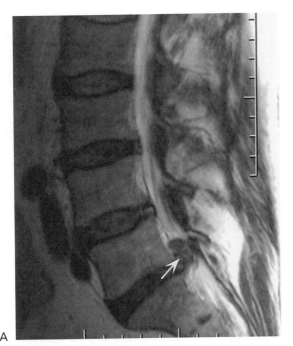

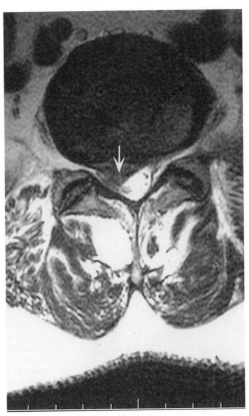

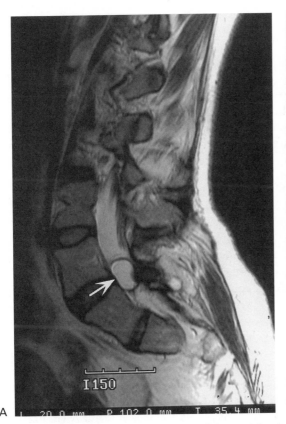

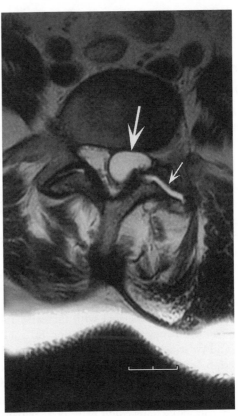

FIGURE 3.6. Sagittal **(A)** and axial **(B)** T$_2$-weighted magnetic resonance imaging of lumbar spine shows a large L5–S1 disc protrusion *(arrows),* which posteriorly displaces and distorts the right S1 nerve root. On the sagittal view, a portion of the disc has migrated upward and lies behind the L5 vertebral body.

FIGURE 3.7. Sagittal **(A)** and axial **(B)** T$_2$-weighted magnetic resonance imaging of lumbar spine shows a large synovial cyst on the patient's left at the L5–S1 level *(large arrows).* On the axial view, fluid can be seen within the facet joint on the side of the synovial cyst *(small arrow).* The thecal sac is shifted to the patient's right.

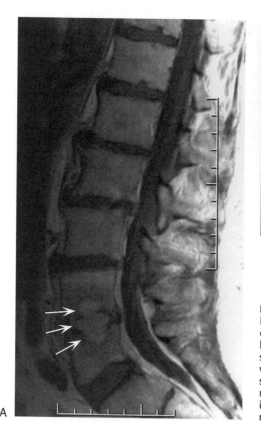

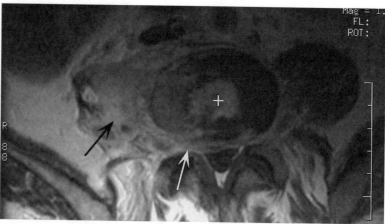

FIGURE 3.8. Sagittal **(A)** T$_1$-weighted magnetic resonance imaging (MRI) scan of lumbar spine with gadolinium shows obliteration of the L4–L5 interspace with enhancement of the disc space and adjoining portions of the L4 and L5 vertebral bodies *(arrows)*. Axial **(B)** T$_1$-weighted MRI scan with gadolinium at the L4–L5 level shows enhancing soft tissue mass involving the right psoas muscle *(black arrow)*, which is contiguous with similarly enhancing tissue that extends into the epidural space through the right L4–L5 neural foramen *(white arrow)*. Contrast enhancement is also seen within the disc space (+). The findings are those of a disc space infection with osteomyelitis within the L4 and L5 vertebral bodies and involvement of the right psoas muscle and epidural space.

Prevention and Therapy

Prevention

Primary prevention includes those measures that are intended to prevent the first-ever occurrence of low back pain, whereas secondary prevention includes those efforts that are meant to prevent a subsequent occurrence of back pain in someone who has sustained an initial event. Most of the evidence and recommendations are directed toward secondary rather than primary prevention of LBP. Acute and chronic LBP are, at best, only partially preventable. Most prevention studies have been conducted in the workplace and focus on injury claims or use interventions that cannot be easily offered by primary care providers (3). Since there is an association between smoking, herniated discs, and LBP, smoking cessation could help to reduce an individual's risk for developing back pain. Work-setting factors associated with increased risk include heavy work, lifting, prolonged sitting or standing, bending and twisting, vibration, monotonous work, job dissatisfaction, and poor relationships with co-workers (1,6). To the extent that these factors can be reduced, occupational low back pain might be diminished to some extent. Primary care physicians could offer their patients instruction in proper lifting techniques and recommend that individuals avoid lifting more than they are capable

of doing, but it is not clear how much benefit this would produce. There is some evidence that low back exercises can help in the primary prevention of LBP, but they are more frequently employed for secondary prevention (see later) (3).

Lumbar corsets and lumbosacral supports used for primary prevention of LBP may be of some benefit in individuals required to do frequent lifting at work (3), but the evidence is weak. Activity alteration and exercise therapy are usually recommended for recurrent and chronic back pain but not for primary prevention. In general, no pharmacologic preventive treatments are available. For patients with recurrent episodes of LBP due to musculoskeletal causes, the regular use of nonsteroidal, antiinflammatory drugs (NSAIDs) may help to blunt if not prevent some episodes. Surgery is never recommended as primary prevention for low back pain and is generally only offered to patients with ongoing symptoms. Nonetheless, in certain circumstances, one could make a case for operative intervention on patients with structural abnormalities and multiple previous recurrent episodes of pain who are virtually certain of experiencing additional attacks in the future (see later). LBP is most common between the ages of 35 and 55. As people age, they are actually less likely to experience new episodes of LBP, which reduces the need for preventive intervention.

Therapy

Treatment for LBP can be divided into patients with acute (less than 6 to 12 weeks' duration) and chronic (greater than 6 to 12 weeks' duration) pain with or without limb radiation. Recurrent episodes of acute pain are approached as episodes of acute pain, but the need for secondary prevention measures is much greater in the patient who has experienced previous acute attacks. The shorter the interval between acute attacks, the greater the need for secondary prevention measures, most of which fall under the realm of "physical therapies," such as exercises and lumbar corsets and supports. The evidence-based practice guidelines (2–4) form the basis for the following recommendations.

Therapy for Acute Low Back Pain

For patients without any of the previously described red flags, both nonpharmacologic and pharmacologic treatments are recommended. First, patients should be reassured that the vast majority of attacks of acute low back pain subside without specific intervention. Patient education is helpful and material can be found by contacting the guideline websites (www.ahcpr.gov or www.ahrq.gov and www.icsi.org). Currently, there is no evidence to support the use of bed rest for acute pain, and patients should be told to be "up and about" as their pain will allow. Short periods of bed rest may provide temporary pain relief for patients who experience severe pain with radiculopathy. Activities and postures that increase pain should be restricted. Lifting should be limited and performed with objects close to the abdomen, with the back kept straight, and twisting, bending, and stooping should be minimized. To avoid debilitation, patients should be encouraged to resume normal activity as soon as possible and to consider aerobic conditioning exercises such as walking, stationary biking, or swimming when they are able to do so. The local use of ice and/or heat may provide some short-term symptomatic benefit. There is no evidence that specific exercises are helpful during the first 4 to 6 weeks of acute back pain. The AHCPR guidelines do recommend manipulation ("manual loading of the spine using short or long leverage methods") during the first month of acute low back symptoms, whereas the ICSI guidelines do not. For pain control, both guidelines recommend the use of acetaminophen and NSAIDs as the mainstay for comfort control, if needed. Short-term use of muscle relaxants can be helpful but can cause drowsiness and dependence. Opioid analgesics are of equivocal efficacy, are rarely indicated, and have a significant potential for producing drowsiness and dependency. The guidelines recommend against the use of acupuncture, injections, corsets, and traction for acute LBP with or without sciatica. Figure 3.9 gives an overview of the treatment of acute LBP at the initial and follow-up visits, and Table 3.10 outlines the AHCPR recommended symptom control methods.

Providers are often asked to prescribe work limitations for patients with acute LBP. Although these will depend on the patient's age, other health factors, and their work, the AHCPR guidelines provide a rough framework (Table 3.11).

Patients whose symptoms continue for more than 4 to 6 weeks should be reassessed (Figs. 3.3, 3.4, and 3.9), especially looking for "red flags." Additional investigations are carried out if indicated for patients with slow-to-recover LBP alone or LBP with sciatica as described earlier. If there is no need for additional investigation or the investigations are negative, then the patient should be referred to a trained spine therapy professional for additional education; limited passive treatments, including manual therapy (manipulation and mobilization); and instruction in self-administered exercises to condition specific trunk (abdominal and back) muscles. The passive treatments are meant to be self-limited; the patient should become self-sufficient in performing the exercises. Conditioning trunk exercises are helpful for persistent acute LBP.

The AHCPR guidelines recommend against the use of oral corticosteroids for acute LBP with or without lower limb pain and against the use of epidural steroids for acute LBP without radiculopathy, but they suggest that epidural steroids might be helpful for patients with low back and lower limb pain in an effort to avoid surgery.

Chronic Low Back Pain

For patients with recurrent bouts of acute LBP and for those with chronic LBP, regular exercises are helpful, but there is no evidence that favors one exercise over another (4). Activities that precipitate attacks of acute pain or provoke chronic back discomfort should be avoided. If not done previously, referral to a spine therapy professional should be considered. "Back school" programs are available that educate patients about their condition, instruct them in a home exercise program, and teach them how to manage their back condition. Acetaminophen and NSAIDs or cyclooxygenase-2 (COX-2) inhibitors can be used for pain control, but muscle relaxants and opioid analgesics should be avoided. Tricyclic agents such as amitriptyline or nortriptyline may be of some help in reducing chronic pain. Injection therapy is frequently employed but has limited benefit and diminishing returns when repeated. Guidelines call for "psychosocial evaluation" of patients with chronic pain. Treatment in pain rehabilitation programs that aim to help patients live and cope better despite their pain can be beneficial.

Indications for Surgery

Fracture with instability, infection, tumor, and cauda equina syndrome requires urgent or emergent surgical

Initial visit

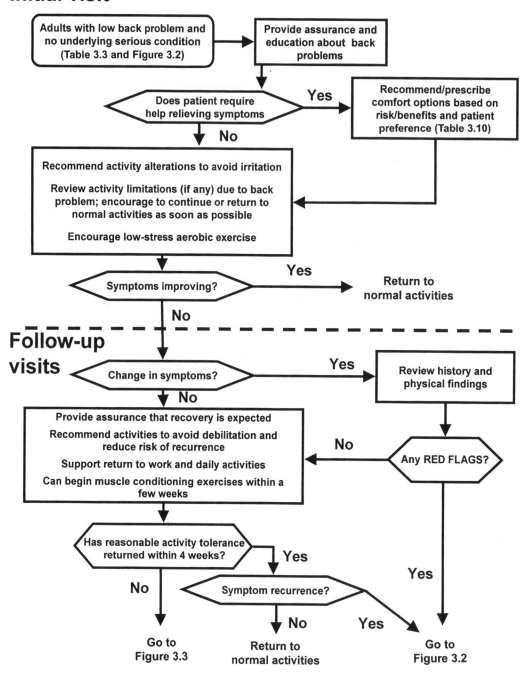

FIGURE 3.9. Treatment of acute low back problem on initial and follow-up visits. (Modified from Bigos S, Bowyer O, Braen G, et al. *Acute low back problems in adults: clinical practice guideline,* Quick Reference Guide Number 14. Rockville, MD: U.S. Department of Health and Human Services, Public Health Service, Agency for Health Care Policy and Research, AHCPR Pub. No. 95-0643. December 1994.)

TABLE 3.10. SYMPTOM CONTROL METHODS

Recommended		

Nonprescription Analgesics

Acetaminophen (safest)
NSAIDs (aspirin,[a] ibuprofen[a])

Prescribed Pharmaceutical Methods	Prescribed Physical Methods	
Nonspecific Low Back Symptoms and/or Sciatica	**Nonspecific Low Back Symptoms**	**Sciatica**
Other NSAIDs[a]	Manipulation (in place of medication or a shorter trial if combined with NSAIDs)	

Options		
Nonspecific Low Back Symptoms and/or Sciatica	**Nonspecific Low Back Symptoms**	**Sciatica**
Muscle relaxants[b–d]	Physical agents and modalities[b] (heat or cold modalities for home programs only)	Manipulation (in place of medication or a shorter trial if combined with NSAIDs)
Opioids[b–d]	Shoe insoles[b]	Physical agents and modalities[b] (heat or cold modalities for home programs only) Few days' rest[d] Shoe insoles[b]

NSAID, nonsteroidal antiinflammatory drugs.
[a]Aspirin and other NSAIDs are not recommended for use in combination with one another due to the risk of gastrointestinal complications.
[b]Equivocal efficacy.
[c]Significant potential for producing drowsiness and debilitation; potential for dependency.
[d]Short course (few days only) for severe symptoms.
From Bigos S, Bowyer O, Braen G, et al. *Acute low back problems in adults: clinical practice guideline,* Quick Reference Guide Number 14. Rockville, MD: U.S. Department of Health and Human Services, Public Health Service, Agency for Health Care Policy and Research, AHCPR Pub. No. 95-0643. December 1994.

TABLE 3.11. GUIDELINES FOR SITTING AND UNASSISTED LIFTING

	Symptoms						
	Severe	→	**Moderate**	→	**Mild**	→	**None**
Sitting[a]	20 min	→	→	→	→	→	50 min
Unassisted lifting[b]							
Men	20 lb	→	20 lb	→	60 lb	→	80 lb
Women	20 lb	→	20 lb	→	35 lb	→	40 lb

[a]Without getting up and moving around.
[b]Modification of National Institute of Occupational Safety and Health Lifting Guidelines, 1981, 1993. Gradually increase unassisted lifting limits to 60 lb (men) and 35 lb (women) by 3 months, even with continued symptoms. Instruct patient to limit twisting, bending, reaching while lifting and to hold lifted object as close to navel as possible.
From Bigos S, Bowyer O, Braen G, et al. *Acute low back problems in adults: clinical practice guideline,* Quick Reference Guide Number 14. Rockville, MD: U.S. Department of Health and Human Services, Public Health Service, Agency for Health Care Policy and Research, AHCPR Pub. No. 95-0643. December 1994.

consultation for possible stabilization, culture, biopsy, or decompression, respectively. These patients should be identified through "red flags" in the history and/or examination. For patients with acute LBP without any of these conditions, surgery should only be considered within the first 3 months after onset of symptoms if (a) the patient has sciatica in addition to LBP, and the sciatica is both severe and disabling; (b) the symptoms of sciatica (pain and/or neurologic deficit) persist without improvement for greater than 4 weeks or progress; and (c) there is strong physiologic evidence of dysfunction of a specific nerve root with confirmation of disc herniation at the appropriate level on an imaging study. Nerve root decompression can be helpful to patients with acute, recurrent, or even chronic LBP with sciatica if these three conditions are present. So long as there is no evidence of severe root dysfunction, there is no evidence that delaying surgery for 1 month after the onset of symptoms worsens eventual outcomes. Surgical intervention speeds pain relief and promotes recovery of lost nerve root function, but 4 to 10 years after onset of herniated disc, the outcomes are the same for operated and nonoperated patients (3). Standard discectomy and microdiscectomy are felt to be of similar efficacy, whereas percutaneous discectomy is less efficacious, and chymopapain injection is no longer available for use. Discectomy includes partial laminectomy, which provides access to the protruding disc. Many surgeons favor the increased exposure afforded by open discectomy over microdiscectomy (6). The risk of first-time back surgery for herniated disc is low with less than 1% of patients experiencing infection, bleeding, or increased neurologic deficit. However, with each successive operation on the same lumbar spine, the risk of complications increases and the benefits of surgery decline. With proper patient selection, 90% or more of patients' sciatica can be relieved with operative intervention, but LBP is less likely to be helped.

There is almost no role for surgery in the treatment of patients with acute LBP without "red flags" and without radiculopathy. For patients with chronic LBP without lower limb pain, decompression of nerve roots is unlikely to be helpful. In this setting, consideration is sometimes given to spinal fusion using autologous or banked bone, or "instrumentation" (various implanted, usually metallic devices) or both. The exact indications for spinal fusion are uncertain. According to one text (6), spinal fusion should be considered only if there is surgical or traumatic instability (as with the removal of facet joints bilaterally), neural arch defects (spondylolysis or spondylolisthesis or both), or symptomatic and radiographically demonstrable segmental instability. Another text states that fusion for LBP is rarely indicated (7). Compared with discectomy with partial laminectomy, spinal fusion is a more involved procedure, has a higher complication rate, and has a longer postoperative recovery period.

LUMBAR SPINAL STENOSIS
Definition and Epidemiology

Lumbar spinal stenosis (LSS) is defined as narrowing of the lumbar spinal canal, its lateral recesses, and neural foramina with associated compression of the lumbosacral nerve roots. The stenosis can be symptomatic or asymptomatic. Although precise incidence and prevalence figures are unavailable, the occurrence of LSS increases with advancing age. Probably because of advancing age of the population, increased recognition of the clinical syndrome, and increased availability and diagnostic capability of imaging studies, there has been a marked increase in the number of operations performed for LSS over time (8). Men and women are affected about equally. Although disability and pain control issues are much less frequent with LSS than with acute and chronic LBP, quality of life is impacted equally.

Pathophysiology and Pathogenesis

LSS can be due to congenital or acquired causes. Frequently, degenerative changes are superimposed upon a congenitally, relatively narrowed lumbar spinal canal (Table 3.12). Hypertrophy of any of the structures that border the spinal canal can lead to stenosis (Fig. 3.10). Facet joint hypertrophy is the leading cause of LSS with contributions from disc degeneration and vertebral body hypertrophy, thickening and bulging of the ligamentum flavum, and degenerative spondylolisthesis. In descending order, the most commonly affected levels are L4–L5, L3–L4, L2–L3, L5–LS1, and L1–L2. Most patients have narrowing at more than one level. In addition to static narrowing, there is a dynamic component that helps to account for the postural relationship of symptoms. When individuals are seated or supine, the lumbosacral spine is relatively straight; however, when they stand or walk, they develop lumbar lordosis with extension of the lower spine. The superior articular facets

TABLE 3.12. FACTORS CONTRIBUTING TO LUMBAR STENOSIS

Degenerative changes
  Hypertrophy of facet joints
  Ligamentum flavum hypertrophy
  Degenerative spondylolisthesis
  Calcium salt deposition
  Synovial cysts
  Scoliosis
Congenital narrowing
  Idiopathic
  Achondroplasia
Less common causes
  Paget disease
  Diffuse idiopathic skeletal hyperostosis
  Fluorosis

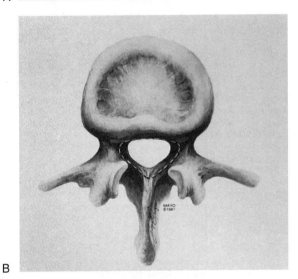

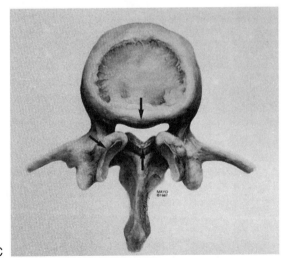

FIGURE 3.10. Types of lumbar spinal canal. **A:** Normal. **B:** Congenital narrowing. *Stippled line* shows normal dimensions. **C:** Narrow lumbar canal due to hypertrophy of ligamentum flavum, enlargement of facet joints, and spondylotic hyperostosis of the vertebral body adjacent to the intervertebral disc (*arrows*). (Floyd Hosmer, artist.) (From Bartleson JD, O'Duffy JD. Spinal Stenosis. In: Koopman WJ, ed. *Arthritis and allied conditions: a textbook of rheumatology,* 14th ed. Philadelphia: Lippincott Williams & Wilkins, 2001:2042–2053, with permission.)

slide backward and downward on the inferior articular facets, while the lumbar discs and posterior longitudinal ligaments may bulge posteriorly into the canal, and the ligamentum flavum may buckle forward into the canal, all of which further narrow the lumbar spinal canal and intervertebral foramina and thus compress the lumbosacral nerve roots. Most authors favor mechanical compression of the lumbosacral nerve roots rather than compromise of the circulation to the nerve roots as the mechanism for the characteristic symptoms and frequent persistent neurologic findings.

Clinical Features

About 70% of patients report a remote history of episodic LBP, and about 20% have had sciatica in the past. In general, LSS is a chronic and gradually progressive condition, so that over time patients note that their tolerance for standing and walking declines. Occasional patients report spontaneous improvement. The cardinal feature of symptomatic LSS is neurogenic claudication or so-called pseudoclaudication. If the canal stenosis is asymmetric or only the lateral recess or neural foramen is affected, the symptoms can be unilateral. Patients report pain, numbness, tingling, and/or weakness in the lower limbs typically brought on by standing and walking and relieved by sitting or flexing forward at the waist. Postures that maintain or increase lumbar flexion (walking behind a cart or lawn mower, using a stationary bicycle, or leaning against an object) help to prevent or relieve pseudoclaudication. Conversely, factors that increase lumbar lordosis such as wearing higher-heeled shoes or walking down an incline can increase symptoms. In advanced cases, patients may experience symptoms when recumbent, especially if lying prone. Typically, the pseudoclaudication affects the entire lower limb, usually the posterior aspect, but can affect the thigh alone or leg alone. About two-thirds of patients have accompanying low back pain, which can occur with or be aggravated by the same postures that increase their lower limb symptoms.

There are few physical signs on examination. Deep tendon reflexes can be reduced at the ankle in up to 50% of patients and at the knee in about 20%. Mild, sometimes unilateral weakness in an L5 and/or S1 distribution can be found in up to one-third of patients. Vibration sense is often reduced in the feet, but this is a common finding in older individuals. SLR is typically negative. The patient may stand and walk flexed at the waist. Pedal pulses should be normal unless there is coexisting atherosclerotic occlusive disease. Provocation of symptoms by having the patient stand or walk and relief of such symptoms by having the patient bend forward at the waist can be helpful office tests. Reexamination when the patient is symptomatic occasionally shows new neurologic findings.

TABLE 3.13. DIFFERENTIAL DIAGNOSIS OF LUMBAR STENOSIS

Vascular claudication–atherosclerotic
Osteoarthritis of hips or knees
Lumbar disc protrusion
Unrecognized neurologic disease
  Multiple sclerosis
  Intraspinal tumor
  Arteriovenous malformation of spinal cord
  Peripheral neuropathy

Evaluation of the Patient with Suspected Lumbar Spine Stenosis

The differential diagnosis of pseudoclaudication is vascular claudication, osteoarthritis of the hips and/or knees, lumbar disc protrusion with radiculopathy, and other neurologic disorders, such as multiple sclerosis, intraspinal mass lesion, arteriovenous malformation of the spinal cord, and peripheral neuropathy (Table 3.13). Differentiating between vascular and neurogenic claudication can be difficult; the main differences between these two conditions are shown in Table 3.14.

If the diagnosis is clear and the provider and patient agree that no intervention is indicated at this time, additional investigation can be deferred. Vascular laboratory evaluation can help confirm or exclude lower limb atherosclerotic occlusive disease. Plain x-rays of the lumbosacral spine are nondiagnostic but can show dense bony struc-

tures, one or more degenerated discs, and degenerative spondylolisthesis, typically L4 on L5. Plain x-rays of the hips and/or knees can help determine if arthritis of these joints is contributing to symptoms.

Electromyography can show neurogenic changes consistent with lumbosacral nerve root injury in 90% of patients (8). Muscles supplied by the L5 and S1 nerve roots are most often affected. A normal EMG does not exclude LSS.

If there is a need to confirm the clinical diagnosis or if surgery is being considered, MRI is the imaging study of choice (Fig. 3.11). Compared with CT, MRI provides superior delineation of the soft-tissue elements of the spinal canal, and the use of the contrast agent gadolinium can help to identify tumors and scar tissue. CT scanning better demonstrates bony pathology, including fractures, and shows if calcification of discs or ligaments is present. Myelography with or without CT scanning can show blockage in the flow of contrast material and, compared with MRI, has the advantage of more easily examining patients with their spine in extension. Surgery can be performed on the basis of MRI alone. Plain CT can be used as a screening test in patients who cannot undergo MRI.

Prevention and Therapy

No measures are known to be effective in preventing LSS. The contribution of a congenitally narrow spinal canal cannot be affected prophylactically. Measures directed at the degenerative, spondylogenic component could in theory help reduce the risk of developing LSS. Thus instruction in

TABLE 3.14. DIFFERENTIAL DIAGNOSIS OF VASCULAR VERSUS NEUROGENIC CLAUDICATION

	Vascular	Neurogenic
Age	Older	Older
Gender	Male > female	Male = female
Current or previous low back pain	Less common	Very common
Lower Limb Symptoms		
Pain	Buttock, thigh, and/or leg	Buttock, thigh, and/or leg
Numbness, tingling	No	Frequent
One or both sides	Yes	Yes
Provoking Factors		
Walking	Yes	Yes
Standing	No	Yes
Bicycle	Yes	No
Up an incline	± More likely	± Less likely
Down an incline	± Less likely	± More likely
Relieving Factors		
Stand still	Helps	No help
Lean	Helps	Helps
Preventive Factor		
Flexed posture (cart, mower)	± No difference	Helps
Time to relief	Slightly quicker	Slightly slower
Pulses	Reduced	Normal
Neurologic examination	Normal	Minor findings
Straight-leg raising test	Negative	Usually negative

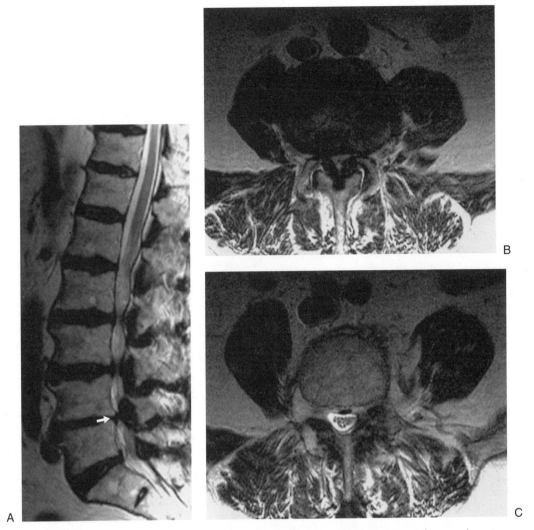

FIGURE 3.11. A: Sagittal T$_2$-weighted MRI of lumbar spine showing severe canal narrowing at L4–L5 (*arrow*) and lesser stenosis at L3–L4 more than at L2–L3. This patient has a congenitally narrow lumbar spinal canal. **B:** Axial T$_2$-weighted image demonstrating marked central canal narrowing. **C:** Axial T$_2$-weighted view at a slightly lower level shows mild to moderate stenosis with white-appearing CSF surrounding the dark lumbosacral nerve roots of the cauda equina. (From Bartleson JD, O'Duffy JD. Spinal Stenosis. In: Koopman WJ, ed. *Arthritis and allied conditions: a textbook of rheumatology,* 14th ed. Philadelphia: Lippincott Williams & Wilkins, 2001:2042–2053, with permission.)

proper lifting technique; limiting one's bending, lifting, stooping, and twisting; and avoiding weight gain might help to lower one's risk of LSS.

Therapy can be divided into physical, pharmacologic, and surgical categories (Table 3.15). Exercises to strengthen abdominal muscles and reduce lumbar lordosis may be helpful (7). A short cane or walker may allow the patient to stand longer and walk further. Corsets and braces may help reduce lumbar lordosis when standing and thereby delay the onset of symptoms. By reducing the degree of lumbar lordosis needed to stand erect and by reducing the axial load on the lumbar spine, substantial weight loss can be very helpful on occasion.

TABLE 3.15. TREATMENT OPTIONS FOR LUMBAR SPINAL STENOSIS

Physical
   Exercises
   Corsets and braces
   Short cane or walker
   Weight loss
Pharmacologic
   Simple analgesics
   Epidural steroids
Surgical
   Decompression alone
   Decompression with fusion

Analgesics are usually not very helpful because the patient's pain is intermittent and can be relieved by change in posture. NSAIDs and acetaminophen are preferred over opioid analgesics. Muscle relaxants are of no benefit. Epidural steroid injections do not provide lasting benefit, may provide some temporary pain relief, and are sometimes difficult to perform because of the degenerative changes and canal stenosis.

The mainstay of effective treatment of LSS is surgical decompression, which may need to be coupled with fusion if there is preoperative or the potential for postoperative spondylolisthesis with instability. Because LSS is frequently a multilevel process, most patients require decompression of more than one spinal level. Foraminotomies for lateral recess or intervertebral foraminal stenosis may be needed, and part or all of one or more facet joints may need to be removed. Complications from surgery are reported in up to 10% to 15% of patients (3). About two-thirds to three-fourths of patients have good to excellent relief of their lower limb symptoms for one to several years (8). Low back pain, even if it is postural and accompanies the pseudoclaudication symptoms, may or may not improve after surgery. In general, surgery is not recommended for patients with postural LBP associated with a narrow lumbar canal if they do not have associated postural pseudoclaudication symptoms. Because of recurrent back and lower limb symptoms, 10% to 20% of patients undergo re-operation over time.

Because of the risk of complications, the less than complete benefit, and the intermittency of symptoms, surgery for LSS is completely elective. The AHCPR guideline states that surgery should not be considered during the first 3 months of symptoms and should only be undertaken if the patient's symptoms interfere enough with daily activities, the patient is otherwise in good health, and surgery is chosen with a full understanding of the potential risks and desired benefits.

ACKNOWLEDGMENT

The author deeply appreciates the superb secretarial assistance of Linda A. Schmidt.

REFERENCES

1. Frymoyer JW, Ducker TB, Hadler NM, et al. *The adult spine: principles and practice,* 2nd ed. Philadelphia: Lippincott Williams & Wilkins, 1997.
2. Bigos S, Bowyer O, Braen G, et al. *Acute low back problems in adults: clinical practice guideline,* Quick Reference Guide Number 14. Rockville, MD: U.S. Department of Health and Human Services, Public Health Service, Agency for Health Care Policy and Research, AHCPR Pub. No. 95-0643. December 1994.
3. Bigos S, Bowyer O, Braen G, et al. *Acute low back problems in adults.* Clinical Practice Guideline No. 14. AHCPR Publication No. 95-0642. Rockville, MD: Agency for Health Care Policy and Research, Public Health Service, U.S. Department of Health and Human Services. December 1994.
4. Institute for Clinical Systems Improvement Health Care Guideline. Adult low back pain. May 2001.
5. Hadler NM. Low back pain. In: Koopman WJ, ed. *Arthritis and allied conditions: a textbook of rheumatology,* 14th ed. Philadelphia: Lippincott Williams & Wilkins, 2001:2026–2041.
6. Borenstein DG, Wiesel SW, Boden SD. *Low back pain: medical diagnosis and comprehensive management,* 2nd ed. Philadelphia: WB Saunders, 1995.
7. McCulloch JA, Transfeldt E. *Macnab's backache,* 3rd ed. Baltimore: Williams & Wilkins, 1997.
8. Bartleson JD, O'Duffy JD. Spinal stenosis. In: Koopman WJ, ed. *Arthritis and allied conditions: a textbook of rheumatology,* 14th ed. Philadelphia: Lippincott Williams & Wilkins, 2001:2042–2053.

THE PAINFUL SHOULDER

DENNIS W. BOULWARE

EPIDEMIOLOGY

Shoulder pain is one of the most common complaints seen in a primary care ambulatory setting and occurs in up to 25% of elderly patients. With most causes of shoulder pain due to intrinsic instability, impingement, or tendinous tears, this clinical situation is seen in a myriad of people. It is a common complaint in older men with an active lifestyle affecting the dominant limb. This chapter addresses the clinical setting of nontraumatic isolated shoulder pain. Shoulder pain due to systemic or generalized diseases such as rheumatoid arthritis or osteoarthritis will not be addressed in this chapter.

PATHOPHYSIOLOGY/PATHOGENESIS

Most causes of shoulder pain can be attributed to soft-tissue structures surrounding the glenohumeral joint, as opposed to those originating from glenohumeral arthritis. An understanding of the anatomy and biomechanics of the shoulder, coupled with a focused physical examination to localize the anatomic source of pain, typically provides the clinician with an accurate diagnosis (Fig. 4.1). Once an accurate diagnosis is made, proper and effective management can be implemented.

The shoulder is the most flexible and mobile joint in the body. This mobility is achieved by having a relatively unstable ball-and-socket joint stabilized by extraarticular structures: the rotator cuff, the bicipital tendon, the coracoacromial ligament, and so on. Shoulder pain is usually due to dysfunction or disruption of the supporting soft-tissue structures, as opposed to glenohumeral arthritis. The most commonly involved structures as a cause of shoulder pain are the rotator cuff, the subacromial bursa, the bicipital tendon, and the synovial capsule.

CLINICAL FEATURES

Symptoms

Localized shoulder pain that is precipitated by use is the most common presenting complaint. The specific location is sometimes helpful, but rarely more helpful than the physical examination. Activity requiring overhead positioning of the arm or rotation of the shoulder is a common exacerbating factor. Nocturnal pain during sleep and the inability to find a restful recumbent position in bed are also common complaints. An efficient use of time for the clinician would be to focus on the physical examination rather than to dwell on the historical details.

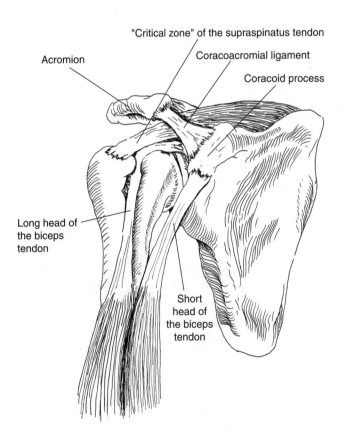

FIGURE 4.1. The glenohumeral joint, illustrating the relationships of the acromion, biceps tendon long and short heads, coracoacromial ligament, and supraspinatus tendon. (From Gispen JG. Painful shoulder and reflex sympathetic dystrophy syndrome. In: Koopman WJ, ed. *Arthritis and allied conditions: a textbook of rheumatology, 14th edition.* Philadelphia: Lippincott Williams & Wilkins, 2001:2095–2142, with permission.)

Signs

A good physical examination of the shoulder is critical in managing shoulder pain. Establishing a systematic routine will help the clinician identify the cause of the shoulder pain quickly and effectively. Since relaxation and cooperation of the patient are critical in examining the shoulder, a prudent clinician will examine the nontender shoulder first to prepare the patient for examination of the painful shoulder.

Start the examination of the shoulder with the examination of the nonpainful side. With the patient sitting on the examination table, passively flex the elbow to 90 degrees and gently use the forearm to rotate the shoulder joint. Passive internal rotation to 90 degrees and passive external rotation to 60 degrees are normal and should be painless. Painless decreased passive rotation may indicate old adhesive capsulitis, or a frozen shoulder; tenderness on passive rotation may indicate an active adhesive capsulitis or active synovitis.

Next, position yourself at the patient's side and stabilize the scapula with one hand, using the other hand to hold the elbow, and passively abduct the shoulder to 90 degrees. Repeat the technique and passively flex the shoulder anteriorly to 120 degrees. A rotator cuff tendinitis may be elicited by tenderness on passive flexing and passive abduction, which will impinge the inflamed tendon. Subacromial bursitis will be tender on only passive abduction and can be confirmed by direct palpation of the subacromial bursa.

Confirmation of rotator cuff tendinitis or a tear can be done by testing for tenderness on isometric testing of shoulder abduction and/or rotation. For isometric rotation, have the patient hold his or her shoulder at the side with the elbow flexed at 90 degrees. Ask the patient to maintain that position as the examiner grasps the patient's wrist and elbow, and attempts to internally, and then externally, rotate the shoulder. For isometric abduction, passively abduct the shoulder to 90 degrees; then ask the patient to actively support the weight of his or her arm. These maneuvers will usually elicit tenderness when the rotator cuff is involved.

If the preceding examination fails to elicit any tenderness, the bicipital tendon should be examined as a possible culprit. Bicipital tenderness can be tested by the presence of tenderness on direct palpation of the tendon within the bicipital groove of the humeral head. Alternatively, it could be tested by Yergason maneuver, which tests the tendon by active isometric loading. Have the patient place his or her fully flexed elbow at the side with the wrist fully supinated. Grasp the patient's hand and ask the patient to resist your attempt to simultaneously extend the elbow and pronate the wrist. This maneuver actively loads the biceps tendon and should elicit tenderness at the shoulder when an active bicipital tendinitis is present.

Occasionally, shoulder pain is not due to dysfunction or disruption of the shoulder joint or its surrounding supportive soft-tissue structures. If the preceding examination fails to reproduce the patient's complaint and identify the source of the pain, then a source of referred shoulder pain should be sought. This should include an assessment of neurologic referred pain from the cervical spine and referred visceral pain from the thorax and the abdomen.

Clinical Evaluation

Initial Evaluation

The laboratory is of no help in evaluating the patient with shoulder pain; the physical examination is the most enlightening. The suspected diagnosis of a rotator cuff tendinitis, rotator cuff partial tears, or subacromial bursitis can be confirmed by injection of a local anesthetic. Instilling 2 to 4 mL of a local anesthetic inferolaterally to the acromial

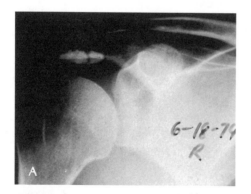 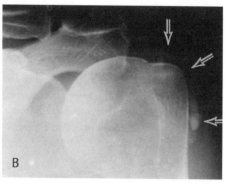

FIGURE 4.2. Plain radiographs of the shoulder in a patient with calcification in the supraspinatus tendon (**A**) and in the subacromial bursa (**B**). Note the calcium extending into the subdeltoid area in **B** (*arrows*). (Courtesy of Dr. Franklin Kozin.) (From Gispen JG. Painful shoulder and reflex sympathetic dystrophy syndrome. In: Koopman WJ, ed. *Arthritis and allied conditions: a textbook of rheumatology, 14th edition.* Philadelphia: Lippincott Williams & Wilkins, 2001:2095–2142, with permission.)

process should provide significant pain relief, reducing the pain with active abduction in subacromial bursitis, and most cases of a rotator cuff partial tear and/or tendinitis. In cases of a complete rotator cuff tear, the pain may be reduced, but active abduction may still be impaired.

In acute shoulder pain, imaging is rarely helpful and should be avoided. In cases of chronic or recurring pain, radiographic findings may help isolate the cause and may sometimes guide therapy. In these cases, plain radiography may reveal calcific tendinitis (Fig. 4.2), signs of chronic impingement with sclerotic and cystic degeneration of the humeral greater tuberosity, a tear of the rotator cuff as evidenced by narrowing or obliteration of the acromiohumeral space, or inferior osteophytes off the acromioclavicular joint as a cause of bony impingement. At the initial evaluation, plain radiography is the only recommended form of imaging.

The differential diagnosis of shoulder pain in the initial evaluation should include glenohumeral arthritis, rotator cuff tendinitis or tears, bursitis, bicipital tendinitis, and referred pain. The examination sequence outlined in the "Clinical Features" section should enable the clinician to identify the cause of the shoulder pain.

SUBSEQUENT EVALUATIONS FOR RECURRENT OR REFRACTORY PAIN

Even with proper treatment, shoulder pain will be recurrent and refractory if an underlying cause of instability or impingement is uncorrected. The patient who returns with recurrent or refractory pain should undergo the same clinical examination initially described under "Clinical Features" to confirm the same diagnosis. If imaging was not performed initially, plain radiographs of the shoulder may reveal the underlying cause.

The following are common causes of recurrent or persistent shoulder pain:

1. *Inferior osteophyte of a degenerative acromioclavicular joint.* The osteophyte will encroach into the acromiohumeral space and result in a bony impingement of the rotator cuff. This finding may indicate the need for a surgical consultation.
2. *Calcific tendinitis.* Calcification of the rotator cuff is a consequence of the chronicity of the inflammation and not a cause of the tendinitis. It should indicate a more chronic condition and the need for continued therapy.
3. *Sclerosis and cystic degeneration of the humeral greater tuberosity.* This implies a chronic and severe impingement of the rotator cuff with consequential joint instability. This finding implies the need for a surgical consultation.
4. *Narrowing or obliteration of the acromiohumeral space.* This finding can only occur with attrition or a complete tear of the rotator cuff, indicating instability of the joint.

If seen on plain radiography, then a surgical consultation may be required.

PREVENTION AND THERAPY

Prevention

Preventive measures can assist in reducing the frequency of refractory or recurrent shoulder pain in some cases of instability. An active and persistent home program in physical therapy is the best preventive measure for shoulder instability due to a rotator cuff problem.

Therapy

For the nontraumatic causes of shoulder pain discussed earlier, a progressive conservative treatment program is usually successful. This program should start with nonpharmacologic management, including rest and judicious physical therapy. Resting the acutely painful shoulder may require the use of a sling when upright to support the arm. Overhead use of the arm with the shoulder in prolonged abduction will certainly aggravate the pain.

Physical therapy in the acutely painful setting should be limited to passive range-of-motion exercises, such as Codman pendulum swinging exercises. This helps avoid adhesive capsulitis and complications of a frozen shoulder. Passive movements after local heat or cold, or after analgesic administration, are advisable. These movements should start slowly, with progressively increased range of motion as symptoms subside. A good starting point is the simple pendulum exercise (Fig. 4.3). Instruct the patient to flex the trunk at the hips and suspend the affected arm at approximately 90 degrees of flexion. The unaffected arm can be placed on a table or chair for support. The patient can swing the body, allowing the suspended affected arm to passively swing like a pendulum. The exercise should be done in the sagittal plane for flexion–extension, and in the coronal plane for abduction–adduction. With time the degrees of swinging can be increased and the passive swinging replaced by active range-of-motion exercise, eventually with resistance (Table 4.1, Fig. 4.4).

Analgesia can be provided through nonpharmacologic measures such as heat and cold packs, or ultrasonic therapy. If ineffective, then simple analgesics and nonsteroidal, antiinflammatory drugs (NSAIDs) are usually adequate. Narcotic analgesics may be necessary for severe pain but should be used on a limited basis.

If the pain is severe or the preceding basic measures have already failed, then local corticosteroids are usually indicated and can be administered into the subacromial bursa or into the glenohumeral joint.

In most cases, there will be significant and satisfactory improvement in 1 to 4 weeks. Pain that persists beyond this

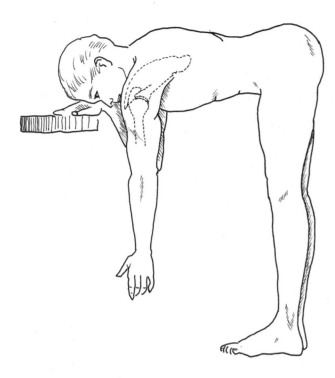

FIGURE 4.3. The position for Codman pendular exercises. The principle of the bent-forward position is that the arm is flexed by gravity, without the need for supraspinatus or deltoid contraction. (From Gispen JG. Painful shoulder and reflex sympathetic dystrophy syndrome. In: Koopman WJ, ed. *Arthritis and allied conditions: a textbook of rheumatology, 14th edition.* Philadelphia: Lippincott Williams & Wilkins, 2001:2095–2142, with permission.)

TABLE 4.1. ROTATOR CUFF–STRENGTHENING EXERCISES

1. Stand with your back and heels against the wall, arms hanging at the sides, palms in. Slowly bring the arm forward, as if you were goose-stepping. Take the arm up to just below shoulder height, hold briefly at the top, then lower slowly. Repeat ten times. A resistive flexion exercise is performed by standing on one end of a long length of tubing or Theraband. The injured arm holds the other end. The arm is slowly raised, with the elbow straight and the palm facing in, to just below shoulder level. Lower. Repeat.
2. Stand sideways to the wall, with the uninjured shoulder next to the wall. The palm of the free outside arm faces in. This arm is slowly abducted, held for an instant just below shoulder level, then lowered. Repeat ten times. This exercise, particularly if done in a plane 20 to 30 degrees anterior to the coronal plane, stresses the supraspinatus muscle. Be careful, especially if using resistive tubing, not to put too much stress on the supraspinatus, exacerbating tendinitis.
3. Lie on your side, and exercise the upper arm as follows. Bend the elbow to 90 degrees and keep the elbow tucked tightly against your waist. Begin with your arm across your chest, like Napoleon Bonaparte, then raise your forearm and hand off your chest until they are parallel to the floor. Hold briefly, lower. Repeat ten times. A resistive exercise to strengthen the infraspinatus (for external rotation) is done standing at right angles to a closed door, with the injured shoulder away from the door. Surgical tubing or Theraband is attached to the door handle. Reach across the front of the body to grasp the tubing with the outside hand. Pull the tubing back across the body, holding the upper arm tight against the lateral chest and the elbow bent, externally rotating against resistance, then passively internally rotating as the stretched tubing pulls the arm back to the starting position. Repeat.
4. Lie on your side as in exercise 3, but it is the underneath arm that exercises, internally rotating, then externally rotating back to the starting position. Again, do ten. To strengthen the subscapularis (for internal rotation) with resistive tubing, stand at right angles to the closed door, but this time the injured shoulder is near the door. Slowly pull the tubing across the body (actively internally rotating against resistance), then return to the beginning position (passively externally rotating). Repeat.

From Gispen JG. Painful shoulder and reflex sympathetic dystrophy syndrome. In: Koopman WJ, ed. *Arthritis and allied conditions: a textbook of rheumatology, 14th edition.* Philadelphia: Lippincott Williams & Wilkins, 2001:2095–2142, with permission.

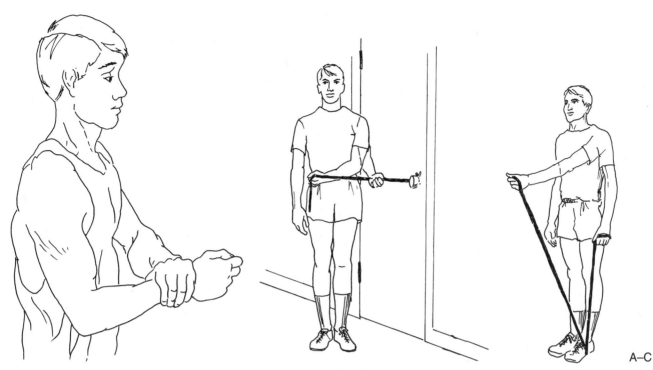

FIGURE 4.4. Stregthening exercises for the rotator cuff. Initially, the exercises are done isometrically. The patient tries to rotate the injured right arm against the resistance of the normal left hand and arm (**A**). The injured left arm rotates internally (**B**) and flexes (**C**) against resistance provided by tubing. (From Gispen JG. Painful shoulder and reflex sympathetic dystrophy syndrome. In: Koopman WJ, ed. *Arthritis and allied conditions: a textbook of rheumatology, 14th edition.* Philadelphia: Lippincott Williams & Wilkins, 2001:2095–2142, with permission.)

time or recurs with a resumption of usual activity suggests an impingement, instability, or alternative cause. At this time, a referral to a rheumatologist may be advisable.

SUMMARY

Most causes of shoulder pain are due to disorders of the periarticular structures: the rotator cuff, the subacromial bursa, and the biceps tendon. Nonsteroidal antiinflammatory drugs, physical therapy, and the judicious use of intraarticular or intralesional steroids will suffice for most cases. Occasionally, recurrent or refractory pain will indi-

cate a more severe problem and require referral to subspecialists.

BIBLIOGRAPHY

Biundo JJ, Torres-Ramos FM. A practical approach to examination of the shoulder and diagnosing common problems. *Primary Care Rheumatol* 1991;4:1–10.

Boulware DW. The painful shoulder. In: Goldman L, Bennett JC, eds. *Cecil textbook of medicine,* 21st ed. Philadelphia: WB Saunders, 2000:1554–1556.

Gispen JG. Painful shoulder and the reflex sympathetic dystrophy syndrome. In: Koopman WJ, ed. *Arthritis and allied conditions,* 14th ed. Philadelphia: Lippincott Williams & Wilkins, 2001:2095–2142.

PAINFUL FEET

JOSEPH J. BIUNDO
PERRY J. RUSH

Foot pain and loss of function may be caused by a multitude of maladies. As with other regions of the musculoskeletal system, the foot can manifest a large number of defined clinical entities. *Foot pain* is a symptom, not a diagnosis. A precise diagnosis should be made to ensure proper treatment, which is specific for that particular problem. Possible treatment may include medications, strategically placed local injections, thoughtfully chosen orthoses, exercise programs, modalities, and corrective surgery. Thus if the physician perceives the problem simply as "foot pain," a successful outcome is unlikely. The complaint of foot pain must be evaluated through a knowledgeable history, a hands-on physical examination, and selected imaging studies. The differential diagnosis takes place cognitively during this active process. Even though foot problems are extremely common, the foot is largely an ignored area. In chronic rheumatoid arthritis, foot deformities occur in approximately 90% of patients (1). Typically, in general medicine, the foot is only examined for the presence of edema and the quality of pedal pulses. Even rheumatologists do not often examine the foot. The physician may be reluctant to ask patients with impaired hand function to remove their shoes and socks because of time constraints. The aesthetics of examining feet also may play a role. The biggest obstacle to a proper foot examination may, however, simply be the lack of expertise in this area.

Foot abnormalities may be clinically significant at any age. The infant can have clubfeet and other developmental defects, the young child can have one of the several osteochondroses, the adolescent can have tarsal coalition, and the young adult can have spondyloarthritis involving the feet. Mechanical and degenerative problems become more prevalent with age, however, including such problems as hallux valgus, hallux rigidus, Morton neuroma, and posterior tibial tendinitis and rupture. The anatomy of the foot is depicted in Fig. 5.1.

GAIT CYCLE AND BIOMECHANICS OF GAIT

To understand foot disorders and the prescription of appropriate foot orthoses, a basic comprehension of the normal gait cycle and of the biomechanics of gait is essential (2,3). The normal gait cycle is divided into two main components, the stance phase, which comprises 60% of the cycle, and the swing phase, which comprises the remaining 40% (Fig. 5.2). The stance phase refers to contact of a limb with the floor.

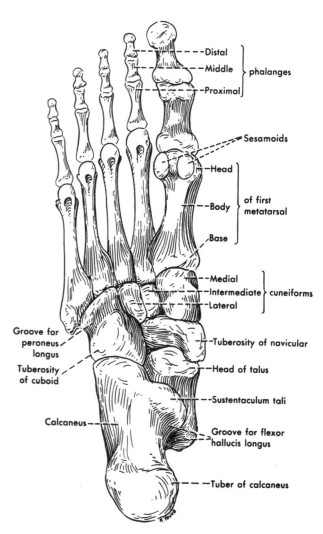

FIGURE 5.1. Plantar view of the bones of the foot. (From Hollinshead WH, Jenkins DB. *Functional anatomy of the limbs and back,* 5th ed. Philadelphia: WB Saunders, 1981:317, with permission.)

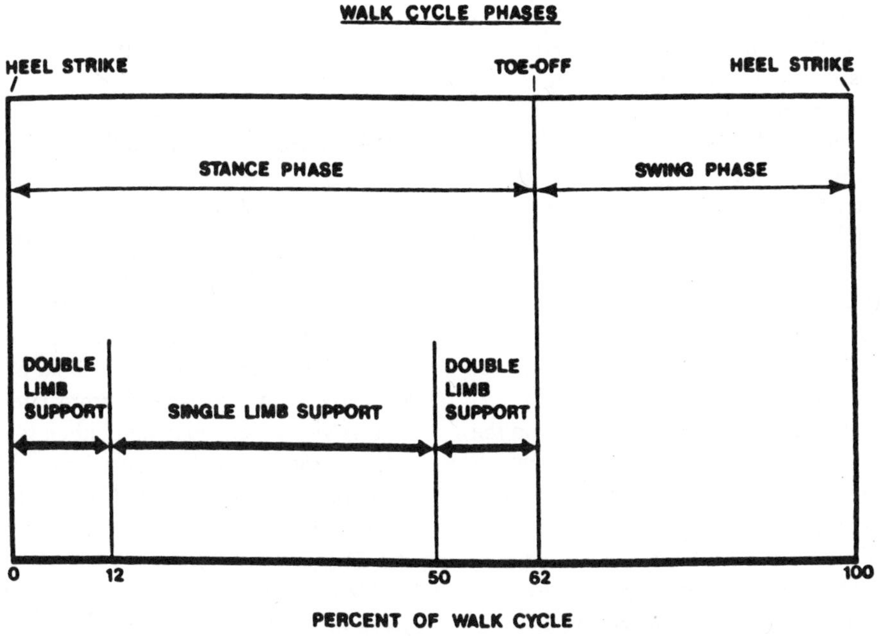

WALK CYCLE PHASES

FIGURE 5.2. Gait cycle. (From Mann RA. Biomechanics of the foot and ankle. *Orthop Rev* 1978; 7:43–48, with permission.)

Five divisions of the stance phase exist: (a) heel-strike, which is the initial contact of the heel with the floor; (b) foot-flat, which is the initial contact of the forefoot with the floor; (c) midstance, which occurs when the greater trochanter is in vertical alignment with the vertical bisector of the foot; (d) heel-off, which begins with plantar flexion and elevation of the heel; and (e) toe-off, the phase that begins with the elevation of the forefoot and ends at the point when the toes have left the floor. Other relevant terms include *single support,* which occurs when only one limb is in contact with the floor; *double support,* which occurs when both feet are simultaneously in contact with the floor; and *push-off,* which is a combination of the phases of heel-off and toe-off.

The swing phase of gait, which comprises 40% of the cycle, is divided into three phases: (a) acceleration, which occurs just as toe-off ends and the leg is posterior to the pelvis but moving anteriorly; (b) midswing, which occurs when the swinging limb passes the opposite limb in the stance phase, and the dorsiflexors of the ankle and foot contract to shorten the limb; and (c) deceleration, which occurs with eccentric contraction of the dorsiflexors to slow the movement of the limb, initiating heel-strike.

The normal biomechanics of the foot and ankle are designed to absorb and direct the force occurring as a result of heel-strike, foot-plant, and toe push-off. The foot is unique in that it is flexible and rigid during different parts of the gait cycle. It becomes supple during the early part of stance and rigid during the latter part of stance phase (4). As the foot is loaded, internal rotation of the tibia, eversion of the subtalar joint, dorsiflexion of the ankle (pronation), and abduction of the foot occur (5). Pronation is the flexi-

ble phase of heel strike in the gait cycle, allowing partial dissipation of the initial contact force. Supination is the stable configuration of the foot where the subtalar joint is inverted and locked.

The key to understanding the foot is to start an evaluation from what is commonly known as the neutral position in which the talus and navicular bones and their related joint are congruous. In pes planus and hyperpronation, the longitudinal arch is depressed in midstance, and the foot does not supinate with toe-off. In pes cavus and limited subtalar motion, a decrease in ability of the foot to pronate and thereby dissipate the contact forces occurs. A tight Achilles tendon will limit ankle dorsiflexion, which leads to excessive pronation and abnormal stretching of the plantar fascia. Biomechanical stressors include running, sudden increase in activity, obesity, inadequate shoes, or prolonged standing or walking.

PHYSICAL EXAMINATION

A proper physical examination of the foot leads to the anatomic localization of the source of the pain symptoms, helps to identify the static and mechanical abnormalities of the foot, and aids in detecting an underlying disease (6–8). Look at the shoes for excessive wear on the heels and soles. Extreme lateral heel wear can signify hindfoot (calcaneal) varus. An examination of gait is valuable in diagnosing and treating many foot problems. The patient walks barefooted with the feet and ankles exposed, and the hindfoot, midfoot, and forefoot are viewed separately.

Observe the foot for swelling, deformity, and erythema or other skin changes. Palpation to detect tenderness is important for diagnosis. Palpate the subtalar joint in the neutral position for tenderness and alignment (9). Look for forefoot varus or forefoot valgus (Fig. 5.3). Examine the midtarsal area for tenderness and mobility. Examine for range of motion and tenderness or swelling of the metatarsophalangeal joints. Check for hammer toes, cocked-up toes, and tenderness or swelling of toes. Observe the toenails for abnormalities. Check the calcaneus on the plantar surface for tenderness. Examine the Achilles tendon, retrocalcaneal bursa, posterior tibial tendon, and peroneal tendon for swelling, tenderness, subluxation, or rupture.

Identify calluses to reveal areas of excessive stresses on the foot. Describe the location of calluses. Identify corns, which are hyperkeratotic lesions secondary to pressure. Hard corns occur over bony prominences and typically are found on the lateral aspect of the fifth toe. Soft corns occur between the toes. Make note of the pulses. Check the spine for scoliosis and spinal mobility. Examine for hamstring and calf tightness, leg length discrepancy, genu varus, genu valgus, patella position, and Q angle.

IMAGING OF THE FOOT

The standard plain radiograph views include the standing anteroposterior, standing lateral, and oblique (pronated), depicting the medial aspect of the foot. It is important to obtain the anteroposterior and lateral radiographs in the standing position to demonstrate the anatomic relationships of the foot in their functional position. In the lateral view, the x-ray beam passes from lateral to medial. Other special views are the lateral oblique (supinated) to visualize an accessory navicular bone; sesamoid view, which is an axial, oblique position (tilted lateral of sesamoids); and axial view of the heel (Harris) for calcaneal fractures and talocalcaneal coalition (10).

Computed tomography (CT) scanning is helpful in imaging the hindfoot, especially for subtalar joint pathology and fractures of the calcaneus. CT is beneficial in the diagnosis of fibrous and cartilaginous coalition, calcaneonavicular bony coalition, and talocalcaneal coalition. Magnetic resonance imaging (MRI) may be used to help diagnose tarsal coalition, osteomyelitis, osteonecrosis, tendinitis, tendon rupture, ligamentous injury, and osteochondral injuries of the talar dome (11). MRI is helpful in identifying soft tissue masses, such as ganglia, fibromatosis, Morton neuroma, and pigmented villonodular synovitis of the tendon sheath (12). Technetium bone scans can be used to determine stress fractures, especially of the metatarsals or calcaneus. Bone scans are also useful to detect inflammation in such sites as the plantar fascia (13). Diagnostic ultrasonography can help identify tendinitis and partial or complete tears of tendons of the foot, especially the Achilles tendon and the posterior tibial tendon (14). Table 5.1 lists indications for the use of diagnostic ultrasonography.

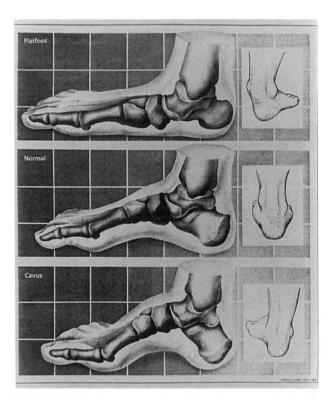

FIGURE 5.3. Feet are grouped into three types according to the way they function. The normal foot is supple on early weight bearing and converts to a rigid structure for push-off. The flat foot is supple and does not reconvert to form a rigid lever for push-off. In a flat foot, the forefoot is typically abducted and in varus and the heel is in valgus. The cavus foot is rigid and does not evert to become supple. In the cavus foot the forefoot is adducted and in valgus. The heel in the cavus foot is in varus, and the first metatarsal is generally plantar flexed. (From Bordelon RL. Practical guide to foot orthoses. *J Musculoskelet Med* 1989;6:71–77, with permission.)

TABLE 5.1. INDICATIONS FOR SONOGRAPHY OF THE ANKLE AND FOOT

1. Tendon pathology: tenosynovitis, tendinosis, tendon tears, subluxation, or dislocation
2. Joint and bursal pathology: joint effusion, intra-articular loose bodies, or bursitis
3. Soft tissue pathology: foreign bodies, or plantar fasciitis, Morton neuroma, ganglions, cellulites, or abscesses
4. Assessment when metallic artifact would limit imaging with magnetic resonance imaging or computed tomography
5. Guidance for intervention: joint aspiration, synovial or soft tissue biopsy, or joint or tendon sheath injection

Adapted from Fessell DP, Vanderschueren GM, Jacobson JA, et al. Ankle ultrasound: technique, anatomy and pathology. *Radiographics* 1998;18:325–340.

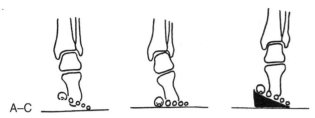

FIGURE 5.4. Demonstration of effect of biomechanical posting for abnormal forefoot and normal hindfoot. **A:** Foot in neutral position showing the hindfoot in normal position and the forefoot in varus position. **B:** Demonstration of what happens when the foot hits the ground with the foot collapsing so that the hindfoot is everted and the entire foot collapses. **C:** Correction of abnormality by placing a "post" beneath the medial side of the foot so that when the foot hits the ground the hindfoot does not collapse and normal function of the subtalar joint complex occurs. (From Bordelon RL. Orthotics, shoes, and braces. *Orthop Clin North Am* 1989;20:751–757, with permission.)

MECHANICAL PROBLEMS

Forefoot Varus

Forefoot varus is an abnormality of the foot in which the forefoot is inverted in relation to the hindfoot when the subtalar joint is in the neutral position. The head of the first metatarsal is more dorsal than the head of the fifth metatarsal. The subtalar joint is in neutral position when the talonavicular joint is congruous. Forefoot varus is a major cause of compensatory subtalar pronation of an abnormal degree during the stance phase of gait. A foot orthosis with a medial wedge (post) may be needed to correct the biomechanical abnormality (Fig. 5.4) (15).

Forefoot Valgus

In forefoot valgus, the forefoot is everted in relationship to the hindfoot when the subtalar joint is in neutral position. The fifth metatarsal head is more dorsal than the head of the first metatarsal head (15). A lateral wedge (post) orthosis may be needed to correct forefoot valgus (Fig. 5.5).

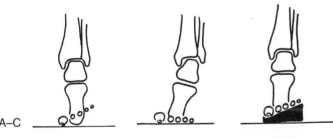

FIGURE 5.5. Demonstration of effect of lateral post. **A:** Examination of foot with foot in neutral position showing valgus deformity of the forefoot. **B:** With weight bearing the foot collapses and twists inward, producing an unstable foot with gait. **C:** Posting of lateral side of forefoot so that the subtalar joint complex remains in neutral during weight bearing and the foot does not twist. (From Bordelon RL. Orthotics, shoes, and braces. *Orthop Clin North Am* 1989;20:751–757, with permission.)

Hindfoot Valgus (Calcaneal Valgus, Rearfoot Valgus, Subtalar Valgus)

A lateral shift of the calcaneus occurs with medial rotation of the talus and a plantar drop of the talar head and navicular. This results in pronation of the foot and is seen in pes planus, rheumatoid arthritis, and posterior tibialis tendon rupture.

Hindfoot Varus

A medial shift of the calcaneus occurs. It is usually congenital and may be associated with pes cavus.

Pes Planus

Pes planus, or flat feet, is often asymptomatic but may cause fatigue of the foot muscles and aching with intolerance to prolonged walking or standing (16). The most common type is the flexible flatfoot (Fig. 5.3). Other causes of flatfoot are tarsal coalition, congenital vertical talus, and rupture of the tibialis posterior tendon, which causes the typical unilateral, acquired flatfoot. In pes planus there is loss of the longitudinal arch on the medial side and prominence of the navicular bone and head of the talus. The calcaneus is everted (valgus), and on ambulation out-toeing can be seen. The tendency for this condition is largely inherited and is seen with generalized hypermobility. A Thomas heel, firm shoes, grasping exercises to strengthen the intrinsic muscles, and toe walking to strengthen the tibialis posterior are helpful. A shoe orthosis may be needed for more severe cases. The asymptomatic flatfoot is left untreated.

Pes Cavus

An unusually high medial arch characterizes pes cavus, or claw foot, and in severe cases, a high longitudinal arch, resulting in shortening of the foot (Fig. 5.3) (16). These abnormally high arches result in some shortening of the extensor ligaments, causing dorsiflexion (extension) of the metatarsophalangeal joints and plantar flexion of the proximal interphalangeal and distal interphalangeal joints, thus giving the clawing appearance of the toes. The plantar fascia may also be contracted. The calcaneus is usually in a varus (inverted) position. Generally, a tendency to pes cavus is inherited, and in a high percentage of cases an underlying neurologic disorder, such as myelomeningocele, Charcot–Marie–Tooth disease, or Friedreich ataxia, is present (17). Although pes cavus can cause foot fatigue, pain, and tenderness over the metatarsal heads with callus formation, it may also be asymptomatic in the milder cases. Calluses may also be present over the dorsum of the toes. Use of metatarsal pads or a metatarsal bar is helpful, and stretching of the toe extensors is usually prescribed. In severe cases, surgical correction may be needed.

CLINICAL ENTITIES

Forefoot

Hallux Valgus

In hallux valgus, deviation of the large toe lateral to the midline and deviation of the first metatarsal medially occur. A bunion (adventitious bursa) of the head of the first metatarsophalangeal joint may be present, often causing pain, tenderness, and swelling. Hallux valgus is more common in women and may result from a genetic tendency or pointed shoes, or it can be secondary to rheumatoid arthritis or osteoarthritis (18). Stretching of shoes, use of bunion pads, or a surgical procedure may be indicated (19). Metatarsus primus varus, a condition in which the first metatarsal is angulated medially, is seen in association with, or secondary to, the hallux valgus deformity.

Hallux Rigidus

In hallux rigidus, immobility of the first metatarsophalangeal (MTP) joint, especially on extension, is present. Limitation of plantar flexion can also occur. Pain is often present at the base of the big toe and is aggravated by walking, especially in high heels. A primary type of hallux rigidus is seen in younger persons, and the acquired form may be secondary to trauma, osteoarthritis, rheumatoid arthritis, or gout. Osteophytes and sclerosis of the first metatarsophalangeal joint may be seen on radiographs. The term *hallux limitus* is sometimes used to denote a milder degree of immobility of the first MTP joint. The treatment of hallux rigidus generally consists of wearing shoes with a wide toe box and a rocker sole, since push-off during gait is limited. Surgery may be needed in some cases.

Bunionette

A bunionette, or tailor's bunion, is a prominence of the fifth metatarsal head resulting from the overlying bursa and a localized callus. The fifth metatarsal has a lateral (valgus) deviation (20). Pressure from shoes can cause pain, and tenderness may be present over the swollen bursa. Treatment consists of wearing a shoe with a wide toe box, stretching the shoe over the involved area, and using a pad. In chronic, painful cases surgical excision of the lateral eminence of the fifth metatarsal can be performed.

Hammer Toe

In hammer toe, the proximal interphalangeal joint is flexed and the tip of the toe points downward (21). The second toe is most commonly involved. Calluses may form at the tip of the toe and over the dorsum of the interphalangeal joint, resulting from pressure against the shoe. Hammer toe may be congenital or acquired secondary to hallux valgus or improper footwear. When hammer toes are associated with hyperextension of the metatarsophalangeal joints, the deformity is known as "cocked-up toes." This may be seen in rheumatoid arthritis.

Metatarsalgia

Pain arising from the metatarsal heads, known as metatarsalgia, is a symptom resulting from a variety of conditions. Pain on standing and tenderness on palpation of the metatarsal heads are present. Calluses over the metatarsal heads are usually seen. The causes of metatarsalgia are many, including foot strain, use of high-heel shoes, everted foot, trauma, sesamoiditis, hallux valgus, arthritis, foot surgery, or a foot with a high longitudinal arch. Flattening of the transverse arch and weakness of the intrinsic muscles occur, resulting in a maldistribution of weight on the forefoot. Treatment is directed at elevation of the middle portion of the transverse arch with an orthotic device, strengthening of the intrinsic muscles, weight reduction, and use of metatarsal pads or a metatarsal bar.

Metatarsal Stress Fracture

Stress fracture is also known as march fracture or fatigue fracture, because it was associated with a spontaneous fracture after long marches in army recruits. Pain, swelling, tenderness, and occasional erythema develop over the metatarsal area, usually without any clear history of trauma. Upon questioning, however, the episode of spontaneous pain related to the onset of the fracture can be identified in some cases. The neck of the second metatarsal bone is most frequently involved, but the other metatarsals are also sites of fracture. Athletic events, including jogging, or other activities stressful to the feet are common causes. Stress fractures may be seen in rheumatoid arthritis or generalized osteoporosis and may occur in the elderly. The key to diagnosis of stress fractures of the foot is to have a high index of suspicion. The difficulty in making the diagnosis is that initial radiographs usually show no abnormalities or, at most, show only a faint fracture line (22). A repeat radiograph

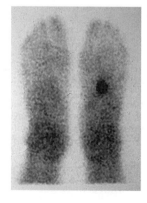

FIGURE 5.6. A plantar view on bone scan shows an intense uptake in metatarsal area of right foot, indicating a stress fracture. (From Biundo JJ, Rush PJ. Painful feet. In: Koopman WJ, ed. *Arthritis and allied conditions,* 14th ed. Philadelphia: Lippincott Williams & Wilkins, 2001: 1996–2008, with permission.)

several weeks later may show healing with callus formation. Bone scans are essential to the early diagnosis and show an increase in uptake over the fracture site (Fig. 5.6) (23). Usually, these fractures heal spontaneously, and rest and strapping of the foot or use of a postoperative shoe are helpful. Occasionally, a cast may be needed.

Flexor Hallucis Longus Tendinitis

This tendon is the most posterior of the three tendons running posterior to the medial malleolus and passes through a fibroosseous tunnel. Inflammation can occur at this site, and triggering or snapping may develop as the tunnel becomes stenotic. In stenosing tenosynovitis, pain occurs during active plantar flexion of the big toe and on passive dorsiflexion. A snapping sensation may occur at the posteromedial aspect of the ankle. Occasionally, flexion of the big toe is impaired. A contracture of the flexor hallucis longus tendon is seen, and the big toe cannot be extended beyond neutral with the foot and ankle in neutral position or be passively extended with the ankle in plantar flexion. Rupture of the tendon can occur. Treatment of the tendinitis is usually conservative. Surgery may be employed in severe cases.

Sesamoid Injuries

Lesions of the sesamoid bones of the big toe may exhibit local pain and tenderness under either the medial or lateral sesamoid (24). Pain may begin gradually or may be more abrupt following acute trauma, and usually increases with dorsiflexion of the digit or upon weight bearing. Recognized causes of sesamoid pain, which has loosely been called sesamoiditis, are repetitive strain from activities such as dancing or long-distance running, stress fracture, traumatic fracture, bipartite sesamoid, and osteochondritis (25). Treatment consists of elimination of the offending activity, avoidance of high heels, an orthosis that decreases weight bearing on the area, nonsteroidal antiinflammatory drugs (NSAIDs), and a local steroid injection. Surgery may be indicated to remove a painful, nonunited fractured sesamoid.

Freiberg Disease

Freiberg disease is an osteochondrosis of the second metatarsal head, primarily affecting girls around 12 years of age (26). Pain, tenderness, and swelling of the metatarsal are present. Radiographs reveal fragmentation, sclerosis, and deformity of the metatarsal head. Treatment is aimed at reducing stress on the metatarsal joint with a metatarsal pad or metatarsal bar. Occasionally, a residual deformity with subsequent degenerative changes of the involved metatarsophalangeal joint occurs.

Midfoot

Sinus Tarsi Syndrome

Lateral foot pain and a feeling of instability of the ankle (27) characterize this syndrome. Marked tenderness is present on pressure over the sinus tarsi area. Prolonged standing, walking on uneven surfaces, or supination or adduction of the foot may initiate the pain. Rest usually alleviates the pain. Most patients with sinus tarsi syndrome have sustained either a single or repeated ankle sprain with an inversion injury (28). Other factors associated with the acquisition of this syndrome are inflammation from rheumatoid arthritis or gout and foot abnormalities such as pes cavus, pes planus with instability of the hindfoot, or forefoot valgus.

Usually, plain radiographs are negative. Subtalar arthrograms have revealed complete disappearance of the microrecesses along the interosseous ligament. MRI is helpful in identifying abnormalities of the interosseous talocalcaneal ligament, which fills the sinus tarsi (29).

Initial treatment often consists of a lidocaine and steroid injection into the sinus tarsi. If a biomechanical abnormality, such as forefoot valgus, is found, a foot orthosis is of benefit (30). In persistent cases, surgical excision of fatty tissue and part of the ligaments in the sinus tarsi may be performed. A triple arthrodesis has been successfully performed in a few reported cases.

Tarsal Coalition

Tarsal coalition is a fusion of two or more tarsal bones, and the connection may be fibrous (syndesmosis), cartilaginous (synchondrosis), or osseous (synostosis). The cause of coalition is congenital, but occasionally may result from trauma, prior foot surgery, inflammatory arthritis, degenerative arthritis, or infection.

The clinical manifestations consist of a dull pain of gradual onset that is perceived as foot fatigue or stiffness. Vigorous activities or prolonged standing may intensify the discomfort. The initial symptoms may follow such activity or begin after an injury such as an ankle sprain. On examination, limited or absent subtalar motion is usually present. Pes planus, tenderness of the medial aspect of the calcaneus (sustentaculum tali), and occasionally, peroneal spasm may be found.

The most common site of involvement is a calcaneonavicular coalition, with 49% of cases in one study occurring at this location, while 37% were reported to have a talocalcaneal coalition (31). Talonavicular and calcaneocuboid coalitions were the next most frequent, and together totaled just under 10%.

On plain radiographs, the anteroposterior and lateral views usually fail to identify any bony union of the calcaneus and navicular or of the talus and calcaneus. A medial-oblique view of the foot, however, may reveal calcaneonavicular coalition, whereas an axial view (Harris-Beath view) of the foot can identify talocalcaneal coalition (32). A talar beak or large bony spur of the distal, dorsal surface of the talus may be seen in tarsal coalition. The subtalar joint may appear narrowed or tilted. CT is very helpful in diagnosis of fibrous and cartilaginous coalition, confirms calcaneonavicular bony coalition, and is excellent in diagnosing talocalcaneal coalition. MRI can also successfully identify tarsal coalition and is the most accurate technique to image fibrous coalitions (33).

Tarsal coalition may not cause symptoms. When present, however, symptoms are initially treated with NSAIDs, steroid injections, and shoe modifications aimed at reducing stress on the talus, including heel wedges and Plastizote inserts. Persistent symptoms may be treated with a walking cast for 3 to 6 weeks. A number of surgical procedures have been used in chronic cases, including resection of the coalition with interposition grafting or triple arthrodesis.

Köhler Disease

Köhler disease is an osteochondrosis of the navicular bone (26). The onset is gradual, beginning at about 5 or 6 years of age and affecting boys more frequently. Occasionally, it is bilateral. Trauma is not thought to be the primary cause, but the initial pathology is that of avascular necrosis. The symptoms are discomfort over the dorsum of the foot and a limp. Tenderness and a mild swelling may be palpable over the affected navicular. A plain radiograph reveals a small, dense, irregular navicular. Treatment is directed toward the pain, and a temporary medial arch support may be used. When more severe symptoms are present, immobilization with a splint may be used for a few weeks. The involved bone usually remodels to a correct form within 2 years.

Hindfoot

A complaint of heel pain is usually quite broad, and since heel pain can emanate from a number of different anatomic sites and from a number of different causes, it is essential to identify the specific location. The potential sites include the plantar surface (subcalcaneal), or posterior, medial, or lateral aspect of the heel.

Achilles Tendinitis

Achilles tendinitis usually results from trauma, athletic overactivity, or improperly fitting shoes with a stiff heel counter, but it can also arise from inflammatory conditions such as ankylosing spondylitis, Reiter syndrome, gout, rheumatoid arthritis, and calcium pyrophosphate deposition disease. Pain, swelling, and tenderness occur over the Achilles tendon at its attachment and in the area proximal to the attachment. Crepitus on motion and pain on dorsiflexion may be present. Management includes NSAIDs, rest, shoe corrections, heel lift, gentle stretching, and some-

times a splint with slight plantar flexion. The Achilles tendon is vulnerable to rupture and the tendon itself must not be injected with a corticosteroid. However, peritendinous steroid injections for achillodynia have been reported (34).

Achilles Tendon Rupture

Spontaneous rupture of the Achilles tendon is well known and occurs with a sudden onset of pain during forced dorsiflexion (35). An audible snap may be heard, followed by difficulty in walking and standing on toes. Swelling and edema over the area usually develop. Diagnosis can be made with the Thompson test, in which the patient kneels on the chair with the feet extending over the edge and the examiner squeezes the calf and pushes toward the knee. Normally, this produces plantar flexion, but in a ruptured tendon no plantar flexion occurs. Achilles tendon rupture is generally due to athletic events or trauma from jumps or falls. MRI can aid in the diagnosis and can distinguish a complete rupture from a partial one (36). The tendon is more prone to tear in those having preexisting Achilles tendon disease or taking corticosteroids (37). Immobilization or surgery may be selected, depending on the situation (38).

Retrocalcaneal Bursitis

The retrocalcaneal bursa is located between the inside surface of the Achilles tendon and the calcaneus. The bursa's anterior wall is fibrocartilage where it attaches to the calcaneus, whereas its posterior wall blends with the epitenon of the Achilles tendon. Manifestations are pain at the back of the heel, tenderness of the area anterior to the Achilles tendon, and pain on dorsiflexion. Local swelling is present, with bulging on the medial and lateral aspects of the tendon. Retrocalcaneal bursitis, also called sub-Achilles bursitis, may coexist with Achilles tendinitis, and distinguishing the two is sometimes difficult. This condition may be secondary to rheumatoid arthritis, spondylitis, Reiter syndrome, gout, and trauma. The treatment consists of NSAIDs, rest, and local injection of a corticosteroid carefully directed into the bursa (39).

Subcutaneous Achilles Bursitis

A subcutaneous bursa posterior to the Achilles tendon may become swollen in the absence of systemic disease. This bursitis, known as "pump-bumps," is seen predominantly in women and results from pressure of shoes, although it can also result from bony exostoses. Other than relief from shoe pressure, no treatment is indicated.

Sever Disease

Sever disease occurs especially in boys between the ages of 8 and 15, and is characterized by pain, tenderness, and mild swelling involving the posterior heel (26). The pathology is a chronic sprain or partial avulsion of the calcaneal apophysis, which is the site where the Achilles tendon attaches to the calcaneus. Radiographs show the epiphyses to be irregular or segmented with areas of increased density. Somewhat problematic, however, is that such changes are seen in asymptomatic children and may be part of the normal ossification. The disorder is self-limiting, with improvement occurring in less than a year. Treatment includes prescription of a heel pad, reduction in activities, and use of a heel lift to reduce the traction of the Achilles tendon at its attachment during walking.

Plantar Fasciitis (Subcalcaneal Pain Syndrome)

Plantar fasciitis occurs primarily between 40 and 60 years of age. A gradual onset of pain in the plantar area of the heel usually occurs but may occur following trauma or from overuse after activities such as taking part in athletics, walking for a prolonged time, wearing improperly fitting shoes, or striking the heel with some force (40–43). The pain characteristically occurs in the morning upon arising. It is most severe for the first few steps. After an initial improvement, the pain may get worse later in the day, especially after prolonged standing or walking. The pain is burning, aching, and occasionally lancinating. Palpation typically reveals tenderness anteromedially on the medial calcaneal tubercle at the origin of the plantar fascia (Fig. 5.7). Less common is central heel tenderness. Passive stretching of the plantar fascia and eversion of the foot may exacerbate symptoms.

The pain is the result of degenerative changes in the origin of the plantar fascia and traction periostitis of the medial calcaneal tubercle resulting from overload. Over time and with repetitive stress, microtears can occur in the origin of the plantar fascia, generating an inflammatory response consisting of collagen necrosis, angiofibroblastic hyperplasia, mucinoid degeneration, chondroid metaplasia, and matrix calcification (41).

Most patients with heel pain have calcaneal spurs, but some do not. The spur itself is not likely to cause pain unless it is directed vertically downward. Calcaneal spurs are commonly seen in patients with spondyloarthropathies, and plantar fasciitis may be the presenting problem is such patients (44). Less common than plantar fasciitis, subcalcaneal pain may also occur from entrapment of the nerve to the abductor digiti quinti muscle, fat atrophy of the heel pad, or calcaneal stress fracture (42).

Treatment includes relative rest with a reduction in stressful activities, NSAIDs, and use of a heel pad or heel cup orthosis (45). A night splint with 5 degrees of dorsiflexion may help (43,46). Stretching of the calf muscles and plantar fascia is very important in the treatment. In some cases, physical therapy with strengthening, modalities with contrast baths, or ultrasound may be prescribed, along with the stretching. A local injection, using a 25-gauge needle, with a corticosteroid is often of help. Ionotophoresis of dexamethasone has also been used to treat plantar fasciitis (47). Surgery may be indicated in chronic cases.

Posterior Tibial Tendinitis

Pain, swelling, and localized tenderness just posterior to the medial malleolus occurs in posterior tibial tendinitis (48). Extension and flexion may be normal, but pain is present on resisted inversion or passive eversion. The discomfort is usually worse after athletic events. Treatment is usually rest, NSAIDs, and possibly a local injection of a corticosteroid (49). Immobilization with a splint is sometimes needed.

Posterior Tibialis Tendon Rupture

Rupture of the posterior tibialis tendon, which is not commonly recognized, is a cause of progressive flatfoot (50–53). It may be caused by trauma, chronic tendon degeneration, or rheumatoid arthritis (54). An insidious onset of pain, swelling, and tenderness occurs along the course of the tendon just distal to the medial malleolus. The unilateral deformity of hindfoot valgus and forefoot abduction is an important finding. The forefoot abduction can be seen best from behind; more toes are seen from this position than would be seen normally. The result of the single heel rise test is positive when the patient is unable to rise onto the ball of the affected foot while the contralateral foot is off the

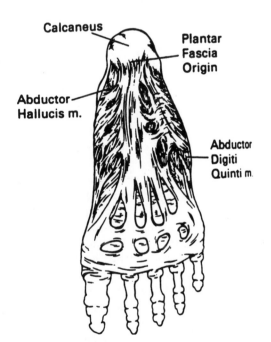

FIGURE 5.7. Anatomy of plantar fascia. (From Schepsis AA, Leach RE, Gorzyca J. Plantar fasciitis: etiology, treatment, surgical results, and review of the literature. *Clin Orthop* 1991;266: 185–196, with permission.)

floor. CT and MRI are helpful in the diagnosis of tendon rupture (52). Orthopedic consultation may help to determine whether the rupture should be treated conservatively with NSAIDs and casting or with a surgical repair.

Peroneal Tendon Dislocation and Peroneal Tendinitis

Dislocation of the peroneal tendon may occur from a direct blow, repetitive trauma, or sudden dorsiflexion with eversion (55,56). Sometimes a painless snapping noise is heard at the time of dislocation. Other patients report more severe pain and tenderness of the tendon area where it lies over the lateral malleolus. The condition may be confused with an acute ankle sprain. Conservative treatment with immobilization is often satisfactory, since the peroneal tendon usually reduces spontaneously. If the retinaculum supporting the tendon is ruptured, however, surgical correction may be required. Peroneal tendinitis is manifested as localized tenderness and swelling over the lateral malleolus (56,57). Conservative treatment is usually indicated.

Neurologic Lesions

The foot is a frequent site of neurologic symptoms, some of which are common and others of which are rare. The usual symptom is numbness of some portion of the foot, but this complaint is often ignored as being nonspecific. The symptoms are often not well described by the patient. Moreover, the patient is often not questioned by the physician in a manner specific enough to elicit a proper description of the problem. As with the upper extremity, numbness is often misinterpreted by the patient, and sometimes by the physician, as being due to "poor circulation." The symptoms of numbness, tingling, paresthesias, burning pain, or pins and needle sensation should first point to a possible neurologic lesion. The most common cause of numbness of the feet is peripheral neuropathy. If suspected, this can be confirmed by electrodiagnostic studies. A number of other local entities causing numbness of the foot, however, should also be considered.

Morton Neuroma

Middle-aged women are most frequently affected by Morton neuroma, an entrapment neuropathy of the interdigital nerve occurring most often between the third and fourth toes (58). Paresthesias and a burning, aching type of pain are usually experienced in the fourth toe. The symptoms are made worse by walking on hard surfaces or wearing tight shoes or high-heel shoes. Tenderness may be elicited by palpation between the third and fourth metatarsal heads. Occasionally, a neuroma is seen between the second and third toes. Compression of the interdigital nerve by the

transverse metatarsal ligament and possibly by an inter-metatarsophalangeal bursa or synovial cyst may be responsible for the entrapment (59). Zanetti et al. illustrated with excellent images the difficulty of diagnosing Morton neuroma only by clinical examination and the value of MRI in influencing diagnostic and therapeutic decisions (60).

Treatment of Morton neuroma is usually with a metatarsal bar or pad, or a local steroid injection into the web space (61). Ultimately, surgical excision of the neuroma and a portion of the nerve may be needed.

Tarsal Tunnel Syndrome

In tarsal tunnel syndrome the posterior tibial nerve is compressed at or near the flexor retinaculum, which is located posterior and inferior to the medial malleolus. Just distal to the retinaculum, the nerve divides into the medial plantar, lateral plantar, and posterior calcaneal branches. Numbness, burning pain, and paresthesias of the toes and sole extend proximally to the area over the medial malleolus (62,63). Nocturnal exacerbation may be reported. The patient usually gets some relief by leg, foot, and ankle movements. A positive Tinel sign is elicited on percussion posterior to the medial malleolus, and loss of pinprick and two-point discrimination may be present. Women are more often affected. Trauma to the foot, especially fracture, valgus foot deformity, hypermobility, occupational factors, and synovitis, may contribute to development of the tarsal tunnel syndrome (64). An electrodiagnostic test may show prolonged motor and sensory latencies and slowing of the nerve conduction velocities (62,63,65). Additionally, a positive tourniquet test and pressure over the flexor retinaculum can induce symptoms. Shoe corrections and steroid injection into the tarsal tunnel may be of benefit, but often surgical decompression is needed (63).

Anterior Tarsal Tunnel Syndrome

Anterior tarsal tunnel syndrome (deep peroneal nerve entrapment) is an entrapment neuropathy of the deep peroneal nerve at the inferior extensor retinaculum on the dorsum of the foot. The symptoms consist of numbness and paresthesias over the dorsum of the foot, especially at the web space (66). A tight feeling may be described over the anterior aspect of the ankle. The symptoms may arise following the wearing of tight shoes or high heels. Other causes include contusion of the dorsum of the foot, metatarsal fracture, talonavicular osteophytosis, and ganglion (67). Symptoms also tend to occur in bed at night and are relieved by standing or walking. Hypesthesia and hypalgesia may be present in the first dorsal web space, and a Tinel sign may be elicited on percussion just anterosuperior to the medial malleolus. The extensor digitorum brevis may be atrophied and weak.

A diagnosis of anterior tarsal tunnel syndrome may be confirmed by electrodiagnostic studies (68). Conservative measures include avoiding shoes that might stretch or compress the nerve. Steroid injections have been used. In persistent cases, the deep peroneal nerve can be decompressed at the retinaculum (66).

Superficial Peroneal Nerve Entrapment

The superficial peroneal nerve bifurcates into the intermediate dorsal cutaneous and the medial dorsal cutaneous terminal nerves. The lateral aspect of the foot is usually innervated by a branch of the sural nerve, the lateral dorsal cutaneous nerve. When this branch is absent, the intermediate branch of the superficial peroneal nerve supplies the innervation to the lateral foot.

The symptoms are pain, numbness, or tingling over the lateral aspect of the dorsum of the foot, worsened by exercise and often becoming more severe at night (69). The intermediate dorsal cutaneous branch, being very superficial, can be observed and palpated upon plantar flexing and inverting the foot. If this branch of the nerve is entrapped, then compression at this site will reproduce symptoms. A Tinel sign is usually present. A decrease in sensation to light touch and pinprick may be present in the cutaneous distribution of the nerve.

The most common cause of this neuropathy is acute and chronic ankle sprains. Other causes include osteoarthritis of tarsal bones and muscle herniation in the anterior compartment. Since the intermediate branch is so superficial, it is very susceptible to trauma and may be the source of chronic posttrauma ankle and foot pain. Electrodiagnostic studies with abnormal sensory conduction velocity and prolonged distal latency help confirm the diagnosis. The treatment is a local steroid injection or, if persistent, surgical decompression.

Sural Nerve Entrapment

Entrapment of the sural nerve, although uncommon, may be overlooked because of its limited cutaneous distribution. This nerve, which is formed from branches of the posterior tibial and common peroneal nerves, descends lateral to the Achilles tendon, and after passing the lateral malleolus the nerve turns anteriorly and continues as the lateral dorsal cutaneous nerve along the lateral side of the foot and the fifth toe.

The manifestations are numbness and a burning pain along the lateral side of the dorsum of the foot, which may be worse at night (70). A decrease in sensation and a Tinel sign may be present. Trauma, scar tissue, and ganglia have been reported as causes of entrapment (71). Local decompression can relieve the symptoms.

FOOT REHABILITATION

Orthoses

Orthotics is the field of correcting foot deformities by means of external support; the name was coined by Nickel in 1953 (72). The devices used for this task are known as orthoses and not orthotics. These orthoses (orthotic devices) are used to relieve and/or cushion an area of pressure, support an area of collapse, or convert a biomechanically abnormal foot into a biomechanically functional foot during the stance phase of gait (15,16,73). In short, these mechanical devices help restore lost function or help maintain optimal function by altering biomechanics. Orthoses may provide pain relief and compensate for muscle and ligament weakness by decreasing forces passing through painful weight-bearing areas, stabilizing or immobilizing subluxing joints, and repositioning toes.

The range of these orthotic devices varies from simple inexpensive pads available in drugstores to complex, expensive, custom-made orthoses. The importance and value of foot orthoses in the treatment of foot disorders is often underrecognized. The physician should establish a relationship with a pedorthotist (an orthotist who is trained in foot devices), an orthotist, or a trained therapist who can fabricate orthoses that are specific for the problem (74).

Foot orthoses can be divided into three types: devices that relieve pressure on various parts of the foot; those that cushion the foot and decrease impact; and those that are custom made to correct abnormal biomechanics and restore better function of the foot (9,16). Orthoses that relieve pressure on specific areas of the foot are generally foam or felt with an adhesive backing. These can be shaped specifically for pressure areas such as under the first, second, or fifth metatarsal heads. The pad is placed just proximal to the area of pressure.

The second type of orthosis, which reduces impact and cushions the foot, is constructed of material such as Spenco, which is composed of microcellular rubber. These are transferable to different shoes and are used in mild cases. Spenco is available in most sporting goods and foot-care product stores. Additional materials used in orthoses that reduce impact and cushion the foot are Plastizote, Pelite, and Aliplast, which are closed-cell thermoplastic, polyethylene foam devices, and Sorbothane, a viscoelastic material. The material can be molded to the contour of the foot.

The third type of orthosis is the biomechanical custom-fabricated type, which attempts to restore the subtalar joint to a neutral position. These may be rigid, semiflexible, or soft, depending upon the need. The thermoplastic materials are the semiflexible types. The rigid type is usually composed of an acrylic, rigid polyurethane foam, or polypropylene (74,75). As part of this type of orthosis, a "post," which is a wedge, can be incorporated to support the foot and correct the abnormality (Figs. 5.4 and 5.5) (15,16,73). If forefoot varus is present, then a medial post is used; and if forefoot valgus is present, then a lateral post is devised. Likewise, a medial post is used to correct pronation (eversion) of the hindfoot, whereas a lateral post is used to correct hindfoot supination (inversion). Typically, a custom-made orthosis may incorporate several features to address the foot problems, and if needed, all three types of foot orthoses can be combined into one orthosis (74). A depression can be made in the orthosis to relieve pressure in a specific area. Larger-than-normal or extra-depth shoes are needed for the orthosis to fit comfortably.

Ligament laxity is common in many inflammatory rheumatic diseases, often resulting in subluxation of joints. Subluxation of the metatarsophalangeal joint results in broadening of the forefoot, clawing of toes, and painful weight bearing on metatarsophalangeal heads. Callous, a protective reaction of the skin to stress, may be seen on the bottom of the foot. An internal or external metatarsal bar or pad can be placed in, or on, the shoes just behind the metatarsal heads to redistribute the weight away from this area to the metatarsal shafts. Alternatively, a metatarsal corset (a metatarsal pad attached directly to a toe with a strap, inside the sock) may be used in any shoe. Joint subluxation also results in loss of foot arches, uneven weight distribution, and pain. Arch supports such as a medial longitudinal arch support placed in the shoe can reform these arches. Spacers can be placed between toes to prevent overlapping and secondary calluses.

Shoe Modification

It is important to have a general understanding of shoe construction and available shoe modifications to help treat foot problems (76,77). As a start, one can simply examine shoe bottoms for wear and tear to determine the abnormal forces involved. A variety of modifications can be made. Extra-depth shoes with a large toebox should be used to accommodate fixed deformities such as clawed toes and to provide room for foot and ankle–foot orthoses (AFOs). Otherwise, corns may develop where the proximal interphalangeal joints of the toes or other parts of the foot rub on the superior part of the shoe. For patients with toe deformities, shoe closures can be modified. Traditional shoelaces can be changed to Velcro closures. Elastic laces can replace regular laces, effectively turning the shoe into a loafer type. Shoes with proper closures are generally preferred over loafers, however, as loafers maintain their place on the foot by tension.

A Thomas heel, which is a medial extension of the heel, may be added to support the longitudinal arch (78). Replacing the regular shoe heel with a "solid ankle cushion heel" may be helpful for heel pain or a fused ankle, as this heel can simulate ankle plantar flexion while walking (78). A rocker bottom sole may be helpful for a fused ankle, hal-

lux rigidus, or other toe deformities by substituting for the push-off and heel-strike phase of walking.

Lighter shoes are easier to wear but have less stability and durability. Heavier shoes may have greater stability and durability but are more difficult to carry. Ultimately, the shoe must be comfortable, have a good fit, and be aesthetically appealing. Otherwise, it will not be used. One can always advise patients to wear their special shoes at home and on the way to work, and to change when they get there.

In a leg length discrepancy, a lift can be attached to the outside of the whole shoe of the short leg, and not just to the sole or heel. The shoe raise should be one-half to three-fourths of the leg length discrepancy. The difference should probably be greater than 1 cm to consider correcting. However, if the leg length discrepancy is not a recent event, and especially if it is asymptomatic, it is probably best left untreated, since changing walking biomechanics after years of compensation may result in new symptoms.

Braces

A patellar tendon–bearing orthosis is helpful for the problem of pain and limitation in ambulation due to destructive

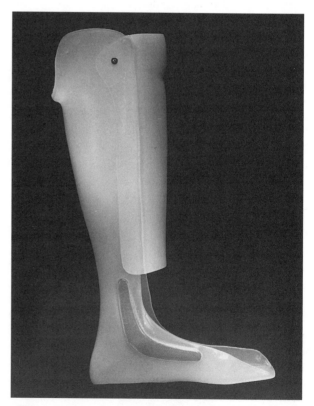

FIGURE 5.8. Patellar tendon–bearing orthosis used to decrease weight on ankle or subtalar joints. (From Biundo JJ, Rush PJ. Painful feet. In: Koopman WJ, ed. *Arthritis and allied conditions,* 14th ed. Philadelphia: Lippincott Williams & Wilkins, 2001: 1996–2008, with permission.)

changes of the ankle or subtalar joint subsequent to rheumatoid arthritis or other inflammatory arthritis (79). This patellar tendon–bearing brace, which provides weight bearing on the patellar tendon and tibial condyles through a molded upper-calf band, has a fixed ankle and a rocker bottom sole. Thus weight of the upper body can be directly transmitted from the knee region and calf to the floor, bypassing the ankle (Fig. 5.8) (80). This patellar tendon–bearing brace is also used to decrease stress on the ankle or subtalar joints in other conditions such as severe osteoarthritis, Charcot joint, and nonunited fractures of the lower limb (81).

Modalities

The most commonly used modalities are heat and cold. Methods of superficial heating for the feet include hot packs, heating pads, hydrocollator packs, hot water bottles, heated whirlpools, and infrared lamps. Hydrotherapy in a whirlpool can provide superficial heat to the whole foot. At home, hot baths and foot soaks, especially in the morning, can be used for relief. Ultrasound may be used to heat tendons and deeper structures.

Cooling of tissues can be obtained with coolant sprays, ice packs, basins of ice water, and frozen food packages. Cooling also causes vasoconstriction, with a reduction of blood flow and a decrease in metabolic activity in the region treated. Generally, patients seem to prefer heat, however. Both heat and cold may be used alternatively as a contrast bath.

Therapeutic Exercises

Therapeutic exercise may be broadly classified into three groups: (a) range of motion or stretching, (b) strengthening (resistive), and (c) aerobic (endurance). In many cases, a simple home exercise program is adequate and may be taught to the patient by the physician. Other cases require the prescription of a more formal physical therapy program. An exercise prescription should include the exercise frequency, intensity, type, and duration (timing), with the eponym FITT.

Range-of-motion exercises are important during the active phase of an inflammatory arthritis to maintain mobility of the ankle, subtalar, tarsal, and metatarsophalangeal joints. Ankle exercises include foot circles, active dorsiflexion, and plantar flexion. Writing the alphabet with the toes and cloth tugs with the toes and foot provide range of motion to the joints of the foot (82). After the acute phase has resolved, strengthening exercises against a resistance can be used (82). The ankle may be stretched with rubber tubing. Patients can be asked to push their feet against a board attached to the bed. Bicycle riding, swimming, and a rowing machine are non–weight-bearing exercises that can help maintain cardiovascular conditioning.

REFERENCES

1. Calabro JJ. A critical evaluation of the diagnostic features of the feet in rheumatoid arthritis. *Arth Rheum* 1962;5:19–29.
2. Mann RA. Biomechanics of the foot and ankle. *Orthop Rev* 1978;7:43–48.
3. Morris JM. Biomechanics of the foot and ankle. *Clin Orthop* 1977;122:10–17.
4. Mann RA. Biomechanics of the foot and ankle. In: Sammarco GJ, ed. *Foot and ankle manual.* Philadelphia: Lea and Febiger, 1991:32–41.
5. Perry J. Anatomy and biomechanics of the hindfoot. *Clin Orthop* 1983;177:9–15.
6. Shereff MJ. Clinical evaluation of the foot and ankle. In: Sammarco GJ, ed. *Foot and ankle manual.* Philadelphia: Lea and Febiger, 1991:42–53.
7. Smith RW. Evaluation of the adult forefoot. *Clin Orthop* 1979;142:19–23.
8. Polly HF, Hunder GG. The ankle and foot. In: *Physical examination of the joints,* 2nd ed. Philadelphia: WB Saunders, 1978: 239–274.
9. Riegler HF. Orthotic devices for the foot. *Orthop Rev* 1987;16: 293–303.
10. Brodsky JW. Radiology of the foot and ankle. In: Sammarco GJ, ed. *Foot and ankle manual.* Philadelphia: Lea and Febiger, 1991: 54–67.
11. Beltran J. Magnetic resonance imaging of the ankle and foot. *Orthopedics* 1994;17:1075–1082.
12. Llauger J, Palmer J, Monill JM, et al.: MR imaging of benign soft-tissue masses of the foot and ankle. *Radiographics* 1998;18: 1481–1498.
13. Graham CE. Painful heel syndrome: rationale of diagnosis and treatment. *Foot Ankle* 1983;3:261–267.
14. Klebo P, Allenmark C, Peterson L, et al. Diagnostic value of ultrasonography in partial ruptures of the Achilles tendon. *Am J Sports Med* 1992;20:378–381.
15. Bordelon RL. Orthotics, shoes, and braces. *Orthop Clin North Am* 1989;20:751–757.
16. Bordelon RL. Practical guide to foot orthoses. *J Musculoskeletal Med* 1989;6:71–87.
17. Ritterbusch JF, Drennan JC. The cavus foot: a review. *Contemp Orthop* 1992;24:525–532.
18. Inman VT. Hallux valgus: a review of etiologic factors. *Orthop Clin North Am* 1974;5:59–66.
19. Mann RA. Bunion surgery: decision making. *Orthopedics* 1990; 13:951–957.
20. Nestor BJ, Kitaoka HB, Illstrup DM, et al. Radiologic anatomy of the painful bunionette. *Foot Ankle* 1990;11:6–11.
21. Coughlin MJ. Lesser toe deformities. *Orthopedics* 1987;10: 63–75.
22. Santi M, Sarttoris DJ, Resnick D. Diagnostic imaging of tarsal and metatarsal stress fractures. *Orthop Rev* 1989;18:178–185.
23. Prather JL, Nusynowitz ML, Snowdy HA, et al. Scintigraphic findings in stress fractures. *J Bone Joint Surgery* 1977;59A: 869–874.
24. Jahss MH. The sesamoids of the hallux. *Clin Orthop* 1981;157: 88–97.
25. Dietzen CJ. Great toe sesamoid injuries in the athlete. *Orthop Rev* 1990;19:966–972.

26. Brower AC. The osteochondroses. *Orthop Clin North Am* 1983; 14:99–117.

27. Kjaersgaard-Andersen P, Andersen K, Soballe K, et al. Sinus tarsi syndrome: presentation of seven cases and review of the literature. *J Foot Surg* 1989;283–286.

28. Taillard W, Meyer J-M, Garcia J, et al. The sinus tarsi syndrome. *Int Orthop* 1981;5:117–130.

29. Klein MA, Spreitzer AM. MR imaging of the tarsal sinus and canal: normal anatomy, pathologic findings, and features of the sinus tarsi syndrome. *Radiology* 1993;186:233–240.

30. Shear MS, Baitch SP, Shear DB. Sinus tarsi syndrome: the importance of biomechanically based evaluation and treatment. *Arch Phys Med Rehabil* 1993;74:777–781.

31. Carson CW, Ginsburg WW, Cohen MD, et al. Tarsal coalition: an unusual cause of foot pain—clinical spectrum and treatment in 129 patients. *Semin Arthritis Rheum* 1991;20:367–377.

32. Sartoris DJ, Resnick DL. Tarsal coalition. *Arthritis Rheum* 1985; 28:331–338.

33. Wechsler RJ, Schweitzer ME, Deely DM. Tarsal coalition: depiction and characterization with CT and MR imaging. *Radiology* 1994;193:447–452.

34. Reed MT. Safe relief of rest pain that eases with activity in achillodynia by intrabursal or peritendinous steroid injection: the rupture rate was not increased by these steroid injections. *Br J Sports Med* 1999;33:134–135.

35. Wills CA, Washburn S, Caiozzo V, et al. Achilles tendon rupture: a review of the literature comparing surgical versus nonsurgical treatment. *Clin Orthop* 1986;207:156–163.

36. Panageas E, Greenberg S, Franklin PD, et al. Magnetic resonance imaging of pathologic conditions of the Achilles tendon. *Orthop Rev* 1990;19:975–980.

37. Holmes GB, Mann RA, Wells L. Epidemiologic factors associated with rupture of the Achilles tendon. *Contemp Orthop* 1991; 23:327–331.

38. Maffulli N. Rupture of the Achilles tendon. *J Bone Joint Surg* 1999; 81:1019–1036.

39. Canoso JJ, Wohgethan JR, Newberg AH, et al. Aspiration of the retrocalcaneal bursa. *Ann Rheum Dis* 1984;43:308–312.

40. Baxter DE, Pfeffer GB, Thigpen M. Chronic heel pain: treatment rationale. *Orthop Clin North Am* 1989;20:563–569.

41. DeMaio M, Paine R, Mangine RE, et al. Plantar fasciitis. *Orthopedics* 1993;16:1153–1163.

42. Karr SD. Subcalcaneal heel pain. *Orthop Clin North Am* 1994; 25:161–175.

43. Michelson JD. Heel pain: when is it plantar fasciitis? *J Musculoskeletal Med* 1995;12:22–29.

44. Sebes JI. The significance of calcaneal spurs in rheumatic diseases. *Arthritis Rheum* 1989;32:338–340.

45. Martin RL, Irrgang JJ, Conti SF. Outcome study of subjects with insertional plantar fasciitis. *Foot Ankle Int* 1998;19: 803–811.

46. Powell M, Post WR, Keener J, et al. Effective treatment of chronic plantar fasciitis with dorsiflexion night splints: a crossover prospective randomized outcome study. *Foot Ankle Int* 1998;19:10–18.

47. Gudeman SD, Eisele SA, Heidt RS, et al. Treatment of plantar fasciitis by iontophoresis of 0.45 dexamethasone: a randomized, double-blind, placebo-controlled study. *Am J Sports Med* 1998; 25:312–316.

48. Conti SF. Posterior tibial tendon problems in athletes. *Orthop Clin North Am* 1994;25:109–121.

49. Cozen L. Posterior tibial tenosynovitis secondary to foot strain. *Clin Orthop Rel Res* 1965;42:101–102.

50. Mann RA, Thompson FA. Rupture of the posterior tibial tendon causing flat foot. *J Bone Joint Surg* 1985;67A:556–561.

51. Supple KM, Hanft JR, Murphy BJ, et al. Posterior tibial tendon dysfunction. *Semin Arthritis Rheum* 1992;22:106–113.

52. Rosenberg ZS, Cheung Y, Jahss MH, et al. Rupture of posterior tibial tendon: CT and MR imaging with surgical correlation. *Radiology* 1988;169:229–235.

53. Churchill RS, Sferra JJ. Posterior tibial tendon insufficiency: its diagnosis, management, and treatment. *Am J Orthop* 1998:27: 339–347.

54. Downey DJ, Simkin PA, Mack LA, et al. Tibialis posterior tendon rupture: a cause of rheumatoid flat foot. *Arthritis Rheum* 1988;31:441–446.

55. Arrowsmith SR, Fleming LL, Allman FL. Traumatic dislocations of the peroneal tendons. *Am J Sports Med* 1983;11:142–146.

56. Sammarco GJ. Peroneal tendon injuries. *Orthop Clin North Am* 1994;25:135–145.

57. Parvin RW, Ford LT. Stenosing tenosynovitis of the common peroneal tendon sheath. *J Bone Joint Surg* 1956;38A:1352–1357.

58. Alexander IJ, Johnson KA, Parr JW. Morton's neuroma: a review of recent concepts. *Orthopedics* 1987;10:103–106.

59. Bossley CJ, Cairney PC. The intermetatarsophalangeal bursa—its significance in Morton's metatarsalgia. *J Bone Joint Surg* 1980; 62B:184–187.

60. Zanetti M, Strehle JK, Kundert HP, et al. Morton neuroma: effect of MR imaging findings on diagnostic thinking and therapeutic decisions. *Radiology* 1999;213:583–588.

61. Strong G, Thomas PS. Conservative treatment of Morton's neuroma. *Orthop Rev* 1987;16:343–345.

62. DeLisa JA, Saeed MA. The tarsal tunnel syndrome. *Muscle Nerve* 1983;6:664–670.

63. Wilemon WK. Tarsal tunnel syndrome: a 50-year survey of the world literature and a report of two new cases. *Orthop Rev* 1979; 8:111–118.

64. Grabois M, Puentes J, Lidsky M. Tarsal tunnel syndrome in rheumatoid arthritis. *Arch Phys Med Rehabil* 1981;62:401–403.

65. Galardi G, Amadio S, Maderna L, et al. Electrophysiologic studies in tarsal tunnel syndrome. *Am J Phys Med Rehabil* 1994;73: 193–198.

66. Dellon AL. Deep peroneal nerve entrapment on the dorsum of the foot. *Foot Ankle* 1990;11:73–80.

67. Gessini L, Jandolo B, Pietrangeli A. The anterior tarsal syndrome: report of four cases. *J Bone Joint Surg* 1984;66A: 786–787.

68. Andressen BL, Wertsch JJ, Stewart WA. Anterior tarsal tunnel syndrome. *Arch Phys Med Rehabil* 1992;73:1112–1117.

69. Sridhara CR, Izzo KL. Terminal sensory branches of the superficial peroneal nerve: an entrapment syndrome. *Arch Phys Med Rehabil* 1985;68:789–791.

70. Pringle RM, Protheroe K, Mukherjee SK. Entrapment neuropathy of the sural nerve. *J Bone Joint Surg* 1974;56B:465–468.

71. Bryan BM. Sural nerve entrapment after injury to the gastrocnemius: a case report. *Arch Phys Med Rehabil* 1999;80: 604–606.

72. Nickel VL. Orthotics in America: past, present and future. *Clin Orthop* 1974;102:10–17.

73. Donatelli R, Hurlbert C, Conaway D, et al. Biomechanical foot orthotics: a retrospective study. *J Orthop Sports Phys Ther* 1988; 10:205–212.

74. Janisse DJ. Indications and prescriptions for orthoses in sports. *Orthop Clin North Am* 1994;25:95–107.

75. Yates G. Molded plastics in bracing. *Clin Orthop* 1974;102: 46–57.

76. Bistevins R. Footwear and footwear modifications. In: Kottke FJ, Lehmann JF, eds. *Handbook of physical medicine and rehabilitation,* 4th ed. Philadelphia: WB Saunders, 1990:967–975.

77. Cowell HR. Shoes and shoe corrections. *Pediatr Clin North Am* 1977;24:791–797.

78. Milgram JE, Jacobson MA. Footgear: therapeutic modifications of sole and heel. *Orthop Rev* 1978;7:57–62.

79. Swezey RL. Below-knee weight-bearing brace for the arthritic foot. *Arch Phys Med Rehabil* 1975;56:176–179.

80. Lehmann JF, Warren CG, Pemberton DR, et al. Load-bearing function of patellar tendon bearing braces of various designs. *Arch Phys Med Rehabil* 1971;52:366–370.

81. Gristina AG, Nicastro JF, Clippinger F, et al. Neuropathic foot and ankle patellar-tendon-bearing orthosis as an adjunct to patient management. *Orthop Rev* 1977;6:53–59.

82. Kisner C, Colby LA. *Therapeutic exercise: foundations and techniques,* 2nd ed. Philadelphia: FA Davis, 1990.

83. From Hollinshead WH, Jenkins DB. *Functional anatomy of the limbs and back,* 5th ed. Philadelphia: WB Saunders, 1981.

84. Schepsis AA, Leach RE, Gorzyca J. Plantar fasciitis: etiology, treatment, surgical results, and review of the literature. *Clin Orthop* 1991;266:185–196.

85. Fessell DP, Vanderschueren GM, Jacobson JA, et al. Ankle ultrasound: technique, anatomy and pathology. *Radiographics* 1998; 18:325–340.

MECHANICAL DISORDERS OF THE KNEE

DENNIS W. BOULWARE

EPIDEMIOLOGY

Mechanical disorders of the knee include clinical conditions caused by malfunction, trauma, or degeneration of a specific component of the knee interfering with normal knee function. Normal knee operation depends on proper function of various intraarticular and extraarticular components. Internal derangement of the knee commonly refers to a disorder of the intraarticular components, such as the articular cartilage, meniscus fibrocartilage, collateral ligaments, or cruciate ligaments. Disorders of extraarticular components of the knee joint include patellofemoral malalignment and insufficiency of the quadriceps or hamstring muscle groups and are considered as mechanical disorders.

Significant mechanical disorders of the knee, if continued unabated, eventually lead to osteoarthritis. Several experimental animal models of osteoarthritis involve an initiating internal derangement of the joint, followed by continued use. The most common models of experimental osteoarthritis include partial medial meniscectomy or transection of the anterior cruciate ligament. As our population ages and becomes more engaged in recreational and sports-related activities, mechanical disorders of the knee will become more prevalent and, if not recognized early, will result in an increased prevalence of osteoarthritis of the knee.

PATHOPHYSIOLOGY/PATHOGENESIS

Most knee pain results from disruption of one of the many components that comprise a functional knee joint. These components include the articular hyaline cartilage, the supporting meniscal fibrocartilage, the various ligaments, and the patella. An understanding of the anatomy and biomechanics of the knee coupled with a complete physical examination will usually identify the cause of pain.

Articular Hyaline Cartilage

Articular cartilage is a firm, resilient tissue capable of absorbing impact, transmitting load, and sustaining tremendous shear forces. Changes in the proteoglycan content or macroscopic structure results in a diminished ability to function and remain resilient. Cartilage is an avascular structure, receiving its nutrients from synovial fluid during compressive loading and unloading. Any condition that affects the anatomic or biochemical integrity of hyaline cartilage of the knee predisposes an individual to a greater potential for a future mechanical disorder and places the knee at greater risk for eventual osteoarthritis. The most common cause of articular cartilage dysfunction is aging and the inability of the body to maintain the integrity of the cartilage.

Meniscal Fibrocartilage

The medial and lateral menisci are crescents of fibrocartilage, triangular in cross section, that modify the flat tibial plateau, creating a concave surface for the convex femoral condyles (Fig. 6.1). The menisci function by stabilizing the knee and limiting mobility into simple flexion and exten-

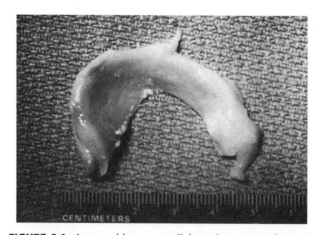

FIGURE 6.1. A normal human medial meniscus. Note the semilunar shape with a thin free edge and considerably thickened marginal attachment site. Menisci increase the stability of the joint and serve as weight-bearing structures in the knee. (From Boulware DW. Mechanical disorders of the knee. In: Koopman WJ. *Arthritis and allied conditions: a textbook of rheumatology,* 14th ed. Philadelphia: Lippincott Williams & Wilkins, 2001: 1988–1995, with permission.)

sion. The composition of fibrocartilaginous menisci differs biochemically and functionally from hyaline articular cartilage. In adulthood, the menisci are predominantly avascular structures with most of their nutrients being acquired from synovial fluid during loading and unloading. A vascular zone in the menisci is adjacent to the bone, which accounts for their ability to undergo repair more easily than articular cartilage. The medial meniscus is essentially attached to the medial collateral ligament, and damage to the ligament usually translates into damage to the medial meniscus.

Ligaments

Ligaments are comprised nearly entirely of collagen and elastin in dense, parallel-organized bundles. They function to constrain knee mobility into desired flexion and extension (Fig. 6.2). The collateral ligaments prevent varus or valgus deviation, and the cruciate ligaments prevent anterior or posterior displacement of the tibial plateau as it pivots about the distal femoral condyles. Ligaments are vascularized structures, and damage to the ligament usually results in a hemarthrosis.

Patellofemoral Alignment

During flexion and extension of the knee, the patella glides superiorly and inferiorly along the femoral intercondylar groove. Patellar tracking malalignment can occur with an imbalance of the quadriceps' vector forces on the patellar

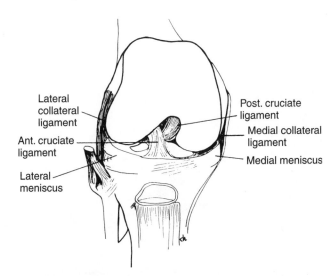

FIGURE 6.2. Diagram of the human knee joint. The patella and capsule have been removed. Note that the distal femur and proximal tibia are covered by hyaline articular cartilage. Affixed to the surface of the tibia are the medial and lateral collateral ligaments, stout collagenous bands, which provide stability in the coronal plane. The cruciate ligaments control stability in the sagittal plane. (From Boulware DW. Mechanical disorders of the knee. In: Koopman WJ. *Arthritis and allied conditions: a textbook of rheumatology,* 14th ed. Philadelphia: Lippincott Williams & Wilkins, 2001:1988–1995, with permission.)

tendon or in varus and valgus deformities. Similarly, the patella will exhibit abnormal tracking when there is significant subluxation of the patella secondary to patellar tendon laxity. All these anatomic aberrations can lead to a mechanical disorder of the knee, with the major impact on the patellofemoral compartment causing pain.

MENISCAL DISORDERS

The medial and lateral menisci are crescent-shaped structures that appear triangular in configuration upon cross-sectional examination. Their structure allows the knee to function with greater stability and improved joint congruity and to transmit 50% to 70% of the load across the knee during axial loading. Disorders of the menisci account for about two-thirds of all derangements of the knee joint. Lesions of the menisci can be divided into acute tears and chronic or degenerative tears. Most acute tears occur following trauma, such as an athletic injury, in which there is abnormal excursion of the articular surfaces under conditions of loading that entrap the menisci. Usually, an acute tear consists of a vertical and longitudinal tear. A chronic or degenerative tear often does not have a recognizable precipitating event. Symptoms are usually less severe in chronic tears, and the lesions often result in a horizontal cleavage, particularly in the posterior third of the meniscus. In a large recent arthroscopic study of symptomatic meniscal lesions by Dandy, 81% of the patients were men, with medial meniscal lesions predominating. Approximately 75% of the medial meniscal tears were vertical, with the remainder being horizontal tears. Similarly, vertical tears were the more common pattern seen in lateral meniscal injuries.

Clinical Features

Clinical History

Acute meniscal injuries generally involve easily identifiable precipitating events, often followed by an associated limited range of motion with the pain. If the acute injury results in a displacement of the torn meniscus, patients often complain of a painful "catching" or "popping" sensation in the knee. Although "buckling" sensations are often associated with meniscal tears, they are more common with anterior cruciate ligament injuries but can be seen in any painful condition of the knee. They are caused by a reflexive muscle relaxation and "giving way."

A chronic tear of the meniscus is usually less painful than an acute tear, and there is frequently a lack of any recognizable precipitating event. Usually associated with osteoarthritis, a precipitating cause may be as simple as a squatting and twisting maneuver or a simple misstep. Complaints usually include chronic pain with use of the knee and occasional swelling. Limitation in range of motion is less of a prominent feature than with acute displaced tears.

Physical Examination

Joint effusions usually correlate with the severity of inflammation within the knee joint. Obviously, acute injuries generally have a greater associated effusion than chronic degenerative tears. A limitation in passive range of motion occurs if there is a displaced tear of the meniscus with entrapment of the meniscus. The entrapped fragment of the meniscus is frequently the culprit in limiting full flexion or full extension. The McMurray test is a specific test to induce entrapment of a meniscal tear. With the patient supine, the examiner grasps the affected leg and passively flexes the knee and hip maximally. At the point of maximal flexion, the knee is rotated forcibly internally and externally to attempt impingement of the torn lateral or medial meniscus. With the knee held in passive internal rotation in flexion, the knee is extended to detect a palpable or audible snap in the joint. The maneuver is repeated with the flexed knee held in full, passive, external rotation. Pain is not always present, particularly in an older degenerative tear. The Apley grind test is also used to detect possible meniscal derangement. This test is performed with the patient in a prone position and the knee flexed at 90 degrees. In this position the examiner manually loads the knee joint while rotating the knee in internal and external rotation. Tenderness elicited during this procedure is not specific for a meniscal injury, as an articular cartilage lesion will also produce tenderness. The combined presence of a "snap" and an abnormal Apley grind test is consistent with a torn meniscus.

Because of the anatomic location of the menisci near the medial and lateral joint lines, joint line tenderness is the hallmark of a meniscal injury. The menisci are in close congruity with the peripheral joint capsule, which has a rich nerve supply, accounting for the localized tenderness. A combination of joint line tenderness with a positive McMurray and/or Apley sign correlates well with a clinically torn meniscus.

Imaging Studies

A clinically suspected torn meniscus is usually confirmed by an imaging study, either noninvasive or invasive. Noninvasive studies include plain radiography, computerized tomography (CT), or magnetic resonance imaging (MRI) (Fig. 6.3). Invasive imaging, including arthroscopy and arthrography, carries a higher accuracy. Plain radiography is a poor diagnostic modality for soft-tissue injury. The only utility of plain radiography would be to assess the severity of coexisting osteoarthritis, a common co-morbid feature of a degenerative or chronic tear. MRI has a high diagnostic accuracy, approaching 70% to 95%, but should not be part of the initial evaluation. An excellent modality to evaluate soft-tissue injuries, MRI is limited by the difficulty in differentiating a degenerative intact meniscus from a chronic or degenerative meniscal tear. The greatest utility of MRI is in a negative study, because of its high negative predictive value. Computerized tomography is of limited value in evaluating meniscal injury when compared with the ability of MRI to differentiate soft-tissue lesions.

Double-contrast arthrography previously had been the gold standard for meniscal tears. Its accuracy, however, is highly dependent upon the experience of the interpreter and the severity of the lesion. Arthroscopy is a major surgical procedure (Fig. 6.4) and at present should be considered

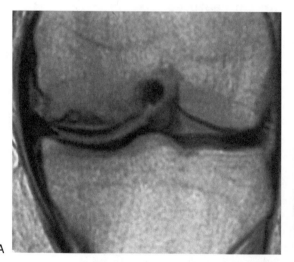
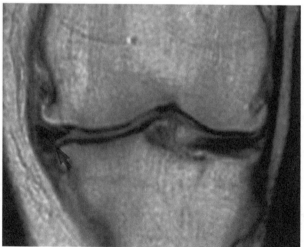

A   B

FIGURE 6.3. A: Magnetic resonance image of the knee of a 74-year-old man demonstrating concomitant spontaneous osteonecrosis of the medial femoral condyle. **B:** Complex degenerative horizontal cleavage tear of medial meniscus (*arrow*). (From Boulware DW. Mechanical disorders of the knee. In: Koopman WJ. *Arthritis and allied conditions: a textbook of rheumatology,* 14th ed. Philadelphia: Lippincott Williams & Wilkins, 2001:1988–1995, with permission.)

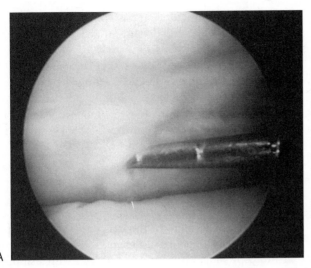 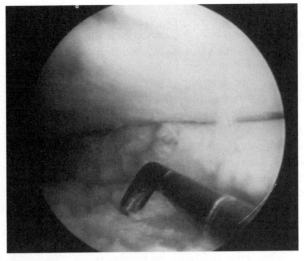

FIGURE 6.4. A: Arthroscopic appearance of the degenerative medial meniscus with probe in substance of tear. **B:** Associated chondral lesion with exposed subchondral bone. (From Boulware DW. Mechanical disorders of the knee. In: Koopman WJ. *Arthritis and allied conditions: a textbook of rheumatology,* 14th ed. Philadelphia: Lippincott Williams & Wilkins, 2001:1988–1995, with permission.)

the gold standard for the diagnosis of a meniscal tears. There is still difficulty in visualizing the posterior horn of the medial meniscus, and the experience and efficiency of the operator limit the test. With a proper physical examination and the diagnostic utility of MRI, there is little need for diagnostic arthroscopy. This technique should be reserved for cases in which surgical intervention is deemed essential for treatment.

Treatment

A conservative versus surgical treatment approach is determined by the displacement of a meniscal tear. A displaced meniscal tear resulting in entrapment and limitation of range of motion warrants surgical intervention. Tears that are nondisplaced or do not result in entrapment can be treated conservatively, including nonsteroidal antiinflammatory drugs for analgesic effect and supervised physical therapy to maintain passive range of motion and muscle strength. If a displaced meniscal tear requires surgical intervention, arthroscopic partial meniscectomy is preferable to open meniscectomy due to the advantage of more rapid recovery. The fraction of meniscus removed during meniscectomy should be minimized to maintain as much meniscal function as possible. Experimental models have found that postmeniscectomy osteoarthritic changes vary directly with the fraction of meniscus removed during meniscectomy. Nonsteroidal antiinflammatory drugs and vigorous supervised physical therapy are also indicated for patients undergoing arthroscopic synovectomy.

LIGAMENTOUS DISORDERS

Normal knee stability and range of motion depend on intact ligaments. Four major ligaments restrict the knee to primary flexion and extension: medial collateral ligament, lateral collateral ligament, anterior cruciate ligament, and posterior cruciate ligament. The collateral ligaments reside on the medial and lateral aspect of the knee and restrict the knee from varus or valgus angulation. The medial collateral ligament is firmly attached to the medial meniscus, and disruption of one structure often leads to injuries to the other structure in the medial compartment. The anterior and posterior cruciate ligaments function to retard anterior and posterior displacement of the tibia relative to the femoral condyles during flexion and extension. Acute injuries to the ligaments of the knee, particularly the anterior cruciate ligament, often result in a brisk hemarthrosis due to the vascularity of the ligaments. Acute injuries to the ligaments often have easily identifiable precipitating injuries.

Clinical Features

Clinical History

Injuries of the ligaments occur during activity and usually involve jumping or rapid changes in direction while running. Painful swelling of the joint, usually due to hemarthrosis, occurs precipitously within the first 2 to 6 hours after injury.

Physical Examination

Most ligamentous disorders can be easily detected by simple physical examination. Medial and lateral collateral ligament injury is best tested by passively placing the knee in 30 degrees of flexion. Applying passive stress that results in a valgus deviation of the knee would indicate a medial collateral ligament tear. Incomplete medial collateral ligament tears often result in *tenderness* over the medial compartment of the knee during this maneuver in the absence of valgus deviation. Conversely, a varus force applied to the knee still held in this position can be used to detect similar signs in the lateral compartment, implicating a lateral collateral ligament injury. Caution should be exercised in interpreting this maneuver because "relative" laxity of the collateral ligaments is often seen in knees with loss of full articular cartilage thickness due to chronic osteoarthritis.

A torn anterior cruciate ligament is best tested by the anterior drawer sign or Lachman test (Fig. 6.5). This maneuver is performed with the knee passively flexed to 25 degrees with an anterior force placed on the tibia relative to the femoral condyles. Anterior displacement of the tibial plateau relative to the femoral condyle indicates a torn or lax anterior cruciate ligament. Tenderness elicited by this maneuver in the absence of displacement suggests an incomplete tear of the anterior cruciate ligament. The posterior cruciate ligament is best tested by the posterior Drawer sign, which is performed with the knee in 90 degrees of flexion. A posterior force is placed on the tibia while looking for posterior displacement of the tibia relative to the femoral condyles. Again, caution should be exercised

in interpreting these tests in patients with chronic osteoarthritis and relative laxity of the ligaments due to articular cartilaginous loss.

Most ligamentous disruptions can be quantified by the degree of laxity or displacement. Using the normal contralateral knee as a reference point, a grade I laxity would represent up to 5 mm of additional motion; grade II, 6 to 10 mm; grade III, 11 to 15 mm; and grade IV, greater than 15 mm of additional displacement.

Imaging Studies

Diagnostic imaging, including plain radiography, CT, and MRI, offers little more to the diagnostic accuracy of the physical examination of ligamentous disorders. Invasive arthroscopy should be considered in cases with a suspected associated torn meniscus or osteochondral fracture, requiring arthroscopic repair.

Treatment

Anterior Cruciate Ligament

The treatment of most ligamentous injuries is based on the severity or grade of the injury, and anticipated or desired future functional capacity of the individual. For injuries to the anterior cruciate ligament, patients with grade I or II severity remain functionally stable after rehabilitation and modification of their activities. The decision to pursue a surgical reconstruction for grade III injuries often depends on the patient's desire to pursue future functional activities that will be demanding of the knee. Individuals with acute injuries resulting in grade IV laxity require surgical reconstruction to remain functional. Nonsteroidal antiinflammatory drugs for analgesia and vigorous supervised physical therapy are warranted for all individuals, whether they are surgical candidates or not.

Collateral Ligaments

The treatment of a medial collateral ligament injury is similar to that of the anterior cruciate ligament. Injuries up to and including grade II can often be treated conservatively without surgery, including supervised physical therapy, nonsteroidal antiinflammatory drugs for analgesia, and use of a hinged cast or brace for 3 to 6 weeks. Injuries with severity of grade III or greater often require surgical intervention for repair due to the likelihood of later problems with osteoarthritis. Lateral collateral ligament tears of grade II or greater severity often require surgical reconstruction.

An isolated disruption of the posterior cruciate ligament is a rare event, but can result from an exaggerated pull of the quadriceps tendon on the patella to stabilize the knee in flexion, or with hyperextension injuries of the knee. Most patients are only modestly impaired from this injury,

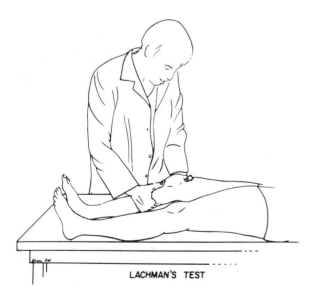

LACHMAN'S TEST

FIGURE 6.5. Lachman's test for anterior cruciate stability done with the knee at 25 degrees of flexion. (From Boulware DW. Mechanical disorders of the knee. In: Koopman WJ. *Arthritis and allied conditions: a textbook of rheumatology,* 14th ed. Philadelphia: Lippincott Williams & Wilkins, 2001:1988–1995, with permission.)

although the incidence of future osteoarthritis remains high. Surgical repair is usually reserved for those cases in which there has been an avulsion of a bone fragment.

Mid-ligamentous tears usually are not successfully repaired. Combined injuries such as a medial collateral ligament disruption *combined with* an anterior cruciate ligament tear often require surgical repair.

Supervised rehabilitation is an important modality of treatment for all knee injuries, but particularly with ligamentous injuries. The goal of strengthening the hamstring muscle relative to the quadriceps depends on the type of ligamentous injury. After anterior cruciate ligament injuries, physical therapy should be directed toward achieving hamstring and quadriceps muscles of relatively equal strength. This is unlike the normal situation where the quadriceps muscle is roughly 50% stronger than the hamstring. In posterior cruciate ligament injuries, the quadriceps muscles are strengthened maximally to ensure knee stability. Each patient must have a physical strengthening regimen specifically tailored to the injury.

PATELLOFEMORAL MALALIGNMENT

Malalignment of the patella as it tracks superiorly and inferiorly in the intercondylar groove of the femur is one of the most common causes of knee pain. Previously called chondromalacia patella, the degenerative process of the patellar cartilage is usually secondary to malalignment of the patella within the intercondylar groove. Unlike the previously described disorders of the meniscus and ligament, patellofemoral malalignment is not associated with an injury. Problems with patellofemoral pain usually correlate with severity of abnormal patellar tilt, alignment, and subluxation.

Clinical Features

Clinical History

The most common complaint of patients with patellofemoral malalignment is exertional knee pain, particularly with activities involving active weight-bearing knee extension or flexion, such as stair climbing, running, jumping, and squatting. Interestingly, in patellofemoral disease, difficulty in descending stairs is often more symptomatic than difficulty in ascending stairs. Prolonged periods of immobility with the knee in flexed positions such as sitting at a desk or riding in an automobile will often cause pain upon resuming a standing position.

Physical Examination

Joint effusions are not commonly seen but correlate with the degree of inflammation and histopathology of the patel-

lar articular cartilage. Passive range of motion is frequently preserved. Crepitus is a common feature of patellofemoral malalignment and usually is confined to the patellofemoral compartment. The patellofemoral compartment as a source of knee pain can be confirmed by reproducing the complaints by patellofemoral compression or patellar inhibition. There is often concomitant tenderness of the peripatellar muscles and iliotibial band.

An abnormal degree of patellar tilt or patellar laxity can be a cause of patellofemoral malalignment and subsequently a mechanical disorder of the knee (Fig. 6.6). The

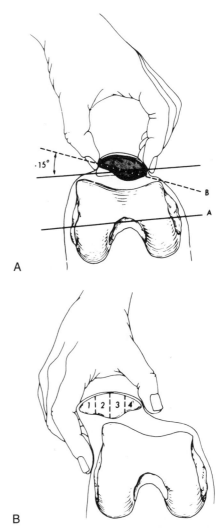

FIGURE 6.6. A: Passive patellar tilt indicates laxity of lateral ligamentous restraints. A patellar tilt of 0 degrees or less indicates tight lateral retinacular ligaments. **B:** Passive lateral glide test demonstrates the ability to displace the patella laterally with the knee in full extension. Subluxation beyond one-half of its width indicates laxity of medial retinacular restraints. (From Boulware DW. Mechanical disorders of the knee. In: Koopman WJ. *Arthritis and allied conditions: a textbook of rheumatology,* 14th ed. Philadelphia: Lippincott Williams & Wilkins, 2001:1988–1995, with permission.)

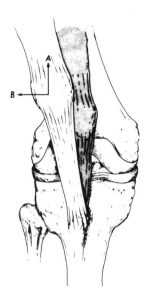

FIGURE 6.7. Increased "functional" Q angle is present if lateral excursion (*B*) exceeds proximal excursion (*A*). (From Boulware DW. Mechanical disorders of the knee. In: Koopman WJ. *Arthritis and allied conditions: a textbook of rheumatology,* 14th ed. Philadelphia: Lippincott Williams & Wilkins, 2001:1988–1995, with permission.)

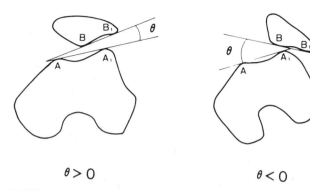

FIGURE   6.8. Angle of Laurin measures the lateral patellofemoral angle, where line *A–A1* passes through the femoral condyles and *B–B1* passes through the lateral patellar facet. The angle is positive if it opens laterally and abnormal if it opens medially. (From Boulware DW. Mechanical disorders of the knee. In: Koopman WJ. *Arthritis and allied conditions: a textbook of rheumatology,* 14th ed. Philadelphia: Lippincott Williams & Wilkins, 2001:1988–1995, with permission.)

passive patellar tilt test measures patellar laxity. The tilting of the lateral patellar edge relative to the lateral femoral condyle tests the degree of lateral retinacular tightness. A zero-degree or a negative-angle tilt usually reflects excessive retinacular tightness. The passive patellar glide test allows the examiner to estimate the degree of lateral patellar deviation. The examiner passively displaces the patella laterally with the knee in passive full extension. The ability to displace the patella greater than one-half of its total width suggests laxity of the medial retinacular restraints. Either medial retinacular laxity or lateral retinacular tightness will result in an abnormal tilt and malalignment of the patella.

Overall malalignment of the lower extremity, particularly angulation of the knee, should be assessed with the patient standing. An increase in the Q angle (Fig. 6.7) results in abnormal patellar tracking. Similarly, vastus medialis muscle atrophy, valgus deformities of the knee, or forefoot pronation problems for any reason will result in patellofemoral malalignment.

Imaging Studies

The clinical suspicion of a patellar tilt can usually be confirmed by plain radiography measuring the angle of Laurin. With the knee in 20 degrees of flexion, the lateral patellofemoral angle is measured (Fig. 6.8). In the normal patellofemoral compartment, the angle will open laterally when the angle of Laurin is positive. In the case of an abnormal patellar tilt, the angle of Laurin is negative and suggests an abnormal medial opening of the compartment.

Computerized tomography and MRI are alternatives to plain radiography in confirming patellofemoral alignment and tilting problems. Although they offer a better view of the soft tissue of the knee compartment, their expense offers little justification for these imaging techniques.

Arthroscopy is invaluable in grading the severity of patellar cartilage pathology but offers little more in confirming the clinical suspicion than does the physical examination and plain radiography.

Treatment

Conservative management should be instituted for all degrees of severity of patellar malalignment. Supervised physical therapy is indicated to stretch the lateral retinaculum, hamstring, and iliotibial band in concert with strengthening exercises of the quadriceps muscles, particularly the vastus medialis. The use of external support such as elastic knee supports and orthotics is also helpful. Quadriceps-strengthening exercises utilizing the last 30 degrees of extension to strengthen the vastus medialis muscle are important. Heavily loaded isotonic exercises with full range of motion (i.e., full squats with weights) should be avoided. Nonsteroidal antiinflammatory drugs are useful, particularly in cases with large effusions and for their analgesic properties.

Surgical management is occasionally required for severe malalignments. In the case of a chronic patellar subluxation, a lateral retinacular release may be helpful, although previous studies have been inconsistently successful when a lateral release is performed alone. Other surgical modalities, including transposition of the vastus medialis insertion, have similarly had equivocal outcomes.

SUMMARY

Mechanical disorders of the knee can eventually lead to the final clinical pathway of osteoarthritis. A severe derangement of any of the intraarticular or extraarticular components required for a normally functioning knee joint can result in osteoarthritis. Early recognition, appropriate treatment, and modification of body habitus and lifestyle may retard the progression of mechanical disorders of the knee to clinical osteoarthritis.

BIBLIOGRAPHY

Boulware DW. Mechanical disorders of the knee. In: Koopman WJ, ed. *Arthritis and allied conditions: a textbook of rheumatology,* 14th ed. Philadelphia: Lippincott Williams & Wilkins, 2001:1988–1995.

Dandy DJ. The arthroscopic anatomy of symptomatic meniscal lesions. *J Bone Joint Surg* 1990;72B:628–633.

Elmer RH, Moskowitz RW, Frankel VH. Meniscal regeneration and postmeniscectomy degenerative joint disease. *Clin Orthop* 1977; 124:304–310.

Guilak F, Ratcliffe A, Lane N, et al. Mechanical and biochemical changes in the superficial zone of articular cartilage in canine experimental osteoarthritis. *J Orthop Res* 1994;12:474–484.

Mehraban F, Kuo SY, Riera H, et al. Prostromelysin and procollagenase genes are differentially up-regulated in chondrocytes from the knees of rabbits with experimental osteoarthritis. *Arthritis Rheum* 1994;37:1189–1197.

Pelletier JP, Mineau F, Raynauld JP, et al. Intra-articular injections with methylprednisolone acetate reduce osteoarthritic lesions in parallel with chondrocyte stromelysin synthesis in experimental osteoarthritis. *Arthritis Rheum* 1994;37:414–423.

NERVE ENTRAPMENT DISORDERS

KENNETH K. NAKANO

The term *peripheral nerve* entrapment describes the mechanical irritation by which a specific peripheral nerve becomes locally compressed or angulated at a vulnerable anatomic site (1,2). Nerve entrapment disorders may result from a number of mechanisms, including pressure (compression), stretch, friction, and angulation. Owing to the variety of mechanisms, the pathophysiology of the peripheral nerve entrapment syndromes differs. In addition, the clinical circumstances, including the patient's age and the presence of certain underlying systemic diseases (e.g., diabetes, thyroid disease, rheumatoid arthritis), influence these peripheral nerve entrapment disorders. Compression on a peripheral nerve within a closed anatomic space can occur wherever a peripheral nerve passes through an opening in fibrous tissue or through an osseofibrous canal (e.g., cubital tunnel), soft-tissue swelling (viz., rheumatoid arthritis), an anomalous or hypertrophied muscle, a constricting scar or ligament, a bony deformity, or a mass (viz., ganglion, synovial cyst) (Table 7.1).

In some peripheral nerve entrapment disorders, the diagnosis is readily established on clinical grounds and confirmed by electrodiagnostic studies (nerve conduction measurements and electromyography). The most frequently diagnosed entrapment neuropathy, the carpal tunnel syndrome is the best example of this situation, where fortunately specific therapy is most successful. However, some nerve entrapment disorders are not clear-cut. Some doubt that the syndrome/disorder exists at all, or its limits are poorly defined, the cause is disputed, the therapy is of unknown efficacy, or the prevalence is so variable from one medical center to another as to shed doubt on the diagnostic criteria. In this category the following can be included: thoracic outlet syndrome; resistant tennis elbow, which is a result of a posterior interosseous nerve compression; the pronator syndrome, causing median nerve entrapment; and the piriformis syndrome, which produces sciatic pain.

Many clinical peripheral nerve entrapment disorders involve mixed peripheral nerves, so both sensory and motor symptoms will be present (3). If autonomic fibers are involved, there may also be sympathetic and parasympathetic dysfunction. An accurate diagnosis depends on a careful history and clinical examination. Since certain peripheral nerve entrapments are caused by friction, pressure, or traction on peripheral nerves from chronic occupational use, an occupational history will provide an important clue in specific situations. In addition to the clinical examination, the evaluation of patients with peripheral nerve entrapments should include electrophysiologic assessment [nerve conduction studies (NCS) and electromyography (EMG)] (4,5). These electrodiagnostic evaluations are useful under four clinical situations: (a) when the clinical diagnosis is uncertain; (b) for following patients with entrapment neuropathies who are being treated conservatively; (c) for detection or exclusion of coexisting conditions, such as a radiculopathy or subclinical polyneuropathy; and (d) before a surgical procedure to correct the entrapment. In certain nerve entrapment disorders computerized neuroimaging technology in the form of mag-

TABLE 7.1. NERVE ENTRAPMENT DISORDERS

Nerve	Entrapment Syndrome
Upper limbs	
Median	Carpal tunnel
	Anterior interosseous nerve
	Pronator teres
	Ligament of struthers
	Digital nerve
Ulnar	Cubital canal
	Guyon canal
	Digital nerve
Radial	Posterior interosseous nerve
	Superficial radial nerve
Suprascapular	Suprascapular foramen
	Infraspinatus branch
Musculocutaneous	Coracobrachialis
Brachial plexus	Thoracic outlet
Lower limbs	
Sciatic	Piriformis
Peroneal	Fibular tunnel
	Anterior tarsal tunnel
Posterior tibial	Posterior tarsal tunnel
	Morton neuroma
Lateral femoral cutaneous	Meralgia paresthetica

netic resonance imaging (MRI), computerized tomography (CT), and ultrasonography has assisted in the diagnosis, localization, and planning of surgical approaches.

Peripheral entrapment neuropathies cause focal disturbances of nerve function. Therefore the differential diagnosis of peripheral nerve entrapments resolves around other conditions that may damage nerves in a focal manner. These disorders include mononeuritis multiplex, brachial plexopathy, radiculopathy, amyotrophic lateral sclerosis, connective-tissue and vasospastic conditions [e.g., Raynaud phenomenon, peripheral neuropathies with vasomotor changes, and reflex sympathetic dystrophy (RSD)].

Nerve entrapment disorders will be discussed here according to the nerves that they involve in the upper and lower limbs and in the order of how commonly they occur in the clinical setting.

UPPER LIMBS

Median Nerve

Carpal Tunnel Syndrome

Clinical Evaluation

The most common peripheral nerve entrapment occurs in the carpal tunnel of the hand, at the point where the median nerve passes in company with nine flexor tendons of the fingers (6,7). In most cases of carpal tunnel syndrome (CTS), the clinical symptoms and the physical findings are specific. Individuals affected with CTS report numbness, tingling, and pain in the hand (palmar thumb, index, middle and part of the ring fingers), which often worsens at night or after use of the hand. Some patients complain of pain that radiates proximally into the forearm and arm. During the early stages of CTS, the clinical examination often reveals no abnormality. With greater severity of median nerve compression, the patient with CTS experiences sensory loss over some or all of the digits innervated by the median nerve and weakness of thumb abduction. The clinical physical evaluation in suspected cases of CTS includes assessment for Tinel sign (paresthesia in the median nerve territory elicited by gentle tapping over the carpal tunnel of the wrist) and positive response to Phalen maneuver (appearance or worsening of paresthesias with maximal passive wrist flexion for 1 minute). The reverse Phalen maneuver (passive wrist and finger extension for 1 minute) may produce higher intracarpal canal hydrostatic pressure and result in prolonged symptoms when compared with a traditional Phalen test.

Trauma and repetitive activities may cause the CTS. The following medical conditions may also be associated with CTS: diabetes mellitus, rheumatoid arthritis, hypothyroidism, gout, pseudogout, acromegaly, pregnancy and lactation, renal failure with chronic hemodialysis, lipoma of the flexor digitorum superficialis, fascia of the flexor digito-

rum superficialis, ganglion cysts, gonococcal tenosynovitis, pigmented villonodular synovitis, Lyme borreliosis, arterial anomalies (including aneurysm of the median nerve), and other previously known inflammatory reactions involving tendons and connective tissues of the wrist. Additionally, CTS may arise in paraplegic patients as a result of repetitive daily hand/wrist activities or athletic pursuits.

Differential Diagnosis

In the differential diagnostic possibilities in a patient suspected of having a CTS, the clinician must exclude a cervical radiculopathy, which often can be identified by the occurrence of proximal radiation of pain above the shoulder, paresthesias with coughing or sneezing, or a pattern of motor or sensory disturbances beyond the territory of the median nerve. Rarely, transient ischemic attacks (TIAs) and pure sensory strokes (lacunar strokes) may present with confusing symptoms, but usually pain is absent during an episode of numbness. Owing to the fact that no more than half of the patients with CTS can reliably report the location of their paresthesias, and because of the anomalous anatomy of peripheral nerves, ulnar neuropathies should be considered in certain clinical presentations. In the occupational setting, the overuse syndrome may become a diagnostic concern. Overall, CTS accounts for a minority of cases of the overuse syndrome. However, the frequency of both CTS and cumulative trauma appears to increase in parallel in workers who are at risk.

Diagnostic Assessment

NCS and EMG will be very useful to confirm the presence of a median neuropathy at the wrist in a patient suspected of having CTS clinically (8,9). Internal control median–ulnar/radial comparison studies substantially increase the sensitivity of conventional electrodiagnosis and should be performed in patients with normal standard motor or sensory nerve testing. Caution should be taken when performing EMG and NCS, because approximately one-half of patients with CTS possess abnormalities of the contralateral median nerve. Thus NCS values in patients should be compared with reference data for normal individuals as well as with the involved patient's own contralateral median and ipsilateral ulnar and radial latency values. In addition, the electromyographer must consider the data of normal control subjects for that lab, limb temperature, age, and body mass index when conducting electrodiagnostic procedures. Needle EMG of the limb muscles as well as the paraspinal cervical muscles should usually be performed in order to consider in the differential diagnosis the presence of coexisting disease (such as radiculopathy due to cervical spine disease, diffuse peripheral neuropathy, proximal nerve lesions). In cases of CTS, no tests provide greater diagnostic accuracy than NCS. However, false-negative and false-positive results occur; many of the apparent false-positive results occur in patients who have measurable abnormalities on NCS but no symptoms (e.g., there exists a high rate of abnormalities in the contralateral hands of patients with CTS). On the other hand, on rare occasions individuals with typical symptoms of CTS have normal EMG and NCS studies yet respond to carpal tunnel surgical procedures.

Treatment

In CTS early diagnosis and treatment will be important, because delay can result in irreversible median nerve damage with persistent symptoms and permanent disability. Conservative nonsurgical treatment would be advised for patients with mild symptoms, intermittent symptoms, or an acute flare-up of CTS from a specific injury. Included among the five types of nonsurgical treatments are (a) patient avoidance of the activities that precipitate the condition; (b) splinting of the wrist firmly in the neutral position for night and day use; (c) local steroid injection by an experienced clinician; (d) administration of a brief course of either oral steroids or nonsteroidal, antiinflammatory drugs (NSAIDs); and (e) a trial of diuretics, particularly when the CTS symptoms appear premenstrually. For the patient with mild nighttime CTS symptoms, a removable volar wrist splint that holds the wrist in a neutral position can often alleviate all symptoms. If CTS symptoms persist or recur, additional treatment is indicated. Local steroid injections or a trial of oral medications is recommended for those with mild persistent symptoms or for patients who complain of pain from their CTS and are elderly or poor surgical risks. Often local steroid injections relieve the pain but may not change the other symptoms of CTS. Individuals with thenar atrophy or muscle weakness or those with advanced sensory loss should not receive local steroid injections. Surgical treatment of CTS demands skill and care, and is one of the most successful operations that can be performed on the hand. Moreover, such hand surgery is reliably successful and may now be performed with low morbidity by means of a variety of minimally invasive techniques that use limited incisions involving less extensive exposure than the classic open procedure. Usually, complications of CTS surgery and poor results are related to suboptimal surgical technique. Indications for hand surgery in CTS cases include (a) failure of nonoperative treatment or clinical evidence of thenar atrophy; (b) persistent sensory loss, and (c) reexploration when the patient fails to respond to CTS release or when recurrent CTS is present.

Anterior Interosseous Nerve Syndromes

Clinical Evaluation

The anterior interosseous nerve (AIN) is a purely motor branch of the median nerve that arises 5 to 8 cm distal to the lateral epicondyle and supplies the flexor pollicis longus (FPL), the pronator quadratus (PQ), and the flexor digito-

rum profundus (FDP) of the index and middle fingers. The AIN contains no fibers of superficial sensation but does supply deep pain and proprioception to some deep tissues, including the wrist joint.

Differential Diagnosis

An anatomic variation, trauma, or inflammation may cause disorders of the AIN. Acute localized neuritis may be more common than compression or trauma. Patients with anterior interosseous nerve syndrome (AINS) often complain of a nonspecific pain in the forearm or elbow and frequently demonstrate weakness of the FPL, PQ, FDP1, and FDP2 on examination. At times only the FPL or FDP1 is involved. In the latter situation, the physician must rule out tendon ruptures of the FPL or the FDP1, which occasionally develop in rheumatoid arthritis. In the diagnostic evaluation of AINS, routine motor and sensory NCS of the radial, median, and ulnar nerves will be normal; however, the latency and duration of the evoked action potential from elbow to PQ will be prolonged, and the EMG demonstrates denervation in the PQ, FPL, and FDP1, and FDP2 muscles (10).

Treatment

Therapy for AINS depends on the cause of the compression. Penetrating wounds require immediate exploration and surgical repair. Impending Volkmann contracture demands urgent surgical decompression. In spontaneous AINS, the initial steps in management include avoiding activity that exacerbates the symptoms, resting the affected upper limb, and taking NSAIDs. If no clinical improvement transpires within 8 to 12 weeks, surgical exploration by an experienced hand surgeon should be considered.

Digital Nerves in the Hand

Prolongations of the median nerve end as interdigital nerves, which provide sensation to the index fingers and to part of the middle fingers. An anastomosis between the median and ulnar nerves forms the interdigital nerve to the middle and ring fingers. An entrapment of the interdigital nerve may occur in the intermetacarpal tunnel of the hand region if trauma or a mass (cyst, osteophyte, tumor) obstructs the passageway. When the finger is hyperextended and spread laterally, the interdigital nerve draws tightly against the edge of the deep transverse metacarpal ligament, causing symptoms. Avoiding recurrent trauma caused by external compression is essential to relieve these conditions.

Median Nerve Compression in the Region of the Elbow

Pronator Teres Syndrome

In the pronator teres syndrome (PTS), entrapment of the median nerve occurs at the level of the pronator teres muscle, producing pain and tenderness of the proximal forearm as well as paresthesias of the hand. The PTS is controversial and rare. Individuals with a PTS demonstrate weakness in the FPL and the abductor pollicis brevis muscles while pronation of the forearm remains normal. Causes of PTS include abnormal vascular structures, muscle hypertrophy, trauma, and fractures. In cases of PTS, NCS reveal median nerve slowing in the proximal forearm but normal distal motor latencies and sensory action potentials at the wrist. Abnormalities in the EMG are found in the median nerve innervated muscles below the level of the pronator teres muscle, but the pronator teres is normal. Nonsurgical therapy is indicated in cases of PTS with mild, intermittent symptoms associated with strenuous use of the involved limb (especially repeated elbow flexion and pronation). NSAIDs plus splints on the elbow and wrist often provide benefit, especially in conjunction with avoidance of exacerbating activities. Surgery (with adequate exploration and decompression both distally and proximally) becomes an option in those PTS cases with persistent or progressive symptoms and signs of nerve dysfunction.

Ligament of Struthers Entrapment

Rarely will the median nerve become entrapped by the ligament of Struthers (LS), a fibrous band from a supratrochlear spur or supracondylar process at the distal anteromedial humerus. The LS encloses a foramen, the other boundaries of which are the median intermuscular septum and the distal and anterior surface of the medial humeral condyle; the brachial artery and median nerve pass through this foramen. When the median nerve is entrapped by a LS in the upper arm area, the clinical symptoms may simulate the PTS. In cases of PTS the innervation to the pronator teres muscle is spared, whereas in the LS entrapment above the elbow the pronator teres muscle is weak. Palpation and routine x-rays will demonstrate a spur about 5 cm above the medial epicondyle in the LS case. EMG of the pronator teres muscle and more distal median innervated muscles as well as NCS from above and below the elbow and from elbow to wrist can localize the deficit as proximal to the pronator teres muscle. Owing to entrapment of the brachial artery along with the median nerve in the LS entrapment, the radial pulse often decreases or disappears when the forearm is fully extended or supinated. Most patients with a focal entrapment by a fibrous band benefit from surgery.

Ulnar Nerve

Ulnar Nerve Compression at the Elbow

Clinical Evaluation

The second most common peripheral nerve entrapment involves the ulnar nerve in the region of the elbow. In the vicinity of the medial epicondyle of the elbow the ulnar nerve passes through the ulnar groove, where it is subject to several types of compressive trauma or injury. Causes of ulnar nerve syndromes at the elbow, in order of frequency, include the cubital tunnel syndrome (CUBTS), external compression, previous fracture and scarring, and recurrent subluxation of the ulnar nerve. The CUBTS occurs where the ulnar nerve passes the aponeurosis of origin of the flexor carpi ulnaris (FCU) muscle. In certain instances, the aponeurosis is drawn taut over the ulnar nerve, particularly with elbow flexion; the point of constriction lies 1.5 to 3.5 cm distal to the medial epicondyle. Compression of the ulnar nerve externally results from repeated resting of the elbow on a flat surface, especially if the ulnar groove is shallow. Individuals subjected to immobility (e.g., in anesthesia, coma, restrained positions) appear at risk for prolonged pressure on the ulnar nerve.

Differential Diagnosis

A previous arm fracture may damage the elbow, and residual scarring can compromise the ulnar nerve. Recurrent ulnar nerve subluxation and rolling over the medial epicondyle may contribute to ulnar neuropathies at the elbow, especially in an athlete who engages in throwing sports (e.g., baseball). Synovial cysts occasionally compress the ulnar nerve in the region of the elbow. Infrequently, a CUBTS will be caused by an abnormal insertion of the medial head of the triceps muscle of the arm onto the medial epicondyle of the elbow. In addition, a high ulnar nerve palsy may be caused by the arcade of Struthers, or entrapments may occur distal to the cubital tunnel (more than 4 cm beyond the medial epicondyle) in the flexor–pronator aponeurosis. Patients with a CUBTS experience one or more of the following symptoms: pain, numbness, or tingling with the elbow flexion test (full elbow flexion with full extension of the wrists for 3 minutes). When weakness occurs, it affects functions of the hand, including finger abduction, thumb abduction, pinching of the thumb and forefinger, and, eventually, power of grip. Performing artists and athletes who require very fine control of their fingers may note a decline in performance with minimal ulnar nerve compression. A C8 cervical radiculopathy can produce radiating paresthesias in the hand. On infrequent occasions a brachial plexus lesion or a thoracic outlet syndrome may mimic symptoms of ulnar neuropathy.

Diagnostic Evaluation

On motor and sensory NCS the site of the ulnar nerve abnormality can be located by sequentially assessing ulnar nerve conduction across the elbow segment (11). EMG should examine the intrinsic muscles of the hand as well as the forearm, arm, and paraspinal cervical muscles to verify that no other condition exists.

Treatment

The cause and severity of the ulnar nerve compression as well as the duration of symptoms dictate therapy. In patients with intermittent symptoms, acute or chronic mild neuropathy, or mild neuropathy associated with an occupational cause, nonsurgical treatment usually suffices (viz., avoiding repetitive flexion and extension of the elbow, resting the elbow, or splinting the elbow in extension). As long as there is no motor involvement or objective sensory loss, surgical intervention will be unnecessary. Development of a motor deficit, atrophy, or weakness warrants a surgical opinion. Various surgical techniques for an ulnar nerve entrapment at the elbow exist and remain controversial; however, the best results of surgery occur in patients with mild signs, and poor results are often seen in patients with severe atrophy.

Ulnar Nerve Entrapment at the Wrist

Entrapments of the ulnar nerve occur less often at the wrist in Guyon canal than at the elbow. A ganglion will be the most likely cause of an entrapment in Guyon canal. However, trauma, rheumatoid arthritis, long-distance bicycling ("handlebar palsy"), masses, anomalies, or inflammation can produce similar clinical symptoms. The diagnosis of an ulnar nerve deficit at the wrist will be confirmed if prolonged motor and sensory terminal latencies are demonstrable on NCS. Treatment will depend on the origin and duration of the condition responsible for the ulnar nerve syndrome. Conservative therapy should be prescribed initially for mild compression associated with a single traumatic event. Avoidance of the trauma and splinting would be an initial step in treatment. In those cases that are unresponsive to nonsurgical care, a surgical opinion relative to exploration, decompression, and neurolysis may be considered.

Isolated neuropathy of the dorsal sensory branch of the ulnar nerve may be associated with either a laceration, blunt trauma, or tight restraints. A careful clinical examination and sensory NCS will confirm the diagnosis. In cases with a painful neuroma after a laceration surgical exploration may be considered, whereas neurolysis may be beneficial in patients with a dorsal sensory ulnar nerve entrapped by scar tissue.

Digital Ulnar Nerve

Prolongations of the ulnar nerve end as interdigital nerves to the ring and little fingers. The nerves to the middle and ring fingers are formed by an anastomosis between the median and ulnar nerves. Mechanisms and causes for ulnar digital entrapment syndromes will be similar to those for the median digital neuropathies. Treatment is similar to that for other interdigital entrapments.

Radial Nerve

Posterior Interosseous Nerve Syndrome

Clinical Evaluation

The posterior interosseous nerve syndrome (PINS) is an entrapment of the deep branch of the radial nerve just distal to the elbow joint. Motor weakness of the extensors of the wrist and fingers occurs. The extensor carpi radialis longus (ECRL) and extensor carpi radialis brevis (ECRB) muscles are spared.

Differential Diagnosis

Patients with the PINS report pain and show limitation of movement along with elbow spasm. In cases with rheumatoid arthritis there is evidence of elbow synovitis as well. In PIN paralysis there is a positive tenodesis effect. When the wrist is passively flexed, the metacarpophalangeal joints extend; this extension demonstrates that the extensor tendons are intact. In cases with ruptured extensor tendons, the ends of the tendons are distal to the wrist, and thus no tenodesis is seen. In the PIN the most important physical finding is radial deviation of the wrist on dorsiflexion, as a result of noninvolvement of the ECRL and ECRB, with paralysis of the extensor carpi ulnaris (ECU). Even in cases with partial paralysis, the digits that extend the fingers show marked weakness.

Diagnostic Evaluation

Owing to denervation in the muscles supplied by the PIN (i.e., extensor digitorum communis, ECU, extensor digiti minimi, extensor indicis proprius, abductor pollicis longus, extensor pollicis brevis, and extensor pollicis longus), EMG will confirm the diagnosis.

Treatment

In most cases of PINS, treatment is surgical. Tumors, ganglions, malformation, and lipomas should be removed surgically, and the PIN should be freed from any compressive bands or other constricting structures. When the PIN becomes entrapped and mimics lateral epicondylitis in the resistant tennis elbow syndrome (12), surgical exploration with release of the ECR tendon origin and removal of any constricting vascular or fibrous band has been reported in certain cases.

Superficial Radial Nerve

Owing to its superficial location, the superficial radial nerve (SRN) can be damaged by lacerations or compression around the wrist. Infrequently, the SRN can be compressed by tightly fitting bands or straps (e.g., wristwatch, handcuffs, bandages) around the wrist. Wartenberg syndrome is an entrapment of the SRN in the forearm. De Quervain disease can be found in association in 50% of these cases (13). In entrapments of the SRN the clinical examination as well as sensory NCS will provide a diagnosis. Both conservative and surgical treatments for Wartenberg syndrome have yielded good results.

Brachial Plexus

Thoracic Outlet Syndrome

Muscular, bony, and fascial structures can interfere with functions of the neurovascular bundle located in the thoracic outlet (14). The rare condition of a neurogenic thoracic outlet syndrome (TOS) is caused by abnormal bands that cross the brachial plexus, often inserting on the rudimentary cervical rib. Paresthesias commonly precede the development of persistent pain, atrophy, or muscle weakness. The anatomic territories affected in the neurogenic TOS include those of the ulnar nerve and the medial cutaneous nerve of the forearm. Electrodiagnostic testing and MRI neuroimaging may be useful diagnostic tools in certain disorders of the brachial plexus. Surgical treatment of TOS carries some risk and should be reserved for the rare patient with documented worsening of neurologic function.

Suprascapular Nerve

The suprascapular nerve (SSN) is a purely motor nerve and arises from the upper trunk of the brachial plexus, which is formed from the roots of C5 and C6 (15). SSN entrapment occurs when the nerve's passage through the suprascapular foramen becomes compromised and produces pain and weakness or atrophy of the supraspinatus and infraspinatus muscles. SSN syndromes may develop from exertion during sports activities, from exertion during (e.g., lifting heavy objects overhead), from masses, as a complication of certain surgeries (e.g., when the patient is placed in predisposing positions during surgery), from certain exercises, from an arthrodetic shoulder, or from primary shoulder dislocations and humeral fractures. Electrodiagnostic testing and MRI studies are helpful in diagnosing the location of the entrapment. When a severe comminuted fracture of the scapula occurs with involvement of the scapular notch, early exploration may be considered in suspected SSN impingement. In addition, whenever persistent signs or symptoms occur or when spontaneous onset occurs without known cause, surgical exploration may be considered.

LOWER LIMBS

Sciatic Nerve

The sciatic nerve arises from undivided primary rami at L4, L5, S1, S2, and S3, and can be divided into component parts: the tibial nerve, the common peroneal nerve, and the nerve to the hamstring muscles. Sciatic nerve entrapments are uncommon. Most patients complaining of symptoms traceable to the sciatic nerve suffer from effects of trauma, fracture, or arthroplasty, or have disease of the lumbosacral spine (e.g., spinal stenosis, degenerative disease, rheumatoid arthritis, osteoarthritis, ankylosing spondylitis). A variation in the course of the sciatic nerve involves its passage between parts of the piriformis muscle. (The division of the nerve that becomes the peroneal trunk is usually the one that deviates.) A careful clinical examination coupled with EMG and NCS often defines and localizes the sciatic neuropathy. In the case of the piriformis syndrome, surgery includes removal of one of the heads of origin of the muscle and release of any constrictions.

Peroneal Nerve

Clinical Evaluation

The most vulnerable location for compression of the peroneal nerve is where the nerve winds around the neck of the fibula near its division into the deep and superficial peroneal nerves (16). The mechanism of damage to the peroneal nerve at the head of the fibula will be compression causing a neuropraxic lesion. In contrast to the CTS and the CUBTS, peroneal entrapment at the fibular tunnel ("fibular tunnel syndrome") is extremely rare. Most cases of the fibular tunnel syndrome are probably caused by abnormal congenital bands in the vicinity of the fibular neck and tunnel.

Differential Diagnosis

Compressive etiologies of peroneal nerve damage include improperly applied plaster casts, tight bandages, constrictive garments, and rarely, extrinsic masses (e.g., ganglion cysts, Baker cysts, lipomas, osteomas, osteochondromas) or intrinsic nerve tumors (e.g., neurofibromas, schwannomas, ganglion cysts). Unconsciousness from anesthesia, drug overdose, or acute illness with stupor or coma may render patients susceptible to a compressive peroneal neuropathy.

Diagnostic Evaluation

The clinical examination and EMG as well as NCS generally provide an accurate diagnosis of the peroneal palsy.

Treatment

Surgical therapy should be considered in those rare patients with a slowly progressive disturbance of peroneal nerve function in whom there is pain and progressive motor and sensory loss due to a suspected mass or congenital bands.

Anterior Tarsal Tunnel Syndrome

Clinical Evaluation

The anterior tarsal tunnel syndrome (ATTS) is a rarely reported entrapment neuropathy of the deep peroneal nerve under the extensor retinaculum at the ankle (17). The roof of the tunnel is the inferior extensor retinaculum, and the floor is the fascia overlying the talus and navicular bone. Within the anterior tarsal tunnel lie four tendons, an artery, a vein, and the deep peroneal nerve.

Differential Diagnosis

Individuals with a peroneal or sciatic neuropathy or an L5 radiculopathy may present with similar symptoms.

Diagnostic Evaluation

Patients with ATTS present with foot pain and dysesthesias. NCS reveal prolonged peroneal distal latencies with reduced amplitude from the extensor digitorum brevis muscle (EDB). EMG abnormalities are confined to the EDB.

Treatment

Ensuring a comfortable foot position by splints, rest, or a combination of both often provides relief for patients with ATTS. If symptoms and findings persist, surgical release should trace the nerve far enough proximally to exclude a lesion in the ankle under the extensor retinaculum.

Posterior Tibial Nerve

Posterior Tarsal Tunnel Syndrome

Clinical Evaluation

In the posterior tarsal tunnel syndrome (PTTS), the posterior tibial nerve becomes entrapped at the level of the medial malleolus, the point from which the nerve supplies sensory innervation to the sole of the foot and motor innervation to the intrinsic muscles of the foot (18). Pain in the sole of the foot will be the primary symptom of a PTTS.

Differential Diagnosis

A sciatic or posterior tibial neuropathy and an S1 radiculopathy may present with symptoms similar to those seen in PTTS.

Diagnostic Evaluation

NCS and EMG studies often localize the site of the posterior tibial nerve entrapment within the tarsal tunnel.

Treatment

Initially, treatment should remove any irritating process plus bracing of the foot with a medial arch support. NSAIDs will assist in treatment of local phlebitis or tenosynovitis. Surgery may be required in as many as 60% of cases with PTTS; the release and dissection of the nerve must be carried as far distally as possible, typically to the level of its bifurcation into the plantar nerve.

Lateral Femoral Cutaneous Nerve

Clinical Evaluation

Meralgia paresthetica is the term employed for the condition caused by entrapment of the lateral femoral cutaneous

nerve (LFCN) as it passes underneath or through the inguinal ligament at its origin on the anterior iliac spine.

Differential Diagnosis

Other etiologies for LFCN dysfunction include complications following laparoscopic procedures and surgery, and rarely in cases of leprosy and tumor of the psoas muscle.

Diagnostic Evaluation

The characteristic sensory symptoms and findings along the lateral thigh as well as changes in the sensory nerve action potentials on NCS are diagnostic.

Treatment

Patients with an LFCN entrapment should avoid any new or recently started exercises and remove constricting garments (binders, corsets, or tight belts). In certain conditions, local nerve blocks may prove beneficial. Surgery should be considered if the symptoms are relatively long-lasting or very painful and consist of release of the entrapment at the level of the nerve's exit under the inguinal ligament. If the LFCN is severed, unpleasant paresthesias may ensue.

MISCELLANEOUS UNCOMMON NERVE ENTRAPMENT DISORDERS

Upper Limbs

Double-Crush Syndrome

The double-crush hypothesis attempts to explain the clinical observation that patients with distal compression neuropathies also frequently have signs of a more proximal nerve injury (19). In addition, this hypothesis suggests that serial constraints to axoplasmic flow, each of which is insufficient to cause changes in function by itself, can be additive in causing ultimate dysfunction of the nerve. Degenerative cervical spine disorders, with variable degrees of spondylosis, are common. When an individual becomes symptomatic from the cervical spine disorder and then develops a concomitant entrapment neuropathy (especially the CTS), confusion may arise with regard not only to diagnosis but also to treatment. Most often the patient with a double-crush syndrome responds when treatment is directed toward both processes (i.e., cervical spine disorder as well as the more distal entrapment neuropathy).

Dorsal Scapular Nerve

The dorsal scapular nerve (DSN) arises primarily from spinal segment C5 and innervates the levator scapulae and rhomboid muscles. Following trauma and in rare instances entrapments of the DSN, weakness of the rhomboideus major and minor and the scapulae occurs as well as a tendency of the vertebral border of the scapula (particularly the lower portion) to be displaced dorsally. This displacement forms a prominence under the skin, and the scapula shifts laterally. Since this syndrome results secondary to scalene hyperactivity caused by inadequacy of the spinal stabilization system, treatment will be directed toward the cervical spine and includes use of muscle relaxants, analgesics, and physical therapy. In unresponsive cases surgical neurolysis may be considered.

Long Thoracic Nerve

The long thoracic nerve (LTN) follows a straight course and becomes fixed by the scalene and muscle slips of the serratus anterior. Owing to the straight anatomic course and fixation of the LTN, it can be stretched; this, in turn, occurs most often with heavy labor or after direct trauma. In this condition the shoulder girdle displaces slightly backward, and the lower scapula demonstrates undue winging. In the vast majority of patients with this syndrome recovery occurs within 6 months of the original stretch injury.

Musculocutaneous Nerve

Infrequently an injury affects the musculocutaneous nerve (MCN) in the vicinity of the lateral cord of the upper trunk of the brachial plexus. With disorders of the MCN, flexion of the forearm at the elbow is weakened because of biceps and brachialis involvement; however, the disability is not severe, since the brachioradialis and pronator teres muscles take part in producing this movement. With the forearm in pronation, flexion at the elbow becomes impossible and sensation is reduced along the lateral border of the forearm. Surgery with exploration may become necessary to differentiate a nerve entrapment from a nerve rupture.

Axillary Nerve

Most disorders of the axillary nerve are due to trauma. The quadrilateral space syndrome (QLSS) manifest by shoulder pain occurs secondary to compression of the axillary nerve by fibrous bands in the quadrilateral space (20). EMG and NCS localize the clinical problem to the axillary nerve, and in the case of the QLSS, MRI confirms atrophy of the teres minor muscle.

Lower Limbs

Femoral Nerve

Femoral nerve lesions produce weakness and atrophy of the quadriceps muscle, reduction in the knee reflex on the affected side, and a sensory loss over the anterior thigh and medial calf. More common causes of femoral neuropathy include trauma, complication of surgery, diabetes, and vascular disease (hemorrhage in either the psoas or iliacus compartments); entrapments of the femoral nerve occur rarely. Most femoral entrapments do not require surgery. Lesions in the femoral triangle at the region of the inguinal ligament can be treated by observation if a vascular process is suspected or by medical management if a tumor or other mass lesion is the cause.

Saphenous Nerve

The saphenous nerve is one of three sensory branches of the femoral nerve possessing a long course through the adductor canal, penetrating fascia above the level of the knee, and supplying the medial calf, the medial malleolus, and a small portion of the medial part of the arch of the foot. Trauma, surgical procedures, or entrapments may produce a saphenous neuropathy. In most cases with a saphenous neuropathy rest, NSAIDs and physical therapy are effective.

Posterior Femoral Cutaneous Nerve

The posterior femoral cutaneous nerve (PFCN) exits from the pelvis in company of the sciatic nerve and then sends branches to the medial posterior buttocks, parts of the scrotum or labia, and posterior thigh (usually to the level of the knee). Rare cases of PFCN entrapments have been reported (e.g., venous malformation surrounding the nerve).

Ilioinguinal Nerve

The point of entrapment of the ilioinguinal nerve is located slightly medial to the anterior iliac spine near its exit from the superficial inguinal ring, where it lies almost directly superior to the pelvic tubercle. In this condition the patient complains of burning pain over the lower abdomen that radiates down into the inner portion of the upper thigh and into the scrotum or labia majora. Causes of an ilioinguinal nerve syndrome include trauma, a surgical incision or procedure, a scar, or rarely, scleroderma. Neurolysis is indicated in severely affected patients who experience persistent pain.

Genitofemoral Nerve

The genitofemoral nerve supplies the skin over the upper thigh below the femoral triangle and the lower lateral scrotum or labia and descends through the pelvis over the iliac muscle near the obturator nerve. This nerve can be affected in retroperitoneal processes, such as tumor, infection, and, rarely, laparoscopic varicocelectomy. In situations where adhesions entrap the genitofemoral nerve, surgery will be indicated.

Obturator Nerve

In an obturator neuropathy the symptoms will be sensory, including paresthesias, sensory loss, and radiating pain in the medial thigh. Most cases involving the obturator nerve suffer some form of trauma (pelvic and acetabular fractures, gunshot wounds, pelvic laparoscopic procedures, extracorporeal shock-wave lithotripsy). Rarely, a benign schwannoma of the retroperitoneal space as well as pelvic cancers can produce an obturator neuropathy. Initial therapy for an obturator neuropathy includes rest, analgesics, and NSAIDs. Infrequently, surgical exploration and epineural repair are considered.

Pudendal Nerve

Temporary penile insensitivity occurs due to compression of the pudendal nerve within the Alcock canal (Alcock syndrome) (21). Other etiologies of a pudendal palsy include a complication of intramedullary nailing of the femur during surgery and induction by fracture table. In cases of pudendal compression, surgery will provide relief. Care should be taken during surgical procedures to avoid trauma to the pudendal nerve.

Sural Nerve

Lacerations or compressive lesions can involve the sural nerve primarily at the level of its exit through fascia and produce paresthesias radiating into the lateral part of the foot. If rest as well as avoidance of continued irritation of the affected area do not produce relief of symptoms, then surgical exploration becomes a consideration.

Interdigital Nerve

The medial and lateral plantar nerves terminate as the interdigital nerves. Morton neuroma may occur at the region of the interdigital nerve in the third and fourth interspaces of the foot and become a source of lower limb pain. Initial treatment consists of padding the metatarsal head of the foot or changing to shoes that cause less lateral pinching. On occasion, surgical excision of the nerve is required.

SUMMARY

In regional musculoskeletal disorders that affect peripheral nerves, patients present with pain, numbness, tingling, or weakness in an extremity. The evaluation of patients with these nerve entrapment disorders remains a clinical discipline for which laboratory, electrophysiologic, and computerized neuroimaging cannot substitute. An emphasis has been placed on the clinical features and evaluation of the various diseases and syndrome, their differential diagnoses, and the results expected from currently accepted treatments.

REFERENCES

1. Nakano KK. Entrapment neuropathies. *Muscle Nerve* 1978;1: 264.
2. Dawson DM, Hallett M, Millender LH. *Entrapment neuropathies,* 2nd ed. Boston: Little, Brown, 1990.
3. Koppel HP, Thompson WAL. *Peripheral entrapment neuropathies.* Baltimore: Williams & Wilkins, 1963.
4. Iyer VG. Understanding nerve conduction and electromyographic studies. *Hand Clin* 1993; 9:2373.
5. Levin KH. Common focal mononeuropathies and their electrodiagnosis. *J Clin Neurophysiol* 1993; 10:181.
6. Dawson DM. Entrapment neuropathies of the upper extremities. *NEJM* 1993;329:2013.
7. Phalen GS. The carpel tunnel syndrome: seventeen years' experience in diagnosis and treatment of six-hundred fifty-four hands. *J Bone Joint Surg Ann* 1966;48:211–228.
8. Stevens JC. AAEE Minimonograph #26. The electrodiagnosis of carpal tunnel syndrome. *Muscle Nerve* 1987;10:99.
9. Preston DC, Ross MH, Kothari MJ, et al. The median-ulnar latency difference studies are comparable in mild carpal tunnel syndrome. *Muscle Nerve* 1994;17:1469.
10. Nakkano KK, Lundergan C, Okihiro MM. Anterior interosseous nerve syndromes. *Arch Neurol* 1977;34:477.
11. Campbell WW, Carroll DJ, Greenberg MK. Practice parameter, electrodiagnostic studies in ulnar neuropathy at the elbow. *Neurology* 1999;52:688.
12. Stewart JD. The radial nerve. *Focal peripheral neuropathies.* New York: Raven Press, 1993.
13. Lanzetta M, Foucher G. Entrapment of the superficial branch of the radial nerve (Wartenberg's syndrome): a report of 52 cases. *Int Orthop* 1993; 17:342.
14. Wilbourn AJ. Thoracic outlet syndromes. *Neurol Clinics* 1999; 17:477.
15. Horiguchi M. The cutaneous branch of some human suprascapular nerves. *J Anat* 1980; 130:191.
16. Katirji B. Peroneal neuropathy. *Neurol Clin* 1999; 17:567.
17. Borges LF, Hallett M, Selkoe DJ, et al. The anterior tarsal tunnel syndrome: report of two cases. *J Neurosurg* 1981; 54:89.
18. Oh SJ, Sarala PK, Kuba T, et al. Tarsal tunnel syndrome: electrophysiological study. *Ann Neurol* 1979; 5:327.
19. Upton RM, McComas AJ. The double crush in nerve entrapment syndromes. *Lancet* 1973; 11:359.
20. Cahill BR, Palmer RE. Quadrilateral space syndrome. *J Hand Surg* 1983; 8:65.
21. Oberpenning F, Roth S, Leusmann DB. The Alcock syndrome: temporary penile insensitivity due to compression of the pudendal nerve within the Alcock canal. *J Urol* 1994; 151:423.

8

TEMPOROMANDIBULAR DISORDERS

M. FRANKLIN DOLWICK

Temporomandibular pain and dysfunction are common problems that occur in about 33% of the general population (1). It has been estimated that 75% of the population have symptoms and 33% have signs of temporomandibular disorders (TMDs). Approximately 5% of the population will require treatment for TMDs (2). Interestingly, most patients seeking treatment are young females (20 to 40 years of age).

Typically, patients present with complaints of orofacial pain, joint noise, and limitations of mandibular movement. Other symptoms such as headache, neck ache, earache, dizziness, and tinnitus also have been associated with this condition. Despite extensive research during the past two decades, the etiology of most cases remains elusive. Proposed etiologies include malocclusion (bad bite), bruxism (clenching or grinding the teeth), and trauma (3).

Because of the nonspecific nature of patients' symptoms, temporomandibular complaints have been difficult to classify. As a result, confusing terminologies have appeared in the literature. These include *temporomandibular joint* (TMJ), *Costen syndrome, temporomandibular joint syndrome* (TMJS), *myofascial pain and dysfunction* (MPD), and *craniomandibular disorders* (CMD). Currently, these complaints are broadly classified as *TMDs*. Collectively, temporomandibular complaints seem to represent an assemblage of disorders that can be divided into subcategories. It has been recognized finally that TMD complaints do represent not a single disease entity, but a family of clinical conditions similar to those involving other joints (4). TMDs have, for the most part, been managed by dentists. Dentists became the primary care providers because the etiology was believed to be associated with abnormalities of the occlusion and therefore treatment was directed at modifying the dentition. In recent years, it has been recognized that the etiology is multifaceted and that malocclusion does not play a central role. It is important that physicians become informed about TMDs in order to facilitate diagnosis and treatment. Although no statistics exist, it is apparent that many patients undergo inappropriate and expensive diagnostic procedures because physicians do not consider TMDs in their differential diagnosis.

Physicians should plan an orderly evaluation of the patient with temporomandibular pain and dysfunction. A differential diagnosis should be established by medical history, physical examination, diagnostic imaging, and laboratory analysis. At the most basic level, the physician should determine whether the patient's complaints are caused by a musculoskeletal condition or some other condition. It is important that such complaints as headache, neck ache, and ear pain be thoroughly evaluated.

Once a diagnosis has been made, a logical treatment plan can be developed. The most common TMJ problems are self-limiting and rarely progress to more serious conditions. Therefore initial treatment should be simple and reversible. Escalation toward nonreversible treatments should be made with caution.

ANATOMY

The TMJ is located anterior to the tragus of the ear and is the articulation between the base of the skull and the condyle of the mandible. The articular surface of the skull is the squamous part of the temporal bone. The bone has a concavity, the articular (glenoid) fossa, and a convexity, the articular eminence. The condyle is convex on surfaces that are load bearing. It is widest in the mediolateral direction.

The articular surfaces of the TMJ are covered with dense fibrous connective tissue instead of hyaline cartilage. Occasionally, cartilage cells occur within this tissue, in which case the surface is termed *fibrocartilage.* The surfaces are nonvascularized and noninnervated.

An articular capsule surrounds the joint. Laterally, the capsule is thickened to form the lateral (temporomandibular) ligament, which reinforces the joint. Capsular tissues are highly vascular and richly innervated.

The TMJ is a synovial joint. The articular space is divided into two synovial compartments by an articular disc (meniscus) (Fig. 8.1). The articular disc consists of dense, fibroelastic connective tissue and encloses the superior surface of the condyle. It attaches to the capsule and lateral pterygoid muscle anteriorly, joins the capsule mediolat-

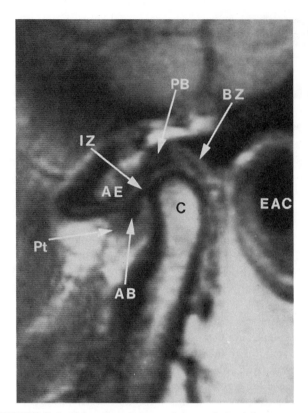

FIGURE 8.1. Magnetic resonance image of the left temporo-mandibular joint in closed position. (*AB*, anterior band of disc; *AE*, articular eminence; *BZ*, bilaminar zone; *C*, condyle; *EAC*, external auditory canal; *IZ*, intermediate zone; *PB*, posterior band of disc; *PT*, lateral pterygoid muscle.) (From Dolwick MF. Temporomandibular disorders. In: Koopman WJ, ed. *Arthritis and allied conditions: a textbook of rheumatology*, 14th ed. Philadelphia: Lippincott Williams & Wilkins, 2001:2019–2025, with permission.)

tions during opening and excursive (protrusion and lateral) movements, and the suprahyoids act during opening of the mandible or with elevation of the hyoid bone. The infrahyoids function during depression of the hyoid bone or elevation of the larynx.

DIFFERENTIAL DIAGNOSIS

The evaluation of the patient with temporomandibular pain and dysfunction is like that of any other diagnostic workup (5). The evaluation should include a thorough history, physical examination of the masticatory system, and some type of plain TMP radiography. Special diagnostic studies such as laboratory tests or advanced imaging techniques should be performed only as indicated and not as routine studies.

History

The patient's history may be the most important part of the evaluation. It begins with the chief complaint, a statement of the patient's reason for seeking consultation or treatment. The history of the present illness should be comprehensive, including an accurate description of the patient's symptoms, chronology of the symptoms, determination of palliative and aggravating factors, description of how the problem affects the patient, and information about any previous treatments. Patients suffering from TMD usually have complaints of orofacial pain that is worse during jaw function such as mastication and mandibular movement. Frequently, patients also have complaints related to decreased mandibular range of motion.

Physical Examination

The physical examination consists of an evaluation of the entire masticatory system. The TMJs are examined for tenderness and noise. The most common forms of joint noise are clicking (a distinct sound) and crepitus (multiple, scraping sounds). Joint sounds occur in 33% to 50% of the population and are not necessarily significant, especially in the absence of pain or dysfunction. The mandibular range of motion is determined, with the normal range of movement of the adult's mandible being about 50 mm opening and 10 mm protrusively and laterally. The normal movement is straight and symmetric.

The masticatory muscles should be systematically examined. The head and neck should be inspected for soft-tissue asymmetry and evidence of muscle hypertrophy. The patient should be observed for signs of jaw clenching or other habits. The muscles should be palpated for the presence of tenderness, fasciculations, spasm, or trigger points.

The dental examination is important. Odontogenic sources of pain should be eliminated. The teeth should be

erally, and attaches to loose, vascular connective tissue posteriorly. The superior compartment is largest and contiguous with the fossa. The inferior compartment is smallest and is reinforced by disc attachments. The condyle articulates with the disc, with rotational movement occurring in the lower compartment between the condyle and disc. Sliding (translation) movement occurs in the upper compartment between the temporal bone and the disc–condyle complex. The disc maintains contact of the joint surfaces at rest and during function, serving important functions of load distribution and lubrication.

The main blood supply to the TMJ is derived from the terminal branches of the external carotid artery, the maxillary, and superficial temporal arteries. The TMJ is innervated primarily by the auriculotemporal nerve.

Movement of the TMJ is produced by the muscles of mastication acting with the suprahyoid and infrahyoid muscle groups. Three large muscles—the masseter, medial pterygoid, and temporalis—function during closing movements of the mandible. The lateral pterygoid muscle func-

examined for wear facets, soreness, and mobility, which may be evidence of bruxism. Although the significance of occlusal (bite) abnormalities is controversial, the occlusion should be evaluated. Missing teeth should be noted, and dental and skeletal classification should be determined.

Finally, examination should be directed to specific areas of complaints. For example, patients complaining of ear symptoms should have an ear examination; patients complaining of neck ache should have a cervical examination.

Routine Imaging

Routine radiography of the TMJ is essential for the diagnosis of intraarticular osseous pathology. Lateral and anteroposterior views are recommended to evaluate the joint structures. A variety of lateral techniques exist, including transcranial, lateral pharyngeal, and panographic studies. Anteroposterior techniques include transorbital and modified Towne views. Currently, no single technique can be recommended as the best screening examination.

Special Imaging Studies

Special imaging studies such as computerized tomography (CT), arthrography, magnetic resonance imaging (MRI), and scintigraphy should be used only when specifically indicated (6). Although TMJ arthrography and MRI have proven to be of value in depicting disc displacement, the clinical symptoms have often failed to correlate with the findings (7,8). Overreliance on the diagnostic value of imaging may lead to overdiagnosis and hence to overtreatment.

CT is indicated for the evaluation of osseous pathology. Condylar erosion, osteophytes, heterotopic bone, and osseous tumors can be seen with more detail than with plain radiography. CT has little role in the evaluation of disc displacement.

TMJ arthrography involves the injection of contrast medium into the synovial joint compartments followed by radiography of the joint. It is used to determine the position and shape of the disc. Arthrography is an invasive procedure and has been replaced for the most part by TMJ MRI.

TMJ MRI is the technique of choice for imaging the articular disc. It has been shown to image the disc and its posterior attachment tissues reliably; however, the clinical symptoms often do not correlate with the imaging findings (Figs. 8.1 and 8.2). Therefore MRI should be used prudently. MRI may also identify joint effusions as well as avascular necrosis.

Although scintigraphy is rarely indicated, it may be helpful in the evaluation of osseous pathology, such as cysts, tumors, or metastatic disease. It can also be useful in evaluating growth disturbances of the mandibular condyles, such as condylar hyperplasia.

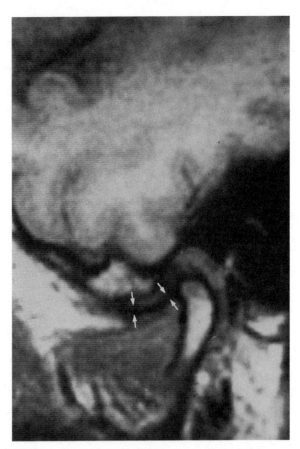

FIGURE 8.2. Magnetic resonance image of the left temporomandibular joint in closed position showing an anteriorly displaced disc (*arrows*). (From Dolwick MF. Temporomandibular disorders. In: Koopman WJ, ed. *Arthritis and allied conditions: a textbook of rheumatology,* 14th ed. Philadelphia: Lippincott Williams & Wilkins, 2001:2019–2025, with permission.)

MYOFASCIAL PAIN AND DYSFUNCTION

MPD is the most common cause of masticatory pain and dysfunction for which patients seek evaluation and treatment (9). This subject is complex, involving several muscular disorders, which, for simplicity, we group together here as MPD. Generally, the source of pain and dysfunction is muscular. The masticatory muscles become tender and painful as a result of abnormal muscular function. This abnormal muscular function is frequently, but not always, associated with bruxism.

The cause of MPD is controversial, although it is generally considered multifaceted. The most commonly accepted cause is bruxism secondary to stress and anxiety.

Clinical Findings

Patients presenting with MPD generally complain of diffuse, poorly localized, preauricular and temporal pain, which may be cyclic (Fig. 8.3). Patients frequently report

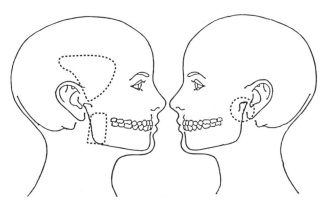

FIGURE 8.3. Facial pain diagram showing diffuse muscular pain associated with myofascial pain and dysfunction **(right)** and localized temporomandibular joint pain associated with internal derangement and osteoarthritis **(left)**. (From Dolwick MF. Temporomandibular disorders. In: Koopman WJ, ed. *Arthritis and allied conditions: a textbook of rheumatology,* 14th ed. Philadelphia: Lippincott Williams & Wilkins, 2001:2019–2025, with permission.)

that they have difficulty sleeping and that their pain is most severe in the morning on awakening. The patient may also complain of sore teeth. Generally, patients describe decreased and painful mandibular opening as well as pain associated with chewing. Headaches, usually bitemporal in location, also occur. Many patients are conscious of bruxing, although others are unaware of it. The pain most often exists or worsens during periods of stress and anxiety.

Examination of the patient reveals diffuse tenderness of the masticatory muscles. The TMJs are either nontender or mildly tender to palpation. Joint noise may be present but is not usually associated with pain or mandibular dysfunction (catching or locking). The range of mandibular movement may be decreased and associated with deviation toward the most affected side. The teeth frequently have wear facets, particularly on the anterior teeth. However, the absence of wear facets does not eliminate bruxism as a cause of the problem.

Radiographic Findings

Radiographs of the TMJ are usually normal. Some patients may have evidence of degenerative joint changes, including altered surface contours, erosion, or osteophytes. These changes, however, may be secondary to or unrelated to MPD problems.

Treatment

The treatment of MPD should initially employ reversible, noninvasive forms of therapy (10). Escalation of treatment to irreversible forms of therapy should be done slowly and only after failure to obtain satisfactory results with reversible methods. Initially, treatment involves a careful explanation of the problem to the patient. It is important to reassure patients that the condition usually resolves with simple treatment and to alleviate concerns they may have about more serious conditions such as tumors or cancer. Home care should include a soft diet, moist heat or cold treatments, muscle massage, and simple exercises consisting of opening and closing, protrusion, and right and left lateral movements of the mandible. Medical therapy should include some type of nonnarcotic analgesic, usually a nonsteroidal antiinflammatory medication, and,

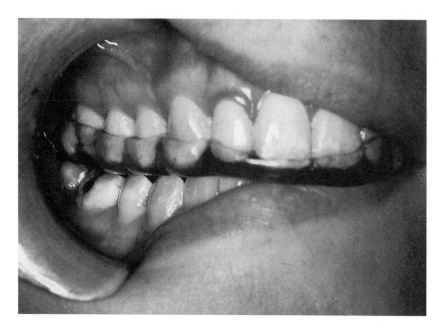

FIGURE 8.4. Maxillary occlusal appliance used for dental treatment of temporomandibular disorders. (From Dolwick MF. Temporomandibular disorders. In: Koopman WJ, ed. *Arthritis and allied conditions: a textbook of rheumatology,* 14th ed. Philadelphia: Lippincott Williams & Wilkins, 2001:2019–2025, with permission.)

if sleep disturbance exists, a low-dose tricyclic antidepressant. The tricyclic antidepressants, particularly amitriptyline, have analgesic properties independent of an antidepressant effect and may be useful for chronic pain patients who have pain and sleep disturbance (11). They decrease the number of awakenings, increase stage IV (delta) sleep, and decrease time in rapid eye movement (REM) sleep. For these reasons, they have potential for treating nocturnal bruxism. Dental treatment involves the use of an occlusal appliance (Fig. 8.4). The reduction of painful symptoms with occlusal appliance therapy has been well documented. Clark reviewed the design, theory, and effectiveness of occlusal appliances and found a 70% to 90% rate of clinical success (12). Although the treatment effects are predictable, the physiologic basis of the treatment response has not been well understood. Patients who initially obtain relief of symptoms with occlusal appliance therapy may benefit from occlusal treatment, including occlusal adjustment, restorative dentistry, or orthodontics. Patients who have significant behavioral problems or who are refractory to treatment may benefit from psychologic evaluation and treatment (13).

It is important to recognize that MPD is usually a chronic problem associated with a behavioral etiology, and the treatment goal should be to manage the pain and dysfunction and not necessarily eliminate them totally. With the exception of dental treatments, MPD is managed in a way similar to that of tension headaches and fibromyalgia. Surgery is not indicated in the treatment of MPD.

INTERNAL DERANGEMENT AND OSTEOARTHRITIS

Internal derangements and osteoarthritis are the most common joint cause of masticatory pain and dysfunction for which patients seek evaluation and treatment. This problem involves both disc derangement and osteoarthritis, which, for simplicity, we group together here. During the past two decades, disc position has been the focus of classification, diagnosis, and treatment of TMJ internal derangement (14). Recent observations have provided new insights into the pathology of TMJ internal derangement, and the evidence indicates that TMJ internal derangement is a complicated pathology involving disc displacement and deformity, synovitis, changes in articular cartilage, alteration in joint pressures and synovial fluid, and probably several yet to be defined factors (15). In fact, the pathologic processes are probably similar to those seen in osteoarthritis of other joints.

The cause of TMJ internal derangement is not well understood. The most commonly proposed etiologies are adverse joint loading secondary to bruxism and traumatic injuries.

Clinical Findings

Patients with internal derangement and osteoarthritis often complain of well-localized pain, predominantly in front of the ear and over the joint structures (5) (Fig. 8.3). The pain is usually constant and increases in severity with jaw movements, particularly chewing. The patients also frequently complain of ear problems and headaches. Joint noise commonly exists and consists of either clicking or crepitus, and is usually associated with pain and interference with mandibular movement. Patients may also experience intermittent or permanent locking.

Examination of the patient reveals localized tenderness over the TMJ. However, diffuse muscle tenderness may also exist. Joint noise is commonly present. Patients with limited opening of less than 30 mm usually do not have joint noise. Crepitus may indicate disc perforation and advanced degenerative changes of the joint components. Mandibular movement is typically decreased and painful. The patient experiences increased joint pain when biting on the opposite side.

Radiographic Findings

Radiographs of the TMJ are normal in early cases and demonstrate degenerative changes (irregularity of the articular surfaces and osteophytes) in more advanced cases. MRI is the preferred diagnostic procedure to demonstrate disc derangement (6) (Fig. 8.2); however, the correlation of the anatomic findings with symptoms is weak. Disc derangement is commonly observed with arthrography or MRI in individuals without pain (8).

Treatment

Clinical experience shows that most patients have a resolution of their symptoms with simple, reversible treatments (16,17). Toller reported that 51% of patients with TMJ osteoarthritis were pain-free after 1 year; 76%, after 2 years; and 98%, after 5 years (18). The treatment of internal derangement and osteoarthritis initially is similar to that for myofascial pain. A careful explanation of the problem emphasizing its self-limiting nature should be given to the patient. Home care should include a soft diet, jaw rest, and application of moist heat. Medical therapy is directed at pain relief and reduction of inflammation by the use of nonsteroidal antiinflammatory medications. Narcotic analgesics should be avoided. Low-dose tricyclic antidepressants may be helpful if the patient is experiencing sleep disturbance. Dental treatment involves the use of occlusal appliances (Fig. 8.4). While the physiologic basis for the effectiveness of occlusal appliances is poorly understood, they seem to reduce pain in 70% to 80% of the patients.

TMJ surgery plays an important but limited role in the treatment of patients whose symptoms are severe and refractory to conservative treatment (19). TMJ arthrocentesis and joint lavage have been shown to be effective in managing acute cases with severe limitation of opening (20). The procedure is simple to perform and has no associated significant morbidity. TMJ arthroscopy has revolutionized the surgical approach to the treatment of internal derangement and osteoarthritis of the TMJ (21,22). Arthroscopic lavage and lysis of adhesions has proven effective in reducing pain and increasing range of motion in approximately 80% of the patients treated. Complications with TMJ arthroscopy are less common than with open surgery (23). Advanced arthroscopic operative techniques utilizing rotary instruments, electrocautery, and lasers are being developed, but their effectiveness compared with simple lavage and lysis of adhesions has not been proven. TMJ arthrotomy procedures, including disc repositioning and arthroplasty or discectomy (meniscectomy), have been used for treating severe symptoms for many years and are successful in reducing symptoms in about 80% of the patients (24). TMJ arthrotomy procedures are indicated for patients who have severe mechanical problems such as intermittent locking or patients who previously have undergone surgery. Complications associated with TMJ arthrotomy include facial nerve injury, malocclusion, and continued or increased symptoms (23). In past years, the use of alloplastic implants in the TMJ was popular; however, experience has shown that most of these patients developed particulation of the implant and foreign-body reactions. Therefore the use of alloplastic implants in the TMJ is not recommended.

In summary, TMJ surgical procedures benefit about 80% of the patients treated. Unfortunately, about 5% of patients who undergo surgery experience a worsening of their symptoms. The decision to proceed with surgery therefore must be carefully considered and made by both the patient and surgeon.

RHEUMATOID ARTHRITIS

Approximately 50% of patients with rheumatoid arthritis (RA) have involvement of the TMJ (25). Affected women outnumber affected men 3 to 1. TMJ involvement usually occurs late during the disease process and is more likely to occur in severe cases. The disease affects both TMJs. RA causes destruction of the mandibular condyles, frequently resulting in the development of a recessive mandible and open-bite malocclusion.

Clinical Findings

Patients with RA with TMJ involvement may experience deep, dull, preauricular pain with exacerbation during function. TMJ tenderness, crepitation, and occasionally swelling over the joint also occur. The patient may notice decreased range of motion, which is usually worse in the morning. In patients with the juvenile form of RA or with severe disease that has caused extensive resorption of the mandibular condyles, a recessive mandible and open-bite malocclusion

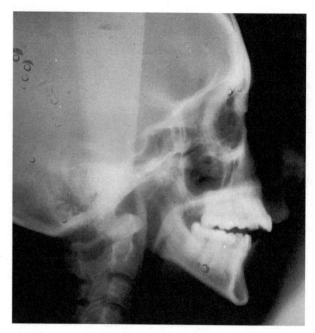

FIGURE 8.5. Lateral head radiograph showing posterior rotation of mandible associated with temporomandibular joint rheumatoid arthritis. (From Dolwick MF. Temporomandibular disorders. In: Koopman WJ, ed. *Arthritis and allied conditions: a textbook of rheumatology,* 14th ed. Philadelphia: Lippincott Williams & Wilkins, 2001:2019–2025, with permission.)

usually is present (Figs. 8.5 and 8.6). Hypomobility from fibrous or bony ankylosis may also occur.

Radiographic Findings

TMJ radiographs may show flattening of the condylar heads. In advanced cases, a spiked appearance of the condyle is observed.

Treatment

Management of the TMJ affected by RA is directed at the systemic disease. This includes medical management of symptoms and physical therapy designed to maintain functional range of motion. Dental therapy is directed at establishing and maintaining stable occlusal relationships. Special oral hygiene programs may have to be developed for the patient who has a decreased ability to brush and floss.

Surgical intervention should be considered when there is persistent pain or significantly altered function manifested by either severe hypomobility or an open-bite malocclusion. Generally, the surgical alternatives are either orthognathic surgery or total joint replacement.

OTHER DISEASES

Any disease involving synovial joints can affect the TMJ. Ankylosing spondylitis, psoriatic arthritis, and crystal-

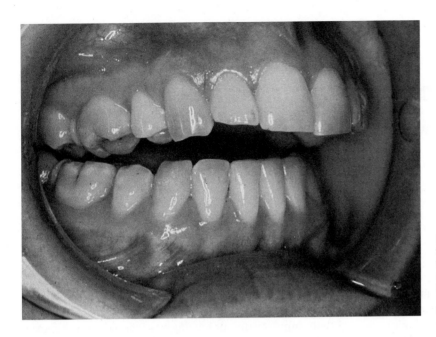

FIGURE 8.6. Open-bite malocclusion secondary to condylar resorption in patient with rheumatoid arthritis. (Dolwick MF. Temporomandibular disorders. In: Koopman WJ, ed. *Arthritis and allied conditions: a textbook of rheumatology,* 14th ed. Philadelphia: Lippincott Williams & Wilkins, 2001:2019–2025, with permission.)

lopathies rarely affect the TMJs. Other conditions affecting the TMJ include hypermobility manifested by subluxation or dislocation of the condyles, fibrous or osseous ankylosis, and growth disturbances such as condylar hyperplasia or hypoplasia. Tumors are rare but do occur and must always be considered in the differential diagnosis. The most common benign tumor seen in the TMJ is osteochondroma, and the most common malignant tumor is osteo- or chondrosarcoma. Metastatic disease may also occur, especially with breast malignancies.

REFERENCES

1. Rugh JD, Solberg WK. Oral health status in the United States. Temporomandibular disorders. *J Dent Educ* 1985;49:398–404.
2. Solberg WK, Woo MW, Houston JB. Prevalence of mandibular dysfunction in young adults. *J Am Dent Assoc* 1979;98:25–34.
3. McNeill C. Craniomandibular (TMJ) disorders—the state of the art: Part II. Accepted diagnosis and treatment and modalities. *J Prosthet Dent* 1983;49:393–397.
4. McNeill C. Diagnostic classification. In: McNeill C, ed. *Temporomandibular disorders, guidelines for classification, assessment and management.* Chicago: Quintessence Publishing, 1993:19–20.
5. Dolwick MF. Clinical diagnosis of temporomandibular joint internal derangement and myofascial pain and dysfunction. *Oral Maxillofac Surg Clin North Am* 1989;1:1–6.
6. Katzberg RW. Temporomandibular joint imaging. *Radiology* 1989;170:297–307.
7. Kaplan PA, Tu HK, Sleder PR, et al. Inferior joint space arthrography of normal TMJ: reassessment of diagnostic criteria. *Radiology* 1986;159:585–589.
8. Kiros LT, Ortendahl DA, Mark AS, et al. Magnetic resonance of the TMJ disc in asymptomatic volunteers. *J Oral Maxillofac Surg* 1987;45:852–854.
9. Laskin DM. Etiology of pain dysfunction syndrome. *J Am Dent Assoc* 1969;79:147–153.
10. Green CS, Laskin DM. Long-term evaluation of treatment for myofascial pain dysfunction syndrome: a comparative analysis. *J Am Dent Assoc* 1983;108:235–238.
11. Kreisberg MK. Tricyclic antidepressants: analgesic effect and indications in orofacial pain. *J Craniomandib Disord Facial Oral Pain* 1988;1:171–177.
12. Clark GT. A critical evaluation of orthopedic interocclusal appliance therapy: design, theory and overall effectiveness. *J Am Dent Assoc* 1984;108:359–364.
13. Rugh JD. Psychological components of pain. *Dent Clin North Am* 1987;31:579–594.
14. Dolwick MF, Katzberg RW, Helms CA. Internal derangements of the temporomandibular joint: fact or fiction? *J Prosthet Dent* 1983;49:415–418.
15. Stegenga B, DeBont LGM, Boering G, et al. Tissue responses to degenerative changes in the temporomandibular joint. *J Oral Maxillofac Surg* 1991;49:1079–1088.
16. Boering G. *Temporomandibular joint arthrosis: an analysis of 400 cases.* Leiden: Stafleu, 1966.
17. DeLeeuw R, Boering G, Stengenga B, et al. Clinical signs of TMJ osteoarthrosis and internal derangement 30 years after nonsurgical treatment. *J Orofacial Pain* 1994;8:18–24.
18. Toller PA. Osteoarthrosis of the mandibular condyle. *Br Dent J* 1973;7:47.
19. Dolwick MF, Dimitroulis G. Is there a role for temporomandibular joint surgery? *Br J Oral Maxillofac Surg* 1994;32:307–313.
20. Nitzan DW, Dolwick MF, Martinez A. Temporomandibular joint arthrocentesis: a simplified treatment for severe, limited mouth opening. *J Oral Maxillofac Surg* 1991;49:1163–1169.
21. Sanders B. Arthroscopic surgery of the temporomandibular joint: treatment of internal derangement with persistent closed lock. *Oral Surg* 1986;62:361–364.
22. McCain JP. Arthroscopy of the human temporomandibular joint. *J Oral Maxillofac Surg* 1988;46:648–652.
23. Vallerand WP, Dolwick MF. Complications of temporomandibular joint surgery. *Oral Maxillofac Surg Clin North Am* 1990;2:481–488.
24. Dolwick MF, Nitzan DW. The role of disc-repositioning surgery for internal derangement of the temporomandibular joint. *Oral Maxillofac Surg Clin North Am* 1994;6:271–275.
25. Ogus H. Rheumatoid arthritis of the temporomandibular joint. *Br J Oral Maxillofac Surg* 1975;12:275–284.

FIBROSING SYNDROMES

WILMER L. SIBBITT, JR.
RANDY R. SIBBITT

FIBROSING DISEASES

Fibrosis is the end stage of a reactive, usually inflammatory process, resulting in the invasion and replacement of normal tissue by connective tissue (1–4). A fibrosing or sclerosing disease is defined by overwhelming fibrosis that interferes with function (Table 9.1).

PATHOGENESIS OF FIBROSIS

Fibrosis is mediated by the same processes (Table 9.2) that are responsible for normal tissue repair, but in fibrosis these processes are exaggerated and detrimental (5,6). Fibrosis is initiated by tissue injury, which is followed by an inflammatory response. During this phase, cytokines, adhesion molecules, and other mediators are released in the injury site, followed by infiltration with inflammatory cells (5–11). Chronic inflammatory processes repeatedly injure tissue, producing vascular ablation, hypoxia, release of TNF-α, and free radicals, which along with TGF-β, stimulate fibroblasts to produce collagen (4,12–15). The contractures and distorted anatomy of fibrosing diseases are largely mediated by the powerful contraction of myofibroblasts in the maturing granulation tissue. Therapeutic interventions focusing specifically on the inflammatory cascade, including blocking or modulating the effects of TNF-α, TGF-β, and other cytokines, hold great promise for the treatment of fibrosing diseases (16–23).

TABLE 9.1. FIBROSING DISEASES

Skin and Musculoskeletal System	Sclerosing cholangitis
Progressive systemic sclerosis	Esophageal stricture
Morphea	Collagenous colitis
Graft–host reaction	Mesenteric fibrosis
Diabetic stiff-hand syndrome	Oral submucous fibrosis
Dupuytren contracture	Diffuse pancreatic fibrosis
Aponeurotic plantar fibrosis	Inflammatory fibroid polyp of the gastrointestinal
Knuckle pads (Garrod nodules)	tract
Plantar fasciitis	Sclerosing peritonitis
Keloids	Genitourinary
Idiopathic fibrosing cervicitis	Nephritis
(neck)	Nephrosclerosis
Focal myositis	Interstitial cystitis
Lungs	Peyronie disease
Pulmonary fibrosis	Renal inflammatory pseudotumor
Chronic pleural reaction	Other
Peribronchial fibrosis	Pseudotumor
Cardiovascular	Calcifying fibrous pseudotumor
Constrictive pericarditis	Retroperitoneal fibrosis
Atherosclerotic plaques	Riedel struma
Intimal proliferation	Cancer, especially sclerosing large-cell lymphoma
Inflammatory abdominal aneurysm	Sjögren syndrome
Chronic fibrosing periaortitis	Systemic idiopathic fibrosis
Gastrointestinal	Multifocal idiopathic fibrosclerosis
Chronic active hepatitis	Polyfibromatosis
Primary biliary cirrhosis	Inflammatory myofibroblastic tumor

TABLE 9.2. THE NORMAL HEALING PROCESS

	Events in Progress	Time After Injury (Days)
Phase 1		
Tissue injury	Exposure of hidden proteins	0
Platelet activation	Release of mediators	0
Coagulation	Release of chemoattractants	0–2
Phase 2		
Secondary inflammation	Neutrophils and eosinophils	1–4
	Monocytes and macrophages	2–6
Phase 3		
Tissue proliferation	Fibroblast migration	1–7
	Vascular ingrowth	2–10
	Collagen secretion	2–21
	Myofibroblast differentiation	7–72
Phase 4		
Tissue remodeling	Modification by proteases	3–21
	Collagen cross-linking	7–72
	Contraction	21–72

DUPUYTREN CONTRACTURE

Pathology and Biochemistry

Dupuytren contracture is characterized by a deforming, nodular fibrosis of the palmar fascia and flexion contracture of the digits (1–24). Plantar fibromatosis is less common but has identical histology, and is probably the same disorder (25). Dupuytren diathesis consists of Dupuytren contracture, nodules in the plantar fascia (Ledderhose disease), Peyronie disease, and pads in the popliteal fossa, shoulder, knuckles, and other areas (Garrod nodules) (26,27).

The early or proliferative stage of Dupuytren contracture begins with the appearance of a palpable palmar nodule. Dermal dendrocytes, contractile myofibroblasts, and T-lymphocytes are present throughout the lesion, and dense connective tissue accumulates in nodules and cords (28). The advanced or residual stage of Dupuytren disease is characterized by rigid, disabling contractures, thickened cords and nodules, and atrophy of the muscles of the hand and forearm (29).

Etiology

Genetic risk factors for Dupuytren contracture include northern European ancestry, family history, and male gender. Dupuytren disease has been associated with increasing age, diabetes mellitus, occupational or repetitive injury to the palmar structures, epilepsy, anticonvulsant therapy, osteoarthritis, peripheral vascular disease, hepatic disease, carpal tunnel syndrome, trigger finger, alcoholism, cigarette smoking, chronic pulmonary tuberculosis, human immunodeficiency virus, eosinophilic fasciitis, rheumatoid arthritis, and hyperlipidemia (1–3,29–33).

Clinical Findings

Patients note decreased mobility in the affected fingers and may complain of pain in the palm or digits. Both hands are often affected, and identical lesions may occur on the palmar surface of the feet. The ring finger is most commonly involved, but the fifth, third, and second digits in decreasing frequency can also be affected. Typically, as the disease progresses, the active fibrotic process entraps the palmar aponeurosis, the flexor tendons, the neurovascular bundles, the skin, and the periarticular structures, resulting in pain, deformity, and progressive loss of function.

Congenital flexion deformity, posttraumatic scar, immobilization contracture, Volkmann ischemic contracture (wrist and proximal interphalangeal joints flexed), primary joint contracture, palmar or plantar tenosynovitis, fibrosarcoma, and plantar fasciitis should be excluded by appropriate history and physical findings. Clinically, a nodular thickening is present in the palmar fascia, but unlike flexor tenosynovitis, the nodule of Dupuytren is less discrete, does not move in the exact track of the tendon, and dimples the overlying skin (skin tethering) (Fig. 9.1). If any question remains concerning the identity of the process, magnetic resonance imaging (MRI) is accurate at delineating the presence and stage of the Dupuytren fibrotic mass (Fig. 9.2).

Therapy

Reassurance, local heat, range-of-motion exercises, splinting, and intralesional injection of a long-acting corticosteroid may alleviate the symptoms and improve function. A new trend in therapy of more advanced Dupuytren contracture has been the forced gradual reduction of digital

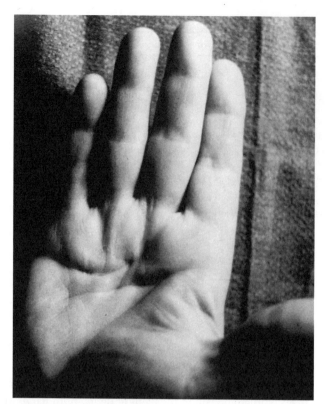

FIGURE 9.1. Dupuytren contracture. This is an early stage of Dupuytren contracture characterized by a puckering of the skin and the presence of a nodular thickening of the palmar fascia. The contracture of the fourth metacarpophalangeal joint is in an incipient stage but should progress with time. Similar lesions may be present in the plantar fascia (plantar fibromatosis). (From Sibbitt WL Jr, Sibbett RR. Fibrosing syndromes: Dupuytren's contracture, diabetic stiff hand syndrome, plantar fasciitis, and retroperitoneal fibrosis. In: Koopman WJ, ed. *Arthritis and allied conditions: a textbook of rheumatology,* 14th ed. Philadelphia: Lippincott Williams & Wilkins, 2001:2054–2066, with permission.)

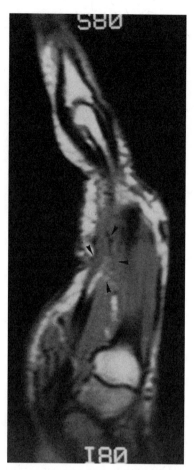

FIGURE 9.2. Dupuytren contracture. This magnetic resonance imaging (MRI) scan of the same patient in Fig. 9.1 demonstrates the invading mass of connective tissue extending along the palmar fascia into the adjoining structures. The contractile mass of tissue has enmeshed itself around the flexor digitorum profundus and superficialis tendons and exerts traction, resulting in a angular deformity of the tendon and a clinical contracture. (From Sibbitt WL Jr, Sibbett RR. Fibrosing syndromes: Dupuytren's contracture, diabetic stiff hand syndrome, plantar fasciitis, and retroperitoneal fibrosis. In: Koopman WJ, ed. *Arthritis and allied conditions: a textbook of rheumatology,* 14th ed. Philadelphia: Lippincott Williams & Wilkins, 2001:2054–2066, with permission.)

flexion contractures using skeletal traction, continuous extension, or elongation techniques, resulting in considerable clinical regression (34). Promising experimental medical therapies include injection of the palmar fascia with interferon-γ, the use of collagenase and other proteolytic enzymes, and oral colchicine (3,35,36). In patients with disabling contractures, surgery may be necessary. Surgical procedures include nodule excision, limited fasciotomy, dermatofasciectomy (radical fasciectomy) with skin grafting, and amputation, but recurrence, extension, and complication rates are high.

THE SYNDROME OF LIMITED JOINT MOBILITY

Definition

The syndrome of limited joint mobility (SLJM) is characterized by decreased range of motion of the joints of the hands and wrists in a patient with diabetes mellitus without an apparent underlying inflammatory joint disease (1–3,37). Synonyms include *cheiroarthropathy, diabetic stiff hand syndrome,* and *waxy contractures of diabetes.* SLJM is associated with increasing age, duration of diabetes, Dupuytren contracture, palmar flexor tenosynovitis, retinopathy, neuropathy, and cigarette smoking. SLJM is most common in patients with type I diabetes, but is also frequent in type II patients. Of all insulin-dependent diabetics, 32% to 40% may eventually be affected. By definition, the SLJM is a complication of diabetes mellitus and must be distinguished from other diabetic and nondiabetic contractures. SLJM should be considered in the context of

TABLE 9.3. DIABETIC COMPLICATIONS INVOLVING THE UPPER EXTREMITY

Condition	Typical Joints Involved	Comments
Syndrome of limited joint mobility	MCP, PIP, wrists, other joints	Decreased range of motion of the small joints. Often associated with sclerodactyly
Diabetic sclerodactyly	Distal digits, but may extend to entire hand	Thickened, waxy skin
Reflex sympathetic dystrophy (RSD)	Contracture and edema of the entire hand, occasionally entire arm	More often bilateral (42%) than in other conditions (5%). Bone scan is positive.
Adhesive capsulitis	Contracture of shoulder	Often associated with RSD or bicipital or supraspinatus tenosynovitis
Dupuytren contracture	Third, fourth, and fifth MCP and PIP contractures	Palpably thickened palmar fascia, dimpling of skin, associated with plantar fibromatosis
Flexor tenosynovitis	Any digit, but especially second, third, and fourth digits	Presence of painful trigger finger, thickened tendon sheath, nodule on tendon
Carpal tunnel syndrome	MCP and PIP contractures	Prominent pain, wasting of thenar musculature, positive Tinel and Phelan sign, slowed nerve conduction
Diabetic neuropathy	Variable contractures	Dysesthesias, pain, loss of proprioception and fine touch. Abnormal nerve conduction
Aseptic necrosis of humoral head	Shoulder contractures	Pain, loss of motion, radiographic changes delayed

MCP, metacarpophalangeal joint; PIP, proximal interphalangeal joint; RSD, reflex sympathetic dystrophy.

other diabetes-associated lesions of the hand and upper extremity (Table 9.3). These musculoskeletal disorders constitute a spectrum of pathology resulting from active fibrosis (Dupuytren contracture, tenosynovitis), passive fibrosis (nonenzymatic glycosylation), motor neuropathy (neuropathic contractures), and autonomic disturbance (reflex sympathetic dystrophy) (37,38).

Clinical Findings

SLJM is characterized by contractures involving the small joints of the hands, including the proximal and distal interphalangeal joints and the metacarpophalangeal joints (Fig. 9.3). However, decreased range of motion in the shoulders and other large joints may also be present. The "prayer sign," formed by apposing the palmar surfaces of both hands, is usually present, indicating the contractures of the interphalangeal and metacarpophalangeal joints. SLJM is often accompanied by diabetic sclerodactyly, a thickening and rigidity of the digital skin that resembles scleroderma (39). Conditions that can be confused with SLJM and diabetic sclerodactyly include true scleroderma, scleredema, reflex sympathetic dystrophy, diabetic neuropathy, Dupuytren contracture, and flexor tenosynovitis. SLJM is closely associated with other diabetic complications, including retinopathy, nephropathy, and neuropathy. Antinuclear antibodies and rheumatoid factor are usually negative.

Pathology

The etiology of SLJM and diabetic sclerodactyly is related to the same underlying mechanisms that induce other diabetic complications resulting in local or systemic fibrosis.

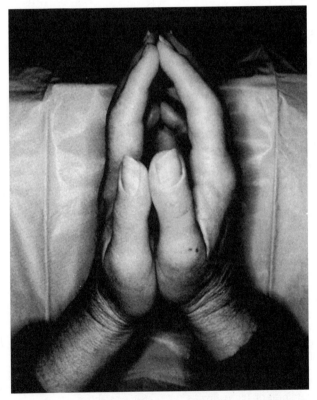

FIGURE 9.3. Syndrome of limited joint mobility (SLJM). This diabetic patient is suffering from contractures of the metacarpophalangeal, proximal interphalangeal, and distal interphalangeal joints, resulting in a prominent "prayer sign." The skin is also thickened and has lost much of the fine wrinkles, simulating true sclerodactyly. (From Sibbitt WL Jr, Sibbett RR. Fibrosing syndromes: Dupuytren's contracture, diabetic stiff hand syndrome, plantar fasciitis, and retroperitoneal fibrosis. In: Koopman WJ, ed. *Arthritis and allied conditions: a textbook of rheumatology,* 14th ed. Philadelphia: Lippincott Williams & Wilkins, 2001: 2054–2066, with permission.)

These potential mechanisms include polyol accumulation, increased cross-linking of collagen, nonenzymatic glycosylation of proteins, accumulation of matrix constituents, endothelial cell degeneration, obliterative microvasculopathy, and release of TGF-β and other factors, resulting in fibrosis, tenosynovitis, and contracture (40,41).

Treatment of SLJM

Treatment of SLJM is controversial and unsatisfactory at this time. Strict control of blood glucose, range-of-motion exercises, forced progressive extension, aldose reductase inhibitor agents, and aminoguanidine have been used (34,37,42–45). However, injection of the affected flexor tendon sheaths with a long-acting corticosteroid may be the safest and most effective therapy at the present (41).

PLANTAR FASCIITIS

The painful heel is one of the most common musculoskeletal complaints (1–3,46). Plantar fasciitis refers specifically to the clinical syndrome of pain, inflammation, and fibrosis of the plantar fascia and its calcaneal insertion. Plantar fasciitis is induced by excessive repetitive stresses applied to the foot, resulting in torsion and tension of the plantar fascia. Stress along the plantar fascia is increased with obesity, overuse, inappropriate footwear, and structural instability (the flexible flat foot) that has a tendency to pronate (evert)

at the talonavicular and naviculocuneiform joints. These factors increase tension across the plantar fascia after heel strike and before toe-off, resulting in microavulsion, microtears, and inflammation of the plantar fascia and calcaneal periosteum.

Pathology

Histopathology of plantar fasciitis is characterized by collagen degeneration, angiofibroblastic hyperplasia, chondroid metaplasia, and calcification of degenerated matrix. Periosteal inflammation is ubiquitous, frequently inducing an anterior calcaneal spur (ostosis) at the insertion of the fascia. The anterior calcaneal ostosis remains after symptoms of pain have resolved, indicating that inflammation and injury, not the ostosis itself, constitute the usual etiology of pain.

Diagnosis of Plantar Fasciitis

Plantar fasciitis is diagnosed with the following findings: (a) pain and morning stiffness involving the heel and plantar surface of the foot and (b) maximum tenderness to palpation localized at the insertion of the plantar fascia on the calcaneal tuberosity. Other causes of heel pain should be excluded, as noted in Table 9.4. The foot and heel should be deeply palpated to determine the site of pain. The structure and motion of the foot, ankle, knee, and hip should be carefully examined with weight bearing and walking for a tendency to pronate (evert).

TABLE 9.4. INTRINSIC CAUSES OF HEEL PAIN

Disorder	Complaints	Diagnostic Sign
Plantar Fasciitis		
	Plantar foot	Tenderness over calcaneal tuberosity
	Anterior heel	Anterior osteophyte
Achilles Tendon		
Tenosynovitis	Tendon; posterior heel	Diffuse pain and swelling along tendon
Tendinitis	Tendon	Diffuse pain along tendon and calcaneal insertion
Subtendinous bursitis	Tendon; posterior heel	Pain, swelling superior calcaneus
Subcutaneous bursitis	Tendon; posterior heel	Pain, swelling inferior calcaneus
Rupture	Weakness; pain variable	Absence of tendon in area of rupture
Flexor Hallucis Longus		
Tendinitis or Tenosynovitis	Anterior superior heel	Pain and swelling posterior to medial malleolus into plantar foot
	Posterior medial malleolus	
Tibialis Posterior		
Tendinitis or Tenosynovitis	Same as above	Same as above
Calcaneus		
Apophysitis	Posterior heel	Tenderness insertion on Achilles tendon, x-ray
Fracture	Heel	Stress fracture, x-ray
Periostitis	Heel	Tenderness, x-ray, systemic arthritis
Erosion	Heel	Same as above
Osteomyelitis	Heel	X-ray, bone scan
Ostosis	Heel	Nonanterior calcaneal ostosis, pain directly over ostosis
Tarsal Tunnel Syndrome		
	Heel or midfoot	Neurologic abnormalities in heel and plantar foot

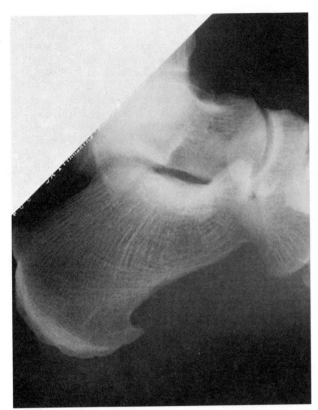

FIGURE 9.4. Plantar fasciitis. This patient was a long-distance runner who continued to run despite severe calcaneal pain secondary to plantar fasciitis. A large calcaneal hyperostosis extends anteriorly, following the plantar fascia. The patient responded to 8 months of abstinence from long-distance running and eventually was able to resume running at reduced distances with the use of antipronator running shoes. (From Sibbitt WL Jr, Sibbett RR. Fibrosing syndromes: Dupuytren's contracture, diabetic stiff hand syndrome, plantar fasciitis, and retroperitoneal fibrosis. In: Koopman WJ, ed. *Arthritis and allied conditions: a textbook of rheumatology,* 14th ed. Philadelphia: Lippincott Williams & Wilkins, 2001:2054–2066, with permission.)

Neurologic dysfunction as an etiology for heel pain should be considered and tarsal tunnel syndrome in particular should be excluded. The patient's footwear should be examined for appropriate heel and midfoot support and for signs of excessive wear, instability, or loss of integrity. Radiologic studies may reveal small calcifications anterior to the calcaneal tuberosity or the presence of an exuberant anterior calcaneal ostosis (spur) (Fig. 9.4). The presence of an anterior heel spur is not necessary for the diagnosis of plantar fasciitis but is confirmatory and implies that the process is chronic.

Therapy

Therapy consists of resting, unloading, and stabilizing the foot. Nonsteroidal antiinflammatory drugs diminish the pain and stiffness but are not curative. Obesity should be

reduced, nonsupportive footwear should be discarded, and stable, comfortable footwear with excellent heel control and padding should be substituted. If greater stability is required, splinting, casting, and orthotics can be considered (47–49). Long-distance running and other activities contributing to overuse should be suspended until the symptoms have completely resolved, a process that typically requires months. Continued abuse of the foot will result in chronic, intractable pain and the development of a hyperostosis on the calcaneus.

If 3 to 6 months of rest, nonsteroidal drugs, and foot stabilization with appropriate shoes or orthotics have not been effective, injection of corticosteroids into the plantar fascia may be considered. Before this is undertaken, an erythrocyte sedimentation rate and imaging consisting of radiographs, and in some instances MRI or radionuclide bone scan, should be considered to exclude confounding conditions, including osteomyelitis, inflammatory joint disease, and stress fracture (50). Corticosteroid injection of the plantar fascia, although moderately effective, should not be undertaken lightly because of potential complications, including infection, plantar fascia rupture, chronic midfoot pain, and foot weakness (51). For cases resistant to a minimum of 12 months of conservative therapy, surgical intervention, including fasciectomy, fasciotomy (fascial release), and exostectomy, may be considered (52,53). Unfortunately, recurrence of foot pain is common.

RETROPERITONEAL FIBROSIS

Retroperitoneal fibrosis is a fibrosing disease of the retroperitoneum that entraps and distorts retroperitoneal structures, including the great vessels, the ureters, nerves, kidneys, and biliary tree (3,27,54–57). Secondary retroperitoneal fibrosis can be caused by drugs and toxins (methylsergide, methyldopa, levodopa, ergot, bromocriptine, pergolide, asbestos), aortic aneurysm, malignant tumors (metastatic carcinomas, carcinoid, lymphoma), retroperitoneal injury (hemorrhage, infection, radiation, surgery, stenting, angioplasty), autoimmune disease, tuberculosis, sarcoidosis, biliary tract disease, gonorrhea, and ascending lymphangitis (3,58–60).

Clinical Signs and Symptoms

Retroperitoneal fibrosis usually presents with pain in the lower abdomen, lumbosacrum, and flank or with signs of visceral obstruction, including vomiting, diarrhea, or dehydration. Hydronephrosis, renal insufficiency, peripheral edema, varicosities, or claudication may follow. Nerve entrapment and epidural cord compression may result in pain, dysesthesias, weakness, or spasticity. Pulmonary emboli, deep venous thrombosis, obstruction of the bowel, bladder, or bronchi can occur. Mediastinal fibrosis may result in a lymphoma-like mass and superior vena caval syndrome with edema and venous dilatation of the arms, neck, and head. Extrahepatic portal vein obstruction, portal hypertension, esophageal varices, and uveitis may occur.

Pathology

Biopsies typically demonstrate irregular masses characterized by fibrosis, granulation tissue, inflammatory cells, spindle-shaped cells expressing macrophage markers, and activated fibroblasts (61–63). Aortic disease resulting from aneurysm, atherosclerosis, aortitis, inherited diseases of collagen, trauma, or infection may be causative and must be suspected in all patients with idiopathic retroperitoneal fibrosis. Lymphoma, crystal-storing histiocytosis, immunocytoma, diffuse retroperitoneal carcinoma (pancreatic, scirrhous gastric, prostate, ovarian, renal, uterine cervix, carcinoid), Wegener granulomatosis, xanthogranulomatous pyelonephritis, chronic pyelonephritis, tuberculosis, sarcoidosis, or aortic graft infection should be excluded by appropriate imaging, by biopsy or aspiration of the retroperitoneal tissues, or by careful examination of affected nonretroperitoneal tissues (64–66).

Diagnosis of Retroperitoneal Fibrosis

A CT or MRI scan will demonstrate diffuse, discrete, unifocal, or multifocal retroperitoneal masses with or without obstruction of ureters, great vessels, biliary tree, or pancreatic ducts (67,68). Indium-111-labeled leukocyte or gallium radionuclide scans are useful to exclude abscess and other intensely inflammatory retroperitoneal processes and have been used to follow disease activity (69,70). After suspicious masses are identified, CT or ultrasound-guided percutaneous needle biopsy, laparoscopy, or retroperitoneal exploration can be undertaken to confirm the diagnosis and exclude confounding conditions, especially neoplasia and infection (71,72).

Treatment of Retroperitoneal Fibrosis

Conventional treatment for obstructive retroperitoneal fibrosis consists of surgery to relieve ureteral and vascular entrapment and subsequent administration of long-term corticosteroids. An alternative approach is the use of ureteral stents to relieve obstruction followed by pulse methylprednisolone therapy and long-term penicillamine, azathioprine, or cyclophosphamide (73,74). Tamoxifen has been used as primary therapy on a limited basis with some success and very little toxicity (70). Lifelong anticoagulation is required for those patients with large vein involvement. Surgical repair of an associated abdominal aortic aneurysm may either exacerbate or ameliorate retroperitoneal fibrosis; thus therapy for these patients must be individualized.

REFERENCES

1. Sibbitt WL, Jr. Fibrosing syndromes: diabetic stiff hand syndrome, Dupuytren's contracture, and plantar fascitis. In: McCarty DJ, ed. *Arthritis and allied conditions*. Philadelphia: Lea & Febiger, 1989:1473–1485.
2. Sibbitt WL, Jr. Fibrosing syndromes: diabetic stiff hand syndrome, Dupuytren's contracture, and plantar fascitis. In: McCarty DJ, ed. *Arthritis and allied conditions: a textbook of rheumatology, 12th edition*. Philadelphia: Lea & Febiger, 1993: 1609–1618.
3. Sibbitt WL, Jr. Fibrosing syndromes: Dupuytren's contracture, diabetic stiff hand syndrome, plantar fascitis, and retroperitoneal fibrosis. In: Koopman W, ed. *Arthritis and allied conditions: a textbook of rheumatology, 13th edition*. Philadelphia: Lippincott Williams & Wilkins, 1997:1847–1866.
4. Border WA, Ruoslahti E. Transforming growth factor-beta in disease: the dark side of tissue repair. *J Clin Invest* 1992;90:1–7.
5. Mutsaers SE, Bishop JE, McGrouther G, et al. Mechanisms of tissue repair: from wound healing to fibrosis. *Int J Biochem Cell Biol* 1997;29:5–17.
6. Trojanowska M, LeRoy EC, Eckes B, et al. Pathogenesis of fibrosis: type 1 collagen and the skin. *J Mol Med* 1998;76:266–274.
7. Gharaee-Kermani M, Phan SH. The role of eosinophils in pulmonary fibrosis. *Int J Mol Med* 1998;1:43–53.
8. Metcalfe DD, Baram D, Mekori YA. Mast cells. *Physiol Rev* 1997;77:1033–1079.
9. Haque MF, Harris M, Meghji S, et al. Immunolocalization of cytokines and growth factors in oral submucous fibrosis. *Cytokine* 1998;10:713–719.
10. Schins RP, Borm PJ. Mechanisms and mediators in coal dust induced toxicity: a review. *Ann Occup Hyg* 1999;43:7–33.
11. Robledo R, Mossman B. Cellular and molecular mechanisms of asbestos-induced fibrosis. *J Cell Physiol* 1999;180:158–166.
12. Wahl SM. Transforming growth factor beta (TGF-beta) in inflammation: a case and a cure. *J Clin Immunol* 1992;12:61–74.
13. Roulot D, Sevcsik AM, Coste T, et al. Role of transforming growth factor beta type II receptor in hepatic fibrosis: studies of human chronic hepatitis C and experimental fibrosis in rats. *Hepatology* 1999;29:1730–1738.
14. Clark DA, Coker R. Transforming growth factor-beta (TGF-beta). *Int J Biochem Cell Biol* 1998;30:293–298.
15. Wardle EN. Modulatory proteins and processes in alliance with immune cells, mediators, and extracellular proteins in renal interstitial fibrosis. *Ren Fail* 1999;21:121–133.
16. Border WA, Okuda S, Languino LR, et al. Suppression of experimental glomerulonephritis by antiserum against transforming growth factor beta$_1$. *Nature* 1990;346:371–374.
17. Shah M, Foreman DM, Ferguson MW. Control of scarring in adult wounds by neutralizing antibody to transforming growth factor beta. *Lancet* 1992; 339:213–214.
18. Giri SN, Hyde DM, Hollinger MA. Effect of antibody to transforming growth factor beta on bleomycin-induced accumulation of lung collagen in mice. *Thorax* 1993;48:959–966.
19. Wilutzky B, Berndt A, Katenkamp D, et al. Programmed cell death in nodular palmar fibromatosis (Morbus Dupuytren). *Histol Histopathol* 1998;13:67–72.
20. Kapanci Y, Desmouliere A, Pache JC, et al. Cytoskeletal protein modulation in pulmonary alveolar myofibroblasts during idiopathic pulmonary fibrosis. Possible role of transforming growth factor beta and tumor necrosis factor alpha. *Am J Respir Crit Care Med* 1995;152:2163–2169.
21. Maish GO 3rd, Shumate ML, Ehrlich HP, et al. Tumor necrosis factor binding protein improves incisional wound healing in sepsis. *J Surg Res* 1998;78:108–117.

22. Cooney R, Iocono J, Maish G, et al. In vivo effects of tumor necrosis factor-alpha on incised wound and gunshot wound healing. *J Trauma* 1996;40(3 Suppl):S140–S143.
23. Thrall RS, Vogel SN, Evans R, et al. Role of tumor necrosis factor-alpha in the spontaneous development of pulmonary fibrosis in viable motheaten mutant mice. *Am J Pathol* 1997;151: 1303–1310.
24. Benson LS, Williams CS, Kahle M. Dupuytren's contracture. *J Am Acad Orthop Surg* 1998;6:24–35.
25. De Palma L, Santucci A, Gigante A, et al. Plantar fibromatosis: an immunohistochemical and ultrastructural study. *Foot Ankle Int* 1999;20:253–257.
26. Classen DA, Hurst LN. Plantar fibromatosis and bilateral flexion contractures: a review of the literature. *Ann Plast Surg* 1992;28: 475–478.
27. Lee YC, Chan HH, Black MM. Aggressive polyfibromatosis: a 10-year follow-up. *Australas J Dermatol* 1996;37:205–207.
28. Wilutzky B, Berndt A, Katenkamp D, et al. Programmed cell death in nodular palmar fibromatosis (Morbus Dupuytren). *Histol Histopathol* 1998;13:67–72.
29. Ross DC. Epidemiology of Dupuytren's disease. *Hand Clin* 1999;15:53–62.
30. Yi IS, Johnson G, Moneim MS. Etiology of Dupuytren's disease. *Hand Clin* 1999;15:43–51.
31. Arkkila PE, Kantola IM, Viikari JS. Dupuytren's disease: association with chronic diabetic complications. *J Rheumatol* 1997;24: 153–159.
32. Burge P, Hoy G, Regan P, et al. Smoking, alcohol and the risk of Dupuytren's contracture. *J Bone Joint Surg Br* 1997;79:206–210.
33. Liss GM, Stock SR. Can Dupuytren's contracture be work-related? Review of the evidence. *Am J Ind Med* 1996;29: 521–532.
34. Citron N, Messina JC. The use of skeletal traction in the treatment of severe primary Dupuytren's disease. *J Bone Joint Surg Br* 1998;80:126–129.
35. McCarthy DM. The long-term results of enzymic fasciotomy. *J Hand Surg [Br]* 1992; 17:356.
36. Dominguez-Malagon HR, Alfeiran-Ruiz A, Chavarria-Xicotencatl P, et al. Clinical and cellular effects of colchicine in fibromatosis. *Cancer* 1992;69:2478–2483.
37. Kapoor A, Sibbitt WL, Jr. Diabetic contractures: the syndrome of limited joint mobility. *Semin Arthritis Rheum* 1889;18:168–174.
38. Chammas M, Bousquet P, Renard E, et al. Dupuytren's disease, carpal tunnel syndrome, trigger finger, and diabetes mellitus. *J Hand Surg [Am]* 1995;20:109–114.
39. Tuzun B, Tuzun Y, Dinccag N, et al. Diabetic sclerodactyly. *Diabetes Res Clin Pract* 1995;27:153–157.
40. Ismail AA, Dasgupta B, Tanqueray AB, Hamblin JJ. Ultrasonographic features of diabetic cheiroarthropathy. *Br J Rheumatol* 1996;35:676–679.
41. Sibbitt WL Jr, Eaton RP. Corticosteroid responsive tenosynovitis is a common pathway for limited joint mobility in the diabetic hand. *J Rheumatol* 1997;24:931–936.
42. Rosenbloom AL, Silverstein JH. Connective tissue and joint disease in diabetes mellitus. *Endocrinol Metab Clin North Am* 1996; 25:473–483.
43. Eaton RP. Aldose reductase inhibition and the diabetic syndrome of limited joint mobility: implications for altered collagen hydration. *Metabolism* 1986;35:119–121.
44. Eaton RP, Sibbitt WL Jr, Harsh A. The effect of an aldose reductase inhibiting agent on limited joint mobility in diabetes mellitus. *JAMA* 1985;253:1437–1471.
45. Eaton RP, Sibbitt WL Jr, Shah VO, et al. A commentary on 10 years of aldose reductase inhibition for limited joint mobility in diabetes. *J Diabetes Complications* 1998;12:34–38.
46. Karr SD. Subcalcaneal heel pain. *Orthop Clin North Am* 1994; 25:S161–S175.
47. Sobel E, Levitz SJ, Caselli MA. Orthoses in the treatment of rearfoot problems. *J Am Podiatr Med Assoc* 1999;89:220–223.
48. Powell M, Post WR, Keener J, et al. Effective treatment of chronic plantar fasciitis with dorsiflexion night splints: a crossover prospective randomized outcome study. *Foot Ankle Int* 1998;19:10–18.
49. Lynch DM, Goforth WP, Martin JE, et al. Conservative treatment of plantar fasciitis. A prospective study. *J Am Podiatr Med Assoc* 1998;88:375–380.
50. DiMarcangelo MT, Yu TC. Diagnostic imaging of heel pain and plantar fasciitis. *Clin Podiatr Med Surg* 1997;14:281–301.
51. Acevedo JI, Beskin JL. Complications of plantar fascia rupture associated with corticosteroid injection. *Foot Ankle Int* 1998;19:91–97.
52. Benton-Weil W, Borrelli AH, Weil LS Jr, et al. Percutaneous plantar fasciotomy: a minimally invasive procedure for recalcitrant plantar fasciitis. *J Foot Ankle Surg* 1998;37.269–272.
53. Sammarco GJ, Helfrey RB. Surgical treatment of recalcitrant plantar fasciitis. *Foot Ankle Int* 1996;17:520–526.
54. Dehner LP, Coffin CM. Idiopathic fibrosclerotic disorders and other inflammatory pseudotumors. *Semin Diagn Pathol* 1998;15: 161–173.
55. Johal SS, Manjunath S, Allen C, et al. Systemic multifocal fibrosclerosis. *Postgrad Med J* 1998;74:608–609.
56. Kaipiainen-Seppanen O, Jantunen E, Kuusisto J, et al. Retroperitoneal fibrosis with antineutrophil cytoplasmic antibodies. *J Rheumatol* 1996;23:779–781.
56a. Moroni G, Farricciotti A, Cappelletti M, et al. Retroperitoneal fibrosis and membranous nephropathy: improvement of both diseases after treatment with steroids and immunosuppressive agents. *Nephrol Dial Transplant* 1999;14:1303–1305.
57. Levey JM, Mathai J. Diffuse pancreatic fibrosis: an uncommon feature of multifocal idiopathic fibrosclerosis. *Am J Gastroenterol* 1998;93:640–642.
58. Shaunak S, Wilkins A, Pilling JB, et al. Pericardial, retroperitoneal, and pleural fibrosis induced by pergolide. *J Neurol Neurosurg Psychiatry* 1999;66:79–81.
59. Sakr G, Cynk M, Cowie AG. Retroperitoneal fibrosis: an unusual complication of intra-arterial stents and angioplasty. *Br J Urol* 1998;81:768–769.
60. Sauni R, Oksa P, Jarvenpaa R, et al. Asbestos exposure: a potential cause of retroperitoneal fibrosis. *Am J Ind Med* 1998;33:418–421.
61. Hughes D, Buckley PJ. Idiopathic retroperitoneal fibrosis is a macrophage-rich process. *Am J Surg Pathol* 1993;17:482–490.
62. Lee I. Human fibroblasts in idiopathic retroperitoneal fibrosis express HLA-DR antigens. *J Korean Med Sci* 1991;6:279–283.
63. Parums DV, Choudhury RP, Shields SA, et al. Characterization of inflammatory cells associated with idiopathic retroperitoneal fibrosis. *Br J Urol* 1991; 67:564–568.
64. Garcia JF, Sanchez E, Lloret E, et al. Crystal-storing histiocytosis and immunocytoma associated with multifocal fibrosclerosis. *Histopathology* 1998;33:459–464.
65. Cuny C, Chauffert B, Lorcerie B, et al. Retroperitoneal fibrosis and infection of an aortic graft prosthesis: diagnosis and therapeutic problems. *Clin Cardiol* 1997;20:810–812.
66. Kaipiainen-Seppanen O, Jantunen E, Kuusisto J, et al. Retroperitoneal fibrosis with antineutrophil cytoplasmic antibodies. *J Rheumatol* 1996;23:779–781.
67. Engelken JD, Ros PR. Retroperitoneal MR imaging. *Magn Reson Imaging Clin North Am* 1997;5:165–178.
68. Kottra JJ, Dunnick NR. Retroperitoneal fibrosis. *Radiol Clin North Am* 1996;34:1259–1275.
69. Fink AM, Miles KA, Wraight EP. Indium-11 labelled leucocyte uptake in aortitis. *Clin Radiol* 1994;49:863–866.

70. Oosterlinck W, Derie A. New data on diagnosis and medical treatment of retroperitoneal fibrosis. *Acta Urol Belg* 1997;65:3–6.

71. Stein AL, Bardawil RG, Silverman SG, et al. Fine needle aspiration biopsy of idiopathic retroperitoneal fibrosis. *Acta Cytol* 1997;41:461–466.

72. Kava BR, Russo P, Conlon KC. Laparoscopic diagnosis of malignant retroperitoneal fibrosis. *J Endourol* 1996;10:535–538.

73. Harreby M, Bilde T, Helin P, et al. Retroperitoneal fibrosis treated with methylprednisolone pulse and disease-modifying antirheumatic drugs. *Scand J Urol Nephrol* 1994;28:237–242.

74. Netzer P, Binek J, Hammer B. Diffuse abdominal pain, nausea and vomiting due to retroperitoneal fibrosis: a rare but often missed diagnosis. *Eur J Gastroenterol Hepatol* 1997;9:1005–1008.

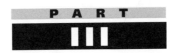

PART

III

SPECIFIC RHEUMATIC DISEASES: DIAGNOSIS AND TREATMENT

RHEUMATOID ARTHRITIS: CLINICAL ASPECTS

JAMES R. O'DELL

Rheumatoid arthritis (RA) is a life-long disease of unknown cause where no cures are currently available. The diagnosis of RA continues to require clinical skills and experience. Management puts a premium on the physician's ability to practice the art, as well as the science, of medicine.

RA is a systemic inflammatory disease with its primary manifestation in the synovium. The hallmark of the disease is a chronic, symmetric polyarthritis (synovitis) that typically affects the hands, wrists, and feet initially, and later may involve any synovial joint. Why RA has a particular predilection for the synovial joints has not been elucidated and remains one of the keys to pathogenesis. Although RA primarily involves the synovium, features of systemic disease are present in almost all patients and range in severity from fatigue to severe multisystemic vasculitis. Fortunately, significant advances in therapy have recently occurred, but despite these advances, RA continues to result in substantial morbidity (1) for most patients and premature mortality in many (1,2).

EPIDEMIOLOGY

RA is a common illness affecting all racial groups worldwide, although it is seen more commonly in some populations than in others; the prevalence in most cohorts averages approximately 1% (3). A recent study in Minnesota found an incidence of 50/100,000 person-years in men and 98/100,000 person-years in women. The preponderance of women was marked in the younger age groups, but nearly equal for patients more than 75 years of age. The incidence of RA increases with age, with female excess in each age range found in most studies (4). Some have suggested that currently not as many people are severely affected as in decades past. It is hoped that new and better treatments will continue to decrease the consequences of RA.

ESTABLISHING THE DIAGNOSIS

The importance of making an accurate diagnosis of RA as early as possible cannot be overemphasized. All modern treatment paradigms stress early aggressive disease-modifying antirheumatic drug (DMARD) therapy (5). It is critical to ensure that effective treatments are begun when they have the maximum chance of making the biggest differences, while at the same time protecting patients who do not have RA from the potential toxicities of therapies. *The diagnosis of RA is a clinical one,* based almost exclusively on the history and physical examination. No single finding, either on examination or from laboratory testing, is pathognomonic for RA. Therefore a set of seven criteria has been established for classification purposes and is useful for diagnostic purposes [Table 10.1 (6)]. The presence of four of seven criteria is required to establish RA for study purposes. It is important to note that in the case of the first four criteria, the patient must have had these present for a minimum of 6 weeks. This is a requirement because there are many other causes of symmetric polyarthritis (viral and others) that may mimic RA but that are of short duration. Unfortunately, this need to wait a minimum of 6 weeks for a definitive diagnosis can be frustrating for the patient and the physician and, worse, often results in significant delays in therapy.

The diagnosis of RA should be considered in any patient with polyarticular inflammatory arthritis of greater than 6 weeks' duration, especially if the hands and feet are involved. The patient's response to the question, "What is the worst time of day for your joints?" is often telling. Patients with inflammatory arthritis such as RA usually report significant morning stiffness (often greater than 1 hour), whereas patients with OA and other mechanical syndromes are usually worse later in the day after activity. In addition, significant fatigue may be present even in early RA. Early physical findings of disease include soft-tissue joint swelling and joint tenderness to palpation. Joint distribution is critical in diagnosis. Initially, RA is often limited to the hands and feet. In the hands, it is the proximal interphalangeal joints (PIPs) and metacarpal phalangeal joints (MCPs) that are most likely to be involved early. Figure 10.1 compares and contrasts the joints most commonly involved in the two most common kinds of arthritis—rheumatoid and OA. In the hand, the distal interphalangeal joints (DIPs) are characteristically involved in OA (Heber-

TABLE 10.1. 1987 AMERICAN COLLEGE OF RHEUMATOLOGY REVISED CRITERIA FOR THE CLASSIFICATION OF RHEUMATOID ARTHRITIS (TRADITIONAL FORMAT)

Criterion	Definition
Morning stiffness	Morning stiffness in and around the joints, lasting at least 1 hour before maximal improvement
Arthritis of three or more joint areas	At least three joint areas simultaneously with soft-tissue swelling or joint fluid observed by a physician; the 14 possible areas are (right or left): PIP, MCP, wrist, elbow, knee, ankle, and MTP joints
Arthritis of hand joints	At least 1 area swollen in a wrist, MCP, or PIP joint
Symmetric arthritis	Simultaneous involvement of the same joint areas on both sides of the body (bilateral involvement of PIP, MCP, or MTP acceptable without perfect symmetry)
Rheumatoid nodules	Subcutaneous nodules over bony prominences or extensor surfaces, or in juxtaarticular regions, observed by a physician
Serum rheumatoid factor	Abnormal amount of serum rheumatoid factor by any method for which the result has been positive in <5% of control subjects
Radiographic changes	Erosions or unequivocal bony decalcification localized in or most marked adjacent to the involved joints (osteoarthritis changes excluded), typical of rheumatoid arthritis on posteroanterior hand and wrist radiographs

For classification purposes, a patient is said to have rheumatoid arthritis if four of seven criteria are satisfied. Criteria 1–4 must have been present for at least 6 weeks. Patients with two clinical diagnoses are not excluded.
MCP, metacarpophalangeal; MTP, metatarsophalangeal; PIP, proximal interphalangeal.
From Arnett FC, Edworth SM, Bloch DA, et al. The American Rheumatism Association 1987 revised criteria for the classification of rheumatoid arthritis. *Arthritis Rheum* 1988;31:315–324, with permission.

den nodes) but seldom involved in RA, the PIPs may be involved with either, whereas MCP involvement is the rule in RA and seldom occurs in OA. The wrist is frequently involved in RA, whereas only the first carpal–metacarpal joint is commonly involved in OA. A remarkable feature of RA is the symmetry of involvement.

If inflammation persists over time, permanent damage—including tendon, ligament, cartilage, and subchondral bone destruction—will occur, with resultant joint deformity and disability. Although inflammation and deformity

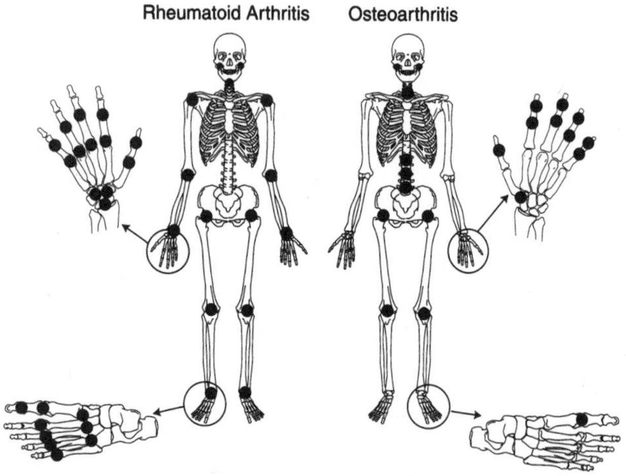

FIGURE 10.1. This figure compares and contrasts the joint distribution of the two most common kinds of arthritis: rheumatoid arthritis and osteoarthritis. *Black circles* over the involved joint areas denote joints involved in these arthritides. (From O'Dell JR. Rheumatoid arthritis: the clinical picture. In: Koopman WJ, ed. *Arthritis and allied conditions: a textbook of rheumatology,* 14th ed. Philadelphia: Lippincott Williams & Wilkins, 2001:1153–1186, with permission.)

are most often seen initially in the hands and feet, later the disease often metastasizes to larger joints, and involvement of the knees, hips, and shoulders accounts for significant morbidity, including work disability in a large percentage of patients. A major difference in the pathophysiology of RA versus OA or mechanical joint problems is the presence of extensive synovial-based inflammation.

Gender and Hormonal Influences

The incidence rate of RA is two to three times higher in women than in men (3). The greatest differences in incidence rates are in patients below 50 years of age, where RA is uncommon in men. Therefore hormonal mechanisms are felt to play a part (7). Somewhat paradoxically, the use of oral contraceptives and pregnancy are protective with respect to the development of RA, and 75% of pregnancies in patients with RA result in a significant decrease in symptoms (8). It is important to note that hormonal replacement therapy in women does not result in an increase in the activity of disease and should be considered in this group of patients who are at high risk for osteoporosis. Some have suggested that males with RA may have mild testosterone deficiencies, and replacement may result in some decrease in symptoms.

Genetics

First-degree relatives of those with RA are at increased risk of developing RA, with siblings of severely affected patients at highest risk (9). Monozygotic twins have a concordance rate of about 12% to 15%, whereas dizygotic twins have a rate about one-quarter of this. In populations of northern European descent, HLA-DR4 is associated with both an increased incidence of RA and more severe disease (9). Monozygosity for HLA-DR4 or this particular DRB1 epitope may predispose for seropositivity, for rheumatoid factor (RF) and more severe disease (10).

CLINICAL PICTURE

Stiffness

Morning stiffness is a hallmark of the inflammatory arthritides. Joint stiffness is a major symptom of most types of arthritis, and RA in particular is often accompanied by significant stiffness early in the day. Prolonged stiffness has been included in RA classification criteria (Table 10.1). Other inflammatory conditions, such as systemic lupus erythematosus, ankylosing spondylitis, and polymyalgia rheumatica, are also accompanied by morning stiffness. The presence of morning stiffness may better discriminate a primary inflammatory process from other joint processes.

Pain

Unfortunately, pain is a major problem for most patients with RA and is often what brings them to the physician's office. Pain is very difficult to quantify, although its relief is a major endpoint used to measure the effectiveness of therapy [Table 10.2 (11)]. RA patients as a group tend to minimize symptoms and often complain very little even when obvious swelling and deformities are present. Joints with rapidly evolving effusions, as seen in early disease, may be extremely painful.

Tenderness

Palpation of the joints may elicit tenderness, and counting the number of tender joints is a major endpoint of clinical

TABLE 10.2. AMERICAN COLLEGE OF RHEUMATOLOGY DISEASE ACTIVITY MEASURES FOR RHEUMATOID ARTHRITIS CORE SET

Disease Activity Measure
1. Tender joint count
2. Swollen joint count
3. Patient's assessment of pain
4. Patient's global assessment of disease activity
5. Physician's global assessment of disease activity
6. Patient's assessment of physical function
7. Acute-phase reactant value

For trial duration ≥1 year and agent being tested as a disease-modifying antirheumatic drug (DMARD), also perform radiography or other imaging technique.
To meet improvement requirement, both 1 and 2 and three of measures 3 through 7 must improve by a specified amount.
From O'Dell JR. Rheumatoid arthritis: the clinical picture. In: Koopman WJ, ed. *Arthritis and allied conditions: a textbook of rheumatology*, 14th edition. Philadelphia: Lippincott Williams & Wilkins, 2001:1153–1186, with permission.

trials to demonstrate the effectiveness of therapies (Table 10.2). A lateral squeeze of the metacarpophalangeal and metatarsophalangeal joint row will detect tenderness in inflamed joints. Tenderness of three or all four of these joint areas occurs almost exclusively in patients with RA (12). Severe muscle tenderness should suggest another diagnosis, such as fibromyalgia.

Swelling

Joint swelling is a seminal finding for the diagnosis of RA and is a major endpoint of therapeutic trials (Table 10.2). Swelling of a joint may result from proliferation of the synovial tissues, effusions, or bony proliferation. In RA the first two processes predominate, whereas bony proliferation around joints should suggest another type of process, such as OA. This soft-tissue swelling is most evident in the small joints of the hands and feet, particularly in the PIPs, MCPs, and MTPs (Fig. 10.2).

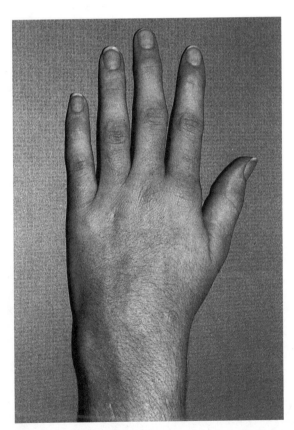

FIGURE 10.2. Fusiform swelling and erythema about the proximal interphalangeal joints, most marked in the long finger. Swelling at the metacarpophalangeal joints has caused loss of definition of joint margins. The extensor carpi ulnaris tendon sheath (sixth dorsal compartment of the wrist) has synovial thickening and swelling. (From O'Dell JR. Rheumatoid arthritis: the clinical picture. In: Koopman WJ, ed. *Arthritis and allied conditions: a textbook of rheumatology,* 14th ed. Philadelphia: Lippincott Williams & Wilkins, 2001:1153–1186, with permission.)

If synovial proliferation is abundant, a doughy texture may be felt due to the resultant soft-tissue mass. Synovial proliferation is also commonly identified in the elbow, ankle, MTP, and knee joints, as well as in the flexor tendons of the fingers, the common extensor compartment of the dorsal wrist, and the extensor carpi ulnaris tendon sheath (Fig. 10.2). Swelling in the hip and shoulder joints may be difficult to ascertain on physical examination, unless it is severe.

Joint effusions also contribute to swelling. When the effusion is put under increased pressure with joint flexion, the synovium may be forced between articular structures and a portion becomes trapped and separated from the rest of the joint, forming a Baker cyst. More fluid is forced into the structure with subsequent loading of the distended joint, and a one-way valve effect may prevent the fluid from returning to the joint. Baker cysts were originally described in the knee, and although a similar phenomenon may be seen in most peripheral joints (13), they are most commonly recognized in the knee, where the larger the effusion, the more likely there will be a painful cyst. Dissection of a Baker cyst most often occurs in the posterior calf and often presents with only mild symptoms, such as a feeling of fullness. However, rupture of a Baker cyst at the knee generally produces significant soft-tissue swelling and pain in the calf, and may resemble acute thrombophlebitis, so-called pseudothrombophlebitis syndrome (14). It is important to differentiate this syndrome from deep vein thrombosis, since anticoagulation of patients with a ruptured Baker cyst will result in increased bleeding into the calf and increased pain.

Deformity

Joint deformities develop over time as the inflammatory process damages articular and supporting structures. Joint effusions, which seem benign, particularly if the patient does not complain of symptoms, lead to stretching of tendons and ligaments and, if allowed to persist, will result in deformities and disability. The small joints of the hands and feet are particularly susceptible to this. Greater than 10% of RA patients develop deformity of the small joints of the hands within the first 2 years of disease, and at least one-third develop such deformities over time (15). This phenomenon may result in the seemingly paradoxical situation where deformities become more pronounced as the synovitis is controlled and the joint effusions resolve.

Unfortunately, once deformities develop they are permanent; therefore initiating treatment early to prevent this is crucial. All too often clinicians wait until obvious deformities are present before effective treatments are pursued.

Effects of Rheumatoid Arthritis on Specific Joints

Fingers

Nonreducible flexion at the proximal interphalangeal joint with concomitant hyperextension of the distal interphalangeal (DIP) joint of the finger (boutonniere deformity, Fig. 10.3) occurs. Hyperextension at the proximal interphalangeal joint with flexion of the distal interphalangeal joint (swan-neck deformity, Fig. 10.4) may also be seen in RA. Lupus has a particular predilection for the proximal interphalangeal joints and often produces reducible swan-neck deformities, but boutonniere deformities are almost never seen in lupus.

"Triggering" of the finger occurs when thickening or nodule formation of the tendon interacts with the concomitant tenosynovial proliferation, trapping the tendon

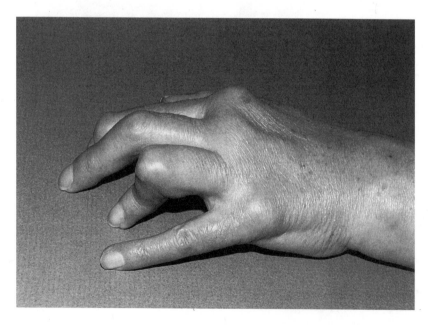

FIGURE 10.3. A boutonniere deformity of the ring finger, flexion deformity of the long finger proximal interphalangeal joint, and mild swan neck deformity of the index finger. Extensive synovitis at the metacarpophalangeal joints obscures the usual definition of joint margins. (From O'Dell JR. Rheumatoid arthritis: the clinical picture. In: Koopman WJ, ed. *Arthritis and allied conditions: a textbook of rheumatology,* 14th ed. Philadelphia: Lippincott Williams & Wilkins, 2001:1153–1186, with permission.)

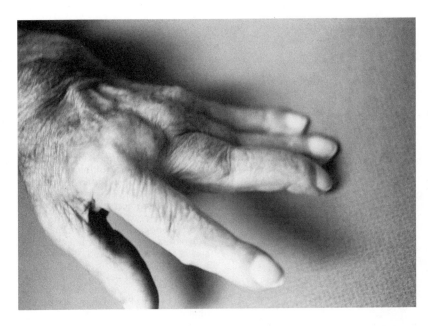

FIGURE 10.4. Swan neck deformities of long, ring, and little fingers, with concomitant subluxation of the metacarpophalangeal joints. (From O'Dell JR. Rheumatoid arthritis: the clinical picture. In: Koopman WJ, ed. *Arthritis and allied conditions: a textbook of rheumatology,* 14th ed. Philadelphia: Lippincott Williams & Wilkins, 2001:1153–1186, with permission.)

(stenosing tenosynovitis). Tendon rupture may occur due to infiltrative synovitis in the digit or bony erosions that produce surfaces that cut the tendon at the wrist (especially the flexor pollicis longus). Arthritis mutilans ("opera glass hands") results if destruction is severe and extensive, with dissolution of bone (Fig. 10.5).

Metacarpophalangeal Joints

Two typical deformities may occur at the metacarpophalangeal (MCP) joints—volar subluxation of the fingers relative to the metacarpal bones and ulnar deviation (Fig.

10.6). Most cases of ulnar deviation are accompanied by radial deviation of the wrist, roughly proportional to the degree of ulnar deviation of the fingers. Although RA is the most common cause of ulnar deviation, other arthritides, as well as certain neurologic deficiencies, may result in ulnar deviation as well.

Wrists

The wrist is the site of multiple problems in patients with RA. The combination of ulnar drift of the fingers and radial deviation of the wrist is known as a "zig-zag" deformity

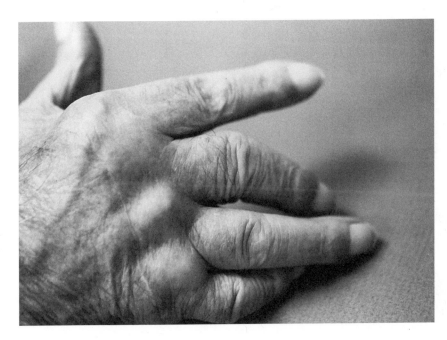

FIGURE 10.5. Arthritis mutilans. Rheumatoid arthritis has destroyed the long proximal interphalangeal joint. Deflection of the distal portion of the phalanx is due to the pull of gravity. (From O'Dell JR. Rheumatoid arthritis: the clinical picture. In: Koopman WJ, ed. *Arthritis and allied conditions: a textbook of rheumatology,* 14th ed. Philadelphia: Lippincott Williams & Wilkins, 2001:1153–1186, with permission.)

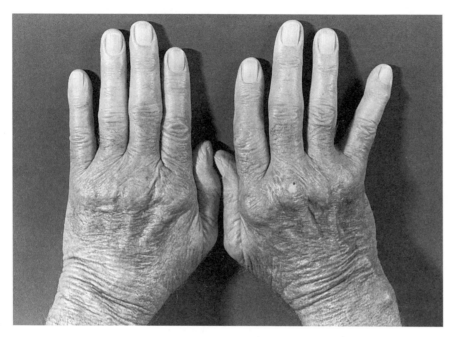

FIGURE 10.6. Subcutaneous tissue atrophy, metacarpophalangeal joint proliferative synovitis with loss of joint definition, and mild proximal interphalangeal joint enlargement. There is slight volar subluxation of the metacarpophalangeal joints and mild ulnar deviation at the metacarpophalangeal joints of the right hand. Involvement of the dominant (right) hand is more pronounced. (From O'Dell JR. Rheumatoid arthritis: the clinical picture. In: Koopman WJ, ed. *Arthritis and allied conditions: a textbook of rheumatology,* 14th ed. Philadelphia: Lippincott Williams & Wilkins, 2001:1153–1186, with permission.)

(Fig. 10.7). Wrist subluxation may lead to rupture of the extensor tendons of the little, ring, and long fingers (Fig. 10.8), as the end of the distal ulna may be roughened secondary to erosion of bone and may abrade the tendons as they move back and forth during normal hand function.

Entrapment of the median nerve as it passes through the carpal tunnel (carpal tunnel syndrome) leads to decreased sensation on the palmar aspect of the thumb, index, long, and radial aspect of the ring fingers, and later to weakness and atrophy of the muscles in the thenar eminence (Fig. 10.9). These symptoms are often most prominent at night and frequently awaken patients. Patients generally report pain, numbness, and/or tingling in the hand. This awakening from sleep may be one reason that patients do not always give a history of the classic cutaneous distribution. In RA, median nerve decompression should be entertained before significant atrophy of the thenar eminence has occurred.

Elbow

Elbow involvement is often detected by palpable synovial proliferation at the radiohumeral joint and commonly is

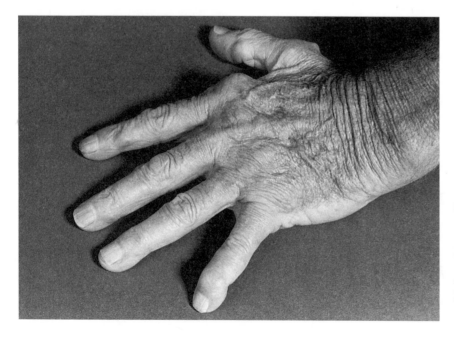

FIGURE 10.7. "Zigzag" deformity with ulnar deviation of the fingers at the metacarpophalangeal joints and clockwise rotation of carpus on distal radius. (From O'Dell JR. Rheumatoid arthritis: the clinical picture. In: Koopman WJ, ed. *Arthritis and allied conditions: a textbook of rheumatology,* 14th ed. Philadelphia: Lippincott Williams & Wilkins, 2001:1153–1186, with permission.)

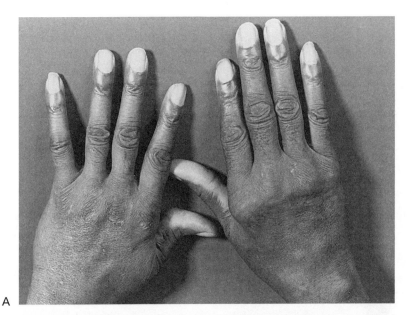

A

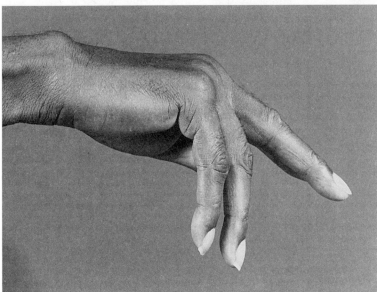

B

FIGURE 10.8. A: More extensive involvement of the dominant (right) hand. Early volar subluxation of the metacarpophalangeal joints and a "doughy" synovitis are present. Subluxation of the right radioulnar joint with dorsal ulnar styloid subluxation is evident. **B:** A lateral view showing the dorsal subluxation of the ulnar styloid. The ability to extend the little and ring fingers fully has been lost due to rupture of the extensor tendons at the ulnar styloid. (From O'Dell JR. Rheumatoid arthritis: the clinical picture. In: Koopman WJ, ed. *Arthritis and allied conditions: a textbook of rheumatology,* 14th ed. Philadelphia: Lippincott Williams & Wilkins, 2001:1153–1186, with permission.)

accompanied by a flexion deformity. If synovitis or effusion is present in the elbow, complete extension will not occur; therefore complete extension is an excellent sign that significant synovitis or effusion is not present. Olecranon bursal involvement is common, as are rheumatoid nodules in the bursa and along the extensor surface of the ulna.

Shoulders

Shoulders are commonly involved, with nocturnal pain being particularly troubling, as it is often difficult for patients with shoulder problems to find a comfortable position for sleep. Swelling occurs initially anteriorly but may

be difficult to detect and is present on examination in a minority of patients at any point in time.

Feet and Ankles

Ankle joint involvement is seldom seen in the absence of midfoot or metatarsophalangeal involvement. Major structural changes occur in the midfoot and foot due to the combination of chronic synovitis and weight bearing. Posterior tibialis tendon involvement or rupture may lead to subtalar subluxation, which results in eversion and migration of the talus laterally. Midfoot disease leads to loss of normal arch contour with flattening of the feet (Fig. 10.10).

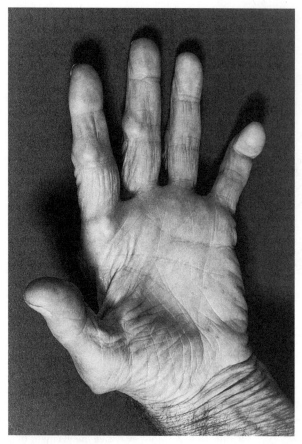

FIGURE 10.9. Sequelae of carpal tunnel syndrome, with thenar eminence atrophy. Rheumatoid nodules are present at the index and long proximal interphalangeal joints. Traumatic disruption of the little finger distal interphalangeal joint has led to a swan neck deformity. (From O'Dell JR. Rheumatoid arthritis: the clinical picture. In: Koopman WJ, ed. *Arthritis and allied conditions: a textbook of rheumatology,* 14th ed. Philadelphia: Lippincott Williams & Wilkins, 2001:1153–1186, with permission.)

Metatarsophalangeal joint inflammation occurs in most patients and is often one of the earliest disease manifestations. The great toe typically develops hallux valgus (bunion). Subluxation of the phalanx at the metatarsophalangeal joint of the other toes is predominantly dorsally (Fig. 10.11). The toes may exhibit compensatory flexion due to a fixed length of the flexor tendons, resulting in "hammer toes" (named because they resemble piano key hammers). When dorsal subluxation occurs, the soft-tissue pad on the plantar surface of the metatarsal heads is displaced, allowing the metatarsal heads to protrude and become the primary weight-bearing surface. This is painful and calluses develop. This results in patients feeling that they are always walking around with pebbles in their shoes.

Knees

Knees may develop large effusions and abundant proliferation of synovium (Fig. 10.12). Persistent effusions may lead to inhibition of quadricep function by spinal reflexes with subsequent atrophy. With chronic effusions the knee is more comfortable in the flexed position, and flexion deformities occur that greatly increase the work expended to walk. Baker cysts are common and have been discussed earlier.

Hips

Limited motion or pain with internal and/or external rotation is the hallmark of hip involvement. Patients with true hip joint pathology have pain in the mid-groin with rotation or with weight bearing.

Cervical Spine

Neck pain on motion and occipital headache are common manifestations of cervical spine involvement and occur in

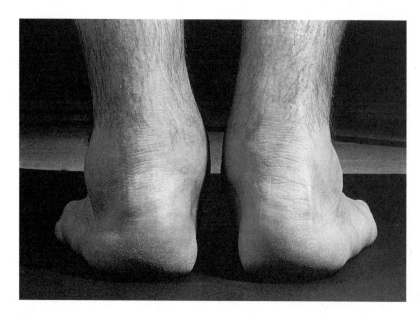

FIGURE 10.10. Marked ankle and midfoot synovitis. There is also loss of definition of the arch and eversion at the subtalar joint. (From O'Dell JR. Rheumatoid arthritis: the clinical picture. In: Koopman WJ, ed. *Arthritis and allied conditions: a textbook of rheumatology,* 14th ed. Philadelphia: Lippincott Williams & Wilkins, 2001:1153–1186, with permission.)

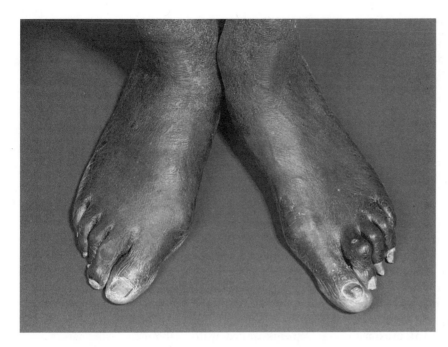

FIGURE 10.11. Mild hallux valgus, with dorsal subluxation of the metatarsophalangeal joints and resultant "hammer toe" deformities of second through fifth toes. Midfoot instability has lead to eversion, with concomitant flattening of the feet. (From O'Dell JR. Rheumatoid arthritis: the clinical picture. In: Koopman WJ, ed. *Arthritis and allied conditions: a textbook of rheumatology,* 14th ed. Philadelphia: Lippincott Williams & Wilkins, 2001:1153–1186, with permission.)

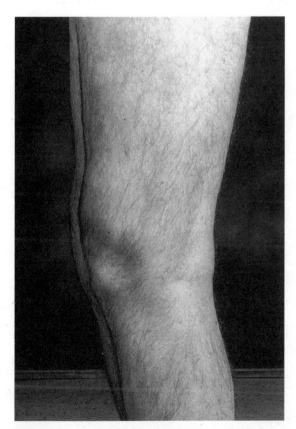

FIGURE 10.12. Lateral view of a patient with rheumatoid arthritis affecting the knees. There is quadriceps atrophy, marked synovial proliferation with joint effusion in the suprapatellar pouch, and fullness in the popliteal space due to a small synovial (Baker) cyst. (From O'Dell JR. Rheumatoid arthritis: the clinical picture. In: Koopman WJ, ed. *Arthritis and allied conditions: a textbook of rheumatology,* 14th ed. Philadelphia: Lippincott Williams & Wilkins, 2001:1153–1186, with permission.)

most patients with persistent disease for more than 10 years (16). The atlantoaxial joint is a synovium-lined joint and is susceptible to the same proliferative synovitis and subsequent instability that are seen in the peripheral joints. Patients generally do fine when they are in control of their neck motion but may experience problems when others try to flex their neck, as when attempting to obtain good flexion x-rays or helping the patient into a fetal position to perform a lumbar puncture. One should consider the possibility of significant C1–C2 instability before a patient with RA undergoes surgical procedures to avoid compromise to the cervical cord or brainstem during intubation or as the patient is transferred while asleep. Patients with severe destruction in the hands (arthritis mutilans) are very likely to have symptomatic cervical spine abnormalities, as are those taking significant amounts of corticosteroids.

Cricoarytenoid Joint

Since synovial tissue is present around the cricoarytenoid joint involvement may occur in up to one-fourth of RA patients. A fullness that is aggravated by speaking or swallowing is usually the initial symptom. Hoarseness and inspiratory symptoms may develop. Severe involvement may produce enough restriction of joint motion to cause acute, life-threatening dyspnea, and emergent tracheotomy may be required.

Extraarticular Manifestations

Rarely, a patient presents with extraarticular manifestations before the onset of arthritis. Extraarticular manifestations clearly demonstrate that RA is a systemic disease that is able to affect multiple organs through chronic inflammation.

TABLE 10.3. EXTRAARTICULAR MANIFESTATIONS OF RHEUMATOID ARTHRITIS

Heart	Pericarditis, premature atherosclerosis, vasculitis, valvular, and valve ring nodules
Lung	Pleural effusions, interstitial lung disease, bronchiolitis obliterans, rheumatoid nodules, vasculitis
Skin	Nodules, fragility, vasculitis
Neurologic	Entrapment neuropathy, cervical myelopathy, mononeuritis multiplex (vasculitis), peripheral neuropathy
Hematopoietic	Anemia, thrombocytosis, lymphadenopathy, Felty's syndrome
Bone	Osteopenia
Eye	Keratoconjunctivitis sicca, episcleritis, scleritis, scleromalacia perforans, peripheral ulcerative keratopathy
Kidney	Amyloidosis, vasculitis

From O'Dell JR. Rheumatoid arthritis: the clinical picture. In: Koopman WJ, ed. *Arthritis and allied conditions: a textbook of rheumatology, 14th edition.* Philadelphia: Lippincott Williams & Wilkins, 2001:1153–1186, with permission.

Vasculitis, serositis, and effects in part due to inflammatory mediators (anemia, osteopenia, and skin fragility) may be seen (Table 10.3). They occur almost exclusively in patients with RF, and their presence suggests a poor prognosis (17).

Rheumatoid nodules occur in about a quarter of RA patients (18). They are most commonly found on extensor surfaces, on sites of frequent mechanical irritation, or over joints. The olecranon process (Fig. 10.13), proximal ulna, back of the heels, occiput, and ischial tuberosities are common periosteal sites for their development. They may also form in subcutaneous tissues of the finger (Fig. 10.14), toe, and heel pads; in tendons; and in viscera. RF is almost invariably present, and if absent, other diagnoses, such as chronic tophus gout, should be entertained.

Patients treated with methotrexate who have a good response to their articular inflammation may have a seemingly paradoxical rapid increase in the number of nodules.

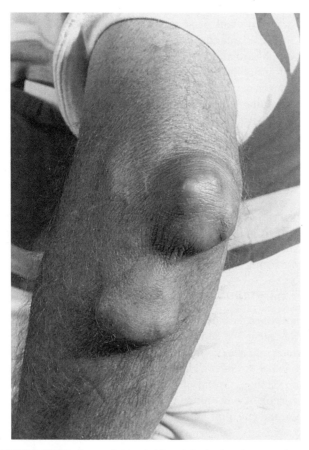

FIGURE 10.13. Large rheumatoid nodules in the olecranon bursa and along the extensor surface of the proximal ulna; each mass is a collection of multiple smaller nodules. A small effusion is present in the olecranon bursa. (From O'Dell JR. Rheumatoid arthritis: the clinical picture. In: Koopman WJ, ed. *Arthritis and allied conditions: a textbook of rheumatology,* 14th ed. Philadelphia: Lippincott Williams & Wilkins, 2001:1153–1186, with permission.)

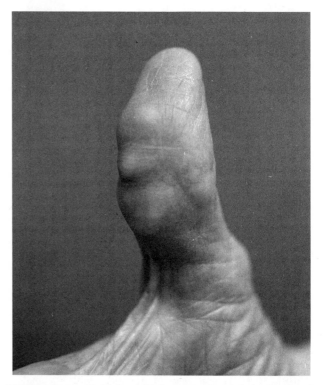

FIGURE 10.14. Multiple small rheumatoid nodule in the thumb pad over sites of use. This patient experienced an increase in the number of nodules after the initiation of methotrexate therapy. (From O'Dell JR. Rheumatoid arthritis: the clinical picture. In: Koopman WJ, ed. *Arthritis and allied conditions: a textbook of rheumatology,* 14th ed. Philadelphia: Lippincott Williams & Wilkins, 2001:1153–1186, with permission.)

IMAGING

Conventional Radiography

Radiologic evaluation of patients with RA may be performed initially to aid in diagnosis but thereafter is used to assess the course of disease, response to therapy, and need for surgical interventions. The ability of therapeutic agents to slow the radiographic progression of RA has been considered the gold standard of efficacy and is therefore a key outcome measure in clinical trials (Table 10.2). Osteopenia is commonly seen in the periarticular regions. Bone mineral density of the lumbar spine assessed by dual-energy absorptiometry can decline within the first few months of disease and is greater with more severe disease. DMARDs can have a significant sparing effect on osteoporosis in RA, indicating that control of synovitis may prevent or reverse the osteopenia (19).

Radiologic changes that are irreversible include erosion of bone, joint space narrowing, ankylosis (rarely seen), and malalignment. Radiologic erosion represents loss of cortical bone and takes place initially at the margin of the joint ["bare area" (20)], where the synovium approximates bone without intervening cartilage (Fig. 10.15).

Table 10.4 compares and contrasts the radiographic features of the two most common kinds of arthritis. Although diffuse joint space narrowing is commonly seen in other

TABLE 10.4. CONTRASTING RADIOGRAPHIC FEATURES

	Rheumatoid Arthritis	Osteoarthritis
Sclerosis	±	++++
Osteophytes	±	++++
Osteopenia	+++	0
Symmetry	+++	+
Erosions	+++	0
Cysts	++	++
Narrowing	+++	+++

From O'Dell JR. Rheumatoid arthritis: the clinical picture. In: Koopman WJ, ed. *Arthritis and allied conditions: a textbook of rheumatology, 14th edition.* Philadelphia: Lippincott Williams & Wilkins, 2001:1153–1186, with permission.

types of chronic inflammatory arthritis, in conjunction with marginal erosion and osteopenia, it is highly characteristic of RA. The small joints of the hands and feet commonly exhibit both erosion and joint space narrowing, whereas the knee and hip have a predominance of joint space narrowing (Fig. 10.16).

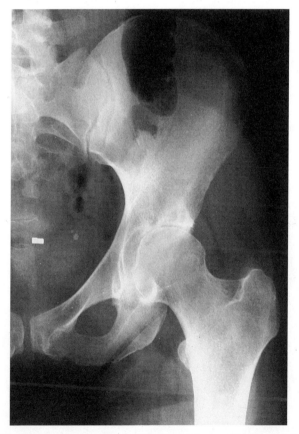

FIGURE 10.16. Hip radiograph of a patient with rheumatoid arthritis. There are diffuse joint space narrowing, small cysts in the femoral head and acetabulum, and little reparative bony change. (From O'Dell JR. Rheumatoid arthritis: the clinical picture. In: Koopman WJ, ed. *Arthritis and allied conditions: a textbook of rheumatology,* 14th ed. Philadelphia: Lippincott Williams & Wilkins, 2001:1153–1186, with permission.)

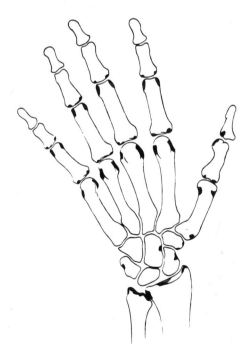

FIGURE 10.15. "Bare areas" in the hand described by Martel et al. These are intraarticular sites of bone not covered with cartilage and susceptible to direct attack by the rheumatoid synovial pannus. (Reprinted by permission from Martel W, Hayes JT, Duff IF. The pattern of bone erosion in the hand and wrist in rheumatoid arthritis. *Radiology* 1965;84:204–214.)

Radiologic evidence of damage (erosion) occurs in almost all patients with RA who are seropositive for RF and are followed for more than 5 years. In one notable study, 99% of RF-positive patients had erosions at follow-up (21). The initial changes may occur early in the course of disease, especially in the hands, where studies show erosion in 20% to 50% of patients in the first 2 or 3 years. Destructive changes of the hip, knee, ankle, shoulder, and elbow joints occur later than those in the hands. Damage in the hands and wrists may be more marked in the dominant hand and in the joints used most heavily (the second MCP more than the fourth MCP), presumably a reflection of increased mechanical stress, as well as increased inflammation that may result from use.

Cervical spine radiographic abnormalities may include atlantoaxial (C1–C2) subluxation, superior migration of the odontoid, subaxial arthritis, and collapse of the lateral masses of C1 from erosion at the facet joints. Erosion of the odontoid (Fig. 10.17) accompanied by invasion and damage of the transverse ligament and alar ligaments (attachments from the odontoid process to the occipital condyles) by pannus lead to instability. Atlantoaxial subluxation is often the initial abnormality and is demonstrated by comparing lateral cervical spine films in extension, when subluxation should be minimal, and in flexion, when the subluxation is maximal with protrusion of the odontoid into the neural canal (Fig. 10.18). Risk for myelopathy increases with progressive C1–C2 subluxation, especially with superior migration of the odontoid (22); those with C1–C2 subluxation over 10 mm are especially at risk. If erosion is severe, the odontoid may fracture or even disappear, allowing posterior subluxation of C1–C2 to occur.

Scintigraphy

Articular inflammation may be documented by increased localization of radionuclide to the joint. Since this is a sensitive technique that may show abnormalities before synovitis is apparent on physical examination, and certainly before radiographic abnormalities occur, it is occasionally used to document the presence of an inflammatory arthropathy in patients with suggestive histories and normal examinations. Scintigraphy is not recommended during the routine workup or monitoring.

Magnetic Resonance Imaging

Studies in hands and wrists have documented the ability of magnetic resonance imaging (MRI) to detect inflammation in tendon sheaths, early abnormalities in carpal bones, and reduction in cartilage thickness before abnormalities appear on conventional radiographs. However, the significance of erosions seen only on MRI (i.e., whether they progress to radiographically detectable lesions) is unknown. MRI results are now appearing in some clinical trials and may provide a way to monitor radiographic progression that is both safe and more rapidly responsive to therapy. However, this is a very costly modality, and currently there is little use for MRI in the routine diagnosis or monitoring of patients with RA.

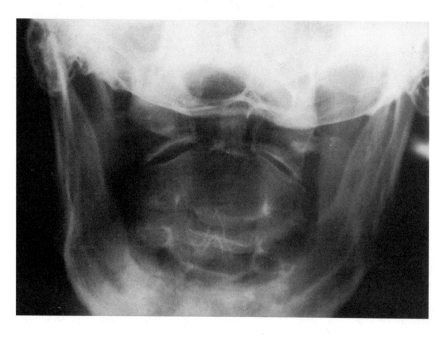

FIGURE 10.17. Anteroposterior radiograph of the C1–C2 articulation showing facet joint space narrowing on the patient's left (patient is facing the observer) and erosion at the base of the odontoid. Both findings are typical for rheumatoid arthritis. (From O'Dell JR. Rheumatoid arthritis: the clinical picture. In: Koopman WJ, ed. *Arthritis and allied conditions: a textbook of rheumatology,* 14th ed. Philadelphia: Lippincott Williams & Wilkins, 2001:1153–1186, with permission.)

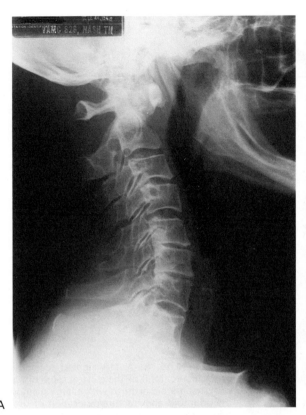 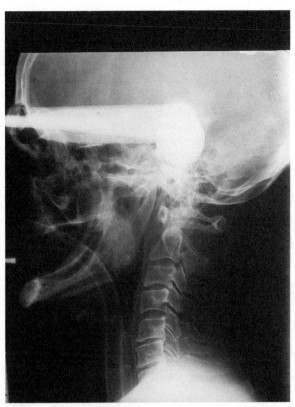

A

B

FIGURE 10.18. A: Lateral flexion view of a rheumatoid arthritis patient with 12 mm of C1–C2 anterior subluxation (distance between the odontoid peg and the C1 arch anterior to the peg). C5–C6 and C6–C7 disc space narrowing is also noted. **B:** The same patient as in **A** after cervical spine stabilization by a "halo," with reduction of the subluxation. (From O'Dell JR. Rheumatoid arthritis: the clinical picture. In: Koopman WJ, ed. *Arthritis and allied conditions: a textbook of rheumatology,* 14th ed. Philadelphia: Lippincott Williams & Wilkins, 2001:1153–1186, with permission.)

MRI of the cervical cord, on the other hand, is superior to other modalities, and its use is routine in the evaluation of patients suspected of serious cervical spine disease. MRI may demonstrate impingement of the cervical cord with synovial pannus about the odontoid, impression of the medulla by upward migration of the odontoid, or impingement of the cervical cord by subaxial subluxations (Fig. 10.19).

LABORATORY MEASURES

Rheumatoid Factor

The term *rheumatoid factor* (RF) is unfortunate; it makes everyone immediately think of RA. *RF is not a diagnostic test.* The presence of RF does not establish the diagnosis of RA, nor does its absence rule out the diagnosis. RF may be seen in many clinical settings other than RA. In most surveys of patients seen in a clinical setting, about three-fourths of RA patients have a positive RF test. Various investigators have found that the presence of RF bears some relationship to the onset of RA. In one series, RF was present in about 33% of patients within 3 months of onset of disease, another 40% developed RF within the next 9 months, and the remainder who developed RF did so after the first 12 months of disease [12% were persistently seronegative in this report (23)].

Many illnesses that induce chronic immune stimulation may lead to the presence of RF. Smoking has been shown to be associated with both a higher incidence of RF and an increased risk of developing RA in males (24). The majority of studies have found that the presence of RF increases with age in the general population.

Acute-Phase Reactants

Systemic inflammation induces the production by the liver of a number of proteins, which are known as acute-phase reactants (24a,24b). These include fibrinogen, C-reactive protein (CRP), amyloid A protein (SAA), amyloid P protein (SAP), haptoglobin, ferritin, ceruloplasmin, and others. Clinical measurement of these proteins is largely restricted to CRP and evaluation of the erythrocyte sedimentation rate (ESR).

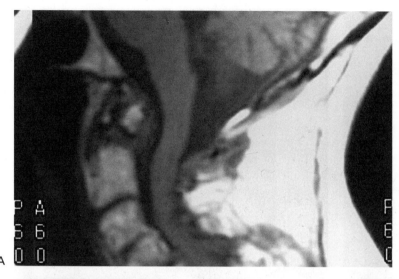

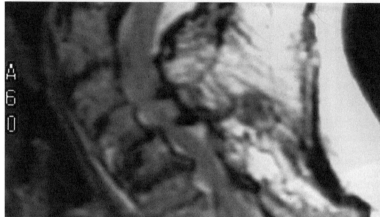

FIGURE 10.19. A: A T1-weighted magnetic resonance image (MRI) of the cervical spine of a patient with rheumatoid arthritis with a large pannus about the odontoid and fracture/dislocation of the odontoid from the body of C2. **B:** Same patient as in **A** demonstrating extensive subluxation with impingement on the spinal canal at C3–C4, C4–C5, and C5–C6. (From O'Dell JR. Rheumatoid arthritis: the clinical picture. In: Koopman WJ, ed. *Arthritis and allied conditions: a textbook of rheumatology,* 14th ed. Philadelphia: Lippincott Williams & Wilkins, 2001:1153–1186, with permission.)

Fibrinogen concentration, the major determinant of the ESR, takes 3 to 5 days to reach maximal levels after an acute stimulus and a comparable time to return to normal levels. CRP levels rise rapidly after a stimulus (within hours) and decay within days after the stimulus resolves.

Sequential monitoring of either the ESR or CRP levels to assess the level of systemic inflammation in RA is reasonable, especially when physical signs may be hard to interpret (e.g., assessing swelling in an obese person, assessing swelling and tenderness in a patient with severely damaged joints, or assessing tenderness in a patient with a very low pain threshold). The magnitude of elevation of the ESR over time (area under the curve) is strongly associated with radiographic erosions (25). While the use of the ESR is more widespread, the CRP may more closely reflect current disease activity.

Anemia and Thrombocytosis

An anemia of chronic disease is commonly seen in patients with RA, and the severity of this anemia correlates with disease activity. Anemia due to iron deficiency may occur secondary to gastrointestinal blood loss. The former is charac-terized by a low serum iron with normal iron stores and a blunted response to erythropoietin. The actions of cytokines commonly elaborated at sites of inflammation in RA, including interleukin-1 (IL-1) and tumor necrosis factor-α (TNF-α), impair iron metabolism and erythropoiesis in the marrow. In general, effective treatment of the disease results in an improvement in the anemia, but many of the drugs used for treatment may also result in bone marrow depression. Interestingly, patients with RA have a significantly reduced mortality from gastrointestinal malignancies (26), possibly because of chronic NSAID therapy.

Platelet counts often parallel acute-phase reactants and are elevated in active RA, usually in association with other extraarticular manifestations. In these instances platelet counts tend to be inversely correlated with the hematocrit.

ASSESSING PATIENT STATUS: SETTING A TREATMENT GOAL

The status of the individual patient at any point in time should always be assessed relative to treatment goals (27).

Specific treatment goals are well accepted and easy to understand in such conditions as hypertension, hyperlipidemia, or diabetes. In RA, goals are more difficult to quantify but no less important. It is impossible to evaluate the effectiveness of treatment without a goal. With improving therapies, remission is becoming a more realistic, although still elusive, goal. No one single measure adequately describes the status of a patient with RA. Rather, combinations of abnormalities detected by laboratory testing, physical examination, radiologic examination, and assessment of pain and functional status are used. The American College of Rheumatology (ACR) has recommended a core set of composite criteria (Table 10.2) for the evaluation of therapies in patients with RA (11). The components of this core set are excellent parameters to follow in individual patients in clinical practice, as well as in clinical research situations. A 20% improvement level has been set as the minimum required to show efficacy of a drug over placebo. This requires that both the tender and swollen joint counts be improved by this amount and that three of the five parameters below the line show similar degrees of improvement. Increasingly, rheumatologists are not satisfied with this modest degree of improvement and are adjusting therapies to achieve ACR 50% or ACR 70% responses (improvement of parameters by 50% and 70%, respectively).

For the short-term management of patients, parameters that assess acute inflammation are the most helpful, since most current medical interventions are aimed primarily at controlling the inflammatory response. Recording the joints that are swollen and tender at each patient encounter will document ongoing inflammation. Acute-phase reactants (ESR or CRP) may also be useful parameters to follow intermittently. Time-integrated ESR has been shown to be strongly correlated with radiographic progression (25). Joints that are persistently swollen over time, as opposed to those that are merely tender, are more likely to become damaged, which emphasizes the need to assess this parameter carefully.

COURSE OF ILLNESS

Remission

Criteria for clinical remission include absence of fatigue, absence of joint pain by history, absence of synovial swelling, absence of joint tenderness, normal sedimentation rate, and morning stiffness of less than 15 minutes. The patient must meet five of these six criteria to be classified as being in remission (28). In population studies, where few patients have RF or radiologic damage (and do not fulfill 1987 ACR classification criteria for RA), the majority of patients are in remission within 3 to 5 years. For patients seen in medical settings, however, only about 15% have a remission or normal functional status a decade later.

Work Disability and Costs

Significant functional declines and work disability occur in RA patients (1). One study reports three-fourths of RA patients changed jobs due to the illness and more than half became disabled within a decade. Another study has shown that one-quarter of RA patients are unable to work just 6.4 years after diagnosis and half cannot work after 20 years (29). The loss of income over time is the greatest financial burden, far surpassing direct medical costs. Lifetime costs of RA are comparable to those for coronary artery disease or stroke. Emerging data show that early consistent use of DMARDs can improve long-term functional outcomes (30).

Factors Affecting Outcome

Age of Onset and Gender

In patients less than 50 years of age, women tend to have a worse prognosis with regard to persistence and severity of disease. *Benign RA of the aged* may include those with RS3PE and polymyalgia rheumatica, as well as mild seronegative RA, and have a relatively good prognosis. Older patients with seropositive RA appear to have immunogenetic profiles and clinical courses similar to those of younger patients. Early aggressive therapy is especially important, as older patients typically have less reserve.

Smoking

Smoking appears to make RA worse (31) and may be a risk factor for developing RA. One study found that smokers are more likely to be seropositive, to have nodules, and to have radiographic erosions (31). Evidence that smoking cessation can ameliorate disease has not yet appeared. RA patients have a significant increased morbidity from cardiovascular disease, from infections (particularly pulmonary infections), and from osteoporosis. The roll of smoking in exacerbating these issues may be significant.

Joint Involvement

Table 10.5 lists the joints involved in a cross section of patients with well-established disease (median duration of 10 years) attending a rheumatology clinic (32). Similar patterns of involvement have also been documented in RA patients participating in clinical trials. Small joints are invariably involved, with metacarpophalangeal involvement most common. Deformities may take years to develop, although in one group of RA patients hand deformities developed in 15% of patients within the first 2 years of disease.

Radiographic Damage

Damage as depicted by radiographs occurs within the first several years of disease in most RA patients followed in

TABLE 10.5. PERCENTAGE OF RHEUMATOID ARTHRITIS PATIENTS WITH ABNORMALITIES IN SPECIFIC JOINTS SEEN IN AN OUTPATIENT SETTING[a]

Joint	Swelling	Tenderness	Pain on Motion	Limitation of Motion	Deformity
Temporomandibular (TM)	3	17	9	21	—
Sternoclavicular (SC)	3	11	1	—	—
Acromioclavicular (AC)	0	22	3	—	—
Shoulder	0	21	52	43	4
Elbow	26	35	25	34	36
Wrist	66	55	58	71	35
Metacarpophalangeal (MCP) index[b]	82	51	24	34	31
Proximal interphalangeal (PIP) index[b]	36	40	23	35	24
Hip	—	5	19	18	1
Knee	33	38	34	11	11
Ankle	40	38	34	29	5
Subtalar	7	5	11	16	3
Tarsometatarsal	11	11	19	23	3
Metatarsophalangeal (MTP) great[b]	24	42	12	6	38

Scoring as in ref. 41 with right side reported. Less than 10% of patients had swollen or tender finger, distal interphalangeal (DIP), or toe PIP joints.
[a]Not evaluated.
[b]Values for index MCP and PIP joints shown as representative joints of these rows of joints; values for great MTP joints shown as representative of this row of joints.
Adapted from Fuchs HA, Brooks RH, Callahan LF, et al. A simplified twenty-eight-joint quantitative articular index in rheumatoid arthritis. *Arthritis Rheum* 1989;32:531–537.

rheumatology clinics. Clinical parameters that predict the development of destructive radiologic changes in the hands and wrists over time include persistently swollen joints, elevation of acute-phase reactants (25), RF, and certain HLA-DR4 subtypes.

Mortality

Mortality rates are increased at least twofold for RA patients and are related to disease severity. Up to one-third of deaths may be directly attributable to the disease itself (2), with increases in the rates of cardiovascular and infectious causes seen as well.

Mortality is correlated with the arthritis itself, in that prognosis is worse in those with the greatest number of abnormal joints (2). Involvement of large joints suggests a worse prognosis than synovitis restricted to hands and feet, and rarely occurs without concomitant involvement of the small joints.

DIFFERENTIAL DIAGNOSIS

When presented with a patient who has joint pain, the first challenge is to discern if the problem is due to mechanical derangements, OA, or inflammation. Stiffness, swelling, tenderness, warmth, and pain with motion are hallmarks of active inflammation in the joint. The presence of severe morning stiffness is indicative of an inflammatory process; gelling of the joints for merely a few minutes in the morning and after rest is more consistent with OA.

The diagnosis of RA is most difficult in early disease or when relatively few joints are involved; unfortunately, diagnosis is usually delayed several months after the onset of symptoms, limiting the initiation of early treatment. Distinguishing RA from other causes of chronic inflammatory arthritis or transient synovitis syndromes (e.g., postviral) early is difficult. Seropositivity for RF and fulfillment of the 1987 ACR criteria for classification of RA increases the likelihood of correct diagnosis (33).

Other Rheumatologic Causes of Inflammatory Arthritis

Signs and symptoms of inflammatory arthritis may be associated with many syndromes other than RA. A history directed at eliciting the associated features of other arthritides is essential. Thus the presence of photosensitivity or nephritis should suggest the possibility of systemic lupus erythematosus (SLE), and conjunctivitis and dactylitis should suggest reactive arthritis. Systemic vasculitis, such as polyarteritis nodosa or Wegener granulomatosis, may be associated with disabling joint pain, although objective signs of arthritis are infrequent. Finally, hypothyroidism can produce rheumatic symptoms, and is seen in increased association with RA.

Spondyloarthropathies

The spondyloarthropathies (reactive arthritis, some types of psoriatic arthritis) may appear similar to RA at presentation. In most cases, differences in the history or on physical examination distinguish them from RA. The nature of the joint inflammation is often different, with a great deal of inflammation found at enthesis or site of tendon insertions (Achilles tendon insertion, plantar fascia, shafts of fingers or toes). Asymmetric oligoarthritis (fewer than four joints), usually of the weight-bearing joints, is common in these disorders with or without sacroiliac and spinal involvement. Recognizing the importance of a focused history, asking about conjunctivitis/iritis, urethritis, and mucocutaneous manifestations is key. In addition, inflammatory symptoms of the axial skeleton strongly suggest the diagnosis of one of the spondyloarthropathies.

Palindromic Rheumatism

Palindromic rheumatism is a remitting, recurring, nondestructive, inflammatory arthritis with recurrences over at least 6 months (34). The accompanying pain has been likened to that of gout, with maximum intensity within hours and pain severe enough to confine patients to bed. A palindrome is a word or a sentence that reads the same backward and forward. Therefore the name was coined to describe the rapid appearance and disappearance of the arthritis, as the attacks may last for hours or days (rarely more than a week) with complete resolution between attacks. Each attack generally involves only a few joints, with the joints ultimately involved being similar to those involved in typical RA.

The disease eventually evolves into typical RA over time in one-quarter to one-half of the patients. Female patients with rheumatoid factor and early hand involvement were eight times more likely to develop RA than patients with only one of these features (35).

Remitting Seronegative Symmetric Synovitis with Pitting Edema

McCarty and colleagues have described a peculiar inflammatory arthritis affecting primarily the elderly (men more than women) called *r*emitting, *s*eronegative, *s*ymmetric *s*ynovitis with *p*itting *e*dema (RS3PE) (36). It is characterized by a very abrupt onset of marked dorsal swelling of the hands with pitting edema, wrist synovitis, and flexor tendinitis of the fingers. Similar swelling and synovitis may also be seen in the feet and ankles. Patients can often precisely pinpoint the time of onset. In general, the prognosis is excellent, although RS3PE occurring with an underlying malignancy as a paraneoplastic syndrome has been reported. For the most part, patients have responded dramatically to low-dose steroids. RF is not generally present and radiographic joint destruction does not occur.

Polymyalgia Rheumatica

Polymyalgia rheumatica (PMR) (37) generally presents with an abrupt onset of pain and stiffness in the shoulder and hip girdles of patients more than 50 years of age. Fever, weight loss, and lethargy can occur and may be severe. Bone scan reveals inflammatory arthritis of the shoulders and hips, although swelling may be difficult to detect. (Any clinical symptoms localize much more to the proximal musculature.) Restriction of shoulder movement secondary to pain and soft-tissue contracture is common. The stiffness and restricted mobility are exquisitely sensitive to treatment with low-dose prednisone, with 10 mg/day often sufficient to control the process. Relapse after discontinuing or reducing the corticosteroid dose is frequent, and up to half of the patients require treatment for more than 2 years.

Persistent small joint synovitis of the hands and feet distinguishes RA from PMR, although morning stiffness may otherwise be identical. RA of acute onset with PMR symptoms in the elderly often has an excellent prognosis.

Viral Arthritis

Polyarthritis may be the presenting feature of viral infections. Clues leading to the etiologic agent may be evident in the history and examination. Fever and the cutaneous manifestations may suggest an infectious process.

Rubella

Rubella virus has been associated with a polyarthritis affecting primarily the metacarpophalangeal and proximal interphalangeal joints of the hands, and wrists, knees, and ankles. The onset usually coincides with cervical adenopathy and fever. The arthritis usually resolves within a few days or weeks, though it may persist for months. As in RA, young women are most susceptible, with about half of those infected with wild virus having arthritis and 14% experiencing arthritis after vaccination. Recurrent arthritis of up to 18 months' duration was seen in 30% of those infected with wild virus (38). There are reports of chronic arthritis developing after rubella infection with both the wild virus and vaccine. NSAIDs are generally used for treatment. Except in these rare cases of chronic arthritis, proliferative synovitis as seen in RA does not occur.

Parvovirus

Human parvovirus B19 causes "fifth disease" in children and adults, bone marrow suppression (including aplastic crisis in those with hemolytic anemias), and hydrops fetalis (39). A macular rash (a "slapped-cheek" appearance) and flu-like symptoms may precede the arthritis. This may present as a symmetric polyarthritis with swelling and tenderness of the small joints of the hands, wrists, and knees, primarily in women and children. The onset of arthritis is often abrupt, with the patient suddenly unable to get out of bed in the morning due to pain. The course is generally limited to less than 2 months, although a chronic arthropathy has been described that can fulfill criteria for seronegative RA with a relatively benign outcome.

Hepatitis B and C

Hepatitis B and C have been reported to cause polyarthritis that is sometimes accompanied by RF but generally only last a few days to a few weeks. Both should be considered in the differential diagnosis of polyarthritis of short duration. Hepatitis C is also associated with RF, cryoglobulinemia, and a nondestructive arthritis (40), and has been reported to cause a chronic polyarthritis resembling RA. In some cases, the arthritis has responded dramatically to treatment of the hepatitis C.

Important Conditions That Often Occur with Rheumatoid Arthritis

Fibromyalgia

Fibromyalgia is a common problem and is often seen in patients with RA. In general, a patient with fibromyalgia is easy to distinguish from a patient with RA. However, when fibromyalgia occurs with RA, as it does in 10% to 20% of patients, it can confuse the clinical situation. The clinician should be on the lookout for this and not treat the aches and pains of fibromyalgia with increasing doses of DMARDs or steroids.

Osteoporosis

Patients of both sexes with RA have a significantly greater risk of osteoporosis. The reasons for this are multifactorial and include the following: active RA, gender (most are women), treatment (especially steroids), and decreased activity. This risk should be recognized early, and all patients should be on calcium and vitamin D, especially if they are on steroids (which decrease gastrointestinal absorption of calcium). Bisphosphanates should be used aggressively in this patient population, particularly in patients on steroids.

SUMMARY

The diagnosis and assessment of RA may be facilitated by laboratory and radiographic examinations; ultimately, however, the diagnosis depends primarily on the clinical skills of the physician. Indeed, few areas are left in medicine in which the physician, relying upon experience, patience, and powers of observation, can make such a difference in the lives of his or her patients.

It is important to remember that the experienced rheumatologist can establish the diagnosis and initiate treat-

ment *early*. With the growing realization that structural damage in RA is a cumulative result of joint inflammation and that irreversible changes occur very early in the course, there is a clear consensus that early initiation of appropriate treatment is desirable. Finally, to manage patients with RA optimally, since there is seldom, if ever, one correct medication for a given situation, the rheumatologist must be skilled in the art and science of medicine.

ACKNOWLEDGMENT

The author wishes to acknowledge Howard A. Fuchs and John S. Sergent for their contribution to this chapter.

REFERENCES

1. Scott DL, Symmons DPM, Coulton BL, et al. Long-term outcome of treating rheumatoid arthritis: results after 20 years. *Lancet* 1987;I:1108–1111.
2. Pincus T, Brooks RH, Callahan LF. Prediction of long-term mortality in patients with rheumatoid arthritis according to simple questionnaire and joint count measures. *Ann Intern Med* 1994; 120:26–34.
3. Gabriel SE, Crowson CS, O'Fallon WM. The epidemiology of rheumatoid arthritis in Rochester, Minnesota, 1955–1985. *Arthritis Rheum* 1999;42:415–420.
4. Dugowson CE, Koepsell TD, Vooigt LF, et al. Rheumatoid arthritis in women—incidence rates in group health cooperative, Seattle, Washington, 1987–1989. *Arthritis Rheum* 1991;34:1502–1507.
5. Kwoh K, Anderson LG, Erlandson DM, et al. Guidelines for the management of rheumatoid arthritis. *Arthritis Rheum* 1996;39: 713–722.
6. Arnett FC, Edworthy SM, Bloch DA, et al. The American Rheumatism Association 1987 revised criteria for the classification of rheumatoid arthritis. *Arthritis Rheum* 1988;31:315–324.
7. Wilder RL. Hormones, pregnancy, and autoimmune diseases. *Ann NY Acad Sci* 1998;840:45–50.
8. Nelson JL, Ostensen M. Pregnancy and rheumatoid arthritis. *Rheum Dis Clin North Am* 1997;23:195–212.
9. Deighton CM, Roberts DF, Walker DJ. Effect of disease severity on rheumatoid arthritis concordance in same sexed siblings. *Ann Rheum Dis* 1992;51:943–945.
10. Olsen NJ, Callahan LF, Brooks RH, et al. Associations of HLA-DR4 with rheumatoid factor and radiographic severity in rheumatoid arthritis. *Am J Med* 1988;84:257–264.
11. Felson DT, Anderson JJ, Boers M, et al. The American College of Rheumatology preliminary core set of disease activity measures for rheumatoid arthritis clinical trials. *Arthritis Rheum* 1993;36: 729–740.
12. Rigby AS, Wood PHN. The lateral metacarpophalangeal/metatarsophalangeal squeeze: an alternative assignment criterion for rheumatoid arthritis. *Scand J Rheumatol* 1991;20:115–120.
13. Palmer DG. Synovial cysts in rheumatoid disease. *Ann Intern Med* 1969;70:61–68.
14. Katz RS, Zizic TM, Arnold WP, et al. The pseudothrombophlebitis syndrome. *Medicine* 1997;56:151–164.
15. Smith RJ, Kaplan EB. Rheumatoid deformities at the metacarpophalangeal joints of the fingers. *J Bone Joint Surg* 1967;49A: 31–47.

16. Komusi T, Munro T, Harth M. Radiologic review: the rheumatoid cervical spine. *Semin Arthritis Rheum* 1985;14:187–195.

17. Gordon DA, Stein JL, Broder I. The extra-articular features of rheumatoid arthritis: a systematic analysis of 127 cases. *Am J Med* 1973;54:445–452.

18. Kaye BR, Kaye RL, Bobrove A. Rheumatoid nodules: review of the spectrum of associated conditions and a proposal of a new classification, with a report of four seronegative cases. *Am J Med* 1984;76:279–292.

19. Kalla AA, Meyers OL, Chalton D, et al. Increased metacarpal bone mass following 18 months of slow-acting antirheumatic drugs for rheumatoid arthritis. *Br J Rheumatol* 1991;30:91–100.

20. Martel W, Hayes JT, Duff IF. The pattern of bone erosion in the hand and wrist in rheumatoid arthritis. *Radiology* 1965;84:204–214.

21. Kaarela K, Luukkainen R, Koskimies S. How often is seropositive rheumatoid arthritis an erosive disease? A 17-year followup study. *J Rheumatol* 1993;20:1670–1673.

22. Weissman BW, Aliabadi P, Weinfield MS, et al. Prognostic features of atlantoaxial subluxation in rheumatoid arthritis patients. *Radiology* 1982;144:745–751.

23. Jacoby RK, Jayson MIV, Cosh JA. Onset, early stages and prognosis of rheumatoid arthritis: a clinical study of 100 patients with 11-year followup. *Br Med J* 1973;2:96–100.

24. Heliovaara M, Aho K, Aromaa A, et al. Smoking and risk of rheumatoid arthritis. *J Rheumatol* 1993;20:1830–1835.

24a. Volkanis JE. Acute-phase proteins in rheumatic disease. In: Koopman WJ, ed. *Arthritis and allied conditions: a textbook of rheumatology*, 14th ed. Philadelphia: Lippincott Williams & Wilkins, 2001:504–514.

24b. Blackburn WD Jr, Chatham WW. Laboratory findings in rheumatoid arthritis. In: Koopman WJ, ed. *Arthritis and allied conditions: a textbook of rheumatology*, 14th ed. Philadelphia: Lippincott Williams & Wilkins, 2001:1202–1222.

25. Wolfe F, Sharp JT. Radiographic outcome of recent-onset rheumatoid arthritis: a 19-year study of radiographic progression. *Arthritis Rheum* 1998;41:1571–1582.

26. Gridley G, McLaughlin JK, Ekborn A, et al. Incidence of cancer among patients with RA. *J Natl Cancer Inst* 1993;85:307–311.

27. Pincus T, Summey JA, Soraci SAJ, et al. Assessment of patient satisfaction in activities of daily living using a modified Stanford Health Assessment Questionnaire. *Arthritis Rheum* 1983;26:1346–1353.

28. Pinals RS, Masi AT, Larsen RA, et al. Preliminary criteria for clinical remission in rheumatoid arthritis. *Arthritis Rheum* 1981;24:1308–1315.

29. Wolfe F, Hawley DJ. The long-term outcomes of rheumatoid arthritis—work disability: a prospective 18-year study of 823 patients. *J Rheumatol* 1998;25:2108–2117.

30. Egsmose C, Lund B, Borg G, et al. Patients with rheumatoid arthritis benefit from early second-line therapy: 5-year follow-up of a prospective double-blind placebo-controlled study. *J Rheumatol* 1995;22:2208–2213.

31. Saag KG, Cerhan JR, Kolluri S, et al. Cigarette smoking and rheumatoid arthritis severity. *Ann Rheum Dis* 1997;56:463–469.

32. Fuchs HA, Brooks RH, Callahan LF, et al. A simplified twenty-eight-joint quantitative articular index in rheumatoid arthritis. *Arthritis Rheum* 1989;32:531–537.

33. Wolfe F, Ross K, Hawley DJ, et al. The prognosis of rheumatoid arthritis and undifferentiated polyarthritis syndrome in the clinic: a study of 1141 patients. *J Rheumatol* 1993;20:2005–2009.

34. Hench PS, Rosenberg EF. Palindromic rheumatism. *Arch Intern Med* 1944;73:293–321.

35. Gonzalez-Lopez L, Gamez-Nava JI, Jhangri GS, et al. Prognostic factors for the development of rheumatoid arthritis and other connective tissue diseases in patients with palindromic rheumatism. *J Rheumatol* 1999;26:540–545.

36. McCarty DJ, O'Duffy JD, Pearson L, et al. Remitting seronegative symmetrical synovitis with pitting edema. RS3PE syndrome. *JAMA* 1985;254:2763–2767.

37. Weyand CM, Goronzy JJ. Polymyalgia rheumatica and giant cell arteritis. In: Koopman WJ, ed. *Arthritis and allied conditions: a textbook of rheumatology*, 14th ed. Philadelphia: Lippincott Williams & Wilkins, 2001: 1784–1798.

38. Tingle AJ, Allen M, Petty RE, et al. Rubella-associated arthritis. I: comparative study of joint manifestations associated with natural rubella infection and RA27/3 rubella immunization. *Ann Rheum Dis* 1986;45:110–114.

39. Torok TJ. Parvovirus B19 and human disease. *Adv Intern Med* 1992;37:431–455.

40. Rivera J, Garcia-Monforte A, Pineda A, et al. Arthritis in patients with chronic hepatitis C virus infection. *J Rheumatol* 1999;26:420–424.

41. O'Duffy JD, Hunder GG, Wahner HW. A follow-up sutdy of polymalgia rheumatica: evidence of chronic axial synovitis. *J Rheumatol* 1980;7:685–693.

JUVENILE IDIOPATHIC ARTHRITIS (JUVENILE RHEUMATOID ARTHRITIS)

ROBERT W. WARREN
ANDREW P. WILKING
MARIA D. PEREZ
MARTHA R. CURRY
BARRY L. MYONES

Juvenile idiopathic arthritis (JIA) is a new name for an old set of diseases, also called *juvenile rheumatoid arthritis* (JRA) and *juvenile chronic arthritis* (JCA). JIA is a group of chronic diseases of childhood that affect joints and other tissues of approximately one in 1,000 children. Although the mortality rate in the United States is less than 1% (7) and only a minority of JIA patients still have inflammatory disease as adults, JIA commonly results in significant functional and/or emotional disability (4–6). It is associated later in life with more pain, more disability, and decreased employment but shows no difference from controls in income, education, and birth rates (6). Important secondary disabilities include psychosocial concerns, such as body image, self-esteem, and dependence (8); suboptimal school achievement due to psychosocial maladjustment and increased absence (9); and family problems, including depression, work loss, separation and divorce, and financial difficulties (10). Of note, these secondary disabilities do not correlate closely with the severity of arthritis (11).

CLASSIFICATION CRITERIA FOR JUVENILE IDIOPATHIC ARTHRITIS

Preceding JIA by 25 years, criteria for JRA were established in 1973 (12) and revised in 1989 (13) as the occurrence of arthritis in a child less than 16 years of age, lasting at least 6 weeks in at least one joint with no other known etiology. Arthritis was defined as swelling or two of the following findings: heat, limited motion, tenderness or pain on motion. JRA was subdivided into three major types, based upon disease onset in the first 6 months of illness. These subgroups were (a) systemic, characterized by spiking fevers, evanescent rash, and other extraarticular disease; (b) pauciarticular, with four or fewer affected joints; and (c) polyarticular, with five or more affected joints. This defini-

tion has been surprisingly effective; at 5-year follow-up, more than 97% of children so identified still carried the diagnosis (14).

Nevertheless, nomenclature has become controversial (15,16). Historically named JRA, and still commonly so in the United States, the illness has been called *juvenile chronic arthritis* (JCA) in Europe. Unfortunately, the American usage of *rheumatoid* recalls for parents the experiences of adults with rheumatoid arthritis, a largely different disease. In addition, the limited subtyping of JRA makes the correlation of research data from across the world difficult. Finally, JRA subtyping of pauciarticular and polyarticular disease reflects the onset of disease, which is far less relevant than the course of the disease. Therefore the new classification of JIA is gaining acceptance and is presented in Table 11.1. Note that only very few clinical studies have utilized the JIA definitions, and thus it is necessary to extrapolate detailed JRA study results to the new diagnostic classification.

EPIDEMIOLOGY AND ETIOLOGY

Joint pain is the chief complaint of about 1% of children seeking acute medical evaluation per year, and about 1% of them will develop chronic arthritis (17,18). The prevalence of JRA has been reported to be as low as 0.16/1,000 (19) but is more typically reported at 1 or 2/1,000 (20–22), and up to 4/1,000 (23). Meanwhile, recent incidence figures for JRA/JCA have been more consistent, ranging from 11.7 to 35/100,000/yr (24–27).

Multiple demographic factors impact JRA prevalence. More than half of all children with JRA present by 5 years of age (21,27–31), but no peak age of onset is observed for systemic disease (29). Similarly, there is no gender preference among children with systemic disease (29), but a female pre-

TABLE 11.1. JUVENILE IDIOPATHIC ARTHRITIS

Disease	Criteria	Exclusions	Descriptors
Systemic arthritis	1. Daily fever lasting at least 2 weeks, documented quotidian for at least 3 days 2. Arthritis (which may trail fever) 3. One or more of Evanescent, erythematous, nonfixed rash Generalized Lymphadenopathy Serositis Liver and/or spleen enlargement	(No specific exclusions, except emphasized importance of excluding infection and malignancy)	1. Age at onset of arthritis 2. Arthritis pattern in first 6 months ("onset") No arthritis Oligoarthritis Polyarthritis 3. Arthritis pattern after first 6 months ("course") No arthritis Oligoarthritis Polyarthritis 4. Systemic features after 6 months 5. Positive RF 6. CRP level
Oligoarthritis	Arthritis of 1–4 joints in first 6 months of disease, of two subcategories: ■ Persistent: affecting no more than four joints during disease course ■ Extended: affecting a total of more than four joints after the first 6 months of disease	1. Confirmed family history[a] of psoriasis 2. Confirmed family history of HLA-B27 associated disease 3. Positive RF 4. HLA-B27 positive male with disease onset after 8 years of age 5. Systemic arthritis	1. Age of onset 2. Patterns of arthritis at 6 months and last clinic visit Large joints only Small joints only Limb predominance Specific joints affected Symmetry 3. Anterior uveitis (acute or chronic) 4. Positive ANA 5. HLA class I and II predisposing and protective alleles
Polyarthritis (rheumatoid factor negative)	1. Arthritis of > four joints in first 6 months of disease 2. Negative RF	1. Positive RF 2. Systemic arthritis	1. Age of onset 2. Symmetry of arthritis 3. Positive ANA 4. Uveitis (acute or chronic)
Polyarthritis (rheumatoid factor positive)	1. Arthritis of > four joints in first 6 months of disease 2. Positive RF, two tests at least 3 months apart	1. Negative RF 2. Systemic arthritis	1. Age of onset 2. Symmetry of arthritis 3. Positive ANA 4. Immunogenetics
Psoriatic arthritis	1. Arthritis and psoriasis, or 2. Arthritis and at least two of Dactylitis Nail pitting or onycholysis Confirmed family history of psoriasis	1. Positive RF 2. Systemic arthritis	1. Age at onset of arthritis/psoriasis 2. Patterns of arthritis 6 months after disease onset, and at last clinic visit Large joints only Small joints only Limb predominance Specific joints Symmetry 3. Disease course Oligoarthritis Polyarthritis 4. Positive ANA 5. Anterior uveitis Chronic anterior Acute 6. HLA descriptors
Enthesitis-related arthritis	1. Arthritis and enthesitis, or 2. Arthritis or enthesitis with at least two of SI tenderness and/or inflammatory spinal pain Positive HLA-B27 Confirmed family history of HLA-B27-associated disease Acute anterior uveitis Arthritis onset in a male after 8 years of age	1. Confirmed family history of psoriasis 2. Systemic arthritis	1. Age of onset of arthritis or enthesitis 2. Patterns of arthritis Large joints only Small joints only Limb predominance Specific joints Symmetry 3. Disease course Oligoarthritis Polyarthritis
Other arthritis	1. Criteria of no other classification fulfilled, or 2. Criteria of more than one classification fulfilled	Fulfilled criteria for single classification	

Note: Classifications of arthritis without known cause, presenting before 16 years of age, and lasting at least 6 weeks (18).
[a]*Confirmed family history* means documentation by physician of disease in a first- or second-degree relative. In the case of psoriasis, confirmation must be by a dermatologist.
ANA, antinuclear antibody; CRP, c-reactive protein; HLA, human leukocyte antigen; RF, rheumatoid factor.

dominance of approximately 3:1 for other subtypes of JRA (29). Ethnicity is clearly an important factor in JRA prevalence. It is similar for blacks and whites in the United States, but higher among Native Americans (32). Finally, there are reported differences by geography (33–36).

The etiology or etiologies of JIA remain mysterious, but the different forms of JIA may well reflect an abnormal immune response to an infection or other environmental stress, strongly influenced by immunogenetic factors. A number of excellent reviews have appeared that deal with the immunogenetics of juvenile arthritis (50–55). Family studies have shown an increased concordance in identical twins. There is also a greater than expected concordance for pauciarticular and polyarticular JRA between sibling pairs. A number of reports over the years have demonstrated associations of JRA with genes of the major histocompatibility complex (MHC). Major associations include pauciarticular JRA [human leukocyte antigen (HLA)-DR5, DR8, DPw2.1, DRB1, A*0202], seronegative [rheumatoid factor (RF)-negative] polyarticular JRA (HLA-DR8, DPw3, DQw4), seropositive (RF-positive) polyarticular JRA (DRB1, the same DR4 subtypes seen in adult RA); and systemic JRA (inconsistent associations). Second, a posttraumatic etiology, possibly exposing "new" autoantigens after injury, is plausible (37). Third, stress may be relevant to the pathogenesis of JIA (38), or infection (39). The data suggesting that enthesitis-related arthritis is related to Gram-negative organisms are relatively strong (40). A number of infectious and postinfectious conditions mimic JIA quite well, including chronic Lyme arthritis (41) and parvovirus-associated arthropathy (42,43).

IMMUNOLOGY

The immunology and immunopathogenesis of JIA are complex and have been reviewed in detail elsewhere (44–48) but are summarized in the following discussion.

The cellular immunopathology in JRA is multifaceted, with CD4+ T cells in synovial tissue, evidence for T-cell activation, and an antigen- or superantigen-driven immune response suggested by an oligoclonal T cell receptor (TCR) V region expansion in JRA synovial fluid. Normal synovial fibroblasts, exposed to synovial fluid from JRA patients, exhibit proliferation, invasiveness of cartilage matrix, and release of matrix metalloproteinases (MMP). Macrophage activation also occurs. Circulating B cells are increased in patients with systemic and polyarticular JRA. A polyclonal gammopathy is common in JIA, and some autoantibodies are typical. Antinuclear antibodies (ANA) occur in 50% to 60% of patients, though the specificity of these antibodies differs from that of lupus and includes nonhistone chromosomal proteins and the nuclear antigen DEK. Classic rheumatoid factors (RF, pentameric IgM antibodies binding IgG) are observed in 5% to 10% of JRA patients by

latex fixation tests (49), but "hidden" 19S RFs detected in special assays are much more common. Other autoantibodies reported in JRA include antineutrophil cytoplasmic and antiphospholipid antibodies; the former correlates with disease activity, but not the latter. Circulating immune complexes (CIC) are often present in patients with JIA and are associated with increased levels of tumor necrosis factor-α (TNF-α), interleukin (IL)-6, and IL-8. Clearance of immune complexes from the circulation may be impaired.

Cytokines play critical roles in intercellular communication and mediate the inflammatory cascade in JIA. Increased synovial and plasma levels of TNF-α and IL-6 are characteristic of active disease of all JRA subtypes. Synovial-fluid T cells from pauciarticular patients have heterogeneous phenotypes but produce interferon (IFN)-γ in a TH1/TH0 pattern. Pro-inflammatory and antiinflammatory cytokines likely modulate joint inflammation. Their ratio may determine the degree of erosive disease. There is an increase in IL-8 and monocyte chemoattractant protein-1 (MCP-1), IL6, IL1, and IL2R in active systemic arthritis patients versus the other subtypes. This correlates with increased systemic symptoms but not with the number of joints or level of inflammation. Soluble IL-6 receptors correlate with fever, and soluble TNF receptors p55 and p75 and IL-12 (p40) correlate with erythrocyte sedimentation rate (ESR) and C-reactive protein (CRP). Antiinflammatory cytokine IL-10 decreases in systemic JRA. Thus the laboratory findings in JIA are those of acute phase reaction, particularly in the systemic arthritis subtype, where elevations in ESR, CRP, C3, C4, serum amyloid A-related protein (SAA), ferritin, platelet count, and white blood cell counts are typical.

DIFFERENTIAL DIAGNOSIS

A history of joint complaints (swelling, pain, limited motion, and/or stiffness) from children should be taken very seriously, since McCarthy found that 82% of such children have objective findings (56). In addition, care should be taken to detail *any* "diffuse" pain and pain or tenderness of extremities, even if *not* at a joint. Change or difficulty in the performance of any age-appropriate motor activities should also be investigated, such as walking, running, crawling, jumping, coloring, writing, buttoning, tying, eating, and holding a cup or spoon. Reported pain may not be as severe as expected (57,58). Since most arthritis in children is posttraumatic or reactive, any report of injury, exposure, or infection in the preceding days to weeks is relevant. Data such as the pattern of arthritis (e.g., asymmetry, number of joints, migration) will be helpful, as well as the symptom duration, intermittency, acceleration, and responsiveness to intervention. Children with oligoarthritis are commonly "normal" after minutes of morning stiffness and limping. Although JIA may present with few or multiple joint disease, children with oligoarthritis are more likely to have infectious, hematologic, or orthopedic (including post-traumatic) conditions, whereas the differential for polyarthritis more typically includes other rheumatic, postinfectious (such as rheumatic fever), and lymphoproliferative diseases. Finally, associated problems, such as growth parameters, gastrointestinal complaints, fever, weakness, and rash may help define the cause of the child's joint complaints.

Physical examination may also suggest a diagnosis, and attention should be paid to other elements besides the musculoskeletal examination. Fever in rheumatic diseases is often spiking and quotidian, as in systemic arthritis (59). Two-thirds of children with rash and arthritis have rheumatic disease, and three-fourths of children with fever and joint complaints have rheumatic disease or bacterial infection and almost never have traumatic or other orthopedic conditions (56). A child with acute monoarthritis should always be considered to have a bacterial infection until proven otherwise.

There are *no* diagnostic laboratory tests for juvenile idiopathic arthritis. A complete blood count and urinalysis, and a metabolic profile may provide information entirely consistent with—or unusual for—the diagnosis. Synovial fluid white blood cell (WBC) counts in clinically active joints have been reported to range between 600 cells/mm^3 (66) to more 100,000 cells/mm^3 (67), although typical counts are about 10,000 cells/mm^3; thus there is no arthrocentesis result that is diagnostic of JIA. Acute-phase reactants are inconsistently elevated in JIA, particularly in children with oligoarthritis, though typically quite elevated in systemic arthritis. Measurements of serum immunoglobulins and total hemolytic complement are often indicated in the evaluation of children with arthritis, because of the possibility of associated immunodeficiency. Particularly since systemic arthritis is the cause of fever of unknown origin in only about 10% of children (60,61), extensive studies may be required to *exclude* diagnoses such as infection, leukemia, and inflammatory bowel disease. Such studies commonly include complete blood counts (CBCs) and liver function tests, bone marrow studies, chest films, abdominal ultrasound and/or computed tomography (CT), bone scan, and small- and/or large-bowel contrast studies, and endoscopy. Wallendal et al. noted that lactate dehydrogenase levels are likely to be significantly higher in patients with malignancy compared with those with systemic arthritis, whereas uric acid levels were not different (62). ANA testing for the diagnosis of JIA is strongly discouraged because 6% of normal children have a positive test (63), though ANA is relevant because of the associated increased risk of uveitis in patients with oligoarthritis. Rheumatoid factor is also a poor diagnostic test for the disease, since RF is present in only about 5% of children with JRA (64). Diagnostic imaging plays an important role in the diagnosis of JIA, generally to help exclude other diagnoses, such as infection, trauma, malignancy, and avascular necrosis; joint erosions on plain film at diagnosis of JIA are extremely rare (65).

PRESENTATION AND COURSE

Systemic Arthritis

Ten percent to 15% of children with JRA (and presumably JIA) have systemic disease. Systemic arthritis typically presents in a previously healthy child, less than 4 years old (68,69) with the acute onset of high-spiking fever, sometimes to 106°F, but often subnormal in the early morning. The associated evanescent rash typically present with fever is usually salmon-colored, macular, and occasionally pruritic, often with clustered lesions on the proximal extremities and trunk (Fig. 11.1). The rash is not diagnostic. Similar exanthems can be seen with viral illnesses. Biopsies of the rash have shown only edema or mild perivascular infiltrates (70,71). Other common presenting systemic signs include fatigue, irritability and drowsiness (72), myalgia (73), generalized adenopathy, and hepatosplenomegaly.

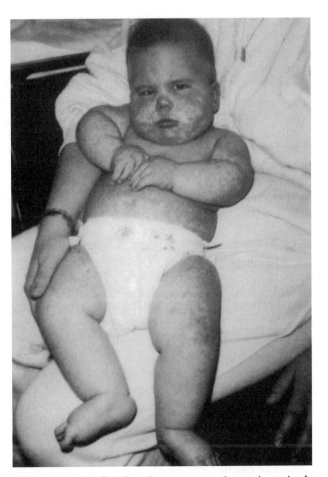

FIGURE 11.1. The florid erythematous maculopapular rash of a child with systemic juvenile rheumatoid arthritis. This rash appeared with fever (daily spike to 103°C) and then faded. [From Warren RW, Perez MD, Curry MR, et al. Juvenile idiopathic arthritis (juvenile rheumatoid arthritis). In: Koopman WJ, ed. *Arthritis and allied conditions: a textbook of rheumatology,* 14th ed. Philadelphia: Lippincott Williams & Wilkins, 2001:1270–1293, with permission.]

Arthritis may occur along with these symptoms or follow weeks to months later, making diagnosis quite difficult. Although patients with systemic arthritis are often uncomfortable, they only rarely have severe pain, a finding that should prompt consideration of malignancy (74). Many patients with systemic arthritis present with serositis, with pericarditis occurring in more than one-third (75), but tamponade is a rare complication (76,77). Pericarditis sometimes recurs (78).

Patients with systemic arthritis commonly present with white blood cell counts of more than 20,000, often severe nonhemolytic anemia (e.g., hgb levels < 6 g/dL) with indices typical of chronic disease, ESRs often greater than 100, negative ANAs, and negative serum RFs. Ferritin levels are often extremely high, particularly in older children (79). Platelet counts at presentation are typically elevated. A low to normal platelet count should raise concern about a different diagnosis (e.g., leukemia, sepsis) or systemic JRA complicated by disseminated intravascular coagulation (DIC). Mild coagulopathy is common in systemic arthritis (80), but only a few patients develop macrophage activation syndrome (MAS), often early in their course (71,82). Children with MAS typically have moderate to severe DIC, a decreasing ESR, severe anemia and leukopenia, and liver dysfunction (83). MAS has also been reported in children with polyarthritis and has been associated with Epstein–Barr virus infection (84).

Although systemic symptoms generally resolve within a year of presentation, some patients have flares of systemic signs thereafter, and a few others continue to have nearly continuous fever and rash. Up to 50% of systemic arthritis patients evolve into a chronic polyarthritis, and in as many as 25% of patients, the arthritis is erosive, particularly in the hips (85). This arthritis is indistinguishable from polyarticular JIA. On the other hand, van der Net et al. reported only mild disability in most children, with a mean disease duration of nearly 6 years (86). Although the mortality rate for JRA as a whole is reported in the United States as less than 1%, 15-year survival for systemic JRA has been reported at only 86% (87).

Other complications noted among patients with systemic arthritis include carditis, with reports of aortic valve regurgitation (88), hepatitis, and infection and sepsis, secondary to therapy or MAS. Uveitis is rare, though yearly screening is still suggested. Amyloidosis is rarely seen in the United States but is reported in about 5% of patients in Europe (90,91). Growth failure is common in patients with systemic disease (92,93), though catch-up growth may occur with disease control.

Oligoarthritis

Children meeting the JIA criteria for oligoarthritis, in both the persistent and extended subcategories, generally fit the old JRA criteria for type I pauciarticular JRA (94). This group comprises about 35% of all JRA patients. Children with persistent oligoarthritis "persist" with arthritis in four or fewer joints, even past the first 6 months of disease, whereas children with extended oligoarthritis have a cumulative number of affected joints over time of more than four. Studies of all children with pauciarticular JRA indicate that up to 20% of that group have a polyarticular course of disease (95).

The typical child with oligoarthritis is a girl, presenting in early childhood. The disease typically begins between 1 and 4 years of age, and uncommonly after 7 years of age (96). Systemic signs and symptoms are absent. Arthritis typically occurs in large joints, with the knee most commonly and initially involved (97). The occurrence of early small joint involvement suggests either extended oligoarthritis or another diagnosis. Presentation of oligoarthritis at the hip is distinctly unusual and should prompt consideration of other diagnoses. In a recent study of pauciarthritis patients, 68% were ANA positive (98). All should be rheumatoid factor negative.

With no reported mortality risk for oligoarthritis, the principal complications are articular and periarticular damage and chronic uveitis; these complications need have no temporal correlation (99). Although commonly perceived as having little permanent impact on the child, oligoarthritis causes articular cartilage and bone destruction in 25% of affected children (100). In addition, contractures and local growth abnormalities occur, particularly in young patients (101) with periarticular osteoporosis but also local bone overgrowth (100). The latter often leads to longer leg length at an affected knee. Finally, only about 20% of patients with oligoarthritis remit within 5 years (102). These outcomes have led recently to more aggressive therapy, including long-acting intraarticular steroid injections.

Children at greatest risk for chronic anterior uveitis include young girls who are ANA positive (103) and HLA-DR5 positive (104). However, in recent studies (98,105), the overall prevalence of uveitis among oligoarthritis patients was 15%. Although uveitis is classically associated with redness of the eye, photophobia, and eye pain, affected children with oligoarthritis and their parents often report no symptoms (106). Moreover, many children with significant uveitis have no findings except on slit lamp examination. Thus routine slit lamp examination, as frequently as every 3 months for the highest-risk group, is recommended (107). Despite care, 21% of patients have recurrent attacks with disease lasting more than 10 years (108), and 11% of children with uveitis develop visual impairment (105).

Polyarthritis

As a group, children with polyarthritis comprise about 30% to 40% of children with JRA and perhaps the same percentage of JIA patients. Approximately 75% of patients are girls, with onset peaks at 1 to 3 and 8 to 10 years of age (109). They often present with mild systemic signs and symptoms, including fatigue; low-grade fever; minimal, if any, weight loss; and mild anemia. Uveitis is reported in 5% (105), and thus slit lamp screening every 6 months is recommended (107). Their arthritis may be symmetrical at onset, involving multiple large and small joints (Fig. 11.2), but more commonly the disease begins in a few joints and then evolves over a few months as an additive polyarthritis.

Twenty-five percent to 35% of children with JIA have rheumatoid factor negative polyarthritis. Children with polyarthritis who are RF negative are generally younger, and they almost never become RF-positive with age. Severe, erosive, and unremitting arthritis has been reported in approximately 15% of patients (110). Extraarticular manifestations of disease are uncommon, except for rheumatoid nodules and low-grade fever. Approximately 25% of children with RF-negative disease are ANA positive (111).

RF-positive polyarthritis accounts for only about 5% of all children with JIA and is most commonly seen in female adolescents. It is apparently identical to adult rheumatoid arthritis. Affected patients have an approximately 50% risk for a severe and deforming arthritis (110), and may have rheumatoid nodules (112) or even vasculitis. About half of patients with RF-positive polyarthritis are ANA positive.

Enthesitis-Related Arthritis

Enthesitis-related arthritis represents 15% to 20% of all JIA, extrapolating from JRA and JCA data (113,114). Affected children are usually more than 8 years of age, are generally male (about 4:1), are often HLA-B27 positive, and typically have an asymmetric, large joint, lower extremity arthritis (115). Juvenile ankylosing spondylitis (JAS), with clear evidence for sacroiliac (SI) (or spinal) disease, represents approximately 20% of children with spondyloarthropathy (74).

The typical child at presentation is a teenage boy with a swollen knee, though the hip may also be affected early. Complaints of low back pain, particularly in the morning and with difficulty sitting and standing for long periods, and poor-quality sleep are common, as well as complaints of other "joint" pain. Examination reveals enthesitis, particularly patellar or calcaneal. Bursal or large joint swelling is often painless. X-rays of the SI joints are typically normal in children at presentation, but bone scans and contrast-enhanced magnetic resonance imaging (MRI) of the SI joints may be positive (116). CBCs and sedimentation rates are rarely significantly abnormal. HLA-B27 is present in about 60% of patients with spondyloarthropathy and the great majority with JAS (74), and is not essential for the diagnosis.

This disease may be complicated by progressive axial skeletal disease and deformity; children with HLA-B27 and evidence for spinal limitation (positive Schober test) are at greatest risk, with nearly 20% developing definite sacroiliitis at 5 years (117). Children with JAS have a low prevalence of mild mitral and/or aortic regurgitation, as do adults (118). Acute anterior uveitis occurs in about 10% to 25% of children with JAS (119,120), with HLA-B27-positive children presumably at greatest risk.

Psoriatic Arthritis

Psoriatic arthritis is addressed elsewhere in this text. It should be noted, however, that arthritis precedes a diagnosis of psoriasis in 40% to 50% of children ultimately diagnosed with psoriatic arthritis (121,122).

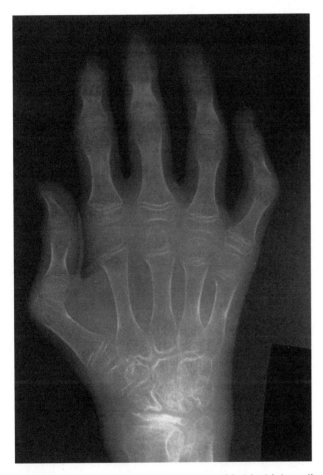

FIGURE 11.2. Hand radiograph in a 9-year-old girl with juvenile rheumatoid arthritis. Note the severe osteopenia with very thin metacarpal cortices. The medullary space is relatively wide. Severe osteopenia is common in severe juvenile rheumatoid arthritis. The carpals are also very irregular, and there are erosions in the carpals, distal radius, metacarpal–carpal joint, and metacarpal–phalangeal joint. There is subluxation of the first metacarpal–phalangeal joint and bulbous enlargement of the distal ends of both the proximal and middle phalanges. The epiphysis of the proximal phalanx of the index finger is irregular, and there is narrowing of that joint space. [From Warren RW, Perez MD, Curry MR, et al. Juvenile idiopathic arthritis (juvenile rheumatoid arthritis). In: Koopman WJ, ed. *Arthritis and allied conditions: a textbook of rheumatology,* 14th ed. Philadelphia: Lippincott Williams & Wilkins, 2001:1270–1293, with permission.]

Other Arthritis

There are children with JIA who do not fit the rules of classification, particularly (a) the occasional child with apparent enthesitis-related arthritis who later develops an erosive rheumatoid factor–positive polyarthritis; and (b) the child classified with persistent or extended oligoarthritis, who does not meet criteria for psoriatic disease, who later develops psoriasis, and has x-ray findings (e.g., "pencil and cup" joints) typical of psoriatic arthritis.

EVALUATION OF DISEASE ACTIVITY AND PROGRESSION OF JUVENILE IDIOPATHIC ARTHRITIS

At a time when the therapeutic options for children with JIA are becoming increasingly complex, objective serial evaluations are very important. Specific attention should be given to the number, severity, and activity of affected joints. Serial diagnostic imaging is useful in following joint erosions (by plain film) and cartilage damage (by MRI). Laboratory studies are not generally useful, because RF and ANA titers are unrelated to disease severity, and the relationship of ESR and CRP to disease activity is weak, except in systemic disease (131–134). A number of quantitative joint evaluations and functional and quality-of-life assessment tools are in use, including the Juvenile Arthritis Functional Assessment Scale [JAFAS (123)], the parent- or child-completed Juvenile Arthritis Functional Assessment Report [JAFAR (124)], and most recently, the JRA Core Set Criteria (125,126), the Childhood Health Assessment Questionnaire (CHAQ) (127), the Childhood Health Questionnaire (CHQ) (128), and the Juvenile Arthritis Quality-of-Life Questionnaire (JAQQ) (129).

THERAPY

General

Education is the initial step in the management of a child with JIA but also part of the ongoing care. Knowledge, patience, and open-mindedness should be the mainstays of the physician-as-educator and other members of the care team.

General health maintenance is especially important in children with JIA so that their bodies may have a firm foundation upon which to depend as they fight the inflammatory process. It is important that health care providers work closely with patients and their parents concerning sleep, nutrition, exercise, and social activity. It is critical that these children, like others with chronic illness, be successful in school and at play. This may require family and child counseling, as well as intensive work with school personnel.

Physical and Occupational Therapy

Physical and/or occupational therapy are critical in managing this disease, maintaining normal joint function if at all possible. The key to this outcome is daily range-of-motion exercises of affected joints, and expert direction by a physical and/or occupational therapist is often necessary, particularly for the child with active and severe disease. Both physical and occupational therapy may be provided at school.

Medications for Oligoarthritis

Nonsteroidal antiinflammatory drugs (NSAIDs) are the mainstay of the pharmaceutical therapy of JIA, and this is especially true of oligoarticular disease. Although effective, aspirin is now uncommonly used for JIA, because of its potential toxicities and qid dosing. Instead, naproxen sodium (15 to 20 mg/kg/d divided b.i.d.), ibuprofen (30 to 50 mg/kg/d divided t.i.d.-q.i.d.), tolmetin sodium (20 to 30 mg/kg/d divided t.i.d.), or other NSAIDs are more commonly used (130–131). Other NSAIDs used include diflunisal, piroxicam, diclofenac, sulindac and indomethacin, celecoxib and rofecoxib, though these are usually not the first medications chosen. All the NSAIDs may cause gastrointestinal, hepatic, and renal toxicity, with variability in the propensity of individual drugs to affect specific organs. Gastrointestinal problems are far less frequently reported with the cyclooxygenase-2 inhibitors.

In patients with a severely affected joint, especially a weight-bearing joint, intraarticular glucocorticoids may be appropriate. Triamcinolone hexacetonide, used in a dose of 10 to 40 mg, is usually the preparation of choice because of its long duration of action (132).

Medications for Polyarticular Disease

Children with polyarticular JIA are almost always treated with an NSAID, but additional medications are usually necessary. Methotrexate is the most frequently prescribed second-line agent because it improves 65% of children treated (133). The drug is usually started at a dose of 10 to 15 mg/M^2, typically given once weekly. Methotrexate toxicity does not not usually limit drug utility; however, monitoring for marrow, gastrointestinal, liver, lung, and kidney effects is important.

Sulfasalazine is also used in the treatment of children with JIA, though it has been especially helpful in older, HLA-B27-positive boys (i.e., those more likely to be identified as having enthesitis-related arthritis or spondyloarthropathy) (134).

Glucocorticoids are frequently used as adjunctive therapy for children with polyarticular JIA. They may be helpful at a low dose (0.2 to 0.35 mg/kg/d) of prednisone between the institution of therapy and demonstration of benefit of methotrexate or sulfasalazine. Often this low dose of prednisone is most effective and demonstrates no deleterious effects when given at bedtime, thereby decreasing morning pain and stiffness. More severely affected children will benefit from pulse intravenous methylprednisolone, 30 mg/kg/dose, not to exceed 1,000 mg (135). The side effects of prolonged use of glucocorticoids are legion and may be devastating.

Most recently, etanercept, an inhibitor of tumor necrosis factor, has been found to be helpful to a large percentage of children who had not responded satisfactorily to, or had unmanageable side effects from methotrexate (136). Etanercept is currently given to children in a dose of 0.4 mg/kg, not to exceed 25 mg subcutaneously twice per week. Infliximab also has been used.

Medications for Systemic JIA

Glucocorticoids are often required to control fevers and serositis, given as prednisone, 1 to 2 mg/kg/d or as intravenous methylprednisolone. Other medications, as discussed earlier, are often needed. A rare child with systemic (or even polyarticular) disease requires even more intensive immunosuppression.

Surgery

Synovectomy, soft-tissue releases, and total joint replacements may benefit severely affected children with JIA, but very careful patient selection and aggressive postoperative therapy are as important as the surgical procedure itself in long-term outcome.

Therapy for Uveitis

Treatment of uveitis usually begins with topical steroids and a mydriatic but may require NSAIDs, methotrexate, and/or intraocular and systemic steroids. Surgery is at times necessary to remove cataracts and to correct other damage caused by the inflammatory process.

SUMMARY

In sum, juvenile idiopathic arthritis is a collection of distinct illnesses, linked principally by the phenomenology of idiopathic joint disease. For the present, JIA is best managed with a team of experts, skilled in disease assessment, medication adjustment, physical and occupational therapy, patient and parent education, family emotional and financial counseling, school liaison, and vocational and transitional assistance.

REFERENCES

1. Builstra JE, Poznanski A, Cerna ML, et al. A case of juvenile rheumatoid arthritis from pre-Columbian Peru: a life in science. In: Buikstra JE, ed. *Papers in honor of J Lawrence Angel.* Kampsville, IL: Center for American Archeology, 1990:99.
2. Cronil V. Méemoire sur les coincidences pathologiques du rhumatisme articulaire chronique. *C R Soc Biol (Paris)* 1864;4:2–25.
3. Diamentberger S. *Du rhumatisme noueux (polyarthrite déformante) chez les enfants.* Paris: Lecrosnier et Babe, 1891:1–148.
4. Levinson JE, Wallace CA. Dismantling the pyramid. *J Rheumatol* 1992;19(Suppl 33):6–10.
5. David J, Cooper C, Hickey L, et al. The functional and psychological outcomes of juvenile chronic arthritis in young adulthood. *Br J Rheumatol* 1994;33:876–881.
6. Peterson LS, Mason T, Nelson AM, et al. Psychosocial outcomes and health status of adults who have had juvenile rheumatoid arthritis. *Arthritis Rheum* 1997;40:2235–2240.
7. Baum J, Gutowska G. Death in juvenile rheumatoid arthritis. *Arthritis Rheum* 1977;20:253.
8. Van Vujm IH, Hoyeraal HM, Fagertun H. Chronic family difficulties and stress life events in recent onset juvenile arthritis. *J Rheumatol* 1989;16:1088–1092.
9. Sturge C, Garralda ME, Boissin M, et al. School attendance and juvenile chronic arthritis. *Br J Rheumatol* 1997;36:1218–1223.
10. Olson DH, Sprenkle D, Russell C. Circumplex model of marital and family systems. I. cohesion and adaptability dimensions. *Family Process* 1979;18:3–28.
11. McAnarney ER, Pless BI, Satterwhite B, et al. Psychological problems of children with chronic juvenile arthritis. *Pediatrics* 1974;53:523–528.
12. Brewer EJ, Base JC, Cassidy JT, et al. Criteria for the classification of juvenile rheumatoid arthritis. *Bull Rheum Dis* 1973;23:712–719.
13. Brewer EJ, Bass J, Cassidy JT, et al. Current proposed revision of JRA criteria. *Arthritis Rheum* 1977;20:195–199.
14. Jacobs JC. *Pediatric rheumatology for the practitioner,* 2nd ed. New York: Springer-Verlag, 1993.
15. Cassidy JT. What's in a name? Nomenclature of juvenile arthritis: North American view. *J Rheumatol* 1993;20(Suppl 40):4–8.
16. Prieur A-M, Kaufman MT, Griscelli C, et al. What's in a name? Nomenclature of juvenile arthritis. A European view. *J Rheumatol* 1993;20(Suppl 40):9.
17. Towner SR, Michael CJ Jr, O'Fallon WM, et al. The epidemiology of juvenile arthritis in Rochester, Minnesota 1960–1979. *Arthritis Rheum* 1983;26:1208–1213.
18. Kunnamo I, Kallio P, Pelkonen P. Incidence of arthritis in urban Finnish children: a prospective study. *Arthritis Rheum* 1986;29:1232–1238.
19. Gewanter HL, Baum J. The frequency of juvenile arthritis. *J Rheumatol* 1989;16:556–557.
20. Pless IB, Satterwhite B, Van Vechten D. Chronic illness in childhood: a regional survey of care. *Pediatrics* 1976;58:37–46.
21. Towner SR, Michet CJ, O'Fallon WM, et al. The epidemiology of juvenile arthritis in Rochester, Minnesota 1960–1979. *Arthritis Rheum* 1983;26:1208–1213.
22. Kiessling U, Doring E, Listing J, et al. Incidence and prevalence of juvenile chronic arthritis in East Berlin 1980–1988. *J Rheumatol* 1998;25:1837–1843.
23. Manners PJ, Diepeveen DA. Prevalence of juvenile chronic arthritis in a population of 12-year-old children in urban Australia. *Pediatrics* 1996;98:84–90.
24. Peterson LS, Mason T, Nelson AM, et al. Juvenile rheumatoid arthritis in Rochester, Minnesota 1960–1993: is the epidemiology changing? *Arthritis Rheum* 1996;39:1385–1390.
25. Anderson GB, Fasth A, Andersson J, et al. Incidence and prevalence of juvenile chronic arthritis: a population survey. *Ann Rheum Dis* 1987;46:277–281.
26. Tower SR, Michet CJ, O'Fallon WM, et al. The epidemiology

of juvenile rheumatoid arthritis in Rochester, Minnesota, 1960–79. *Arthritis Rheum* 1983;26:1208–1213.

27. Gare A, Fasth A, Anderson J, et al. Incidence and prevalence of juvenile chronic arthritis: a population survey. *Ann Rheum Dis* 1987;45:277.

28. Kunnamo I, Kallio P, Pelkonen P. Incidence of arthritis in urban Finnish children. *Arthritis Rheum* 1986;29:1232–1238.

29. Sullivan DB, Cassidy JT, Petty RE. Pathogenic implication of age of onset in juvenile rheumatoid arthritis. *Arthritis Rheum* 1975;18:251–255.

30. Hanson H, Kornreich HK, Bernstein B, et al. Three subtypes of juvenile rheumatoid arthritis: correlations of age at onset, sex, and serologic factors. *Arthritis Rheum* 1977;20(Suppl):184.

31. Sullivan DB, Cassidy JT, Petty RE. Pathogenic implications of age of onset in juvenile rheumatoid arthritis. *Arthritis Rheum* 1975;18:251–255.

32. Lawrence RC, Hochberg MC, Kelsey JL, et al. Estimates of the prevalence of selected arthritic and musculoskeletal diseases in the Unites States. Report of the National Arthritis Data Workgroup. *J Rheumatol* 1989;16:427–441.

33. Prieur AM, LeGall E, Karman F. Epidemiologic survey of juvenile chronic arthritis. *Clin Exp Rheumatol* 1987;5:217–223.

34. Anderson Gäre B, Fasth A. The natural history of juvenile chronic arthritis: a population based cohort study: I. Onset and disease process. *J Rheumatol* 1995;22:295–307.

35. Arguedas O, Porras O, Fasth A. Juvenile chronic arthritis in Costa Rica: a pilot referral study. *Clin Exp Rheumatol* 1995;13: 119–123.

36. Pongpanich B, Daengroongroj P. Juvenile rheumatoid arthritis: clinical characteristics in 100 Thai patients. *Clin Rheumatol* 1988;7:257–261.

37. Cassidy JT, Petty RE. *Juvenile rheumatoid arthritis: textbook of pediatric rheumatology,* 3rd ed. Philadelphia: WB Saunders, 1995:138.

38. Heisel JS. Life changes as etiologic factors in juvenile rheumatoid arthritis. *J Psychosom Res* 1972;16:411–442.

39. Phillips PE. Evidence implicating infectious agents in rheumatoid arthritis and juvenile rheumatoid arthritis. *Clin Exp Rheumatol* 1988;6:87–94.

40. Sieper J, Braun J, Doring E, et al. Aetiological role of bacteria associated with reactive arthritis in pauciarticular juvenile chronic arthritis. *Ann Rheum Dis* 1992;51:1208–1214.

41. Steere AC, Gibofsky A, Pattarroyo ME, et al. Chronic Lyme arthritis: clinical and immunogenetic differentiation from rheumatoid arthritis. *Ann Intern Med* 1979;90:896–901.

42. Naides SJ, Scharosch LL, Foto F, et al. Rheumatologic manifestations of human parvovirus B19 infection in adults: initial two-year clinical experience. *Arthritis Rheum* 1990;33:1297–1309.

43. Nocton JJ, Miller LC, Tucker LB, et al. Human parvovirus B19–associated arthritis in children. *J Pediatr* 1993;122: 186–190.

44. Gallagher KT, Bernstein B. Juvenile rheumatoid arthritis. *Curr Opin Rheumatol* 1999;11:372–376.

45. Moore TL. Immunopathogenesis of juvenile rheumatoid arthritis. *Curr Opin Rheumatol* 1999;11:377–383.

46. De Benedetti F, Martini A. Is systemic juvenile rheumatoid arthritis an interleukin 6 mediated disease? [editorial] *J Rheumatol* 1998;25:203–207.

47. Mangge H, Schauenstein K. Cytokines in juvenile rheumatoid arthritis (JRA). *Cytokine* 1998;10:471–480.

48. Jarvis JN. Pathogenesis and mechanisms of inflammation in the childhood rheumatic diseases. *Curr Opin Rheumatol* 1998;10: 459–467.

49. Moore TL. Rheumatoid factors. *Clin Immunol Newsletter* 1998;18:89–96.

50. Albert ED, Scholz S. Juvenile arthritis: genetic update. *Baillieres Clin Rheumatol* 1998;12:209–218.

51. Graham TB, Glass DN. Juvenile rheumatoid arthritis: ethnic differences in diagnostic types [editorial]. *J Rheumatol* 1997;24: 1677–1679.

52. Ploski R, Forre O. Non-HLA genes and susceptibility to juvenile chronic arthritis. *Clin Exp Rheumatol* 1994;12(Suppl 10): S15–S17.

53. Fernandez-Vina M, Fink CW, Stastny P. HLA associations in juvenile arthritis. *Clin Exp Rheumatol* 1994;12:205–214.

54. Nepom B. The immunogenetics of juvenile rheumatoid arthritis. *Rheum Dis Clin North Am* 1991;17:825–842.

55. Nepom B, Glass D. Juvenile rheumatoid arthritis and HLA: Report of the Park City III workshop. *J Rheumatol* 1992;19 (Suppl 33):70–74.

56. McCarthy PL, Wasserman D, Spiesel SZ, et al. Evaluation of arthritis and arthralgia in the pediatric patient. *Clin Pediatr (Phila)* 1980;19:183–190.

57. Scott PJ, Ansell BM, Huskisson EC. Measurement of pain in juvenile chronic polyarthritis. *Ann Rheum Dis* 1977;36:186–187.

58. Varni JW, Wilcox KT, Hanson V, et al. Chronic musculoskeletal pain and functional status in juvenile rheumatoid arthritis: an empirical model. *Pain* 1988;32:1–7.

59. Callen JP. Myositis and malignancy. *Curr Opin Rheumatol* 1989;1:468–472.

60. Pizzo PA, Lovejoy FH Jr, Smith DH. Prolonged fever in children: Review of 100 cases. *Pediatrics* 1075;55:468–473.

61. Lohr JA, Hendley JO. Prolonged fever of unknown origin. *Clin Pediatr* 1977;16:768–773.

62. Wallendal M, Stork L, Hollister JR. The discriminating value of serum lactate dehydrogenase levels in children with malignant neoplasms presenting as joint pain. *Arch Pediatr Adolesc Med* 1996;150:70–73.

63. McCune WJ, Wise PT, Cassidy JT. A comparison of antibody tests in children with juvenile rheumatoid arthritis on Hep-2 cell and mouse liver substrates. *J Rheumatol* 1986;13:198.

64. Eichenfield AH, Athreya BH, Doughty RA, et al. Utility of rheumatoid factor in the diagnosis of juvenile rheumatoid arthritis. *Pediatrics* 1986;78:480–484.

65. Pachman LM, Poznanski AK. Juvenile (rheumatoid) arthritis. In: Koopman WJ, ed. *Arthritis and allied conditions: a textbook of rheumatology,* 13th ed. Baltimore: Williams & Wilkins, 1997:1155–1178.

66. Cassidy JT, Petty RE. *Juvenile rheumatoid arthritis: textbook of pediatric rheumatology,* 3rd ed. Philadelphia: WB Saunders, 1995:176.

67. Baldassare AR, Chang F, Zuckner J. Markedly raised synovial fluid leukocyte counts not associated with infectious arthritis in children. *Ann Rheum Dis* 1978;37:404–409.

68. Grokoest AW, Snyder AI, Schlaeger R. *Juvenile rheumatoid arthritis.* Boston: Little, Brown, 1962.

69. Petty RE, Epidemiology of juvenile rheumatoid arthritis. In: Miller JJ III, ed. *Juvenile rheumatoid arthritis.* Littleton, MA: PSG, 1979:135.

70. Calabro JJ, Marchesano JM. Rash associated with juvenile rheumatoid arthritis. *J Pediatr* 1968;72:611–619.

71. Schlesinger BE, Forsyth CC, White RHR, et al. Observations on the clinical course and treatment of one hundred cases of Still's disease. *Arch Dis Child* 1961;36:65–76.

72. Jan JE, Hill RH, Low MD. Cerebral complications in juvenile rheumatoid arthritis. *Can Med Assoc J* 1972;1073:623–625.

73. Schaller JG: The diversity of JRA. *Arthritis Rheum* 1977; 20 (Suppl):52–63.

74. Cabral DA, Malleson PN, Petty RE. Spondyloarthropathies of childhood. *Pediatr Clin North Am* 1995;42:1051.

75. Bernstein B, Takahashi M, Hanson V. Cardiac involvement in juvenile rheumatoid arthritis. *J Pediatr* 1985;85:313–317.

76. Brewer E. Juvenile rheumatoid arthritis-cardiac involvement. *Arthritis Rheum* 1977;20:231–236.

77. Miller JJ III. Carditis in JRA. In: Miller JJ III, ed. *Juvenile rheumatoid arthritis.* Littleton, MA: PSG, 1979:165–173.

78. Svantesson H, Bjorkhem G, Elborgh R. Cardiac involvement in juvenile rheumatoid arthritis: a follow-up study. *Acta Paediatr Scand* 1983;72:345–350.

79. Schwarz-Eywill M, Heilig B, Bauer H, et al. Evaluation of serum ferritin as a marker for adult Still's disease activity. *Ann Rheum Dis* 1992;51:683–685.

80. Bloom BJ, Tucker LB, Miller LC, et al. Fibrin D-dimer as a marker of disease activity in systemic onset juvenile rheumatoid arthritis. *J Rheumatol* 1998,25:1620–1625.

81. Morris JA, Adamson AR, Holt PJL, et al. Still's disease and the virus-associated haemophagocytic syndrome. *Ann Rheum Dis* 1985;44:349–353.

82. Heaton DC, Moller PW. Case report: Still's disease associated with Coxsackie infection and haemophagocytic syndrome. *Ann Rheum Dis* 1985;44:341–344.

83. Stephan JL, Zeller J, Hubert P, et al. Macrophage activation syndrome and rheumatic disease in childhood: a report of four new cases. *Clin Exp Rheumatol* 1993;11:451–456.

84. Davies SV, Dean JD, Wardrop CA, et al. Epstein-Barr virus-associated haemophagocytic syndrome in a patient with juvenile chronic arthritis. *Br J Rheumatol* 1994;33:495–497.

85. Ansell BM, Wood PHN. Prognosis in juvenile chronic arthritis. *Clin Rheum Dis* 1976;2:397–412.

86. Van der Net J, Kuis W, Prakken ABJ, et al. Correlates of disablement in systemic onset juvenile chronic arthritis. *Scand J Rheumatol* 1997;26:188–196.

87. Svantesson H, Akesson A, Eberhardt K, et al. Prognosis in juvenile rheumatoid arthritis with systemic onset. *Scand J Rheumatol* 1983;12:139–144.

88. Heyd J, Glaser J. Early occurrence of aortic valve regurgitation in a youth with systemic-onset juvenile rheumatoid arthritis. *Am J Med* 1990;89:123–124.

89. Brewer EJ, Giannini E, Person D. *Juvenile rheumatoid arthritis,* 2nd ed. Philadelphia: WB Saunders, 1982.

90. Schnitzer TJ, Ansell BM. Amyloidosis in juvenile chronic polyarthritis. *Arthritis Rheum* 1977;20(Suppl):245–252.

91. Calabro JJ. Amyloidosis and juvenile rheumatoid arthritis. *J Pediatr* 1969;75:521.

92. Bernstein BH, Stobie D, Singsen BH, et al. Growth retardation in juvenile rheumatoid arthritis (JRA). *Arthritis Rheum* 1977;20:212–216.

93. Polito C, Strano CG, Olicieri AN, et al. Growth retardation in non-steroid treated juvenile rheumatoid arthritis. *Scand J Rheumatol* 1997;26:99–103.

94. Schaller JG. The diversity of JRA. *Arthritis Rheum* 1977;20(Suppl):52–63.

95. Prieur AM, Ansel BM, Bardfeld R, et al. Is onset type evaluated during the first three months of disease satisfactory for defining the sub-groups of juvenile chronic arthritis? A EULAR cooperative study (1983–1986). *Clin Exp Rheumatol* 1990;8:321–325.

96. Sullivan DB, Cassidy JT, Petty RE. Pathogenic implications of age of onset in juvenile rheumatoid arthritis. *Arthritis Rheum* 1975;18:251–255.

97. Sherry DD, Bohnsak J, Salmonson K, et al. Painless juvenile rheumatoid arthritis. *J Pediatr* 1990;116:921–923.

98. Sharma S, Sherry DD. Joint distribution at presentation in children with pauciarthritis. *J Pediatr* 1999;134:642–643.

99. Rosenberg AM, Oen KG. The relationship between ocular and articular disease activity in children with juvenile rheumatoid arthritis and associated uveitis. *Arthritis Rheum* 1986;29:797–800.

100. Cassidy JT, Martel W. Juvenile rheumatoid arthritis: clinicoradiologic correlations. *Arthritis Rheum* 1977;20(Suppl):207–211.

101. Vostrejs M, Hollister JR. Muscle atrophy and leg length discrepancies in pauciarticular juvenile rheumatoid arthritis. *Am J Dis Child* 1988;142:343–345.

102. Cassidy JT, Levinson JE, Brewer EJ Jr. The development of classification criteria for children with juvenile rheumatoid arthritis. *Bull Rheum Dis* 1989;38:1–7.

103. Kanski JJ. Uveitis in juvenile chronic arthritis: incidence, clinical features and prognosis. *Eye* 1988;2:641–645.

104. Suciu-Foca N, Jacobs J, Godfrey M, et al. HLA-DR5 in juvenile rheumatoid arthritis confined to a few joints. *Lancet* 1980;2:40.

105. Candell Chalom E, Goldsmith DP, Koehler MA, et al. Prevalence and outcome of uveitis in a regional cohort of patients with juvenile rheumatoid arthritis. *J Rheumatol* 1997;24:2031–2034.

106. Kanski JJ. Screening for uveitis in juvenile chronic arthritis. *Br J Ophthalmol* 1989;73:225–228.

107. Kanski JJ. Screening for uveitis in juvenile chronic arthritis. *Br J Ophthalmol* 1989;73:225–228.

108. Kanski JJ. Screening for uveitis in juvenile chronic arthritis. *Br J Ophthalmol* 1989;73:225–228.

109. Sullivan DB, Cassidy JT, Petty RE. Pathogenic implications of age of onset in juvenile rheumatoid arthritis. *Arthritis Rheum* 1975;18:251–255.

110. Schaller JG. Juvenile rheumatoid arthritis. *Arthritis Rheum* 1977;20:165–170.

111. Jacobs JC. *Pediatric rheumatology for the practitioner,* 2nd ed. New York: Springer-Verlag, 1993:276.

112. Kaye BR, Kaye RL, Bobrove A. Rheumatoid nodules. Review of the spectrum of associated conditions and proposal of a new classification, with a report of four seronegative cases. *Am J Med* 1984;76:279–292.

113. Schaller JG. The diversity of JRA. *Arthritis Rheum* 1977;20(Suppl):52–63.

114. Denardo BA, Tucker LB, Miller LC, et al. Demography of a regional pediatric rheumatology patient population. *J Rheumatol* 1994;21:1553–1561.

115. Schaller JG. The diversity of JRA. *Arthritis Rheum* 1977;20(Suppl):53.

116. Braun J, Bollow M, Eggens U, et al. Use of dynamic magnetic resonance imaging with fast imaging in the detection of early and advanced sacroiliitis in spondyloarthropathy patients. *Arthritis Rheum* 1994;37:1039–1045.

117. Jacobs JC, Berdon ED, Johnston WE. HLA-B27-associated spondyloarthritis and enthosopathy in childhood: clinical, pathologic, and radiographic observations in 58 patients. *J Pediatr* 1982;100:521.

118. Stamato T, Laxer RM, de Freitas C, et al. Prevalence of cardiac manifestations of juvenile ankylosing spondylitis. *Am J Cardiol* 1995;75:744–746.

119. Ansell BM. Juvenile spondylitis and related disorders. In: Moll JMH, ed. *Ankylosing spondylitis.* Edinburgh: Churchill Livingstone, 1980:120.

120. Schaller J. Ankylosing spondylitis of childhood onset. *Arthritis Rheum* 1977;20(Suppl):398–401.

121. Lambert JR, Ansell BM, Stephenson E, et al. Psoriatic arthritis in childhood. *Clin Rheum Dis* 1976;2:339.

122. Shore A, Ansell BM. Juvenile psoriatic arthritis: an analysis of 60 cases. *J Pediatr* 1982;100:529–535.

123. Lovell DJ, Howe S, Shear E, et al. Development of a disability measurement tool for juvenile rheumatoid arthritis: the Juvenile Arthritis Functional Assessment Scale. *Arthritis Rheum* 1989;32:1390–1395.

124. Howe S, Levinson J, Shear E, et al. Development of a disability measurement tool for juvenile rheumatoid arthritis: The Juvenile Arthritis Functional Assessment Report for children and their parents. *Arthritis Rheum* 1991; 34:873–880.

125. Giannini EH, Ruperto N, Ravelli A, et al. Preliminary definition of improvement in juvenile arthritis. *Arthritis Rheum* 1997; 40:1202–1209.

126. Ruperto N, Ravelli A, Falcini F, et al. Performance of the preliminary definition of improvement in juvenile chronic arthritis patients treated with methotrexate. *Ann Rheum Dis* 1998;57: 38–41.

127. Singh G, Atherya B, Fried J, et al. Measurement of health status in children with juvenile rheumatoid arthritis. *Arthritis Rheum* 1994;37:1761–1769.

128. Landgraf JM, Abetz L, Ware JE. *The CHQ user's manual.* Boston: The Health Institute, New England Medical Center, 1996.

129. Duffy CM, Arsenault L, Watanabe Duffy KN, et al. The juvenile Arthritis Quality of Life Questionnaire: development of a new responsive index for juvenile rheumatoid arthritis and juvenile spondyloarthritides. *J Rheumatol* 1997;24:738–746.

130. Steans A, Manners PJ, Robinson IG. A multicentre, long-term evaluation of the safety and efficacy of ibuprofen syrup in children with juvenile chronic arthritis. *Br J Clin Pract* 1990;44: 172–175.

131. Levinson JE, Baum J, Brewer E Jr, et al. Comparison of tolmetin sodium and aspirin in the treatment of juvenile rheumatoid arthritis. *J Pediatr* 1977;91:799–804.

132. Bird HA, Ring ED, Bacon PA. A thermographic and clinical comparison of three intra-articular steroid preparations in rheumatoid arthritis. *Ann Rheum Dis* 1979;38:36.

133. Giannini EH, Brewer EJ, Kuzmina N, et al. Methotrexate in resistant juvenile rheumatoid arthritis. Results of the USA-USSR double-blind, placebo-controlled trial. *N Engl J Med* 1992;326:1043–1049.

134. Ansell BM, Hall JK, Loftus P, et al. A multicentre pilot study of sulfasalazine in juvenile chronic arthritis. *Clin Exp Rheumatol* 1991;9:201–203.

135. Miller JJ. Prolonged use of large intravenous steroid pulses in the rheumatic diseases of children. *Pediatrics* 1980;65:989–994.

136. Lovell DJ, Giannini EH, Whitmore JB, et al. Safety and efficacy of tumor necrosis factor receptor P7S FC fusion protein (TNFR:FC; ENBREL) in polyarticular course juvenile rheumatoid arthritis. *Arthritis Rheum* 1998;41:S130.

THE SERONEGATIVE SPONDYLOARTHROPATHIES

DENNIS W. BOULWARE
FRANK C. ARNETT, JR.
JOHN J. CUSH
PETER E. LIPSKY
ROBERT M. BENNETT
HERMAN MIELANTS
FILIP DE KEYSER
ERIC M. VEYS

For many years the seronegative spondyloarthropathies were confused with rheumatoid arthritis, but now they are known to be clinically and etiologically distinct (1–4). As a group, they share the following characteristics: rheumatoid factor negativity, sacroiliitis, axial involvement, peripheral arthritis, enthesopathy, eye involvement, familial clustering, and frequent presence of human leukocyte antigen B27 (HLA-B27). This chapter discusses the four main types of seronegative spondyloarthropathies: ankylosing spondylitis, Reiter or reactive arthritis, psoriatic arthritis, and arthritis associated with inflammatory bowel disease (IBD).

ANKYLOSING SPONDYLITIS

Ankylosing spondylitis (AS) (from the Greek *angkylos,* meaning "bent," and *spondylos,* meaning "spinal vertebrae") is an inflammatory disease of unknown etiology characterized by prominent inflammation of spinal joints and adjacent structures leading to progressive and ascending bony fusion of the spine. Peripheral joints are less often affected, but hips and shoulders may become involved in one-third of cases, and inflammatory lesions of extraarticular organs, such as the eye and heart, may occur (5,6).

By definition, idiopathic AS implies exclusion of the other spondyloarthropathies and is typically a disease involving predominantly the axial skeleton. A definite diagnosis of AS is dependent on the radiographic demonstration of grade 3 or 4 sacroiliitis, usually bilateral, and one or more clinical symptoms or signs, as indicated by internationally established diagnostic criteria (7,8) (Table 12.1). Sacroiliitis alone, whether symptomatic or not, should not be implied as representing definite AS, although it may represent a mild form of AS. Previously used synonyms for AS include Marie–Strüm-

pell disease, Bechterew disease, pelvospondylitis ossificans, and the misnomer rheumatoid spondylitis.

Epidemiology and Genetics

Males appear to be disproportionately affected by AS compared with females (3:1) (9). Ages of onset typically range from adolescence to age 35 and peak around 28 years. Approximately 15% of adult American and European cases have been found to have a childhood onset, whereas a higher proportion (40%) of juvenile-onset cases has been reported from developing countries (10).

The prevalence of AS has been most rigorously estimated in white populations and varies from 0.2% in white Americans to 0.9% in Berliners to 1.4% in northern Norwegians (11,12). Because disease susceptibility is strongly linked to HLA-B27 (more than 90% of AS cases are positive in most groups), disease prevalence tends to parallel the frequency of this genetic polymorphism in different ethnic populations, accounting for the low disease expression in Africans (13–17) and Japanese (18,19) and the high prevalence in certain Native American tribes, Inuits (20,21), and Siberian Chukotkas (22,23). The disease develops in approximately 2% to 6% of unrelated HLA-B27+ white individuals (12,24) (Table 12.2). However, the proportion of nonwhite HLA-B27+ individuals who develop the disease has not been estimated.

A positive family history of AS can be found in 15% to 20% of cases (25). The risk of AS for an HLA-B27+ relative is approximately 20% (24), whereas almost no risk exists for HLA-B27–negative relatives (Table 12.2). Patients with AS who are negative for HLA-B27 show similar articular manifestations as HLA-B27+ individuals. However, they differ in that they typically have an older age of onset, absence of

TABLE 12.1. CRITERIA FOR DIAGNOSING ANKYLOSING SPONDYLITIS (AS)

Rome, 1961
  Clinical Criteria
    1. Low back pain and stiffness for more than 3 months that is not relieved by rest
    2. Pain and stiffness in the thoracic region
    3. Limited motion in the lumbar spine
    4. Limited chest expansion
    5. History or evidence of iritis or its sequelae
  Radiographic Criterion
    6. Radiograph showing bilateral sacroiliac changes characteristic of AS (this would exclude bilateral osteoarthritis of the sacroiliac joints)
New York, 1966
  Clinical Criteria
    1. Limitation of motion of the lumbar spine in all three planes—anterior flexion, lateral flexion, and extension
    2. Pain at the dorsolumbar junction or in the lumbar spine
    3. Limitation of chest expansion to 1 inch (2.5 cm) or less measured at the level of the fourth intercostal space
  Grading of Radiographs
    Normal, 0; suspicious, 1; minimal sacroiliitis, 2; moderate sacroiliitis, 3; ankylosis, 4
  Definite AS
    1. Grade 3–4 bilateral sacroiliitis with at least one clinical criterion
    2. Grade 3–4 unilateral or grade 2 bilateral sacroiliitis with clinical criterion 1 or with both clinical criteria 2 and 3
  Probable AS
    Grade 3–4 bilateral sacroiliitis with no clinical criteria
Modified New York Criteria
    1. Low-back pain of at least 3 months' duration improved by exercise and not relieved by rest
    2. Limitation of lumbar spine in sagittal and frontal planes
    3. Chest expansion decreased relative to normal values for age and sex
    4. Bilateral sacroiliitis, grade 2–4
    5. Unilateral sacroiliitis, grade 3–4
    Definite AS if unilateral grade 3 or 4 or bilateral grade 2–4 sacroiliitis and any clinical criteria

From Arnett FC. Ankylosing spondylitis. In: Koopman WJ, ed. *Arthrtitis and allied conditions: a textbook of rheumatology: a textbook of rheumatology,* 14th edition, Philadelphia: Lippincott Williams & Wilkins, 2001:1311–1323, with permission.

a positive family history of AS, and significantly lower frequencies of iritis and spondylitic heart disease (26). Concordance for the disease is 63% to 75% in monozygotic twins, compared with 12.5% in all dizygotic twins and 27% in HLA-B27–positive dizygotic twins (27). Another HLA-class I allele, HLA-B60, increases the risk of AS threefold in both HLA-B27–positive and HLA-B27–negative

individuals (27), and additional MHC effects from the class II alleles HLA-DR1 and HLA-DR8 (28), and possibly class III TNF promoter alleles (29,30) have been reported.

Etiology and Pathogenesis

The cause of the ascending spinal inflammation that characterizes AS is unknown. Because of its many clinical and genetic similarities to Reiter syndrome (or reactive arthritis), etiologic models requiring both bacteria and HLA-B27 are favored (2,31). Unlike reactive arthritis, no obvious triggering bacterial pathogens have been identified. *Klebsiella pneumoniae,* a common colonizer of the gut, has been implicated as a causative microbe in a number of clinical and experimental studies (32). However, attempts to confirm these observations have been unsuccessful (33,34). *Klebsiella* shares a six–amino acid homology with HLA-B27, suggesting that molecular mimicry could play a role (35). Observations of occult bowel inflammation in a high percentage of AS patients (36), as well as a favorable therapeutic response to sulfasalazine (discussed later), also support the possibility of an enteric pathogen.

TABLE 12.2. HLA-B27 AND AS IN WHITE POPULATIONS

Population	Percent
Frequency of HLA-B27 in normal individuals	8–14
Frequency of HLA-B27 in AS patients	≥90
Prevalence of AS in populations	0.2–1.4
Prevalence of AS in random B27⁺ individuals	2–6
Prevalence of AS in B27⁺ relatives of AS patients	20
Prevalence of AS in B27⁻ relatives of AS patients	0

AS, ankylosis spondylitis.
From Arnett FC. Ankylosing spondylitis. In: Koopman WJ, ed. *Arthritis and allied conditions: a textbook of rheumatology: a textbook of rheumatology,* 14th ed. Philadelphia: Lippincott Williams & Wilkins, 2001:1311–1323, with permission.

The recent demonstration of persisting bacterial antigens and possibly dormant, but viable, microorganisms in the peripheral joints of patients with reactive arthritis has led to speculation concerning bacterial antigens and microorganisms in the spinal joints in AS (2,37). To date, one study of sacroiliac joint biopsies using nested polymerase chain reaction (PCR) found no evidence of bacterial DNA from *Klebsiella* or the organisms implicated in reactive arthritis (38). Additionally, elevated serum levels of IgA antibodies to the causative bacteria in reactive arthritis have been reported that probably reflect increased mucosal immunity to persisting infection (39,40). Recent searches for increased serum levels of antibodies to a variety of bacteria in AS patients have been largely unrewarding (2,41,42).

Clinical Features and Diagnosis

Modes of Presentation

Chronic low back pain and stiffness are typically the first symptoms of AS (43–45). Onset is usually insidious rather than abrupt, and patients often cannot date when symptoms first began, or precisely localize the areas affected. Complaints of alternating pain, first in one buttock and then the other, occasionally with radiation down the posterior thigh, can be elicited from some patients and probably represent sacroiliac involvement. Often these symptoms are incorrectly ascribed to hip disease or sciatica by the patient. Because low back discomfort is such a common malady in the population at large, much attention has been directed at attempting to differentiate inflammatory from noninflammatory back pain (43). Characteristically, inflammatory back symptoms are suggested by prominent stiffness and pain in the morning or following other periods of rest (gel phenomenon) that improve with exercise. Such symptoms are most likely to reflect AS in a young person under 40 years of age. Additional historic data suggesting AS include back pain that forces the individual out of bed at night or is unrelieved by lying down, as well as concomitant chest wall pain (44). Although symptoms of inflammatory back disease are often useful in raising the likelihood of AS, it must be emphasized that some patients with AS will have only nonspecific or even no low back complaints despite typical radiographic changes (45). Less commonly, patients with AS may present with a peripheral arthritis, typically mono- or oligoarticular, and often affecting one or both knees (46). Enthesitis, especially involving Achilles or plantar tendon insertions and causing heel pain, may present alone or with arthritis (47,48). Such presentations should prompt a consideration of Reiter syndrome or reactive arthritis in adults. However, juvenile AS or the SEA (seronegative enthesopathy and arthritis) syndrome of children, especially boys, typically presents in this fashion (49–51). Other patterns of AS onset in children have been described, including ankylosing tarsitis (52), symmetric polyarthritis, and dominant cervical spine involvement (53).

Physical Examination and Disease Course

The earliest abnormality on physical examination in AS is usually tenderness in the sacroiliac joints or pain in the same areas elicited by hip hyperextension. The straight-leg-raising test, often used to detect sciatic nerve irritation by a ruptured disc, is typically negative, and deep tendon reflexes in the lower extremities are normal (44,46). More objective findings occur with longer disease duration and include flattening of the normal lordotic curvature and restriction of movement in all planes of the lumbar spine. With lumbar involvement, Schober test of lumbar flexion is significantly reduced (<3 cm), and the patient is unable to touch fingers to floor by a considerable distance. When the disease has advanced to the thoracic spine, a restricted chest expansion (<2.5 cm) due to costovertebral joint fusion is a reasonably specific sign of AS, especially in a young individual (46). Additionally, the normal kyphosis of the dorsal spine becomes accentuated, and the patient assumes a "stooped-shoulder" appearance (Fig 12.1). Cervical spine involve-

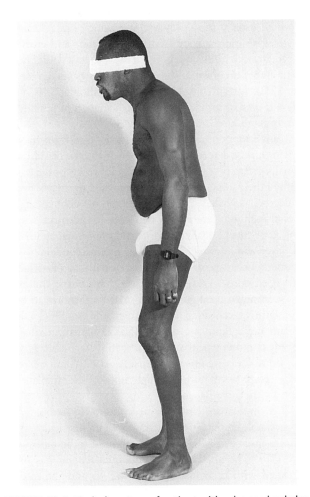

FIGURE 12.1. Typical posture of patient with advanced ankylosing spondylitis. Note loss of normal lumbar lordosis, presence of dorsal kyposis, cervical fixation in mild flexion, and compensatory flexion of the knees. (From Arnett FC. Ankylosing spondylitis. In: Koopman WJ, ed. *Arthritis and allied conditions: a textbook of rheumatology,* 14th ed. Philadelphia: Lippincott Williams & Wilkins, 2001:1311–1323, with permission.)

ment is usually the last manifestation to appear. Pain and stiffness in cervical joints and surrounding muscles are followed by a decreased ability to extend the neck fully. The extent of this deformity can be measured by the occiput-to-wall distance in which the standing patient places the back of the heels against a wall and attempts to touch the wall with the back of the head. Loss of lateral rotation also occurs, and eventually the neck may lose all motion and become fixed in a flexed position. If this deformity is extreme, forward vision may be compromised, as an upward gaze is limited. Depending on the severity of both cervical and thoracic kyphosis, the patient may need to stand with knees voluntarily flexed to maintain a center of gravity.

Radiographic Abnormalities

Sacroiliitis, usually bilateral, is the most frequent and earliest radiographic manifestation of AS (54). The first radiographic signs of sacroiliitis include "pseudowidening" of the joint and sclerosis at one or both joint margins (grades 1 and 2), usually in the lower third, which has a synovial lining. With more advanced disease, sclerosis and erosions appear at both joint margins (grade 3), and later, bony fusion across the joint and loss of sclerosis occur (grade 4) (Fig. 12.2). Interpretation of sacroiliac radiographs is difficult, and there is much interobserver variation, especially in its early stages of disease (55).

An anteroposterior view of the pelvis is usually not an adequate means of detecting early sacroiliac disease because the normal forward tilt of the pelvis precludes a view of the entire length of these joints. Rather, radiographs of the pelvis aimed 30 degrees cephalad (Ferguson views) or oblique-angled views of each joint are usually necessary for adequate assessment. Care must be taken to disregard congenital anomalies and degenerative changes, as well as osteitis condensans ilii (symmetric sclerosis on the iliac sides of both sacroiliac joints without erosions seen in women who have borne children) (54). Computed tomography (CT) has been shown to be a more sensitive technique for detecting early sacroiliitis when standard radiographs are normal (56). Magnetic resonance imaging is more expensive and probably as reliable as CT (57). Bone scans are not at all reliable, especially in bilateral disease, because of normally high uptakes of radiolabeled tracers by the sacroiliac joints.

When evaluating children, plain sacroiliac radiographs are unreliable in detecting sacroiliitis in children; however, contrast-enhanced MRI has been reported to be more sensitive (58). The appearance of hip involvement has been correlated with early age of onset for AS and indicates a poor prognosis (59).

Other pelvic abnormalities that may occur in AS include osteitis pubis (sclerosis and bony irregularities at the symphysis pubis), as well as bony erosions or "whiskering" along the margins of ischial tuberosities, iliac crests, or proximal trochanters indicative of enthesitis (54).

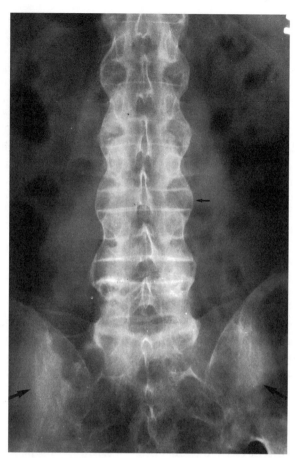

FIGURE 12.2. Anteroposterior radiograph of the upper pelvis and lumbar spine. Both sacroiliac joints (*large arrows*) are fused (grade IV sacroiliitis), and there are bilateral, symmetric syndesmophytes (*small arrow*) resulting in the typical "bamboo" appearance of AS. (From Arnett FC. Ankylosing spondylitis. In: Koopman WJ, ed. *Arthritis and allied conditions: a textbook of rheumatology,* 14th ed. Philadelphia: Lippincott Williams & Wilkins, 2001:1311–1323. Used with permission.)

The most characteristic radiographic changes of AS in the lumbar, dorsal, and cervical spine include "squaring" of the vertebral bodies due to erosions of their normally concave anterior superior and inferior surfaces and often appearing as "shiny corners" (Romanus lesions) (Fig. 12.3) (60). Additionally, ossification of spinal ligaments, which bridge the intervertebral discs, results in the characteristic "syndesmophytes" (Figs. 12.2 and 12.3). When many syndesmophytes are present bilaterally, the radiographic appearance is that of a "bamboo spine" (Fig. 12.2). In general, the syndesmophytes seen in AS, as well as in enteropathic spondylitis, are symmetric and bilateral, and have their insertions at the upper and lower margins of adjacent vertebral bodies. In contrast, syndesmophytes occurring in Reiter syndrome and psoriatic spondylitis tend to be asymmetric and have nonmarginal vertebral insertions (61,62). In addition, zygapophyseal joints in AS are obliterated by bony fusion. The presence of bony fusion of cervical apophyseal joints may be particularly discriminating for AS in some atypical cases described in children and women (Fig. 12.4) (53). Less commonly, erosions

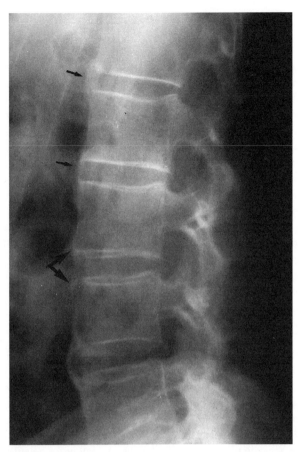

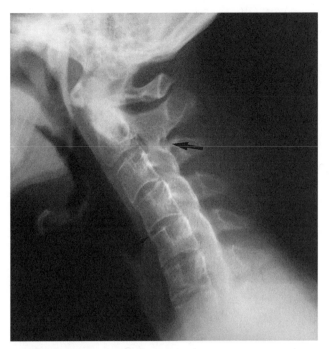

FIGURE 12.4. Lateral radiograph of the cervical spine in anky-losing spondylitis. *Large arrow* points to bony fusion of apophy-seal joint between C2 and C3. All other apophyseal joints below this level are also fused. *Small arrow* indicates a marginal syn-desmophyte. (From Arnett FC. Ankylosing spondylitis. In: Koop-man WJ, ed. *Arthritis and allied conditions: a textbook of rheumatology,* 14th ed. Philadelphia: Lippincott Williams & Wilkins, 2001:1311–1323, with permission.)

FIGURE 12.3. Lateral radiograph of the lumbar spine in anky-losing spondylitis. *Large arrows* indicate "shiny corners" (Romanus lesions) due to marginal erosions of vertebral bodies. *Small arrows* indicate typical marginal syndesmophytes. (From Arnett FC. Ankylosing spondylitis. In: Koopman WJ, ed. *Arthritis and allied conditions: a textbook of rheumatology,* 14th ed. Philadelphia: Lippincott Williams & Wilkins, 2001:1311–1323, with permission.)

Involved peripheral joints may show osteopenia and ero-sions similar to those of rheumatoid arthritis. More often in AS, however, are findings of bony ankylosis in wrists, tarsal bones, hips, or small joints of the fingers and toes.

Diagnosis and Differential Diagnosis

Although symptoms of inflammatory back disease, espe-cially in a young man, and the typical spinal abnormalities on physical examination, when present, should strongly suggest the diagnosis of AS, the most specific diagnostic findings are the characteristic radiographic changes. Sacroiliitis, especially when bilateral, is a virtual prerequisite for definite diagnosis. Both the New York (7) and modified New York (8) Diagnostic Criteria for AS require the pres-ence of radiographic sacroiliitis and one or more of the clin-ical symptoms or signs (Table 12.1). In fact, radiographic sacroiliitis, when properly interpreted, has a very limited differential diagnosis, with the most common causes being the spondyloarthropathies and infectious processes (Table 12.3).

More problematic are patients with characteristic spinal symptoms in whom radiographic studies are normal or equivocal, or patients with atypical presentations, including children or women, who present with predominantly peripheral arthritis, enthesitis, and cervical spine symptoms. Although CT or MRI of the sacroiliac joints may be an

of upper cervical structures such as the transverse ligament or odontoid process may lead to subluxation (63), similar to what is seen in rheumatoid arthritis, or even upward migra-tion of the odontoid into the brainstem (platybasia), result-ing in a neurologic catastrophe (64). Generalized spinal osteopenia is common in AS, probably due to immobility and local cytokine release (65,66), and spinal fractures, espe-cially of the neck, may occur after minor trauma (67,68). As segments of the spine become progressively fused, pain often disappears. The appearance of renewed pain may indicate a complicating fracture, which may not be apparent on stan-dard radiographs (69). In this circumstance, a bone scan may show increased uptake of tracer in the fracture site, which may then require further elucidation by CT (70). Another cause of renewed spinal pain, usually sharply localized and exacerbated by exercise, is spondylodiscitis (Andersson lesion), a sterile, circumscribed, destructive process involving one vertebral body and adjacent intervertebral disc that may mimic and must be discriminated from an infectious discitis or osteomyelitis (71,72).

TABLE 12.3. CAUSES OF SACROILIITIS

Spondyloarthropathies
 AS
 Reiter syndrome (reactive arthritis)
 Psoriatic arthritis
 Inflammatory bowel disease
 Acne-associated arthritis or SAPHO syndrome
 Intestinal bypass arthritis
Infectious
 Pyogenic infections
 Tuberculosis
 Brucellosis
 Whipple disease
Others
 Hyperparathyroidism
 Paraplegia
 Sarcoidosis (rare)

AS, ankylosing spondylitis; SAPHO,
synovitis–acne–pustulosis–hyperostosis–osteitis.
From Arnett FC. Ankylosing spondylitis. In: Koopman WJ, ed.
*Arthrtitis and allied conditions: a textbook of rheumatology: a
textbook of rheumatology,* 14th ed. Philadelphia: Lippincott
Williams & Wilkins, 2001:1311–1323, with permission.

option in some of these patients, a less expensive approach may be a blood test for HLA-B27. Although diagnostic testing for HLA-B27 was previously discouraged (73), subsequent studies have demonstrated its potential usefulness as an adjunct in diagnosis, especially if the patient has inflammatory back symptoms (12,74). The frequency of HLA-B27 is more than 90% in AS patients and approximately 8% in most normal white populations. Thus a "false-positive"' result (HLA-B27 positivity unrelated to the patient's symptoms) would be expected to occur approximately 8% of the time, and a "false-negative" (patient has HLA-B27 negative AS), less than 10% of the time. As with any other test, the predictive value of HLA-B27 is greatest when the physician has reason to believe that the disease is present (74). The finding of HLA-B27 is even more predictive of disease in ethnic populations in which the normal frequency of this genetic marker is low, such as African (2%) or Japanese patients (<1%). In Native Americans and other groups with high normal background levels of HLA-B27, it is much less useful as a diagnostic aid.

Causes other than AS for spinal pain and restriction can usually be excluded by standard radiographs. An exception may be diffuse idiopathic skeletal hyperostosis (DISH), or Forestier disease, in which prominent syndesmophytes and enthesopathy may mimic AS. DISH, however, can usually be differentiated from AS by its later age-of-onset, larger and more flowing ligamentous ossifications (syndesmophytes), and most important, absence of sacroiliitis (54). Also, DISH is not associated with HLA-B27 (75). A DISH-like syndrome has been described in patients, often young, receiving long-term retinoid therapy. Again, sacroiliitis should be absent in such patients, although one case report suggests otherwise (76).

Extraarticular Manifestations

Ocular

Episodes of acute anterior uveitis or iritis occur in approximately 25% of AS patients at some time during the course of their disease (77). Usually, one eye is affected at a time, and there are often long intervals between attacks. Typical symptoms include the sudden onset of ocular pain, redness, and photophobia. Unless inflammation is promptly suppressed, debris may accumulate in the anterior chamber, causing pupillary and lens dysfunction and blurring of vision. In some cases, the posterior chamber becomes inflamed, causing macular edema and further visual compromise. Permanent blindness is unusual but may occur in some patients, especially those not treated promptly and aggressively. Acute anterior uveitis of this type shows a strong association with HLA-B27 regardless of whether the patient has spondyloarthropathy.

Cardiac Manifestations

Aortic regurgitation and variable degrees of atrioventricular or bundle branch block occur in approximately 5% of patients with AS, usually after long-standing disease, but occasionally preceding arthritis symptoms (78). Less often, mitral regurgitation accompanies aortic disease (79). Nearly all such patients are HLA-B27+. Once the murmur of aortic regurgitation is heard, the disease follows a relentless course to heart failure, usually over several years. There is no effective therapy except for valvular replacement. Similarly, complete heart block requires implantation of a cardiac pacemaker.

Bergfeldt and colleagues (80) have conducted extensive clinical studies of spondylitic heart disease. Of 223 patients, 28 (12.5%) were found to have clinical and radiographic evidence of AS or Reiter syndrome, often undiagnosed (81). The combination of heart block and aortic insufficiency found in 91 pacemaker recipients was associated with a spondyloarthropathy in 15% to 20% and with HLA-B27 in 88% (82). Moreover, HLA-B27 was positive in 17% of 83 patients with complete heart block who had no clinical or radiographic evidence of arthritis as compared with 6% in a normal control population, a statistically significant difference (83).

Pulmonary

Lung involvement in AS is unusual (84–86). Despite a diminished chest expansion due to costovertebral joint fusion, patients with AS rarely have significant reductions in total lung and vital capacities because diaphragmatic function is not impaired. Bilateral apical pulmonary fibrosis occurs in approximately 1% of patients, usually after many years of disease, and cavitation mimicking tuberculosis occurs in one-third of these. Rarely, colonization of these cavities by *Aspergillus* occurs, which requires consideration of antifungal therapy.

Renal

Secondary amyloidosis complicates the course of AS and other spondyloarthropathies in 1% to 3% of cases and occurs more commonly in Europe than in the United States. Proteinuria, often in the nephrotic range, is the usual presentation, and progression to renal failure is common. Abdominal fat pad or rectal biopsies for amyloid may be found in approximately 7% of unselected cases of AS, but most do not develop clinically significant disease (87). Proteinuria, with or without renal function impairment, may also indicate the presence of IgA nephropathy, which is of considerable interest in view of serum elevations of IgA in AS patients (88). Renal dysfunction and proteinuria can result from use of nonsteroidal antiinflammatory drugs or large amounts of analgesic use.

Neurologic

Besides cervical spine fractures and dislocations, a slowly progressive cauda equina syndrome may appear late in the disease course (89). Usual symptoms include sensory loss in lumbar and sacral dermatomes and, less often, lower-extremity weakness and pain, and loss of urinary and rectal sphincter tone. MRI is the most reliable means of demonstrating the characteristic enlarged dural sacs and arachnoid diverticula and excluding other potentially surgically correctable myelopathies (90,91). There may be an increased frequency of multiple sclerosis in AS patients, but this has not been proven by definitive epidemiologic studies (90).

Gastrointestinal Tract

Asymptomatic areas of both macroscopic and microscopic inflammation in the proximal colon and terminal ileum have been demonstrated by ileocolonoscopy in up to 60% of patients with AS (36). Although of considerable pathogenetic interest, these findings do not indicate a high likelihood of developing overt Crohn disease or ulcerative colitis. Rarely, patients with long-standing AS develop typical symptoms and findings of IBD.

Laboratory Features

The most characteristic laboratory abnormalities are elevations of the erythrocyte sedimentation rate (ESR) and other acute-phase reactants. Similarly, the platelet count may be slightly or moderately elevated, or there may be mild anemia, depending on the severity of the inflammatory process. Serum IgA levels are elevated in most patients, but whether these represent antibodies to causative bacteria is unknown. Tests for rheumatoid factors and antinuclear antibodies are

negative, and serum complement levels are normal or high. HLA-B27 is positive in more than 90% of patients, and its frequency approaches 100% in those with acute anterior uveitis or spondylitic heart disease. Modest elevations of bone alkaline phosphatase and creatine kinase (CK) occur in some patients, but their significance is unclear (92).

Treatment

The major aims of management include (a) the pharmacologic relief of pain and stiffness; (b) a physical therapy and lifestyle modification program aimed at preserving spinal mobility or, at least, preventing spinal deformity and disability; and (c) the prompt recognition and management of articular and extraarticular complications. It is essential that the patient be well educated in the natural history of this disease and the rationale for each treatment modality.

Pharmacologic

Nonsteroidal antiinflammatory drugs (NSAIDs) are usually necessary, at least initially, to relieve the pain and stiffness before a patient can satisfactorily perform the proper exercises. Indomethacin is now most commonly used, having largely replaced the highly effective but more toxic drug phenylbutazone (93). The dosage of indomethacin should be geared to the severity of symptoms and degree of relief, but nightly administration of the 75-mg sustained-release preparation may be particularly useful in preventing night pain and morning stiffness (94). Many other NSAIDs—including tolmetin, piroxicam, and diclofenac—may prove more effective in individual patients. The recent addition of selective cyclooxygenase-2 inhibitors with less potential for gastrointestinal toxicity offers additional potentially useful NSAIDs. In general, aspirin is usually inadequate. Of course, patients on NSAIDs require monitoring for the usual gastrointestinal and renal complications inherent to these agents.

Multiple controlled clinical trials have demonstrated the effectiveness of sulfasalazine (usually 2 to 3 g daily) for AS, especially early in the disease (95–97). Such studies have shown improvement in spinal symptoms, and perhaps spinal mobility, peripheral arthritis, and, impressively, reduction of the levels of acute-phase reactants, thus suggesting that sulfasalazine might be a "disease-modifying" agent. One recent study demonstrated that the sulfapyridine, rather than the salicylate, moiety accounted for its therapeutic effects (98). It remains unclear, however, whether sulfasalazine improves disease through its antibiotic effect on intestinal bacteria or through other immunomodulatory or antiinflammatory properties.

Immunosuppressive drugs, including methotrexate, azathioprine, and cyclophosphamide, may be effective in some severe cases, but this has not been established by controlled studies. Pulse high-dose methylprednisolone has proved temporarily effective in acute flares (99). The potential effectiveness of newer antirheumatic therapies, such as the anti-TNF agent etanercept, has been demonstrated recently (100). Chronic low-dose corticosteroids may be necessary at times, especially for refractory peripheral arthritis. However, drug-related osteoporotic effects should be considered.

Acute anterior uveitis requires prompt treatment by an ophthalmologist (77). Local corticosteroid and mydriatic drops are the usual first approach. Patients with more refractory eye disease, however, may require retrobulbar injections or even systemic corticosteroids for short periods. Currently, there is no known medical treatment for the cardiac, pulmonary, and renal lesions of AS.

Physical Therapy

Formal instruction in proper posture and exercises emphasizing spinal mobility and strengthening of spinal extensors should be provided to every patient initially and reemphasized periodically. Range-of-motion exercises for the neck, shoulders, and hips, as well as deep-breathing exercises to maintain chest expansion, should also be emphasized (101,102). Swimming is an excellent modality for achieving all these goals. Canes or walkers may be necessary for patients with severe spinal kyphosis or lower-extremity arthritis. Patients with neck fusion or subluxation should use soft cervical collars in situations where they are liable for injury. Adaptive devices such as prism glasses may be necessary to ensure forward vision in those with severe cervical flexion, and special mirrors in automobiles may help those with decreased spinal rotation (103).

Surgical Approaches

Total hip replacement is the most common orthopedic surgical procedure needed by patients with AS, and the results are usually satisfactory (104). Occasionally, heterotopic bone formation around the implant may mimic complicating infection, and at times new bone may encase the prosthesis and restrict motion (105). Osteotomy of the spine has been used to correct severe spinal deformity but is fraught with hazard (106). Moreover, for any surgical procedure requiring general anesthesia, intubation must be approached cautiously because of cervical spine fragility and limitation of mouth opening (107).

Prognosis

Several long-term studies indicate that the prognosis of AS is good in most patients (6,103,108,109). Only 10% to 20% became significantly disabled over long periods (20 to 38 years), and 85% to 90% are able to pursue full-time employment, despite progression to severe spinal restriction in approximately one-half. A predictable pattern of disease usually emerges after the first 10 years. Hip disease, which typically begins early and in the youngest patients, is the surest indicator of a poor functional outcome.

Mortality from the disease itself occurs in less than 5% of patients, most commonly from cervical fractures and dislocations, spondylitic heart disease, and amyloid nephropathy. Malignancies are increased only in those who have received spinal irradiation and include a fivefold increase in leukemias and a 62% excess of other cancers (108,110–112).

REITER SYNDROME AND REACTIVE ARTHRITIS

Reactive arthritis refers to the occurrence of an acute, non-suppurative, sterile, inflammatory arthropathy arising after an infectious process but at a site remote from the primary infection (113). Reiter syndrome is one of the most common examples of reactive arthritis (114,115). Although these terms have been used interchangeably, *Reiter syndrome* refers to a specific complex of organ pathology with typical extraarticular features within the larger group of patients with reactive arthritis. Whereas reactive arthritis describes a variety of conditions in which inflammatory arthritis is a dominant manifestation, typical extraarticular features of Reiter syndrome may not be present. Both Reiter syndrome and reactive arthritis are pathogenically related by virtue of their documented or presumed postinfectious onset, which is followed by persistent inflammation and occurs in individuals inheriting HLA-B27. Numerous reactive arthropathies initiated by a variety of arthritogenic organisms have been described (113–115).

The reactive arthritides share several distinctive clinical and laboratory characteristics. In a substantial number of cases, an identifiable infectious event precedes, by 1 to 4 weeks, the onset of an asymmetric oligoarthritis, often involving the large joints. Commonly, the triggering infectious process subsides before the onset of arthritis. This temporal sequence, along with the presence of microbial material, but not living microorganisms, in the affected joint indicates that these disorders are triggered by the infectious process. In many patients, an identifiable infectious trigger is not apparent, yet these patients manifest a similar constellation of signs and symptoms. The findings of sterile, inflammatory synovial effusions, lymphocytes at sites of tissue inflammation, responsiveness to antiinflammatory regimens, and association with the class I major histocompatibility complex (MHC) antigen HLA-B27 suggest that these disorders share a common immunopathogenesis.

Another distinctive feature of this group of reactive arthropathies is the associated inflammatory symptomatology at extraarticular sites, including the eye, mucosal surfaces, and entheses (tendon insertion sites onto the bone). Although frequently self-limiting, these disorders have the potential for chronicity and articular damage to the peripheral or axial joints.

In 1916, Professor Hans Reiter described a Prussian officer with urethritis, conjunctivitis, and arthritis following an episode of bloody diarrhea (116). In the same year, Fiessinger and Leroy described a similar patient with a post-dysenteric "oculo-urethro-synovial syndrome." Although this syndrome bears Reiter's name, there are earlier descriptions of a similar syndrome.

Reiter Syndrome

Classification

The classic triad of Reiter syndrome requires the presence of arthritis, urethritis, and conjunctivitis, and occurs in only one-third of all patients. The American College of Rheumatology (ACR) established less stringent criteria for the classification of Reiter syndrome (114,115). ACR criteria require the presence of peripheral arthritis of more than 1 month's duration, occurring in association with urethritis and/or cervicitis (117). The ACR criteria exhibit a sensitivity of 84.3% and specificity of 98.2% when used to distinguish patients with Reiter syndrome from those with ankylosing spondylitis, psoriatic arthritis, seronegative rheumatoid arthritis, or gonococcal arthritis. These criteria have not been universally accepted, however, largely because a substantial number of patients at the outset of their disease may not meet these criteria. Such "unclassified" patients may be more numerous than those meeting ACR criteria (118). The European Spondyloarthropathy Study Group (ESSG) (119) and the French Society of Rheumatology (FSR) (120) have each proposed more generic criteria for the diagnosis of the spondyloarthropathies (Table 12.4). These criteria recognize that numerous clinical features are shared by the HLA-B27-

TABLE 12.4. ALTERNATIVE CRITERIA FOR THE DIAGNOSIS OF THE SPONDYLOARTHROPATHIES

European Spondyloarthropathy[a] Study Group Criteria for Spondyloarthropathy

Inflammatory spinal pain *or* Peripheral Synovitis—asymmetric or lower limb *and one or more of the following:*

Positive family history
Psoriasis
Inflammatory bowel disease
Urethritis or cervicitis or acute diarrhea within 1 month of arthritis onset
Alternate buttock pain
Enthesopathy
Sacroiliitis

Classification for Spondyloarthropathy[b]

Parameter	Score
Clinical symptoms or past history of	
1. Lumbar or dorsal pain at night or morning stiffness of lumbar **or** dorsal spine	1
2. Asymmetric oligoarthritis	2
3. Buttock pain or	1
if bilateral or if alternating buttock pain	2
4. Sausage-like toe(s) or digit(s)	2
5. Heel pain or other well-defined enthesiopathic pain	2
6. Iritis	2
7. Nongonococcal urethritis or cervicitis within 1 month before onset of arthritis	1
8. Acute diarrhea within 1 month before onset of arthritis	1
9. Psoriasis, balanitis, or inflammatory bowel disease (IBD)	2
Radiographic findings:	
10. Sacroiliitis (bilateral grade 2 or unilateral grade 3)	2
Genetic background:	
11. Presence of HLA-B27 or family history of ankylosing spondylitis, reactive arthritis, uveitis, psoriasis, or IBD	2
Response to treatment:	
12. Clearcut, rapid (within 48 hours) improvement after NSAID intake or rapid relapse of pain after discontinuation of agent	2
Diagnosis of spondyloarthropathy requires a score ≥6	

[a]Dougados M, Vander Linden S, Juhlin R, et al. The European Spondyloarthropathy Study Group preliminary criteria for the classification of spondyloarthropathy. *Arthritis Rheum* 1991;34:1218–1227.
[b]Reproduced by permission from Amor B, Dougados M, Mijiyawa M, et al. Critères de classification de spondyloarthropathies. *Rev Rhum* 1990;57:85–89.
NSAID, nonsteroidal anti-inflammatory drug.

related spondyloarthropathies and that patients often demonstrate incomplete features of a particular spondyloarthropathy.

Epidemiology

Epidemiologic estimates of the prevalence and incidence of Reiter syndrome are limited because of (a) the lack of consensus regarding diagnostic criteria, (b) the nomadic nature of a young target population, (c) the underreporting of venereal disease, and (d) the asymptomatic and/or milder course in affected women. A survey of patients in Olmstead County, Minnesota, between 1950 and 1980, found that the age-adjusted incidence rate for males under the age of 50 years was 3.5 cases per 100,000 men (121). Similarly, a 2-year survey of reactive arthritis in Oslo, Norway, reported a minimum incidence rate of 4.6 and 5.0 cases per 100,000 for reactive arthritis caused by *Chlamydia* and Enterobacteriaceae (*Salmonella, Yersinia, Campylobacter*), respectively (122).

Reiter syndrome has its peak onset during the third decade of life, but has been reported in children and octogenarians (115,118,123,124). Despite the consistency of these findings, many have noted the decreasing prevalence of Reiter syndrome (114,125). Men are most commonly affected, with some estimates suggesting a male/female ratio of more than 25:1 (115,123). However, the male predominance is likely to be overestimated because Reiter syndrome in women may be associated with occult genitourinary disease. Moreover, disease expression is usually less severe in women (115). Recent estimates have suggested that the male/female ratio in Reiter syndrome is closer to 5:1 or 6:1 (114). Postvenereal Reiter syndrome is more common in males, whereas postdysenteric Reiter syndrome affects men and women equally (115,121,122).

Etiopathogenesis

Infectious Agents
Table 12.5 lists the agents implicated in triggering Reiter syndrome. In most instances, however, no infectious etiology can be identified. The most common microbial pathogens known to induce Reiter syndrome are *Shigella, Salmonella, Yersinia, Campylobacter,* and *Chlamydia* (113–115,126).

Enteric Infections Predisposing to Reiter Syndrome
Shigella. The occurrence of reactive arthritis following epidemics of *Shigella* dysentery has established the arthritogenicity of this organism (127,128). Several reports suggest that 0.2% to 2% of infected individuals develop Reiter syndrome following epidemic shigellosis (121,127,128). Infections with *S. flexneri* 2a and 1b trigger Reiter syndrome, whereas the more frequent *S. sonnei* does not (114,115,123).

TABLE 12.5. INFECTIOUS ORGANISMS ASSOCIATED WITH THE ONSET OF REITER SYNDROME

Enteric Pathogens
Shigella flexneri, serotype 2a, 1b
Salmonella typhimurium
S. enteritidis
S. paratyphi
S. Heidelberg
S. abony
S. blocley
S. schwarzengrund
S. Haifa
S. manila
S. newport
S. bovismorbificans
Yersinia enterocolitica (serotypes 0:3, 0:8, 0:9)
Y. pseudotuberculosis
Campylobacter jejuni
C. fetus
Vibrio parahemolyticus

Urogenital Pathogens
Chlamydia trachomatis
C. psittaci
C. pneumoniae
Ureaplasma urealyticum

From Cush JJ, Lipsky PE. Reiter's syndrome and reactive arthritis. In: Koopman WJ, ed. *Arthrtitis and allied conditions: a textbook of rheumatology,* 14th ed. Philadelphia: Lippincott Williams & Wilkins, 2001:1324–1344, with permission.

Arthritis most commonly affects infected HLA-B27$^+$ individuals and has its peak onset 10 to 30 days following the onset of diarrhea. In most cases, the diarrheal illness resolves before the articular inflammation appears. The clinical manifestations of *Shigella*-related Reiter syndrome are described later.

Salmonella. *Salmonella typhimurium* is the most common species inducing a reactive arthropathy. Although previous reports have suggested that 1% to 3% of infected individuals develop a sterile arthropathy following *Salmonella* outbreaks (114, 115, 129), two studies have suggested that the incidence rate may be as high as 6.4% to 12% (128,130,131). Arthritis usually develops within 3 to 4 weeks of infection with *S. typhimurium*. Reactive arthritis also has been associated with less common infections secondary to *S. paratyphi, S. enteridis, S. heidelberg, S. abony, S. blocley, S. schwarzengrund, S. haifa, S. manila, S. newport,* and *S. bovismorbificans* (114,115,131).

Yersinia. *Yersinia* is a common cause of reactive arthritis in certain endemic areas, especially Scandinavian countries. Although rarely encountered in England or America,

Yersinia enterocolitica is the most frequent isolate in northern Europe. *Y. enterocolitica* 0:3 has most commonly been implicated, but arthritis has also been documented after infections with serotypes 0:9 and 0:8 (113,115,132). *Y. pseudotuberculosis,* an uncommon pathogen, has been reported outside of the Scandinavian countries (114–115,132).

HLA-B27 is present in 60% to 80% of patients with *Yersinia* arthritis (115,133). The associated arthritis is predominantly oligoarticular, affecting the lower extremities and hands. The arthritis pursues a chronic or relapsing course in some patients, with chronic low back pain and chronic sacroiliitis developing in one-third of patients. Five percent of patients exhibit recurrent attacks of reactive arthritis, often resulting from infections with other arthritogenic microbes such as *Salmonella* or *Chlamydia* (133). Rarely, such patients progress to a clinical state indistinguishable from ankylosing spondylitis. Extraarticular features, including urethritis, ocular inflammation, mucocutaneous disease, and carditis, occur in 20% to 30% of individuals, most of whom are HLA-B27+. Uncommon findings, including erythema nodosum and glomerulonephritis, are seen more frequently in HLA-B27−- individuals. Active infection is associated with elevated anti-*Yersinia* antibodies of the IgA and IgG isotypes. Sustained elevations of IgA antibody titers have been shown to correlate with persistent infection, chronic arthritis, and occult enteritis (134,135). *Yersinia* is commonly cultured from the stool during the acute infection; however, synovial fluid or tissue cultures are uniformly negative. Nonetheless, *Yersinia* antigens have been identified in both synovial fluid and tissue (115,132,136), suggesting that a persistent immune response to microbial antigens might play a role in the induction of inflammation.

Yersinia arthritis is usually mild and most often without long-term sequelae. However, chronicity, severity, sacroiliitis, and ocular inflammation are more likely in HLA-B27+ individuals (133). Treatment is similar to that used in other reactive arthropathies. Appropriate antibiotic therapy should be considered, however, for patients with persistently positive stool cultures.

Campylobacter. Gastrointestinal infections with *Campylobacter jejuni* and *C. fetus* are also associated with the development of reactive arthritis that may occasionally manifest as Reiter syndrome (114,115,132).

Sexually Acquired Infections Predisposing to Reiter Syndrome

Chlamydia. *Chlamydia trachomatis* is a common urogenital pathogen that can trigger Reiter syndrome. Although positive cultures are seldom observed in patients with active arthritis, more than 50% of patients with Reiter syndrome have antibodies to *C. trachomatis* (114,115). An equivalent percentage of patients with sexually acquired reactive arthritis or nongonococcal urethritis exhibit antichlamydial antibodies. These are presumably directed at *Chlamydia* antigens (chlamydial elementary bodies) that have been identified in the synovial fluid and synovial tissue of patients with Reiter syndrome, particularly in early disease (115).

Chlamydial infection is thought to be responsible for 10% of all cases of early inflammatory arthritis (137); as many as 1% to 4% of those individuals with chlamydial urethritis will ultimately develop arthritis (115,126). Of the chlamydial species responsible for Reiter syndrome, *C. trachomatis* (serotypes D to K) is the most common, with primary infection involving either the urogenital or ocular tract in men and women. *C. psittaci* and *C. pneumoniae* (Table 12.5) also have been reported to produce a reactive arthropathy (114,115,138–140). *C. pneumoniae* may be associated with erythema nodosum, pneumonia, and myocarditis. The rheumatic manifestations of chlamydial infections are similar to those described in classic Reiter syndrome (i.e., asymmetric oligoarthritis, enthesitis, ocular inflammation, low back pain, and sacroiliitis), although less than 50% of affected individuals are HLA-B27+ (121,137). Diagnosis is suggested by the presence of persistent arthritis in at least one joint, symptoms of genitourinary infection, laboratory evidence of chlamydial infection, and response to antibiotic therapy. Chlamydial infection may be documented by detecting IgG or IgA antichlamydial antibodies [by enzyme immunoassay (EIA) or direct fluorescent antibody (DFA) tests], finding *Chlamydia* RNA using DNA probes, or demonstrating chlamydial infection through genitourinary swabs or urine culture.

Ureaplasma. *Ureaplasma urealyticum* has rarely been implicated as a pathogenic trigger in Reiter syndrome, especially in cases of nonchlamydial sexually acquired reactive arthritis (114,115,136,138a,141).

Acquired Immunodeficiency Syndrome and Reactive Arthritis. In 1987 a group of patients who developed both acquired immunodeficiency syndrome (AIDS) and Reiter syndrome was described (142). The manifestations of Reiter syndrome were especially aggressive in these individuals (142–146). Of note, many developed Reiter syndrome after they became profoundly immunosuppressed (142–145,147). Despite the occurrence of reactive arthritis, no cases of ankylosing spondylitis in AIDS patients have been reported.

Like classic Reiter syndrome, most AIDS patients with reactive arthritis are HLA-B27+ and present with incomplete symptoms and signs of Reiter syndrome (142–147). Although observed in asymptomatic HIV+ individuals, reactive arthritis appears to be more common in individuals with established AIDS or in those progressing from HIV-

TABLE 12.6. FEATURES OF AIDS-ASSOCIATED REACTIVE ARTHRITIS

HLA-B27[+] in 75% of cases
Severe/chronic asymmetric oligoarthritis
Prominent enthesitis and extraarticular features
More rapid progression and deformities
Rarely associated with uveitis or axial disease
Poorly responsive to standard NSAID therapy

NSAID, nonsteroidal anti-inflammatory drug.
From Cush JJ, Lipsky PE. Reiter's syndrome and reactive arthritis. In: Koopman WJ, ed. *Arthrtitis and allied conditions: a textbook of rheumatology*, 14th ed. Philadelphia: Lippincott Williams & Wilkins, 2001:1324–1344, with permission.

positivity to AIDS. The arthritis evolves in two main patterns: (a) an additive, asymmetric polyarthritis, or (b) an intermittent oligoarthritis that most commonly affects the lower extremities (143,145). Dactylitis, conjunctivitis, urethritis, enthesitis, and fasciitis are commonly observed and sometimes predominate (143,145,147). Although sacroiliitis does occur, HIV-associated reactive arthritis rarely occurs with axial ankylosis or uveitis (147). Several investigators have noted that HIV-associated reactive arthritis differs from Reiter syndrome (Table 12.6) in terms of the severity and chronicity of disease, poor response to conventional antiinflammatory therapy, and tendency for fulminant progression of AIDS with administration of immunosuppressive drugs such as methotrexate.

Clinical Features

The clinical triad of urethritis, conjunctivitis, and arthritis is observed in only 33% of patients with Reiter syndrome. The remaining individuals can often be identified on the basis of an acute, additive lower-extremity oligoarthritis accompanied by one or more of the following extraarticular features: diarrhea, urethritis, cervicitis, ocular inflammation, low back pain, enthesitis, keratoderma blennorrhagica, or other mucocutaneous lesions. A detailed history is often necessary to reveal the antecedent infectious event or associated extraarticular features that may suggest the diagnosis of Reiter syndrome. The relative incidence of postdysenteric, postvenereal, and idiopathic Reiter syndrome is highly variable and depends on the geographic locale and on environmental and social conditions. Despite careful questioning, a large number of patients do not have documented prodromal enteric or urethral symptomatology. A postdysenteric onset may occur sporadically or as a sequel to epidemic outbreaks of bacterial enteritis. Although many patients with postvenereal Reiter syndrome report recent sexual contact(s), no relationship with gonococcal infection has been substantiated. There are, however, several reports of Reiter syndrome occurring in patients with a common sexual contact (115,147).

Onset

The earliest features of Reiter syndrome usually appear within 1 to 4 weeks of exposure. The onset of disease is usually heralded by the development of one or more of the extraarticular features of Reiter syndrome. The onset of *genitourinary tract involvement* may manifest as dysuria, urethral discharge, or prostatitis in men and cervicitis or vaginitis in women. Fever as high as 39°C, prominent constitutional complaints (i.e., malaise, fatigue, and weight loss), and ocular symptoms are also common. The arthritis is often the last feature to appear but is usually evident within 1 to 4 weeks of the triggering event.

Arthritis

The arthropathy of Reiter syndrome is typically an acute, asymmetric, additive, and ascending inflammatory oligoarthritis. Reiter syndrome can be confused with septic and gouty arthritis because of the intensity and pattern of articular presentation. At the onset, involvement of the joints of the lower extremity (knees, ankles, and toes) is most common. The arthritis may progress in an additive fashion to involve the joints of the upper extremities and axial spine. Involvement of the digits is sometimes accompanied by the presence of *dactylitis,* resulting in the so-called sausage digit that may involve either the toes or fingers of these patients. Dactylitis is the net result of inflammatory changes affecting the joint capsule, entheses, periarticular structures, and periosteal bone. In addition to the spondyloarthropathies, dactylitis may be seen in sarcoidosis, gout, and juvenile (but not adult) rheumatoid arthritis. Upper-extremity involvement in Reiter syndrome is characterized by asymmetry, dactylitis, and involvement of the fingers and wrist. Less commonly, widespread polyarthritis may be indistinguishable from rheumatoid arthritis. In such patients, however, the diagnosis of Reiter syndrome is suggested by the evolution, pattern of involvement, associated extraarticular features, clinical course, and absence of serum rheumatoid factor.

At onset, there may be symptomatic evidence of axial involvement in approximately 50% of individuals (115, 148). This most frequently manifests as inflammatory low back pain, sometimes with signs of sacroiliac inflammation or limited spinal mobility. Alternatively, low back pain may also be a consequence of muscle spasm, insertional inflammation (enthesitis), and inflammation of intervertebral joints. However, radiographic abnormalities of the sacroiliac joint or axial skeleton are not a routine feature of Reiter syndrome and are only seen in about 20% of affected individuals (115). Nevertheless, sacroiliitis and spondylitis are most common in the most severely affected individuals with chronic Reiter syndrome.

Enthesopathy

Enthesopathy or enthesitis is a distinctive feature of the spondyloarthropathies and refers to inflammation at the sites of tendinous or ligamentous insertions onto bone (124,149,150). Clinically, enthesitis most often manifests as pain, with or without swelling, at the entheses. The most common site of involvement is at the insertion of the posterior and inferior os calcis (Achilles tendon and plantar fascia insertions, respectively). Other common sites include the toes and fingers (sausage digits), symphysis pubis, ischium, iliac crest, greater trochanter, and anterolateral ribs. Enthesitis involving the insertion of the serratus anterior on the anterolateral ribs may be mistaken for pleuritic chest pain. Radiographically, enthesopathy is suggested by the development of erosions and reactive new bone formation at the previously mentioned sites.

Mucocutaneous

Mucous membrane inflammation involving the genitourinary or gastrointestinal tract is observed in up to one-third of patients with Reiter syndrome. *Urethritis* with a sterile, *mucopurulent* discharge may be difficult to detect, as it is transient in men and can be occult in women. Genitourinary symptoms are often seen early in the disease, regardless of whether the syndrome is associated with a postdysenteric or postvenereal trigger. Other common findings include circinate balanitis, cervicitis, and painless, lingual, or palatal *oral ulcerations*. *Circinate balanitis* often presents as vesicles that rupture to form large, shallow ulcerations or plaques on the glans or shaft of the penis. A serpiginous border is characteristic and the ulcerations are nearly always painless.

Keratoderma blenorrhagica is the most common cutaneous manifestation and presents as a painless, papulosquamous eruption frequently found on the soles or palms (Fig. 12.5), although lesions also have been reported on the penis, trunk, extremities, and scalp. The histopathology is indistinguishable from that of pustular psoriasis (3). Patients have been reported with overlapping features of Reiter syndrome and psoriatic arthritis, suggesting a common etiopathogenic mechanism in some patients (151). Nail changes are common in those individuals who develop a chronic arthropathy and include onycholysis, yellowish discoloration, or subungual hyperkeratosis.

Ocular

Ocular manifestations of *conjunctivitis, uveitis,* or *keratitis* are seen in most patients (152,153). Conjunctivitis occurs in up to two-thirds of patients and is often an early manifestation. It tends to be bilateral or unilateral; is recurrent; is symptomatic with pain, burning, or injection; and lasts days rather than weeks. Uveitis can occur in Reiter syndrome; however, the presence of uveitis does not necessarily imply that the patient has a spondyloarthropathy. Of 236 consecutive ophthalmic patients presenting with uveitis, 13% were found to have an underlying spondyloarthropathy (7.2% with Reiter's and 5.5% with ankylosing

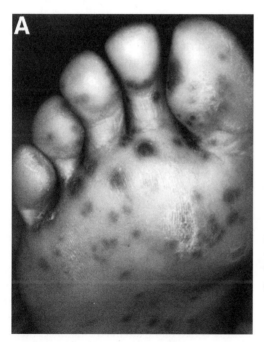
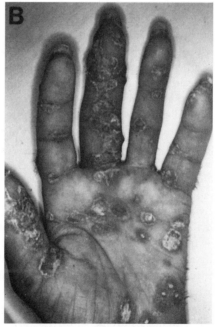

FIGURE 12.5. A. Early lesions of keratoderma blenorrhagica on the sole in Reiter syndrome. **B.** Chronic lesions on the palms and digits in Reiter syndrome. (From Cush JJ, Lipsky PE. Reiter's syndrome and reactive arthritis. In: Koopman WJ, ed. *Arthritis and allied conditions: a textbook of rheumatology,* 14th ed. Philadelphia: Lippincott Williams & Wilkins, 2001:1324–1344, with permission.)

spondylitis) (153). In this subset of uveitis patients, the uveitis was uniformly acute in onset, unilateral, anterior in location, and associated with the presence of HLA-B27 but not chorioretinitis. Nongranulomatous inflammation of the uveal tract may occur with established disease and pursues a chronic or relapsing course. If untreated, this may lead to progressive intraocular damage and visual loss. Keratitis has been rarely reported.

Other Features

Fever is common at the outset of disease and may be hectic enough to suggest an underlying septic process. Patients may present with other systemic manifestations of inflammation, including anorexia, weight loss, fatigue, and morning stiffness. *Cardiac involvement* in Reiter syndrome is seen in less than 10% of patients and most frequently presents as a conduction disturbance that is asymptomatic but detected on electrocardiogram. Common findings include a prolonged PR interval, complete heart block, nonspecific ST segment alterations, and Q waves. Symptomatic conduction disturbances, such as myocarditis and aortitis, are rarely seen. *Aortic regurgitation* is a late complication that is indistinguishable from that seen in ankylosing spondylitis. Amyloidosis, central nervous system involvement, serositis, and pulmonary infiltrates also have been reported rarely (114,115), most often in patients with chronic, severe disease.

Laboratory Abnormalities.

Laboratory results are consistent with an inflammatory process. There are moderate to marked elevations of the erythrocyte sedimentation rate (ESR) and acute-phase reactants, including C-reactive protein. C-reactive protein levels may correlate with disease activity and be a better gauge of therapeutic response than the ESR (154). Other common features are thrombocytosis, leukocytosis, and a modest hypoproliferative anemia. With uncontrolled disease, it is not uncommon to detect mild to moderate elevations of hepatic enzymes indicative of hepatocellular inflammation rather than cholestasis.

Isolation of a microbial agent after reactive arthritis has developed is an unusual event, although this may be the case in some patients with *Shigella*-induced Reiter syndrome. Serologic evidence of an antecedent *Chlamydia* or *Yersinia* infection is frequently present in individuals with reactive arthritis related to these organisms. Serologic proof of infection is unnecessary for diagnosis but in selected instances may provide useful diagnostic information and can be helpful in choosing antibiotic therapy. Despite the reported association of Reiter syndrome with AIDS, HIV testing is unlikely to be sensitive enough or predictive enough to warrant the expense in patients suspected of having Reiter syndrome or reactive arthritis. Nevertheless, HIV testing should be considered in those individuals engaged in high-risk behavior or situations. Antineutrophil cytoplasmic antibodies against lactoferrin or myeloperoxidase have rarely been reported in patients with reactive arthritis (155).

The strong association of HLA-B27 with Reiter syndrome has led to the temptation to utilize this test as a diagnostic aid (115,156). However, ascertainment of the patient's MHC status is seldom necessary. Moreover, because only a relatively small number of B27+ individuals develop Reiter syndrome, the predictive value of this test is low when used as a screening test. In selected circumstances, a positive test result may prove useful, especially in confirming the diagnosis in those patients with early or incomplete Reiter syndrome.

Radiography.

Radiographic abnormalities are observed in up to 70% of patients with established Reiter syndrome and may be characterized by (a) asymmetric involvement of the lower-extremity diarthroses, amphiarthroses, symphyses, and entheses; (b) ill-defined bony erosions with adjacent bony proliferation; and (c) tendency to produce heterotopic bone, as exemplified by findings of paravertebral ossification (114,115,157,158). Inflammatory arthropathy is suggested by the findings of soft-tissue swelling (especially sausage digits), joint space narrowing, and erosions in the small joints of the feet, hands, knees, and sacroiliac joints. Erosions tend to be marginal or central in position and may be accompanied by adjacent bony proliferation, which tends to obscure erosive margins (Fig. 12.6). Whereas juxtaarticular osteopenia may be observed during early disease or acute episodes of peripheral arthritis, chronic arthropathy of Reiter syndrome differs from rheumatoid arthritis because of the slow return of juxtaarticular mineralization to normal in affected joints that have gone into remission.

The formation of reactive new bone is characteristic of the seronegative spondyloarthropathies. Bony proliferation in Reiter syndrome usually develops in one of several sites, including (a) the periosteum, with a linear or fluffy appearance adjacent to cortical margins, especially along the shafts of the metacarpals, metatarsals, phalanges, distal femur (Fig. 12.6), and malleolar regions; (b) the entheses, especially calcaneal, ischial, and trochanteric attachments, often with a poorly defined or frayed osseous appearance (Fig. 12.7); and (c) sites of intraarticular erosions that also tend to have an irregular or poorly defined appearance, often in association with subchondral sclerosis or periostitis. Tendinous and ligamentous calcification has also been observed in Reiter syndrome, especially in the collateral ligaments of the knee, metacarpophalangeal, and interphalangeal joints. Although ankylosis is common in the axial skeleton, bony ankylosis of peripheral articulations is rarely observed.

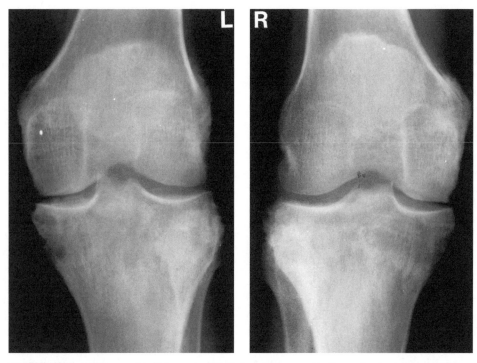

FIGURE 12.6. A 27-year-old white man with Reiter syndrome. Radiographs depict marginal erosions, with adjacent reactive bone, condylar periostitis, and normal juxtaarticular mineralization. (From Cush JJ, Lipsky PE. Reiter's syndrome and reactive arthritis. In: Koopman WJ, ed. *Arthritis and allied conditions: a textbook of rheumatology,* 14th ed. Philadelphia: Lippincott Williams & Wilkins, 2001:1324–1344, with permission.)

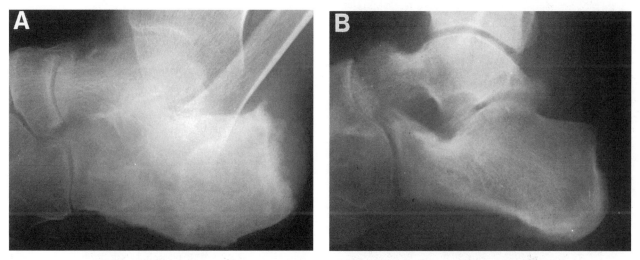

FIGURE 12.7. Enthesitis involving the os calcis with (**A**) severe, chronic, erosive changes at the insertion of the Achilles tendon and (**B**) mild erosive changes with "fluffy" reactive bone at the insertion of the plantar aponeurosis. (From Cush JJ, Lipsky PE. Reiter's syndrome and reactive arthritis. In: Koopman WJ, ed. *Arthritis and allied conditions: a textbook of rheumatology,* 14th ed. Philadelphia: Lippincott Williams & Wilkins, 2001:1324–1344, with permission.)

Appendicular Disease

Peripheral radiographic abnormalities are often most striking in the forefoot (especially the metatarsophalangeal and interphalangeal joints of the first toe), calcaneus, tarsus, ankle, and knee. Calcaneal abnormalities appear as erosive changes on the posterior and plantar surfaces, sometimes associated with thickening of the Achilles tendon. Spurs are commonly found at the insertion of the plantar aponeurosis, accompanied by erosive and osseous changes with poorly defined outlines (Fig. 12.7). Involvement of the upper extremity is uncommon in Reiter syndrome and may present as focal or asymmetric oligoarticular involvement without resultant deformity. Erosions and/or reactive bone formation may occur in the manubriosternal joint and symphysis pubis (115).

Axial Disease

Radiologic involvement of the axial spine may also be seen in Reiter syndrome. The sacroiliac joint is most commonly involved, with the lower half of the joint—the true synovium-lined portion of the articulation—being the site of inflammation. The incidence of sacroiliac involvement increases with the chronicity and duration of disease; 40% to 60% of individuals with chronic Reiter syndrome have radiographic evidence of sacroiliitis (115). Although bilateral sacroiliac involvement is common, asymmetric or unilateral sacroiliitis also occurs, especially early in the disease (Fig. 12.8). Initially, erosions are most evident on the ileal side of the synovial portion of the joint. These progress to "pseudowidening" with eventual bony proliferation, sclero-

sis, and ankylosis. When compared with ankylosing spondylitis, axial abnormalities in Reiter syndrome are less common and less extensive. Whereas the spondylitis of ankylosing spondylitis is an ascending process, isolated involvement of the thoracic or lumbar spine may be the initial radiographic finding in the spine in Reiter syndrome. Asymmetry and skip lesions involving the spine are common. Axial disease often manifests as paravertebral ossification with the appearance of nonmarginal syndesmophytes or bulky osteophytes that are often unilateral or asymmetric and tend to spare the anterior surface of the spine. Involvement of the cervical spine is uncommon.

Other Imaging Modalities

Scintigraphy can be used as an adjunctive imaging modality because of its greater sensitivity in detecting early sacroiliac involvement in the absence of radiographic abnormalities. Moreover, scintigraphy is better suited for complete skeletal surveys and the identification of enthesitis that may not be apparent by physical examination (Fig. 12.9). Likewise, computerized tomography (CT) can assess the extent of sacroiliac and spondylitic involvement accurately. Magnetic resonance imaging has been used with increasing frequency because of its superior ability to identify abnormalities of synovium, cartilage, tendon, and entheses, especially in difficult-to-image joints such as the sacroiliac joint.

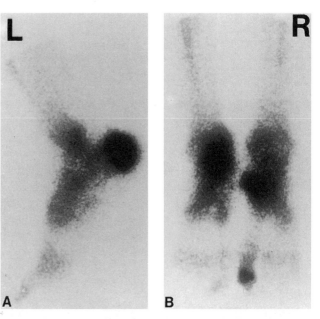

FIGURE 12.9. A 30-year-old black man with Reiter syndrome manifest as sacroiliitis, urethritis, and enthesitis demonstrated by isotopic uptake on ^{99m}Tc-phosphate scintigraphy involving the left calcaneus (**A**) and right navicular with synovitis of the right first interphalangeal joint (**B**). (From Cush JJ, Lipsky PE. Reiter's syndrome and reactive arthritis. In: Koopman WJ, ed. *Arthritis and allied conditions: a textbook of rheumatology,* 14th ed. Philadelphia: Lippincott Williams & Wilkins, 2001:1324–1344, with permission.)

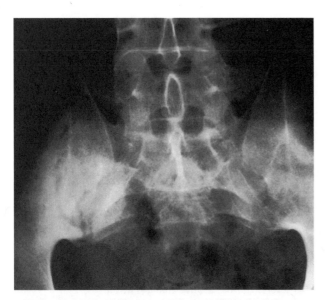

FIGURE 12.8. Bilateral asymmetric sacroiliitis in Reiter syndrome. (From Cush JJ, Lipsky PE. Reiter's syndrome and reactive arthritis. In: Koopman WJ, ed. *Arthritis and allied conditions: a textbook of rheumatology,* 14th ed. Philadelphia: Lippincott Williams & Wilkins, 2001:1324–1344, with permission.)

When compared with CT and scintigraphy, MRI is most sensitive at detecting sacroiliitis (158). However, the prohibitive cost of MRI has tempered the use of this modality in establishing a diagnosis of sacroiliitis, and its use may only be necessary when imaging children, women, and those participating in research protocols.

Diagnosis

Reiter syndrome must be distinguished from septic arthritis (especially gonococcal arthritis), crystal-induced arthritis, sarcoidosis, erythema nodosum, acute rheumatic fever, and seronegative rheumatoid arthritis on clinical grounds and after appropriate laboratory and synovial fluid analyses. More difficult is the distinction of Reiter syndrome from the other spondyloarthropathies, such as ankylosing spondylitis, psoriatic arthritis, or IBD, and other reactive arthritides, such as *Yersinia, Chlamydia,* or AIDS-associated reactive arthritis. In such instances, a diagnosis of Reiter syndrome is made after a careful history, identification of extraarticular features, appropriate use of serologic testing, response to therapy (i.e., NSAIDs or antibiotics) and prolonged follow-up.

Therapy

As Reiter syndrome targets a young population with the potential for recurrence and chronicity, its management poses a therapeutic challenge. Interventions should be directed at optimum joint protection, maintenance of function, patient education, relief of pain, suppression of inflammation, and when appropriate, eradication of infection (115,120,159,160). Patient education is a priority, as it is likely to improve compliance and enhance active participation of the patient in the therapeutic program. Inactivity and immobilization should be discouraged. Each therapeutic regimen should be tailored to the individual patient's limitations and should incorporate the generous use of exercise, including those addressing stretching and range of motion. The physician should utilize the expertise of the physical and occupational therapist to maintain function and to alleviate gait disturbances.

NSAIDs are the mainstay of therapy (115,159,160). Treatment with these agents can suppress signs and symptoms of the disease, although few data suggest that they alter the course of the disease. Reliance on salicylates has been replaced by the use of other ·NSAIDs that are better tolerated and easier to take. Although there are few differences in clinical efficacy among currently available NSAIDs, several of these agents seem to be more effective than others in the management of Reiter syndrome (115). Of the numerous NSAIDs available in the United States, the Food and Drug Administration has approved indomethacin, sulindac, naproxen, diclofenac, phenylbutazone, and enteric-coated salicylate for use in ankylosing spondylitis and Reiter syndrome. Of these, long-acting phenylbutazone has been tested most extensively and has proved effective in the management of Reiter syndrome and ankylosing spondylitis. However, the advent of newer and safer NSAIDs coupled with the concern about the serious toxicity associated with phenylbutazone therapy, particularly with regard to aplastic anemia, has made this a seldom-used agent. Phenylbutazone is no longer marketed in the United States, but may be found in special compounding pharmacies. Because of its known toxicity, its use should be reserved for those with intractable disease. Indomethacin has replaced phenylbutazone in the management of most patients with Reiter syndrome and ankylosing spondylitis. An effective antiinflammatory dose of indomethacin (2 to 3 mg/kg) is often recommended as initial therapy in patients with Reiter syndrome. The 75-mg long-acting formulation of indomethacin is particularly useful in the management of severe morning stiffness and other inflammatory symptoms. If gastrointestinal or central nervous system side effects prevent treatment with indomethacin, other NSAIDs also have been used effectively (159,160). The newer COX-2 inhibitors (i.e., celecoxib, rofecoxib) have not been studied in spondyloarthropathy patients. Prolonged NSAID therapy is indicated as long as clinical and laboratory evidence of ongoing inflammation is present. Therapeutic benefit should always be judged against the well-known toxicity associated with their use. For those patients who have not responded to multiple attempts at conventional NSAID therapy, additional second-line therapies should be considered.

Systemic corticosteroids are relatively ineffective in the routine management of patients with the seronegative spondyloarthropathies. Whereas several uncontrolled studies have suggested the efficacy of corticosteroids in the management of NSAID-resistant patients, most clinicians agree that corticosteroids are not indicated for the treatment of Reiter syndrome (120,159,160). Nonetheless, locally administered corticosteroids may be important adjuncts in the management of some patients. Intraarticular or perilesional (tendons or entheses) corticosteroid injections may be effective in some patients. Likewise, topical or intraocular corticosteroids may be necessary for the management of the ocular or mucocutaneous manifestations associated with Reiter syndrome.

Second-line therapy should be considered for those who demonstrate chronic inflammation that is incompletely responsive to antiinflammatory therapy. Recommended options for NSAID-resistant patients include azathioprine, methotrexate, and sulfasalazine, all of which have exhibited some efficacy, primarily in uncontrolled trials or reports (120,159–165). Azathioprine at doses of 1 to 2 mg/kg was effective in a single placebo-controlled, crossover trial in a majority of individuals (162). In Reiter syndrome, methotrexate has been the subject of a number of reports and appears to be effective at doses currently recommended for rheumatoid arthritis (7.5 to 20 mg/week) (160,163). Sulfasalazine has been reported to be clinically efficacious in several uncontrolled trials (120,159) and has been shown to correct the subclinical intestinal inflammation often associated with active disease (166). Several studies have determined that sulfasalazine may have limited efficacy in controlling the axial manifestations of Reiter syndrome and ankylosing spondylitis (120,159,160,164).

The identification of "triggering" infections may be of value in patients with either sexually acquired or reactive arthritis. Many of these patients have *Chlamydia*-induced arthritis or, in certain endemic areas, recurrent reactive arthritis caused by *Yersinia*. It appears that the early use of antibiotic therapy results in microbial eradication, thereby curtailing a chronic immunologic response and chronic or recurrent arthritis. Clinical efficacy may also be the result of tetracycline-induced suppression of metalloproteinase activity (167). However, not all reactive arthritides respond to antibiotic therapy. Locht et al. (168) demonstrated that antibiotics administered to control *Salmonella* enteritis were ineffective in altering the duration or incidence of subsequent arthritis. In addition, several investigators have demonstrated the lack of efficacy when ciprofloxacin was employed in patients with chlamydial arthritis (138a,169). Prolonged antibiotic therapy in most patients with idiopathic Reiter syndrome appears unlikely to be beneficial.

For AIDS patients with Reiter syndrome, initial therapy with NSAIDs is advised for those with unrelenting arthritis or enthesitis, although such patients frequently fail to respond completely. Whereas additional therapy with sulfasalazine is thought to be safe and efficacious (160,170, 171), the use of high-dose corticosteroids, methotrexate, and other cytotoxic agents should be discouraged because of the risk of precipitating more severe immunosuppression (142,143). Therapy with zidovudine (AZT) may improve the cutaneous manifestations of Reiter syndrome but appears to have little impact on the articular disease (147). A few uncontrolled studies have indicated the potential utility of etretinate in HIV+ patients with Reiter syndrome (172,173).

Clinical Course

The prognosis and course of individual patients with Reiter syndrome are varied and unpredictable, regardless of whether they present with the classic triad, ACR criteria, or incomplete Reiter syndrome (114,115,126,133,137,148, 159). Disparate reports of chronicity and relapse rates among Reiter patients may be confounded by inadequate definition and classification of these patients, inconsistent follow-up, selection bias, differences in postdysenteric and postvenereal populations, and differences in race or genetic factors. Most patients demonstrate an initial episode of arthritis (with or without extraarticular disease), with a mean duration of 2 to 3 months, but which may last up to a year. Many patients experience recurrent attacks, often after prolonged disease-free intervals. Approximately 20% to 50% of patients demonstrate a chronic course of peripheral arthritis with a greater potential for progressive spondylitis (115,159). It has been suggested that patients with the classic triad are more likely to have a relapsing clinical course, whereas those without the classic triad are more likely to demonstrate a chronic course (115). Factors that may influence the outcome in the spondyloarthropathies include hip arthritis, ESR > 30 mm/hr, poor response to NSAIDs, limitation of lumbar spine, sausage digits, oligoarthritis, or onset before 16 years of age (174). Despite the potential for chronicity, several prospective longitudinal studies have shown that patients with Reiter syndrome and reactive arthritis maintain a higher level of continued employment than individuals with other inflammatory arthritides (175). Severe disability occurs in less than 15% of patients and is frequently secondary to unrelenting lower-extremity disease, aggressive axial involvement, or blindness. Death is rare and is usually attributed to cardiac complications or amyloidosis (115).

Other Postinfectious Reactive Arthropathies

Infrequently, additional infectious agents have been reported to be associated with a reactive arthropathy. In each instance, an identifiable infectious event was followed by a sterile inflammatory synovitis. Although these conditions occur after particular infections and their pattern resembles the spondyloarthropathies, they appear to differ from idiopathic Reiter syndrome based on genetic or clinical associations. A variety of clinically similar disorders manifesting reactive osteitis and arthritis in the setting of chronic cutaneous pustular lesions has been reported under a number of designations (Table 12.7). Poststreptococcal reactive arthritis represents an incomplete form of acute rheumatic fever, which is a form of a postinfectious reactive arthritis. Other bacterial organisms besides streptococci have been implicated as causative agents in reactive arthritis: *Brucella abortus* (cow), *B. melitensis* (goat), or *B. suis* (pig), *Clostridium difficile*, certain strains of *Staphylococcus aureus*, *Borrelia burgdorferi*, the *human immunodeficiency virus* (HIV), *Mycobacterium tuberculosis*, *M. avium intracellulare*, *Strongyloides stercoralis*, *Giardia lamblia*, and *Cryptosporidium*.

Lastly, reactive arthritis has also been documented as a result of treatment and immunization. Numerous cases of reactive arthritis bearing features similar to the spondyloarthropathies have been reported following treatment for bladder cancer with intravesical bacillus Calmette–Guérin (BCG). Such cases have presented with inflammatory peripheral arthritis, back pain, and dactylitis following BCG exposure (176,177). More than 50% of these patients were HLA-B27 positive. In addition, sporadic reports of patients

TABLE 12.7. HYPEROSTOTIC SYNDROMES ASSOCIATED WITH CUTANEOUS PUSTULAR LESIONS

SAPHO (synovitis–acne–pustulosis–hyperostosis–osteitis)
Palmoplantar pustulosis with arthroosteitis
Sternocostoclavicular hyperostosis
Pustulotic arthoosteitis
Chronic recurrent multifocal osteomyelitis
Intersternocostoclavicular ossification
Acne arthritis or acne-associated spondyloarthropathy
Arthritis associated with hidradenitis suppurativa
Pustular psoriasis with arthroosteitis

Derived from Jurik AG, Helmig O, Graudal H. Skeletal disease, arthro-osteitis, in adult patients with pustulosis palmoplantaris. *Scand J Rheumatol* 1988;70(Suppl):3–15; Kahn MF, Chamot AM. SAPHO syndrome. *Rheum Dis Clin N Amer* 1992;18:225–246; Olafsson S, Khan MA. Musculoskeletal features of acne, hidradenitis suppurativa, and dissecting cellulitis of the scalp. *Rheum Dis Clin N Amer* 1992;18:215–224; Sartoris DJ, et al. Sternocostoclavicular hyperostosis: a review and report of 11 cases. *Radiology* 1986;158:125–128; Trotta F, et al. Hyperostosis and multifocal osteitis: a purely rheumatological subset of the SAPHO syndrome. *Clin Exp Rheumatol* 1990;8:401–405; Vasey FB. Acne, hydradenitis suppurativa, and arthritis. In: Espinosa L, Goldenberg D, Arnett F, et al., eds. *Infections in the rheumatic diseases: a comprehensive review of microbial relations to rheumatic disorders.* Orlando: Grune and Stratton, 1988:357–360.

developing inflammatory, reactive arthritis have resulted following immunization with the hepatitis A vaccine (178).

PSORIATIC ARTHRITIS

Psoriasis is a chronic autoimmune skin disease that afflicts about 2% of whites. Some 10% to 40% of patients with psoriasis develop a chronic inflammatory arthritis. Psoriatic arthritis (PSA) has a superficial resemblance to rheumatoid arthritis but is considered to be clinically and genetically distinct with a different pathogenesis. It was not until an association of rheumatoid factor and rheumatoid arthritis was described in 1948 that a clearer classification became possible (179). The observation that most patients with an erosive arthritis and psoriasis were seronegative (180), coupled with the introduction of criteria for the diagnosis of rheumatoid arthritis (181), provided a new impetus for reexamining the concept of PSA. Baker noted that seronegative polyarthritis was associated with psoriasis in 20% of patients; in comparison, only 1.2% of patients with seropositive arthritis had psoriasis (180). This suggested that the prevalence of psoriasis was increased 10-fold when associated with seronegative arthritis. Family studies revealed a strong association between psoriasis and arthritis (182).

Clinical Features

In most cases the diagnosis of PSA is readily made based on characteristic findings that occur in combination (Table 12.8).

TABLE 12.8. CLINICAL FEATURES OF PSORIATIC ARTHRITIS IN PATIENTS FROM TWO CENTERS

Features	Jones et al. (213) (%)	Veale et al. (215) (%)
Oligoarticular	22	43
Polyarticular	63	33
Predominant DIP	1	16
Spondyloarthropathy	6	2
Arthritis mutilans	4	2
SAPHO	1	2
Nail involvement	67	57
Monoarthritis	4	NG
Back pain	NG	44

DIP, distal interphalangeal; NG, not given; SAPHO, synovitis–acne–pustulosis–hyperostosis–osteitis.
From Bennett RM. Psoriatic arthritis. In: Koopman WJ, ed. *Arthrtitis and allied conditions: a textbook of rheumatology,* 14th ed. Philadelphia: Lippincott Williams & Wilkins, 2001:1345–1361, with permission.

Age of Onset

Whereas uncomplicated psoriasis usually appears in the second and third decades, the onset of associated arthritis does not occur commonly for another two decades (183). A juvenile onset of PSA is well recognized; the age of onset is usually between 9 and 12 years (184,185). There appears to be a bimodal age of onset, with a stronger familial tendency, a history of antecedent skin lesions, and fewer actively inflamed joints in the early-onset group (186).

Sex Ratio

The reported male/female ratio in PSA has varied widely in different surveys. Data pooled from 10 different studies indicated a male-to-female ratio of 1:1.04 (187). This contrasts with the approximately 3:1 female preponderance in seropositive RA.

Patterns of Onset and Distribution

In most patients there is a lag of approximately two decades between the onset of psoriasis and the evolution of PSA. In a large study of 647 patients with psoriasis, of whom 138 developed PSA (193), psoriasis antedated the arthritis in 68% of patients and followed it in 21% (188); a synchronous onset occurred in 11%. There is a well-recognized association between trauma to a joint and a flare of PSA in that same joint (189–194). An explosive onset of severe skin disease and arthritis, or a dramatic change in the severity of skin disease with an associated arthritis, is accepted as a clue to an associated HIV infection (195–199).

Although PSA is readily recognized on presentation as an oligoarticular arthritis with predominant involvement of distal interphalangeal (DIP) joints and flexor tenosynovitis, this is not the most common presentation (200).

Several large surveys have indicated that an oligoarticular distribution occurs only in 16% to 30% of patients, whereas a polyarticular pattern appears in 40% to 60% (201,202).

Two recent studies, each with 100 patients, found somewhat different patterns of presentation (Table 12.8). Five clinical patterns of PSA are recognized:

- Group 1. *Predominant involvement of distal interphalangeal joints.* As an isolated finding in the absence of other joint involvement, distal interphalangeal changes in PSA occur only in about 8% to 16% of patients.
- Group 2. *Arthritis mutilans.* Arthritis mutilans is due to osteolysis of the phalanges and metacarpals. It occurs in about 5% of patients and is often associated with sacroiliitis. The designation of arthritis mutilans is usually applied to the hands (Fig. 12.10), but this condition may also occur in the feet.
- Group 3. *Symmetric polyarthritis.* The presentation with symmetric polyarthritis is similar to that of RA, and several studies have noted this to be the most common pattern of joint involvement in psoriasis (Fig. 12.11). Compared with RA, there is a higher frequency of distal interphalangeal involvement and a tendency for bony ankylosis of the distal interphalangeal and proximal interphalangeal (PIP) joints leading to claw deformities of the hands (Fig. 12.12).
- Group 4. *Oligoarticular arthritis.* This is the most characteristic pattern of joint involvement in psoriasis. It is an asymmetric arthritis usually involving scattered distal

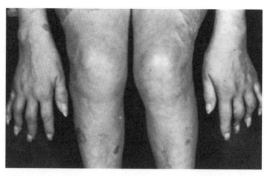

FIGURE 12.11. Asymmetric polyarthritis resembling rheumatoid arthritis in a patient with psoriasis. (From Bennett RM. Psoriatic arthritis. In: Koopman WJ, ed. *Arthritis and allied conditions: a textbook of rheumatology,* 14th ed. Philadelphia: Lippincott Williams & Wilkins, 2001:1345–1361, with permission.)

interphalangeal, proximal interphalangeal, metacarpal phalangeal (MCP), and metatarsal phalangeal (MTP) joints. Involvement of a metacarpophalangeal and proximal interphalangeal joint with an associated flexor tenosynovitis is common, presenting as a "sausage" digit (Fig. 12.13). This pattern of joint involvement occurs in approximately 15% to 40% of patients.

- Group 5. *Axial involvement.* Both sacroiliitis and spondylitis are associated with PSA; however, this is seldom the presenting complaint and usually occurs after several years of peripheral joint disease (203–205). Unlike AS, there is a tendency for the sacroiliac involvement to be asymmetric and a predilection for atypical syndesmophytes that affect random segments of the spine. A spondylitis-like picture occurs in 20% to 40% of patients with PSA (202). In comparison with classic AS, psoriatic patients often display discordance between the occurrence of sacroiliitis and spondylitis. Lambert and Wright found spondylitis in 40% of 130 patients

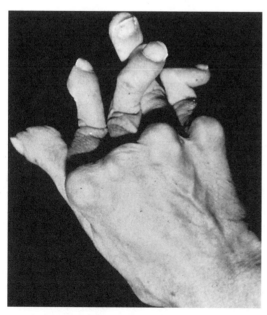

FIGURE 12.10. Severe resorptive arthropathy resulting in arthritis mutilans. (From Bennett RM. Psoriatic arthritis. In: Koopman WJ, ed. *Arthritis and allied conditions: a textbook of rheumatology,* 14th ed. Philadelphia: Lippincott Williams & Wilkins, 2001:1345–1361, with permission.)

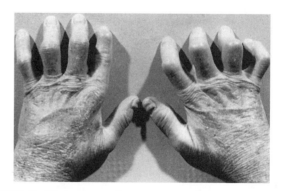

FIGURE 12.12. Long-standing psoriatic arthritis with a symmetric distribution. This patient had a "claw deformity" due to bony ankylosis of the proximal and distal interphalangeal joints. (From Bennett RM. Psoriatic arthritis. In: Koopman WJ, ed. *Arthritis and allied conditions: a textbook of rheumatology,* 14th ed. Philadelphia: Lippincott Williams & Wilkins, 2001:1345–1361, with permission.)

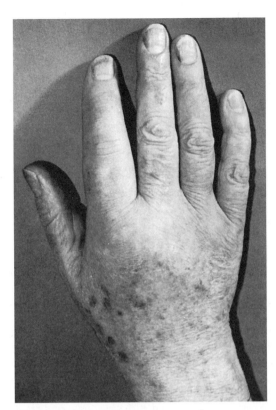

FIGURE 12.13. Psoriatic arthritis involving the metacarpophalangeal and proximal–interphalangeal joints of the index finger with an associated flexor tenosynovitis. This combination gives rise to the "sausage digit." (From Bennett RM. Psoriatic arthritis. In: Koopman WJ, ed. *Arthritis and allied conditions: a textbook of rheumatology,* 14th ed. Philadelphia: Lippincott Williams & Wilkins, 2001:1345–1361, with permission.)

with PSA but only 21% had sacroiliitis (206). Sixty percent of patients with syndesmophytes had normal sacroiliac joints, and they had no more symptoms or signs of spinal disease than those with normal spinal radiographs. Axial involvement occurred mostly in men (male/female ratio 6:1), and the onset of psoriasis was somewhat later in life.

Gladman and co-workers (207) compared PSA spondyloarthropathy and classic AS. Patients with AS had more symptoms of inflammatory back and neck pain, and a greater limitation of lumbar and cervical spine motion. Radiologically, they had more grade IV sacroiliitis and classic syndesmophytes. Salvarani (208) described two major forms of cervical spine involvement in psoriatic spondyloarthropathy: (a) an inflammatory erosive-subluxing presentation resembling RA occurred in 26% of patients, of whom 53% had subaxial subluxations; and (b) an AS-like picture that occurred in 44%. There was no sacroiliac joint involvement in 36% (all this latter group were B27⁻). Predictors of an inflammatory RA presentation included HLA-B39, HLA-DR4, and radiocarpal erosions. Cervical spine involvement may rarely cause neurologic compromise. In

one case, a patient with both atlantoaxial subluxation and multiple subaxial subluxations developed neurologic compromise at several levels and required surgery (209).

Psoriatic Arthritis and Trauma

Reports linking PSA with trauma to the involved joint continue in the literature (189,190). Scarpa (194) reviewed the occurrence of environmental triggers in 138 patients with PSA and compared them with 138 patients with RA. Specific triggering events were described in 9% of PSA patients, but only 1% of RA patients. The initiating events in PSA were the following: operations (four patients); trauma (three patients); abortions (three patients); and one patient each with myocardial infarction, thrombophlebitis, and drug toxicity.

Pregnancy and Hormonal Issues

The effects of pregnancy and the menopause were studied in relation to the expression of PSA in 33 patients (210); 33% had onset of arthritis within 3 months postpartum and 15% had a perimenopausal flare. Ostensen (211) noted that PSA either improved or remitted in 80% of pregnancies, with a postpartum flare noted in 70%. An interesting case study reported cyclical flares of PSA associated with menstruation (212). When estrogen production was suppressed, symptoms and joint count improved markedly.

Skin and Nail Findings

Skin lesions usually antedate the appearance of PSA by one or two decades. Biondi et al. (188) reported the following patterns of psoriasis in association with PSA: vulgaris, 85%; eruptive, 11%; erythrodermic, 2.5%; and pustular, 1.2%. The evolution of mild skin disease to a widespread erythrodermic pattern with an associated flare in arthritis may represent a clue to an associated HIV infection. In a minority of patients, in which the arthritis appears first, it is difficult to make a definitive diagnosis of PSA. Indeed verification of the correct diagnosis is only apparent retrospectively. In the assessment of such patients, it is important to search carefully for the psoriatic lesions in hidden areas (e.g., scalp, perineum, natal cleft, or umbilicus). When attempting to ascertain the presence of minimal psoriasis, there are several pitfalls to be avoided, and it is useful to bear in mind the criteria laid down by Baker (Table 12.9).

Nail involvement is often a useful clue in diagnosing PSA. Jones et al. (213) found psoriatic nail changes in 63% of PSA patients, compared with 37% of patients with psoriasis alone. In those patients in whom arthritis preceded skin lesions, 88% had psoriatic nail changes. In another study, nails were involved in 86.5% of patients with PSA (214). The most common findings are pitting in the fingernails and subungual hyperkeratosis in the toenails. Other

TABLE 12.9. CRITERIA FOR DIAGNOSIS OF BORDERLINE PSORIASIS

1. Psoriasis of the scalp must be palpable.
2. Presumed scalp psoriasis, simulating dandruff, must exhibit normal skin between plaques.
3. In the presence of eczema or seborrheic states, lesions other than classic plaques cannot be accepted as psoriasis.
4. Toenail lesions alone cannot be accepted as evidence of psoriasis.
5. In the absence of psoriasis elsewhere, only classic nail changes (i.e., pitting, onycholysis, and discoloration of the lateral nail edge) can be accepted as unequivocal psoriasis. In such cases fungal infection should be excluded by microscopy and culture.
6. Flexural lesions can only be accepted if they have the classic appearance of a psoriatic plaque. In such cases microscopy of scrapings must be done to exclude *Tinea* or *Candida* infection.
7. Pustular lesions of the palms and soles are not acceptable unless accompanied by classic skin or nail lesions elsewhere.

From Bennett RM. Psoriatic arthritis. In: Koopman WJ, ed. *Arthrtitis and allied conditions: a textbook of rheumatology,* 14th ed. Philadelphia: Lippincott Williams & Wilkins, 2001:1345–1361, with permission.

types of nail involvement include onycholysis (Fig. 12.14), transverse ridges, leukonychia, and crumbling. There is a moderate correlation between distal interphalangeal involvement and nail changes (215). Interestingly, nail lesions have been reported as favoring a better prognosis (216). Abnormal nail findings are not specific for psoriasis, and the differential diagnosis includes fungal and bacterial infections, alopecia areata, lichen planus, and trauma. Fungal infections that frequently cause hyperkeratosis and onycholysis are *Trichophyton rubrum* and *T. mentagrophytes.* When in doubt, nail clippings should be examined for fungus using potassium hydroxide preparations and cultures. It is important to note that normal individuals often have a few nail pits, but these are usually shallow and more irregular than those found in psoriatic patients. Wright and Moll (217) state that 20 pits are suggestive of PSA and more than 60 are diagnostic.

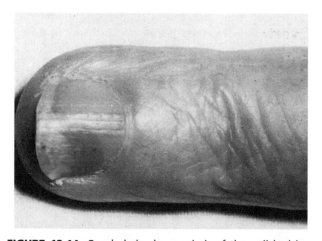

FIGURE 12.14. Onycholysis plus psoriasis of the nail bed in a patient who had an oligoarticular pattern of arthritis. (From Bennett RM. Psoriatic arthritis. In: Koopman WJ, ed. *Arthritis and allied conditions: a textbook of rheumatology,* 14th ed. Philadelphia: Lippincott Williams & Wilkins, 2001:1345–1361, with permission.)

Extraarticular Associations

In contradistinction to RA, vasculitis and its clinical correlates are not seen in PSA. Inflammatory eye disease occurs in about 30% of patients with PSA. The diagnoses made in one report were conjunctivitis 19.6%; iritis, 7.1%; episcleritis, 1.8%; and keratoconjunctivitis sicca, 2.7% (218). Of those patients with iritis, 43% had sacroiliitis and 40% were positive for HLA-B27. Tests for antinuclear antibodies were negative in all patients with iritis (218). Only one study described an increased prevalence (11%) of renal involvement in PSA; the major features were hematuria, proteinuria, or cylindruria (219). Mitral valve prolapse was reported in 14 out of 25 patients with PSA (56%), compared with only 6.4% of psoriatic patients without arthritis (220). Aortic regurgitation has also been noted (221). A well-documented, but inexplicable, association with myopathy has been described (222), and reports exist of an occasional association with Sjögren syndrome (223,225).

Laboratory Findings

Other than the finding of a negative rheumatoid factor, no laboratory tests exist to aid in the diagnosis of either psoriasis or PSA (225). Positive tests for rheumatoid factor in psoriatic patients with coexistent erosive arthritis most likely reflect the concurrent presence of RA and psoriasis. Analysis of synovial fluid usually reveals an inflammatory picture with elevated leukocytes—predominantly neutrophils. The occasional occurrence of antinuclear antibodies in patients with PSA has a prevalence comparable to that of the normal population. Circulating immune complexes have been detected in up to 50% of patients with both psoriasis and PSA; one report indicates these are predominantly of the IgA isotype (226). Hyperuricemia occurs in 10% to 20% of patients and has been related to the severity of the skin disease (227).

Radiographic Findings

Radiographs of patients with PSA exhibit several discriminatory features in comparison to RA. Marginal erosions often have proliferative new bone formation, and there may be joint fusion, acroosteolysis, and periostitis (195). In contradistinction to RA, bone density in PSA is usually preserved (228). Distinctive radiographic features of PSA include asymmetric oligoarticular distribution, relative absence of oligoarticular osteopenia, involvement of the distal interphalangeal joints, and involvement of the sacroiliac joints (229,230). Less common findings include the following:

1. Erosion of terminal phalangeal tufts (acroosteolysis) (Fig. 12.15)
2. Whittling of phalanges and of metacarpal and metatarsal joints (Fig. 12.16).
3. Cupping of the proximal portion of the phalanges (Fig. 12.16).
4. Bony ankylosis (Fig. 12.17).

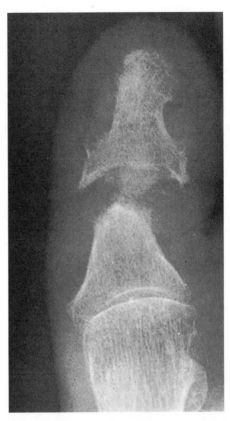

FIGURE 12.16. "Whittling" of the middle phalanx and expansion of the base of the distal phalanx—the "pencil-in-cup" deformity. (From Bennett RM. Psoriatic arthritis. In: Koopman WJ, ed. *Arthritis and allied conditions: a textbook of rheumatology,* 14th ed. Philadelphia: Lippincott Williams & Wilkins, 2001: 1345–1361, with permission.)

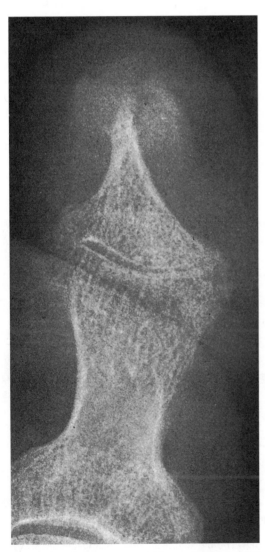

FIGURE 12.15. Psoriatic arthritis with acroosteolysis of the terminal phalanx of the great toe. (From Bennett RM. Psoriatic arthritis. In: Koopman WJ, ed. *Arthritis and allied conditions: a textbook of rheumatology,* 14th ed. Philadelphia: Lippincott Williams & Wilkins, 2001:1345–1361, with permission.)

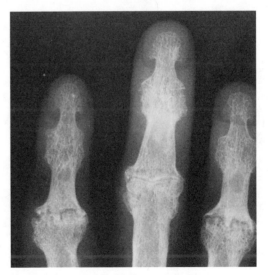

FIGURE 12.17. Bony ankylosis of distal interphalangeal joints in a patient with psoriatic arthritis. (From Bennett RM. Psoriatic arthritis. In: Koopman WJ, ed. *Arthritis and allied conditions: a textbook of rheumatology,* 14th ed. Philadelphia: Lippincott Williams & Wilkins, 2001:1345–1361, with permission.)

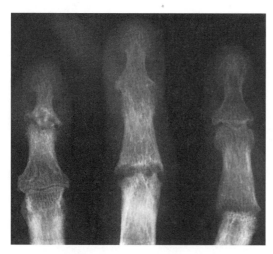

FIGURE 12.18. Complete destruction of middle proximal interphalangeal joint. Also note bony ankylosis of corresponding distal interphalangeal joint. (From Bennett RM. Psoriatic arthritis. In: Koopman WJ, ed. *Arthritis and allied conditions: a textbook of rheumatology,* 14th ed. Philadelphia: Lippincott Williams & Wilkins, 2001:1345–1361, with permission.)

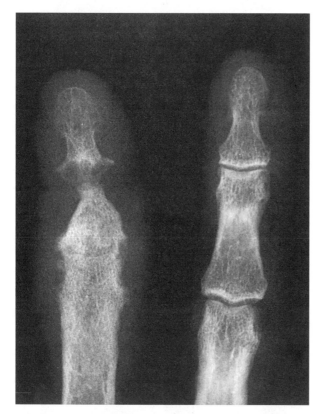

FIGURE 12.19. Destructive arthritis of an isolated distal interphalangeal joint with osteolysis of the proximal phalanx. (From Bennett RM. Psoriatic arthritis. In: Koopman WJ, ed. *Arthritis and allied conditions: a textbook of rheumatology,* 14th ed. Philadelphia: Lippincott Williams & Wilkins, 2001:1345–1361, with permission.)

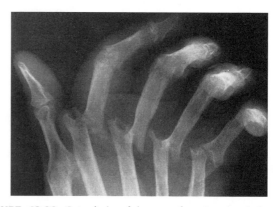

FIGURE 12.20. Osteolysis of bones of metacarpophalangeal joints with resulting subluxations. (From Bennett RM. Psoriatic arthritis. In: Koopman WJ, ed. *Arthritis and allied conditions: a textbook of rheumatology,* 14th ed. Philadelphia: Lippincott Williams & Wilkins, 2001:1345–1361, with permission.)

5. Destruction of isolated small joints (Fig. 12.18).
6. Predilection for distal interphalangeal and proximal interphalangeal joints with relative sparing of metacarpophalangeal and metatarsophalangeal joints (Figs. 12.19 and 12.20).
7. Osteolysis of bones (arthritis mutilans), particularly the metatarsals (Fig. 12.21).
8. Relative lack of osteoporosis when compared with a similar degree of joint involvement in RA.

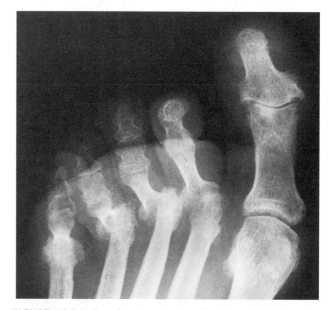

FIGURE 12.21. Prominent metatarsophalangeal joint involvement with subluxation and cupping of the base of the proximal phalanges. The big toe distal interphalangeal joint shows characteristic marginal erosions. (From Bennett RM. Psoriatic arthritis. In: Koopman WJ, ed. *Arthritis and allied conditions: a textbook of rheumatology,* 14th ed. Philadelphia: Lippincott Williams & Wilkins, 2001:1345–1361, with permission.)

Findings in the axial skeleton include the following:

1. Paravertebral ossification (231) [this is not unique to psoriasis, as it is seen in senile ankylosing hyperostosis (DISH)]; paraplegia, fluorosis, hypoparathyroidism, familial hypophosphatemia, and hereditary/familial articular and vascular calcification.
2. Atypical syndesmophytes—often present without sacroiliitis (206) (Fig. 12.22).
3. Asymmetric sacroiliitis (232).
4. Solid fusion of thoracic vertebrae (233).
5. Rarity of the typical bamboo spine of AS (233).
6. A tendency for cervical spine disease to exhibit intervertebral disc-space narrowing and ankylosis (Fig. 12.23).
7. Apophyseal sclerosis and interspinous or anterior ligamentous calcification (229).

Upper cervical spine disease occurs with both atlantoaxial fusion and subluxation (234–236). Involvement of the upper cervical spine can be associated with either ankylosis or atlantoaxial subluxation—as observed in RA (234,235). Temporomandibular joint involvement with condylar erosions and condylar osteolysis is a well-recognized problem (237,238).

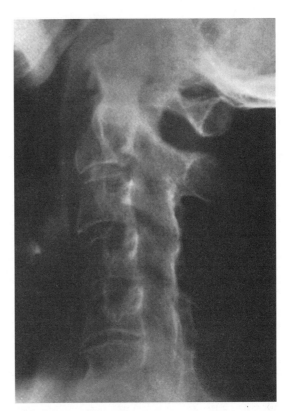

FIGURE 12.23. Ankylosis of cervical apophyseal joints in a patient with psoriatic spondylitis in association with bilateral sacroiliitis. (From Bennett RM. Psoriatic arthritis. In: Koopman WJ, ed. *Arthritis and allied conditions: a textbook of rheumatology*, 14th ed. Philadelphia: Lippincott Williams & Wilkins, 2001:1345–1361, with permission.)

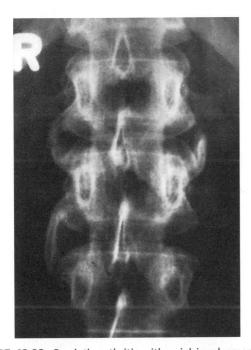

FIGURE 12.22. Psoriatic arthritis with axial involvement. The patient was HLA-B27+ and had no radiologic evidence of sacroiliitis, but atypical syndesmophytes are observed. (From Bennett RM. Psoriatic arthritis. In: Koopman WJ, ed. *Arthritis and allied conditions: a textbook of rheumatology*, 14th ed. Philadelphia: Lippincott Williams & Wilkins, 2001:1345–1361, with permission.)

Differential Diagnosis

A diagnosis of PSA is usually obvious in a patient with inflammatory arthritis in association with unequivocal psoriasis (Table 12.10). Problems arise when the evidence for psoriasis is lacking or ambiguous. In such cases it is useful to follow the guidelines for the diagnosis of borderline psoriasis (Table 12.9). Seborrheic dermatitis resembles scalp psoriasis, whereas fungal infections may mimic nail involvement. Nail pitting alone lacks specificity in differentiating between psoriasis and other conditions such as exfoliative dermatitis and eczema. Isolated nail pitting is a normal occurrence, 20 fingernail pits suggests psoriasis, and more than 60 pits are virtually never found in the absence of psoriasis (217). Keratoderma blenorrhagicum, as seen in Reiter syndrome, is indistinguishable both clinically and histologically from pustular psoriasis. Because mild conjunctivitis may occur in psoriasis, it cannot be relied upon to differentiate Reiter syndrome from PSA (218). Primary osteoarthritis bears a superficial resemblance to distal interphalangeal involvement in PSA. In such instances the presence of Heberden and Bouchard nodes and involvement of the first carpometacarpal joint may help establish a diagnosis of

TABLE 12.10. CLINICAL CHARACTERISTICS SUGGESTIVE OF PSORIATIC ARTHRITIS

Involvement of distal interphalangeal (DIP) joints in absence of primary osteoarthritis
Asymmetric joint involvement
Absence of rheumatoid factor and subcutaneous nodules
Flexor tenosynovitis and "sausage" digits
A family history of psoriatic arthritis
Significant nail pitting (>20 pits)
Axial radiographs showing one or more of the following: (a) sacroiliitis, (b) syndesmophytes (often "atypical"), and (c) paravertebral ossification
Peripheral radiographs showing an erosive arthritis with a relative lack of osteopenia—in particular, DIP erosions with expansion of the base of the terminal phalanx and terminal phalangeal osteolysis

From Bennett RM. Psoriatic arthritis. In: Koopman WJ, ed. *Arthrtitis and allied conditions: a textbook of rheumatology,* 14th ed. Philadelphia: Lippincott Williams & Wilkins, 2001:1345–1361, with permission.

osteoarthritis. Erosive osteoarthritis may be mistaken for PSA, but in typical cases the "mouse ear" radiologic findings of psoriatic involvement are readily distinguished from the "gull wing" appearance of osteoarthritis. Acute-onset PSA, involving the knee and big toe, may resemble gout. In such cases joint aspiration for the detection of urate crystals is advised. Occasionally, both gout and pseudogout occur in association with well-defined PSA. Psoriatic arthritis may flare following trauma to a joint. Persistence of "traumatic arthritis," in association with an inflammatory joint fluid, should suggest early PSA (180,189).

Prognosis

For most patients PSA is a nuisance rather than a significant cause of persistent dysfunction (239,240). In a 10-year follow-up of 227 patients, only 5% developed a deforming arthritis, and 97 lost less than a year from work (241). However, Gladman and co-workers (201) have challenged the concept that PSA is generally benign. In a study of 220 patients with PSA, they found a 40% incidence of deforming erosive arthropathy, with 17% of patients having five or more deformed joints. Stage III and IV radiographic changes occurred in 28% and 14% of patients, respectively. Eleven percent of patients had class III or IV functional impairment. The same group has reported that certain HLA antigens may act as markers for disease progression, with HLA-B39 and DQw3 conferring a worse prognosis and HLA-B22 conferring a better prognosis (216). Wong (242) documented 53 deaths in a group of 428 patients with PSA. Cardiorespiratory disease accounted for 48% of deaths, and cancer, for 17%. Prognostic indicators for death were an ESR >15 mm/hr, radiologic evidence of joint destruction, and a history of prior medications for psoriasis. Death resulting from psoriasis itself is rare but may be asso-

ciated with either exfoliative dermatitis or amyloidosis. Other rare problems associated with morbidity are the development of aortic valve incompetence (221) or atrioventricular conduction defects. These complications usually are seen in association with spondylitis. There has been recent interest about the effects of coping strategies and learned helplessness in chronic disease as possible predictors of functional outcome. A comparison of patients with RA and PSA found that mood and coping strategies correlated with concurrent functional status and were *not* predictors of future function (243).

Management

Patients with PSA have to bear the burden of two chronic and currently incurable diseases. Furthermore, there is a heightened probability that their offspring will be afflicted. An important general principle in managing patients with chronic disease is the establishment of a productive dialogue, which allows the patient to express fears and obtain enlightened answers. One can be optimistic that most patients with PSA will follow a relatively benign course without serious systemic complications; however, such a generalization is of little solace to patients developing arthritis mutilans.

Mild Disease

The general principles espoused in the treatment of patients with RA are pertinent to the management of patients with PSA. Many patients with mild disease need only antiinflammatory doses of a nonsteroidal antiinflammatory drug (NSAID). Flares that usually affect only one or two joints can be effectively treated with local corticosteroid injections. A relative contraindication to joint injections is the presence of psoriatic lesions in the overlying skin (244), as these lesions are often colonized with staphylococci and streptococci.

Progressive Disease

At tertiary referral centers, polyarticular joint involvement has been noted in 30% to 60% of patients with PSA and arthritis mutilans, in about 5%. Compared with RA, there have been few controlled trials of disease-modifying agents in PSA. Most studies have not adequately separated the response of patients with relatively mild oligoarticular disease from those with polyarticular destructive disease (245).

As there is often a correlation between the aggressiveness of skin involvement and the severity of arthritis, it seems logical to maximize the therapy of skin lesions. Photochemotherapy using 8-methoxypsoralens followed 2 hours later by photosensitization using ultraviolet-light type A (PUVA) resulted in a 49% improvement in peripheral synovitis (246). The potential for analogs of 1,25-dihydroxy vitamin D to improve psoriatic lesions (through a down-regulation of keratinocyte responsiveness to growth factors) has provided an important new therapeutic option for treating psoriasis (247–249). Whether treatment with 1,25-dihydroxy vitamin D analogs will also be effective in PSA remains to be documented.

There is a general agreement that systemic corticosteroid treatment should be avoided in PSA. This advice is based not on their lack of efficacy, but on the exacerbation of the skin lesions observed with attempted tapering.

Many of the "classic" disease-modifying agents used in the treatment of RA are also used in treating PSA. Some investigators have used antimalarials with enthusiasm. One study claimed a 75% response rate to hydroxychloroquine in a dose of 200 to 400 mg/day (250). In a controlled trial of chloroquine (251), 75% of the patients on chloroquine had a greater than 30% reduction in active joint inflammation over 6 months, compared with 58% of controls. Six patients on chloroquine suffered a flare of their psoriasis (but there was no exfoliative dermatitis), and six of the controls experienced a flare of their skin disease (251). Another study reported that antimalarials did not cause flares of skin disease (252).

Several reports suggest that chrysotherapy is of benefit in PSA. In one study of intramuscular gold, significant improvement occurred in 71% of patients with PSA compared with 60% of patients with RA (253). Gold therapy has been linked to an exacerbation of skin disease (239), but other studies have failed to corroborate this impression (253).

Sulfasalazine has been used with varied results in treating PSA (254–256). A common problem with sulfasalazine is hypersensitivity to the sulfonamide component. Clegg (257) found no significant difference in efficacy between sulfasalazine (2,000 mg/day) and placebo in a 36-week study. Rahman (258) reported a similar failure of sulfasalazine in a 24-month study and noted a 38% drop-out rate due to side effects.

Etretinate was evaluated in an open study of 40 patients where the tender joint count fell by approximately 50% and morning stiffness improved by approximately 60%. Side effects were common; most patients treated with etretinate developed mucocutaneous problems, with dry, cracked lips being a particularly persistent aggravation (259). Other problems encountered with retinoid therapy include arthralgias, myalgias, hyperlipidemia, and extra spinal calcification.

Colchicine (1.5 mg orally per day) was found to result in significant improvement in 15 patients with PSA (260); however, in another study colchicine was found to be of no value (261).

There is a general consensus that cytotoxic agents are of benefit in destructive PSA. The most widely studied and commonly used agent is methotrexate (262). Studies using weekly oral methotrexate have reported a benefit similar to that observed in RA (263–267). The doses of methotrexate used in PSA are comparable to those in RA (e.g., 15 to 25 mg/week). The risk of liver toxicity with methotrexate increases with the total cumulative dose and an alcohol consumption of greater than 100 g/week. A study of 13 patients with PSA reported good results with 6-mercaptopurine in a relatively low dose (0.36 to 2.4 mg/kg/day). Improvement began within 3 weeks, and remission lasted up to 10 months after treatment stopped (268).

Cyclosporine A (CSA) has been used in patients with severe PSA that is refractory to other treatments (269,270). Salvarani et al. found that seven of 12 PSA patients had a greater than 50% reduction in active joints as well as skin improvement. Responders exhibited decreased serum levels of the soluble IL-2 receptor (sIL-2R) (271). In a 12-month head-to-head comparison trial, methotrexate and CSA were of similar efficacy, but methotrexate was better tolerated (272).

A caveat to the treatment of PSA with cytotoxic agents is the use of these agents in HIV+ patients. Maurer et al. (273) reported on three HIV+ patients with PSA treated with methotrexate; one developed an opportunistic infection. In patients with large-joint proliferative synovitis resistant to other treatments, Yttrium-90-induced synovectomy may be of benefit (274,275). Other therapies include extracorporeal phototherapy (276), gamma interferon (277), cascade apheresis (278), and autologous stem cell transplantation (279). Recently, the FDA has approved etanercept for treating psoriatic arthritis, which adds another potent form of treatment.

Indications for surgical interventions in PSA are similar to those for RA, yet wound infection resulting from the skin colonization with pathogenic bacteria is of concern (245). However, it has been shown that the standard procedure for preoperative skin preparation is as effective in sterilizing psoriatic plaques as uninvolved skin (280). Although a tendency for increased fibrosis and ankylosis in PSA has been suggested, a surgical study did not confirm the tendency to fibrosis and recommended that appropriate reconstructive surgery be withheld (281). In a review of hand surgery in PSA, two of the most useful procedures were found to be metacarpophalangeal joint arthroplasty and fusion of fixed flexion contractures of the proximal interphalangeal and distal interphalangeal joints in positions of maximum function (282). There is an increasing awareness that the temporomandibular joint may be involved in PSA, and several references have dealt with indications for surgical intervention (283).

THE ARTHRITIS ASSOCIATED WITH INFLAMMATORY BOWEL DISEASES

The inclusion of IBD in this group of diseases emphasizes the relationship between gut inflammation and joint inflammation. This relationship is corroborated by ileo-colonoscopic evidence of subclinical gut inflammation in other forms of spondyloarthropathy (284–289). Other gut diseases, such as celiac disease, and intestinal bypass surgery are also occasionally accompanied by joint inflammation, but these are not considered spondyloarthropathies.

Clinical Entities

Idiopathic Inflammatory Bowel Disease

Crohn disease and ulcerative colitis are discussed together because they have comparable rheumatologic and other associated features that cannot be easily differentiated.

Epidemiology

The prevalence of ulcerative colitis ranges from 50 to 100 individuals per 100,000 in the general population. The disease seems to be more frequent in whites than in nonwhites, and more frequent in the Jewish population. The prevalence of Crohn disease has increased during the last few decades to about 75 per 100,000. In a screening study for colorectal cancer involving 37,000 individuals without intestinal symptoms (290), the combined prevalence of ulcerative colitis and Crohn disease was 56 per 100,000, whereas the prevalence of symptomatic IBD is estimated as 90 to 150 per 100,000. Ongoing epidemiologic studies suggest that the true prevalence may have been underestimated by 27% to 35%. These studies also suggest the existence of patients with subclinical IBD. Arthritis is the most common extraintestinal manifestation of IBD and appears in 2% to 20% of patients with either ulcerative colitis or Crohn disease. However, the occurrence of peripheral arthritis is more frequent in patients with colonic involvement and more extensive bowel disease.

Peripheral Arthritis

The frequency of peripheral arthritis in IBD ranges from 17% to 20% of patients, with a higher prevalence in Crohn disease (291). In an extensive retrospective study in the Oxford Inflammatory Bowel Disease Clinic (292) involving 1,459 patients with IBD, arthritis was described in 6% of patients with ulcerative colitis and 10% of patients with Crohn disease. In a recent study from the gastrointestinal clinic (293), actual synovitis was seen in 10% of IBD patients and enthesitis, in 7%, but 29% of the patients reported a history of swollen joints.

The sex ratio in IBD is equal and peak age is between 25 and 44 years. In both Crohn disease and ulcerative colitis, the arthritis is pauciarticular, generally asymmetric, and frequently transient and migratory. Large and small joints, predominantly of the lower limbs, are involved. The arthritis usually is nondestructive, and many attacks subside within 6 weeks. Recurrences are common. Sausage-like fingers and toes may occur. Enthesopathies, especially inflam-

mation of the Achilles tendon or of the insertion of the plantar fascia, are known manifestations (Fig. 12.24) and may involve the knee or other sites. Clubbing and, rarely, periostitis may occur in Crohn disease. The peripheral arthritis becomes chronic in some cases, and destructive lesions of small joints and hips may occur.

In most cases of Crohn disease, intestinal symptoms antedate or coincide with the joint manifestations, but the articular symptoms may precede the intestinal symptoms by years. In some cases of spondyloarthropathies, Crohn disease remains subclinical, with joint and tendon inflammation being the only clinical manifestations (294). In a prospective study of 123 patients with spondyloarthropathy, eight (6%) patients developed Crohn disease 2 to 9 years after the appearance of joint symptoms (295). In ulcerative colitis, there is a more distinct temporal relationship between attacks of arthritis and flares of bowel disease. Surgical removal of diseased colon can induce remission of peripheral arthritis. In Crohn disease, colonic involvement increases the susceptibility to peripheral arthritis, but surgical removal has little effect on the joint disease (296).

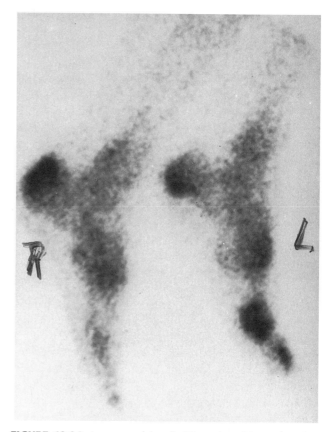

FIGURE 12.24. In a spondyloarthritic patient 99m-technetium DMP scan discloses inflammatory enthesopathies of the feet, including insertion of Achilles tendon of the right foot and plantar fascia of the left foot. (From Mielants H, de Keyser F, Veys EM. Enteropathic arthritis. In: Koopman WJ, ed. *Arthritis and allied conditions: a textbook of rheumatology,* 14th ed. Philadelphia: Lippincott Williams & Wilkins, 2001:1362–1382, with permission.)

In the Oxford study (292) enteropathic peripheral arthropathy without axial involvement was subdivided into pauciarticular large-joint arthropathy and bilateral symmetric polyarthropathy. In the pauciarticular type, joint symptoms were mostly acute and self-limiting. The arthritis coincided with relapses of IBD, and the disease was strongly associated with extraintestinal manifestations such as erythema nodosum and uveitis. Interestingly, 31% of these patients developed arthropathies up to 3 years before diagnosis of IBD. The polyarticular joint symptoms persisted for months to years, ran a course independent of IBD, and were not associated with other extraintestinal manifestations except uveitis.

Axial Involvement

Axial involvement occurs in both diseases. The true prevalence of sacroiliitis in IBD is unclear, since the onset frequently is insidious. Prevalence rates of 10% to 20% for sacroiliitis and 7% to 12% for spondylitis have been reported, although the actual figures are probably higher because of the existence of subclinical axial involvement. In a recent study (293) from an IBD clinic, 30% of the patients with IBD had inflammatory low back pain, and 33% had a Shober index of less than 3 cm. One-third of the patients had unilateral or bilateral sacroiliitis stage II, and in 18% of the patients the sacroiliitis was asymptomatic.

Spondyloarthropathy fulfilling the European Spondyloarthropathy Study Group (ESSG) criteria (297) could be diagnosed in 35% of the patients, and ankylosing spondylitis, in 10%. These frequencies are probably underestimates, since IBD patients attending the rheumatologic clinic were excluded. The same prevalence of spondyloarthropathy (28%) was found in patients with ulcerative colitis followed in an Italian gastrointestinal unit (298).

In review studies of ankylosing spondylitis, IBD occurred in 4% (299) to 6% (300) of patients. Although it is generally accepted that men are more likely to develop ankylosing spondylitis than women, in these studies the male-to-female ratio of patients with IBD and ankylosing spondylitis was 1:1, which is different from the ratio in uncomplicated ankylosing spondylitis (3:1). However, women with IBD and ankylosing spondylitis were shown to have a younger age at onset of ankylosing spondylitis and more severe disease than males with IBD (especially when IBD and ankylosing spondylitis are present in other members of the family). In general, joint disease was more severe, as defined by the intake of nonsteroidal antiinflammatory drugs and decrease of spinal mobility, in patients with combined IBD and ankylosing spondylitis than in those with uncomplicated ankylosing spondylitis.

However, the clinical picture may be indistinguishable from that of uncomplicated ankylosing spondylitis. The patient complains of low back pain, thoracic or cervical pain, buttock pain, and chest pain. Limitation of lumbar or cervical motion and reduced chest expansion are characteristic clinical signs. Peripheral arthritis may be present. The onset of axial involvement does not parallel that of bowel disease but frequently precedes it. The course is also totally independent of the course of the intestinal disease. Bowel surgery does not alter the course of associated sacroiliitis or spondylitis.

In a prospective clinical study, essentially all the patients with spondyloarthropathy who developed Crohn disease after 2 to 9 years also developed axial involvement and fulfilled criteria for ankylosing spondylitis (295).

Extraintestinal and Extraarticular Features

A variety of cutaneous, mucosal, serosal, and ocular manifestations occur in IBD (Table 12.11). Skin lesions are observed in 10% to 25% of patients. Erythema nodosum parallels the activity of bowel disease, tends to occur in patients with active peripheral arthritis, and is probably a disease-related manifestation (301). Pyoderma gangrenosum is a more severe but less common extraarticular manifestation, which is unrelated to the activity of the bowel and joint disease. Leg ulcers and thrombophlebitis also may occur.

TABLE 12.11. EXTRAINTESTINAL MANIFESTATIONS OF CROHN DISEASE AND ULCERATIVE COLITIS

Extraintestinal Manifestations	IBD (%)	Related to Intestinal Manifestations
Peripheral arthritis	11–20	+
Pauciarticular	7	+
Polyarticular	4.5	−
Clubbing periostitis	2	−
Enthesitis	7–15	+
Inflammatory low back pain	10–30	−
Sacroiliitis	10–35	−
Spondylitis	2–10	−
Erythema nodosum	3–7	+
Pyoderma gangrenosum	2	−
Uveitis	6–13	±
Aphthous ulceration	?	+
Amyloidosis	1 (25?)	+
Nephrolithiasis	3	−
Primary sclerosing cholangitis	?	−
Diagnosis spondyloarthropathy	35	
Diagnosis ankylosing spondylitis	10	

IBD, inflammatory bowel disease.
Prevalence (%) of different extraintestinal manifestations in Crohn disease and ulcerative colitis and their relationship with the intestinal manifestations (the prevalence of amyloidosis in Crohn disease between parentheses was found in a postmortem study).
From Mielants H, de Keyser F, Veys EM. Enteropathic arthritis. In: Koopman WJ, ed. *Arthrtitis and allied conditions: a textbook of rheumatology,* 14th ed. Philadelphia: Lippincott Williams & Wilkins, 2001:1362–1382, with permission.

Ocular manifestations, especially anterior uveitis, frequently accompany IBD (3% to 11%). Uveitis is often acute in onset, unilateral, and transient, but recurrences are common (302). It generally spares the choroid and retina. However, a chronic course with lesions in the posterior part of the eye has been described. Granulomatous uveitis is rare but may be present in Crohn disease. Acute anterior uveitis is associated with axial involvement and the presence of HLA-B27. Conjunctivitis and episcleritis also have been observed. In an ileocolonoscopic study involving patients with acute uveitis, inflammatory gut lesions were found in 66% (303), predominating in patients with acute anterior uveitis and associated spondyloarthropathy. Aphthous ulcerations, mainly affecting the buccal mucosa and tongue, are frequent in Crohn disease and can parallel disease activity. Amyloidosis is a well-recognized cause of death in Crohn disease. The incidence in clinical series is approximately 1% (304), but postmortem studies have revealed evidence of amyloid in 25% of patients with Crohn disease. Nephrolithiasis has been reported in 6% of patients with Crohn disease and 3% of patients with ulcerative colitis.

Laboratory and Radiologic Findings

There are no diagnostic laboratory tests for the arthritis or spondylitis of IBD. Elevated serum acute-phase reactants (especially C-reactive protein), thrombocytosis (especially in Crohn disease), and hypochromic anemia due to chronic blood loss or chronic inflammation are common findings. Rheumatoid factor is absent.

Synovial fluid analysis is consistent with an inflammatory arthritis with leukocyte counts ranging from 1,500 to 50,000/mm^3, predominantly neutrophils. Synovial histology reveals only nonspecific inflammation, although granulomas have been described.

Radiographs of the peripheral joints generally do not exhibit erosions. Erosive lesions, mainly of the metacarpophalangeal and metatarsal joints, occasionally have been described, differing from rheumatoid arthritis only by their pauciarticular and asymmetric distribution.

Destructive lesions of the hip have been reported and related to the presence of HLA-W62 and to Crohn disease–like lesions on gut biopsy in undifferentiated spondyloarthropathies (305). The axial joint involvement of IBD is indistinguishable from that of uncomplicated ankylosing spondylitis, although the frequency of asymmetric sacroiliitis is probably higher (306). Enthesopathies do not differ radiologically from those seen in the spondyloarthropathies.

Therapy

The treatment of peripheral arthritis and spondylitis in patients with IBD is the same as in ankylosing spondylitis. NSAIDs are the first choice, although they may cause an exacerbation of intestinal symptoms in ulcerative colitis. Intraarticular corticosteroid injections may be beneficial in monoarticular flares. Sulfasalazine, which has been successfully used to treat colonic inflammation in ulcerative colitis and Crohn disease, has been found to be effective in the treatment of the peripheral arthritis accompanying the spondyloarthropathies (307), especially if intestinal inflammation is present (308). It may also have a favorable effect on the peripheral arthritis of IBD. Although frequently inducing a clinical remission in spondyloarthropathies, sulfasalazine does not prevent the development of IBD (308). Oral corticosteroids may reduce peripheral synovitis, but have no effect on axial symptoms. Their systematic use is only justified if they are required to control the bowel disease. Gold, D-penicillamine, and antimalarial drugs are ineffective. Low-dose methotrexate (MTX), successfully used in the treatment of rheumatoid arthritis and in some cases of refractory IBD (309), has not yet proven effective in joint inflammation associated with Crohn disease or ulcerative colitis.

Recently, infliximab has been approved by the FDA for the intestinal treatment of Crohn disease. The effect of this treatment on the extraintestinal complications of Crohn disease has been encouraging.

Intestinal surgery is occasionally indicated in the treatment of IBD, but only favorably influences the peripheral arthritis in ulcerative colitis.

REFERENCES

1. Arnett FC. Anklosing Spondylitis. In: Koopman WJ, ed. *Arthritis and allied conditions: a textbook of rheumatology,* 14th ed. Philadelphia: Lippincott Williams & Wilkins, 2001:1311-1323.
2. Cush JJ, Lipskey PE. Reiter's syndrome and reactive arthritis. In: Koopman WJ, ed. *Arthritis and allied conditions: a textbook of rheumatology,* 14th ed. Philadelphia: Lippincott Williams & Wilkins, 2001:1324–1344.
3. Bennett RM. Psoriatic arthritis. In: Koopman WJ, ed. *Arthritis and allied conditions: a textbook of rheumatology,* 14th ed. Philadelphia: Lippincott Williams & Wilkins, 2001: 1345–1361.
4. Mielants H, De Kyser F, Veys E. Enteropathic arthritis. In: Koopman WJ, ed. *Arthritis and allied conditions: a textbook of rheumatology,* 14th ed. Philadelphia: Lippincott Williams & Wilkins, 2001:1362–1382.
5. Moll JMH. *AS.* Edinburgh: Churchill Livingstone, 1980.
6. Khan MA. AS and related spondyloarthropathies. Spine: state of the art reviews. *Rheum Dis Clin North Am* 1990; 4:497–688.
7. Gofton JP. Report from the subcommittee on diagnostic criteria for AS. In: Bennett PH, Wood PHN, eds. *Population studies of the rheumatic diseases.* New York: Excerpta Medica, 1968: 314–316.
8. Van der Linden S, Valkenburg HA, Cats A. Evaluation of diagnostic criteria for AS. *Arthritis Rheum* 1984; 27:361–367.
9. Will R, Edmunds L, Elswood J, et al. Is there sexual inequality in AS? A study of 498 women and 1202 men. *J Rheumatol* 1990;17:1649–1652.
10. Burgos-Vargas R, Naranjo A, Castillo J, et al. AS in the Mexican mestizo: patterns of disease according to age at onset. *J Rheumatol* 1989;16:186–191.
11. Lawrence RC, Helmick CG, Arnett FC, et al. Estimates of the

prevalence of arthritis and selected musculoskeletal disorders in the United States. *Arthritis Rheum* 1998;41:778–799.

12. Braun J, Bollow M, Remlinger G, et al. Prevalence of spondyloarthropathies in HLA-B27 positive and negative blood donors. *Arthritis Rheum* 1998;41:58–67.

13. Baum J, Ziff M. The rarity of AS in the black race. *Arthritis Rheum* 1971;14:12–18.

14. Chalmers IM. AS in African blacks. *Arthritis Rheum* 1980;23:1366–1370.

15. Khan MA, Braun WE, Kushner I, et al. HLA-B27 in AS: differences in frequency and relative risk in American blacks and Caucasians. *J Rheumatol* 1977;4:39–43.

16. Mbayo K, Mbuyi-Muamba JM, Lurhuma AZ, et al. Low frequency of HLA-B27 and scarcity of AS in a Zairean Bantu population. *Clin Rheumatol* 1998;17:309–310.

17. Brown MA, Jepson A, Young A, et al. AS in West Africans: evidence for a non-HLA-B27 protective effect. *Ann Rheum Dis* 1997;56:68–70.

18. Sonozaki H, Seki H, Chang S, et al. Human lymphocyte antigen, HL-A27, in Japanese patients with AS. *Tissue Antigens* 1975;5:131–136.

19. Tsujimoto M. Epidemiological research on the prevalence of AS. *Med J Osaka Univ* 1978;28:363–381.

20. Gofton JP, Chalmers A, Price GE, et al. HL-A27 and AS in B.C. Indians. *J Rheumatol* 1975;2:314–318.

21. Boyer GS, Templin DW, Cornoni-Huntley JC, et al. Prevalence of spondyloarthropathies in Alaskan Eskimos. *J Rheumatol* 1994;21:2292–2297.

22. Alexeeva L, Krylov M, Vturin V, et al. Prevalence of spondyloarthropathies and HLA-B27 in the native population of Chukotka, Russia. *J Rheumatol* 1994;21:2298–2300.

23. Felson DT. Epidemiology of the rheumatic diseases. Infectious agents in chronic rheumatic diseases. In: Koopman WJ, ed. *Arthritis and allied conditions: a textbook of rheumatology*, 14th ed. Philadelphia: Lippincott Williams & Wilkins, 2001:3–38.

24. Van der Linden SM, Valkenburg HA, de Jongh BM, et al. The risk of developing AS in HLA-B27 positive individuals: a comparison of relatives of spondylitis patients with the general population. *Arthritis Rheum* 1984;27:241–249.

25. Hochberg MC, Bias WB, Arnett FC. Family studies in HLA-B27 associated arthritis. *Medicine* 1978;57:463–473.

26. Khan MA, Kushner I, Braun WE. Comparison of clinical features of HLA-B27 positive and negative patients with AS. *Arthritis Rheum* 1977;60:909–912.

27. Brown MA, Kennedy LG, MacGregor AJ, et al. Susceptibility to AS in twins. *Arthritis Rheum* 1997; 40:1823–1828.

28. Brown MA, Kennedy LG, Darke C, et al. The effect of HLA-DR genes on susceptibility to and severity of AS. *Arthritis Rheum* 1009;41:460–465.

29. Hohler T, Schaper T, Schneider PM, et al. Association of different tumor necrosis factor promoter allele frequencies with AS in HLA-B27 positive individuals. *Arthritis Rheum* 1998;41:1489–1492.

30. Kaiijzel EL, Brinkman BM, van Krugten MV, et al. Polymorphism within the tumor necrosis factor alpha (TNF) promoter region in patients with AS. *Hum Imunol* 1999;60:140–144.

31. Inman RD, Perl A, Philips PE. Infectious agents in chronic rheumatic diseases. In: Koopman WJ, ed. *Arthritis and allied conditions: a textbook of rheumatology*, 14th ed. Philadelphia: Lippincott Williams & Wilkins, 2001:635–659.

32. Ebringer A. AS is caused by *Klebsiella*. *Rheum Dis Clin North Am* 1992;18:105–121.

33. Russell AS, Suarez-Almazor ME. AS is not caused by *Klebsiella*. *Rheum Dis Clin North Am* 1992;18:95–104.

34. Lahesmaa R, Skurnik M, Granfors K, et al. Molecular mimicry in the pathogenesis of spondylarthropathies: a critical appraisal of cross-reactivity between microbial antigens and HLA-B27. *Br J Rheumatol* 1992;31:221–229.

35. Schwimmbeck PL, Yu DTY, Oldstone MBA. Autoantibodies to HLA B27 in the sera of HLA B27 patients with AS and Reiter's syndrome. Molecular mimicry with *Klebsiella pneumoniae* as potential mechanism of autoimmune disease. *J Exp Med* 1987;166:173–181.

36. Mielants H, Veys EM, Goemaere S, et al. Gut inflammation in the spondyloarthropathies: clinical, radiologic, biologic and genetic features in relation to the type of histology: a prospective study. *J Rheumatol* 1991;18:1542–1551.

37. Granfors K. Do bacterial antigens cause reactive arthritis? *Rheum Dis Clin North Am* 1992;18:37–48.

38. Braun J, Tuszewski M, Ehlers S, et al. Nested polymerase chain reaction strategy simultaneously targeting DNA sequences of multiple bacterial species in inflammatory joint diseases. Examination of sacroiliac and knee joint biopsies of patients with spondyloarthropathies and other arthritides. *J Rheumatol* 1998;24:1101–1105.

39. Granfors K, Toivanen A. IgA-anti-yersinia antibodies in yersinia triggered reactive arthritis. *Ann Rheum Dis* 1986;46:561–565.

40. Wollenhaupt HJ, Drech T, Schneider C, et al. Specific serum IgA-antibodies in Chlamydia-induced arthritis. *Z Rheumatol* 1989;48:86–88.

41. Maki-Ikola O, Lehtinen K, Granfors K, et al. Bacterial antibodies in AS. *Clin Exp Rheumatol* 1991;84:472–475.

42. Ahmadi K, Wilson C, Tiwana H, et al. Antibodies to *Klebsiella pneumoniae* lipopolysaccharide in patients with AS. *Br J Rheumatol* 1998;37:1330–1333.

43. Calin A, Porta J, Fries JF, et al. Clinical history as a screening test for AS. *JAMA* 1977;237:2613–2614.

44. Blackburn WD, Jr, Alarcón GS, Ball GV. Evaluation of patients with back pain of suspected inflammatory nature. *Am J Med* 1988;85:766–770.

45. Hochberg MC, Borenstein DG, Arnett FC. The absence of back pain in classical AS. *Johns Hopkins Med J* 1978;143:181–183.

46. Gran JT. An epidemiologic survey of the signs and symptoms of AS. *Clin Rheum Dis* 1985;4:161–169.

47. Ball J. The enthesopathy of AS. *Br J Rheumatol* 1983;22(Suppl):25–28.

48. Olivieri I, Barozzi L, Padula A. Enthesopathy: clinical manifestations, imaging and treatment. *Baillieres Clin Rheumatol* 1998;12:665–681.

49. Edmonds J, Morris RI, Metzger AL, et al. Follow-up study of juvenile chronic polyarthritis with particular reference to histocompatibility antigen W.27. *Ann Rheum Dis* 1974;33:289–292.

50. Jacobs JC. Spondyloarthritis and enthesopathy. *Arch Intern Med* 1983;143:103–107.

51. Rosenberg AM, Petty RE. A syndrome of seronegative enthesopathy and arthropathy in children. *Arthritis Rheum* 1982;25:1041–1047.

52. Burgos-Vargas R, Petty RE. Juvenile AS. *Rheum Dis Clin North Am* 1992;18:123–143.

53. Arnett FC, Bias WB, Stevens MB. Juvenile-onset chronic arthritis: clinical and roentgenographic features of a unique HLA-B27 subset. *Am J Med* 1980;69:369–376.

54. Resnick D, Niwayama G. AS. In: Resnick D, ed. *Diagnosis of bone and joint disorders*. Philadelphia: WB Saunders, 1981:1040–1102.

55. Hollingsworth PN, Cheah PS, Dawkins RL, et al. Observer variation in grading sacroiliac radiographs in HLA-B27 positive individuals. *J Rheumatol* 1983;10:247–254.

56. Fam AG, Rubenstein JD, Chin-Sang H, et al. Computed tomography in the diagnosis of early AS. *Arthritis Rheum* 1985;28:930–937.

57. Yu W, Feng F, Dion E, et al. Comparison of radiography, com-

puted tomography and magnetic resonance imaging in the detection of sacroiliitis accompanying AS. *Skeletal Radiol* 1998; 27:311–320.

58. Bollow M, Braun J, Biedermann T, et al. Use of contrast-enhanced MR imaging to detect sacroiliitis in children. *Skeletal Radiol* 1998;27:606–616.

59. Amor B, Santos RS, Nahal R, et al. Predictive factors for the long-term outcome of spondyloarthropathies. *J Rheumatol* 1994;21:1883–1887.

60. Aufdermaur M. Pathogenesis of square bodies in AS. *Ann Rheum Dis* 1989;48:628–631.

61. McEwen C, DiTata D, Lingg C, et al. AS and spondylitis accompanying ulcerative colitis, regional enteritis, psoriasis and Reiter's disease. A comparative study. *Arthritis Rheum* 1971;14: 291–318.

62. Helliwell PS, Hickling P, Wright V. Do the radiological changes of classic AS differ from the changes found in the spondylitis associated with inflammatory bowel disease, psoriasis, and reactive arthritis? *Ann Rheum Dis* 1998;57:135–140.

63. Sorin S, Askari A, Moskowitz RW. Atlantoaxial subluxation as a complication of early AS. Two case reports and a review of the literature. *Arthritis Rheum* 1979;22:273–276.

64. Little H, Swinson DR, Cruickshank B. Upward subluxation of the axis in AS. *Am J Med* 1976;60:279–285.

65. Lee YS, Schlotzhauer T, Ott YSM, et al. Skeletal status of men with early and late AS. *Am J Med* 1997;103:233–241.

66. Bronson WD, Walker SE, Hillman LS, et al. Bone mineral density and biochemical markers of bone metabolism in AS. *J Rheumatol* 1998;25:929–935.

67. Murray GC, Persellin RH. Cervical fracture complicating AS. A report of eight cases and review of the literature. *Am J Med* 1981;70:1033–1041.

68. Cooper C, Carbone L, Michet CJ, et al. Fracture risk in patients with AS: a population based study. *J Rheumatol* 1994;21: 1877–1882.

69. Dunn N, Preston B, Jones KL. Unexplained back pain in longstanding AS. *Br Med J* 1985;291:1632–1634.

70. Resnick D, Williamson S, Alazraki N. Focal spinal abnormalities on bone scans in AS: a clue to the presence of fracture or pseudoarthrosis. *Clin Nucl Med* 1995;6:213–217.

71. Dihlmann W, Delling G. Disco-vertebral destructive lesions (so-called Andersson lesions) associated with AS. *Skeletal Radiol* 1983;3:10–16.

72. Kabaskal Y, Garrett SL, Calin A. The epidemiology of spondylodiscitis in AS, a controlled study. *Br J Rheumatol* 1996;35: 660–663.

73. Calin A. HLA-B27: to type or not to type? *Ann Intern Med* 1980;92:208–211.

74. Khan MA, Khan MK. Diagnostic value of HLA-B27 testing in AS and Reiter's syndrome. *Ann Intern Med* 1982;96:70–76.

75. Yagon R, Khan MA. Confusion of roentgenographic differential diagnosis of ankylosing hyperostosis (Forestier's disease) and AS. *Spine: State of Art Rev* 1990;4:561–575.

76. Kaplan G, Haettich B. Rheumatological symptoms due to retinoids. *Baillieres Clin Rheumatol* 1991;5:77–97.

77. Rosenbaum JT. Acute anterior uveitis and spondyloarthropathies. *Rheum Dis Clin North Am* 1992;18:143–151.

78. Stewart SR, Robbins DL, Castles JJ. Acute fulminant aortic and mitral insufficiency in AS. *N Engl J Med* 1978;299:1448–1449.

79. Roberts WC, Hollingsworth JF, Bulkley BH, et al. Combined mitral and aortic regurgitation in AS. *Am J Med* 1974;56: 237–242.

80. Bergfeldt L. HLA-B27 associated cardiac disease. *Ann Intern Med* 1997;127:621–629.

81. Bergfeldt L, Edhag O, Vedin L, et al. AS: an important cause of severe disturbances of the cardiac conduction system. *Am J Med* 1982;73:187–191.

82. Bergfeldt L, Insulander P, Lindblom D, et al. HLA-B27: an important genetic risk factor for lone aortic regurgitation and severe conduction system abnormalities. *Am J Med* 1988;85: 12–18.

83. Bergfeldt L, Moller E. Complete heart block—another HLA-B27 associated disease manifestation. *Tissue Antigens* 1983;21: 385–390.

84. Boushea DK, Sundstrom WR. The pleuropulmonary manifestations of AS. *Semin Arthritis Rheum* 1989;18:277–281.

85. Campbell AH, MacDonald CB. Upper lobe fibrosis associated with AS. *Br J Chest Dis* 1965;59:90–100.

86. Fisher LR, Cawley MID, Holgate ST. Relation between chest expansion, pulmonary function and exercise tolerance in patients with AS. *Ann Rheum Dis* 1990;9:921–925.

87. Gratacos J, Orellana C, Sanmarti R, et al. Secondary amyloidosis in AS. A systematic survey of 137 patients using abdominal fat aspiration. *J Rheumatol* 1997;24:912–925.

88. Lai KN, Li PKT, Hawkins B, et al. IgA nephropathy associated with AS: occurrence in women as well as in men. *Ann Rheum Dis* 1989;48:435–437.

89. Russell ML, Gordon DA, Ogryzlo MA, et al. The cauda equina syndrome of AS. *Ann Intern Med* 1973;78:551–554.

90. Sparling MJ, Bartleson JD, McLeod PA, et al. Magnetic resonance imaging of the arachnoid diverticulae associated with cauda equina syndrome in AS. *J Rheumatol* 1989;16: 1335–1337.

91. Charlesworth CH, Savy LE, Stevens J, et al. MRI demonstration of arachnoiditis in cauda equina syndrome of AS. *Neuroradiology* 1996;38:462–465.

92. Calin A. Raised serum creatine phosphokinase activity in AS. *Ann Rheum Dis* 1975;34:244–248.

93. Calin A, Elswood J. A prospective nationwide cross-sectional study of NSAID usage in 1331 patients with AS. *J Rheumatol* 1990;17:801–803.

94. Calabro JJ. Sustained-release indomethacin in the management of AS. *Am J Med* 1985;79:39–51.

95. Ferez MB, Tugwell P, Goldsmith CH, et al. Meta-analysis of sulfasalazine in AS. *J Rheumatol* 1990;17:1482–1486.

96. Dougados M, van der Linden S, Leirisalo-Repo M, et al. Sulfasalazine in spondyloarthropathy: a randomized, multicentre, double-blind, placebo-controlled study. *Arthritis Rheum* 1995; 38:618–627.

97. Clegg DO, Reda DJ, Weisman MH, et al. Comparison of sulfasalazine and placebo in the treatment of AS. *Arthritis Rheum* 1996;39:2004–2112.

98. Taggart A, Gardiner P, McEvoy F, et al. Which is the active moiety of sulfasalazine in AS? *Arthritis Rheum* 1996;39:1400–1405.

99. Mintz G, Enriquez RD, Mercado U, et al. Intravenous methylprednisolone pulse therapy in severe AS. *Arthritis Rheum* 1981; 24:734–736.

100. Gorman JD, Sack KE, Davis, JC. *N Engl J Med* 2002;346: 1349–1356.

101. Kraag G, Stokes B, Groh J, et al. The effects of comprehensive home physiotherapy and supervision of patients with AS—a randomized controlled trial. *J Rheumatol* 1990;17:229–233.

102. Santos H, Brophy S, Calin A. Exercise in AS: how much is optimum? *J Rheumatol* 1998;25:2156–2160.

103. Wordsworth BP, Mowat AG. A review of 100 patients with AS with particular reference to socioeconomic effects. *Br J Rheumatol* 1986;25:175–180.

104. Calin A, Elswood J. The outcome of 130 total hip replacements and 2 revisions in AS: high success rate after a mean followup of 7.5 years. *J Rheumatol* 1989;16:955–958.

105. Sundaram NA, Murphy JCM. Heterotopic bone formation following total hip arthroplasty in AS. *Clin Orthop* 1986;207: 223–226.

106. Camargo FP, Cordeiro EN, Napoli MMM. Corrective osteotomy of the spine in AS. Experience with 66 cases. *Clin Orthop* 1986;208:157–167.

107. Sinclair JR, Mason RA. AS: the case for awake intubation. *Anesthesia* 1984;39:3–11.

108. Carette S, Graham D, Little H, et al. The natural disease course of AS. *Arthritis Rheum* 1983;266:186–190.

109. Gran JT, Skomsvoll JF. The outcome of AS: a study of 100 patients. *Br J Rheumatol* 1997;36:766–771.

110. Kaprove RE, Little AH, Graham DC, et al. AS: survival in men with and without radiotherapy. *Arthritis Rheum* 1980;23:57–61.

111. Smith PG, Doll R. Mortality among patients with AS after a single treatment course with x-rays. *Br Med J* 1982;284:449–460.

112. Lehtinen K. Cause of death in 79 patients with AS. *J Rheumatol* 1980;9:145–147.

113. Ahvonen P, Sievers K, Aho K. Arthritis associated with *Yersinia enterocolitica* infection. *Acta Rheumatol Scand* 1969;15: 232–253.

114. Amor B. Reiter's syndrome: diagnosis and clinical features. *Rheum Dis Clin North Am* 1998;24:677–695.

115. Cush JJ, Lipsky PE. Reiter's syndrome and reactive arthritis. In: Koopman WJ, ed. *Arthritis and allied conditions: a textbook of rheumatology,* 13th ed. Baltimore: Williams & Wilkins, 1997: 1209–1227.

116. Reiter H. Uber eine bisher unerkannte Spirochaeteninfektion (Spirochaetosis Arthritica). *Dtsch Med Wochenschr* 1916;42: 1535–1536.

117. Willkens RF, Arnett FC, Bitter T, et al. Reiter's syndrome; evaluation of preliminary criteria for definite disease. *Arthritis Rheum* 1981;24:844–849.

118. Khan MA, van der Linden SM. A wider spectrum of spondyloarthropathies. *Semin Arthritis Rheum* 1990;20:107–113.

119. Dougados M, van der Linden S, Juhlin R, et al. The European Spondyloarthropathy Study Group preliminary criteria for the classification of spondyloarthropathy. *Arthritis Rheum* 1991;34: 1218–1227.

120. Amor B, Dougados M, Khan MA, et al. Management of refractory ankylosing spondylitis and related spondyloarthropathies. *Rheum Dis Clin North Am* 1995;21:117–128.

121. Michet CJ, Machado EB, Ballard DJ, et al. Epidemiology of Reiter's syndrome in Rochester, Minnesota: 1950–1980. *Arthritis Rheum* 1988;31:428–431.

122. Kvien TK, Glennaås A, Melby K, et al. Reactive arthritis: incidence, triggering agents and clinical presentation. *J Rheumatol* 1994;21:115–122.

123. Taurog JD, Lipsky PE. Ankylosing spondylitis, reactive arthritis, and undifferentiated spondyloarthropathy. In: Fauci AS, Braunwald E, Isselbacher KJ, et al., eds. *Harrison's principles of internal medicine,* 14th ed. New York: McGraw-Hill, 1998: 1904–1909.

124. Cuttica RJ, Schennes EJ, Garay SM, et al. Juvenile onset Reiter's syndrome: a retrospective study of 26 patients. *Clin Exp Rheumatol* 1992;10:285–288.

125. Iliopoulos A, Karras D, Ioakimidis D, et al. Changes in the epidemiology of Reiter's syndrome (reactive arthritis) in the post-AIDS era? An analysis of cases appearing in the Greek army. *J Rheumatol* 1995;22:252–254.

126. Rich E, Hook EW, Alarcon GS, et al. Reactive arthritis in patients attending an urban sexually transmitted diseases clinic. *Arthritis Rheum* 1996;39:1172–1177.

127. Noer HR. An experimental epidemic of Reiter's syndrome. *JAMA* 1966;198:693–698.

128. Thomson GTD, DeRubeis DA, Hodge MA, et al. Post-salmonella reactive arthritis: late clinical sequelae in a point source cohort. *Am J Med* 1995;98:13–21.

129. Nikkari S, Rantakokko K, Edman P, et al. Salmonella-triggered reactive arthritis: use of polymerase chain reaction, immunocytochemical staining, and gas chromatography-mass spectroscopy in the detection of bacterial components from synovial fluid. *Arthritis Rheum* 1999;42:84–89.

130. Mattila L, Leirisalo-Repo M, Koskimies S, et al. Reactive arthritis following an outbreak of *Salmonella* infection in Finland. *Br J Rheumatol* 1994;33:1136–1141.

131. Mattila L, Leirisalo-Repo M, Pelkonen P, et al. Reactive arthritis following an outbrak of *Salmonella Bovismorbificans* infection. *J Infect* 1998;36:289–295.

132. Wuorela M, Granfors K. Infectious agents as triggers of reactive arthritis. *Am J Med Sci* 1998;316:264–270.

133. Leirisalo-Repo M, Suoranta H. Ten-year followup study of patients with *Yersinia arthritis*. *Arthritis Rheum* 1988;31: 533–537.

134. Toivanen A, Lahesmaa-Rantala R, Vuento R, et al. Association of persisting IgA response with *Yersinia* triggered reactive arthritis: a study on 104 patients. *Ann Rheum Dis* 1987;46: 898–901.

135. Gronberg A, Fryden A, Kihlstrom E. Humoral immune response to individual *Yersinia enterocolitica* antigens in patients with and without reactive arthritis. *Clin Exp Immunol* 1989;76: 361–365.

136. Granfors K, Jalkanen S, van Essen R, et al. *Yersinia* antigens in synovial-fluid cells from patients with reactive arthritis. *N Engl J Med* 1989;320:216–221.

137. Zeidler H. Chlamydial-induced arthritis: the clinical spectrum, serology and prognosis. In: Lipsky P, ed. *Proceedings of the second Simmons Center International Conference on HLA–B27 related disorders.* New York: Elsevier, 1991:175–187.

138. Cooper SM, Ferriss JA. Reactive arthritis and psittacosis. *Am J Med* 1986;81:555–557.

138a. Inman RD, Chiu B. Synoviocyte-packaged *Chlamydia trachomatis* induces a chronic aseptic arthritis. *J Clin Invest* 1998; 15:1776–1782.

139. Gran JT, Hjetland R, Andreassen AH. Pneumonia, myocarditis and reactive arthritis due to *Chlamydia pneumoniae*. *Scand J Rheumatol* 1993;22:43–44.

140. Braun J, Laitko S, Treharne J, et al. *Chlamydia pneumoniae*: a new causative agent of reactive arthritis and undifferentiated oligoarthritis. *Ann Rheum Dis* 1994;53:100–105.

141. Horowitz S, Horowitz J, Taylor-Robinson D, et al. *Ureaplasma urealyticum* in Reiter's syndrome. *J Rheumatol* 1994;21: 877–882.

142. Winchester R, Bernstein DH, Fischer HD, et al. The co-occurrence of Reiter's syndrome and acquired immunodeficiency. *Ann Intern Med* 1987;106:19–26.

143. Winchester R. AIDS and the rheumatic diseases. *Bull Rheum Dis* 1990;39:1–10.

144. Calabrese LH, Kelley DM, Myers A, et al. Rheumatic symptoms and human immunodeficiency virus infection: the influence of clinical and laboratory variables in a longitudinal cohort study. *Arthritis Rheum* 1991;34:257–263.

145. Altman EM, Centeno LV, Mahal M, et al. AIDS-associated Reiter's syndrome. *Ann Allergy* 1994;72:307–316.

146. Kellner H, Fuessl HS, Herzer P. Seronegative spondyloarthropathies in HIV-infected patients: further evidence of uncommon clinical features. *Rheumatol Int* 1994;13: 211–213.

147. Keat A, Rowe I. Reiter's syndrome and associated arthritides. *Rheum Dis Clin North Am* 1991;17:25–42.

148. Paronen I. Reiter's disease: a study of 344 cases observed in Finland. *Acta Med Scand* 1948;131;212(Suppl):1–112.

149. Shichikawa K, Takenaka Y, Yukioka M, et al. Polyenthesitis. *Rheum Dis Clin North Am* 1992;18:203–213.

150. McGonagle D, Gibbon W, O'Conner P, et al. Characteristic MRI entheseal changes of knee synovitis in Spondyloarthropathy. *Arthritis Rheum* 1998;41:694–700.

151. Ingram GJ, Scher RK. Reiter's syndrome with nail involvement: is it psoriasis? *Cutis* 1985;36:37–40.

152. Banares A, Hernandez-Garcia C, Fernandex-Gutierrez, et al. Eye involvement in the spondyloarthropathies. *Rheum Dis Clin North Am* 1998;24:771–784.

153. Rosenbaum JT. Characterization of uveitis associated with spondyloarthropathies. *J Rheumatol* 1989;16:792–796.

154. Nashel DJ, Petrone DL, Ulmer CC, et al. C-reactive protein: a marker for disease activity in ankylosing spondylitis and Reiter's syndrome. *J Rheumatol* 1986;13:364–367.

155. Locht H, Peen E, Skogh T. Antineutrophil cytoplasmic antibodies in reactive arthritis. *J Rheumatol* 1995;22:2304–2306.

156. Reveille JD. HLA-B27 and the seronegative spondyloarthropathies. *Am J Med Sci* 1998;316:239–249.

157. Braun J, Bollow M, Sieper J. Radiologic diagnosis and pathology of the spondyloarthropathies. *Rheum Dis Clin North Am* 1998;24:697–735.

158. Helliwell PS, Hickling P, Wright V. Do the radiological changes of classic ankylosing spondylitis differ from the changes found in the spondylitis associated with inflammatory bowel disease, psoriasis and reactive arthritis? *Ann Rheum Dis* 1998;57:135–140.

159. Leirisalo-Repo M. Prognosis, course of disease, and treatment of the spondyloarthropathies. *Rheum Dis Clin North Am* 1998;24:737–751.

160. Cush JJ, Lipsky PE. The spondyloarthropathies. In: Bennett JC, et al., eds. *Cecil textbook of internal medicine,* 21st ed. Philadelphia: WB Saunders, 2000:1499–1506.

161. Creemers MCW, van Riel PLCM, Franssen MJAM, et al. Second-line treatment in seronegative spondyloarthropathies. *Semin Arthritis Rheum* 1994;24:71–81.

162. Calin A. A placebo-controlled, crossover study of azathioprine in Reiter's syndrome. *Ann Rheum Dis* 1986;45:653–655.

163. Owen ET, Cohen ML. Methotrexate and Reiter's disease. *Ann Rheum Dis* 1979;38:48–50.

164. Clegg DO, Reda DJ, Weisman MH, et al. Comparison of sulfasalazine and placebo in the treatment of reactive arthritis (Reiter's syndrome): a Department of Veterans Affairs Cooperative Study. *Arthritis Rheum* 1996;39:2021–2027.

165. Egsmose C, Hansen TM, Andersen LS, et al. Limited effect of sulphasalazine treatment in reactive arthritis. A randomised double blind placebo controlled trial. *Ann Rheum Dis* 1997;56:32–36.

166. Mielants H, Veys EM, Goemaere S, et al. A prospective study of patients with spondyloarthropathy with special reference to HLA-B27 and to gut histology. *J Rheumatol* 1993;20:1353–1358.

167. Alarcon G, Mikhail IS. Antimicrobials in the treatment of rheumatoid arthritis and other arthritides: a clinical perspective. *Am J Med Sci* 1994;308:201–209.

168. Locht H, Kihlstrom E, Lindstrom FD. Reactive arthritis after salmonella among medical doctors: study of an outbreak. *J Rheumatol* 1993;20:845–848.

169. Sieper J, Fendler C, Laitko S, et al. No benefit of long-term ciprofloxacin treatment in patients with reactive arthritis and undifferentiated oligoarthritis: a three month, multicenter, double-blind, randomized, placebo-controlled study. *Arthritis Rheum* 1999;42:1386–1396.

170. Youssef PP, Vertouch JV, Jones PD. Successful treatment of human immunodeficiency virus–associated Reiter's syndrome with sulfasalazine. *Arthritis Rheum* 1992;35:723–724.

171. Disla E, Rhim HR, Reddy A, et al. Improvement in CD4 lymphocyte count in HIV-Reiter's syndrome after treatment with sulfasalazine. *J Rheumatol* 1994;21:662–664.

172. Louthrenoo W. Successful treatment of severe Reiter's syndrome associated with human immunodeficiency virus infection with etretinate. Report of 2 cases. *J Rheumatol* 1993;20:1243–1246.

173. Williams HC, Du Vivier AWP. Etretinate and AIDS-related Reiter's disease. *Br J Dermatol* 1991;124:389–392.

174. Amor B, Silva Santos R, Nahal R, et al. Predictive factors for the long-term outcome of spondyloarthropathies. *J Rheumatol* 1994;21:1883–1887.

175. Kaarela K, Lehtinen K, Luukkainen R. Work capacity of patients with inflammatory joint diseases: an eight-year follow-up study. *Scand J Rheumatol* 1987;16:403–406.

176. Clavel G, Grados F, Cayrolle G, et al. Polyarthritis following intravesical BCG immunotherapy. Report of a case and review of 26 cases in the literature. *Rev Rheum Engl Ed* 1999;66:115–118.

177. Schwartzenberg JM, Smith DD, Lindsley HB. Bacillus Calmette-Guerin associated arthropathy mimicking undifferentiated spondyloarthropathy. *J Rheumatol* 1999;26:933–935.

178. Ferrazzi V, Jorgensen C, Sany J. Inflammatory joint diseases after immunizations. A report of two cases. *Rev Rheum Engl Ed* 1997;64:227–232.

179. Rose HM, Ragan C, Pearce E, et al. Differential agglutination of normal and sensitized sheep erythrocytes by sera of patients with RA. *Proc Soc Exp Biol Med* 1948;68:1–6.

180. Baker H. Epidemiological aspects of psoriasis and arthritis. *Br J Dermatol* 1966;78:249–261.

181. Ropes MW, Bennett EA, Cobb S, et al. Diagnostic criteria for RA. *Bull Rheum Dis* 1959;9:175–176.

182. Moll JM, Wright V. Familial occurrence of psoriatic arthritis. *Ann Rheum Dis* 1973;32:181–201.

183. Lombolt G. *Psoriasis, prevalence, spontaneous course, and genetics; a census study on the prevalence of skin disease in the Faroe Islands.* Copenhagen: GEC Gad, 1963.

184. Shore A, Ansell BM. Juvenile psoriatic arthritis—an analysis of 60 cases. *J Pediatr* 1982;100:529–535.

185. Southwood TR, Petty RE, Malleson PN, et al. Psoriatic arthritis in children. *Arthritis Rheum* 1989;32:1007–1013.

186. Rahman P, Schentag CT, Gladman DD. Immunogenetic profile of patients with psoriatic arthritis varies according to the age at onset of psoriasis. *Arthritis Rheum* 1999;42:822–823.

187. Prens E, Debets R, Hegmans J. T lymphocytes in psoriasis. *Clin Dermatol* 1995;13:115–129.

188. Biondi Oriente C, Scarpa R, Pucino A, et al. Psoriasis and psoriatic arthritis. Dermatological and rheumatological co-operative clinical report. *Acta Derm Venereol Suppl (Stockh)* 1989;146:69–71.

189. Langevitz P, Buskila D, Gladman DD. Psoriatic arthritis precipitated by physical trauma. *J Rheumatol* 1990;17:695–697.

190. Doury P. Psoriatic arthritis with physical trauma. *J Rheumatol* 1993;20:1629.

191. Olivieri I, Gemignani G, Christou C, et al. Trauma and seronegative spondyloarthropathy: report of two more cases of peripheral arthritis precipitated by physical injury. *Ann Rheum Dis* 1989;48:520–521.

192. Olivieri I, Gherardi S, Bini C, et al. Trauma and seronegative spondyloarthropathy: rapid joint destruction in peripheral arthritis triggered by physical injury. *Ann Rheum Dis* 1988;47:73–76.

193. Pages M, Lassoued S, Fournie B, et al. Psoriatic arthritis precipitated by physical trauma: destructive arthritis or associated

with reflex sympathetic dystrophy? *J Rheumatol* 1992;19: 185–186.

194. Scarpa R, della Valle G, Del Puente A, et al. Physical trauma triggers psoriasis in a patient with undifferentiated seronegative spondyloarthropathy. *Clin Exp Rheumatol* 1992;10:100–102.

195. Winchester R, Brancato L, Itescu S, et al. Implications from the occurrence of Reiter's syndrome and related disorders in association with advanced HIV infection. *Scand J Rheumatol* 1988; 74:89–93.

196. Berman A, Espinoza LR, Aguillar JL, et al. Rheumatic manifestations of human immunodeficiency virus infection. *Am J Med* 1988;85:59–64.

197. Duvic M, Johnson TM, Rapini RP, et al. Acquired immunodeficiency syndrome-associated psoriasis and Reiter's syndrome. *Arch Dermatol* 1987;123:1622–1632.

198. Brancato L, Itescu S, Skovron ML, et al. Aspects of the spectrum, prevalence and disease susceptibility determinants of Reiter's syndrome and related disorders associated with HIV infection. *Rheum Int* 1989;9:137–141.

199. Johnson TM, Duvic M, Rapini RP, et al. AIDS exacerbates psoriasis. *N Engl J Med* 1985;313:1415.

200. Helliwell P, Marchesoni A, Peters M, et al. A re-evaluation of the osteoarticular manifestations of psoriasis. *Br J Rheumatol* 1991;30:339–345.

201. Gladman DD, Shuckett R, Russell ML, et al. Psoriatic arthritis (PSA)—an analysis of 220 patients. *Q J Med* 1987;62:127–141.

202. Scarpa R, Oriente P, Pucino A, et al. Psoriatic arthritis in psoriatic patients. *Br J Rheumatol* 1984;23:246–250.

203. O'Donnell BF, O'Loughlin S, Codd MB, et al. HLA typing in Irish psoriatics. *Ir Med J* 1993;86:65–68.

204. Troughton PR, Morgan AW. Laboratory findings and pathology of psoriatic arthritis. *Baillieres Clin Rheumatol* 1994;8:439–463.

205. Mullen RH, Farber EM. Some thoughts on psoriatic arthritis. *Cutis* 1985;36:388–390.

206. Lambert JR, Wright V. Psoriatic spondylitis: a clinical and radiological description of the spine in psoriatic arthritis. *Q J Med* 1977;46:411–425.

207. Gladman DD, Brubacher B, Buskila D, et al. Differences in the expression of spondyloarthropathy: a comparison between ankylosing spondylitis and psoriatic arthritis. *Clin Invest Med* 1993;16:1–7.

208. Salvarani C, Macchioni P, Cremonesi T, et al. The cervical spine in patients with psoriatic arthritis: a clinical, radiological and immunogenetic study. *Ann Rheum Dis* 1992;51:73–77.

209. Spadaro A, Riccieri V, Sili Scavalli A, et al. Multiple cervical cord compressions in psoriatic arthritis. *Clin Rheumatol* 1992; 11:51–54.

210. McHugh NJ, Laurent MR. The effect of pregnancy on the onset of psoriatic arthritis. *Br J Rheumatol* 1989;28:50–52.

211. Ostensen M. The effect of pregnancy on ankylosing spondylitis, psoriatic arthritis, and juvenile rheumatoid arthritis. *Am J Reprod Immunol* 1992;28:235–237.

212. Stevens HP, Ostlere LS, Black CM, et al. Cyclical psoriatic arthritis responding to anti-oestrogen therapy. *Br J Dermatol* 1993;129:458–460.

213. Jones SM, Armas JB, Cohen MG, et al. Psoriatic arthritis: outcome of disease subsets and relationship of joint disease to nail and skin disease. *Br J Rheumatol* 1994;33:834–839.

214. Lavaroni G, Kokelj F, Pauluzzi P, et al. The nails in psoriatic arthritis. *Acta Derm Venereol Suppl (Stockh)* 1994;186:113.

215. Veale D, Rogers S, Fitzgerald O. Classification of clinical subsets in psoriatic arthritis. *Br J Rheumatol* 1994;33:133–138.

216. Gladman DD, Farewell VT, Wong K, et al. Mortality studies in psoriatic arthritis: results from a single outpatient center. II. Prognostic indicators for death. *Arthritis Rheum* 1998;41: 1103–1110.

217. Wright V, Moll JMH. *Seronegative polyarthritis.* Amsterdam: North Holland, 1976.

218. Lambert JR, Wright V. Eye inflammation in psoriatic arthritis. *Ann Rheum Dis* 1976;35:354–356.

219. Omdal R, Husby G. Renal affection in patients with ankylosing spondylitis and psoriatic arthritis. *Clin Rheumatol* 1987;6: 74–79.

220. Pines A, Ehrenfeld M, Fisman EZ, et al. Mitral valve prolapse in psoriatic arthritis. *Arch Intern Med* 1986;146:1371–1373.

221. Muna WF, Roller DH, Craft J, et al. Psoriatic arthritis and aortic regurgitation. *JAMA* 1980;244:363–365.

222. Thomson GT, Johnston JL, Baragar FD, et al. Psoriatic arthritis and myopathy. *J Rheumatol* 1990;17:395–398.

223. Rodriguez de la Serna A, Casas Gasso F, Diaz Lopez C, et al. Association of Sjögren's syndrome with psoriatic arthritis. *Can Med Assoc J* 1984;131:1329–1332.

224. Whaley K, Chisholm DM, Williamson J, et al. Sjögren's syndrome in psoriatic arthritis, anklyosing spondylitis and Reiter's syndrome. *Acta Rheumatol Scand* 1971;17:105–114.

225. Partsch G. Laboratory features of psoriatic arthritis. *Z Rheumatol* 1987;46:220–226.

226. Hall RP, Gerber LH, Lawley TJ. IgA-containing immune complexes in patients with psoriatic arthritis. *Clin Exp Rheumatol* 1984;2:221–225.

227. Taccari E, Gigante MC, Sorgi ML, et al. Serum uric acid levels in psoriatic arthritis. *Scand J Rheumatol* 1985;14:94.

228. Porter GG. Plain radiology and other imaging techniques. *Baillieres Clin Rheumatol* 1994;8:465–482.

229. Gold RH, Bassett LW, Seeger LL. The other arthritides. Roentgenologic features of osteoarthritis, erosive osteoarthritis, ankylosing spondylitis, psoriatic arthritis, Reiter's disease, multicentric reticulohistiocytosis, and progressive systemic sclerosis. *Radiol Clin North Am* 1988;26:1195–1212.

230. Sherman M. Psoriatic arthritis: observations on the clinical, roentgenographic and radiological changes. *J Bone Joint Surg* 1952;34A:831–852.

231. Bywaters EGL, Dixon ASJ. Paravertebral ossification in psoriatic arthritis. *Ann Rheum Dis* 1965;24:313–331.

232. Jajic I. Radiological changes in the sacroiliac joints and spine of patients with psoriatic arthritis and psoriasis. *Ann Rheum Dis* 1968;27:1–6.

233. Leonard DG, O'Duffy JD, Rogers RS. Prospective analysis of psoriatic arthritis in patients hospitalized for psoriasis. *Mayo Clin Proc* 1978;53:511–518.

234. Dzioba RB, Benjamin J. Spontaneous atlantoaxial fusion in psoriatic arthritis. A case report. *Spine* 1985;10:102–103.

235. Blau RH, Kaufman RL. Erosive and subluxing cervical spine disease in patients with psoriatic arthritis. *J Rheumatol* 1987;14: 111–117.

236. Lee ST, Lui TN. Psoriatic arthritis with C-1–C-2 subluxation as a neurosurgical complication. *Surg Neurol* 1986;26:428–430.

237. Toussirot E, Dupond JL, Wendling D. Spondylodiscitis in SAPHO syndrome. A series of eight cases. *Ann Rheum Dis* 1997;56:52–58.

238. Kononen M. Radiographic changes in the condyle of the temporomandibular joint in psoriatic arthritis. *Acta Radiol* 1987; 28:185–188.

239. Coulton BL, Thomson K, Symmons DP, Popert AJ. Outcome in patients hospitalised for psoriatic arthritis. *Clin Rheumatol* 1989;8:261–265.

240. Anonymous. Prognosis of psoriatic arthritis [Editorial]. *Lancet* 1988;2:375–376.

241. Roberts ME, Wright V, Hill AG, et al. Psoriatic arthritis. Follow-up study. *Ann Rheum Dis* 1976;35:206–212.

242. Wong K, Gladman DD, Husted J, et al. Mortality studies in psoriatic arthritis: results from a single outpatient clinic. I.

Causes and risk of death [see comments]. *Arthritis Rheum* 1997; 40:1868–1872.

243. Stewart MW, Knight RG, Palmer DG, et al. Differential relationships between stress and disease activity for immunologically distinct subgroups of people with rheumatoid arthritis. *J Abnorm Psychol* 1994;103:251–258.

244. Noble WC, Sarin JA. Carriage of *Staphylococcus aureus* in psoriasis. *Br Med J* 1968;1:417–418.

245. Daunt AO, Cox NL, Robertson JC, et al. Indices of disease activity in psoriatic arthritis. *J Roy Soc Med* 1987;80:556–558.

246. Perlman SG, Gerber LH, Roberts RM, et al. Photochemotherapy and psoriatic arthritis. A prospective study. *Ann Intern Med* 1979;91:717–722.

247. Kragballe K. Treatment of psoriasis with calcipotriol and other vitamin D analogues. *J Am Acad Dermatol* 1992;27:1001–1008.

248. Araugo OE, Flowers FP, Brown K. Vitamin D therapy in psoriasis. *DICP* 1991;25:835–839.

249. El-Azhary RA, Peters MS, Pittelkow MR, et al. Efficacy of vitamin D3 derivatives in the treatment of psoriasis vulgaris: a preliminary report. *Mayo Clin Proc* 1993;68:835–841.

250. Kammer GM, Soter NA, Gibson DJ, et al. Psoriatic arthritis: a clinical, immunologic and HLA study of 100 patients. *Semin Arthritis Rheum* 1979;9:75–97.

251. Gladman DD, Blake R, Brubacher B, et al. Chloroquine therapy in psoriatic arthritis. *J Rheumatol* 1992;19:1724–1726.

252. Sayers ME, Mazanec DJ. Use of antimalarial drugs for the treatment of psoriatic arthritis. *Am J Med* 1992;93:474–475.

253. Dorwart BB, Gall EP, Schumacher HR, et al. Chrysotherapy in psoriatic arthritis: efficacy and toxicity compared to rheumatoid arthritis. *Arthritis Rheum* 1978;21:513–515.

254. Farr M, Kitas GD, Waterhouse L, et al. Sulphasalazine in psoriatic arthritis: a double-blind placebo-controlled study. *Br J Rheumatol* 1990;29:46–49.

255. Fraser SM, Hopkins R, Hunter JA, et al. Sulphasalazine in the management of psoriatic arthritis. *Br J Rheumatol* 1993;32: 923–925.

256. Newman ED, Perruquet JL, Harrington TM. Sulfasalazine therapy in psoriatic arthritis: clinical and immunologic response. *J Rheumatol* 1991;18:1379–1382.

257. Clegg DO, Reda DJ, Mejias E, et al. Comparison of sulfasalazine and placebo in the treatment of psoriatic arthritis. A Department of Veterans Affairs Cooperative Study. *Arthritis Rheum* 1996;39:2013–2020.

258. Rahman P, Gladman DD, Cook RJ, et al. The use of sulfasalazine in psoriatic arthritis: a clinic experience. *J Rheumatol* 1998;25:1957–1961.

259. Hopkins R, Bird HA, Jones, et al. A double-blind controlled trial of etretinate (Tigason) and ibuprofen in psoriatic arthritis *Ann Rheum Dis* 1985;44:189–193.

260. Seideman P, Fjellner B, Johannesson A. Psoriatic arthritis treated with oral colchicine. *J Rheumatol* 1987;14:777–779.

261. McKendry RJ, Kraag G, Seigel S, et al. Therapeutic value of colchicine in the treatment of patients with psoriatic arthritis. *Ann Rheum Dis* 1993;52:826–828.

262. Cuellar ML, Espinoza LR. Methotrexate use in psoriasis and psoriatic arthritis. *Rheum Dis Clin North Am* 1997;23:797–809.

263. Espinoza LR, Zakraoui L, Espinoza CG, et al. Psoriatic arthritis: clinical response and side effects to methotrexate therapy. *J Rheumatol* 1992;19:872–877.

264. Kummerle K, Wessinghage D, Schweikert CH. Risk of alloplastic replacements in degenerative and inflammatory diseases of joints. *Acta Orthop Belg* 1971;37:541–548.

265. Goupille P, Soutif D, Valat JP. Treatment of psoriatic arthropathy. *Semin Arthritis Rheum* 1992;21:355–367.

266. Zachariae H, Zachariae E. Methotrexate treatment of psoriatic arthritis. *Acta Derm Venereol (Stockh)* 1987;67:270–273.

267. Willkens RF, Williams HJ, Ward JR, et al. Randomized, double-blind, placebo controlled trial of low-dose pulse methotrexate in psoriatic arthritis. *Arthritis Rheum* 1984;27:376–381.

268. Baum J, Hurd E, Lewis D, et al. Treatment of psoriatic arthritis with 6-mercaptopurine. *Arthritis Rheum* 1973;16:139–147.

269. Wagner SA, Peter RU, Adam O, et al. Therapeutic efficacy of oral low-dose cyclosporin A in severe psoriatic arthritis. *Dermatology* 1993;186:62–67.

270. Kokelj F, Lavaroni G, Stinco G. Psoriatic arthritis treated with cyclosporin A. *Allerg Immunol (Paris)* 1992;24:393–394.

271. Salvarani C, Macchioni P, Boiardi L, et al. Low dose cyclosporine A in psoriatic arthritis: relation between soluble interleukin 2 receptors and response to therapy. *J Rheumatol* 1992;19:74–79.

272. Spadaro A, Riccieri V, Sili-Scavalli A, et al. Comparison of cyclosporin A and methotrexate in the treatment of psoriatic arthritis: a one-year prospective study. *Clin Exp Rheumatol* 1995;13:589–593.

273. Maurer TA, Zackheim HS, Tuffanelli L, et al. The use of methotrexate for treatment of psoriasis in patients with HIV infection. *J Am Acad Dermatol* 1994;31:372–375.

274. Stucki G, Bozzone P, Treuer E, et al. Efficacy and safety of radiation synovectomy with Yttrium-90: a retrospective long-term analysis of 164 applications in 82 patients. *Br J Rheumatol* 1993;32:383–386.

275. Will R, Laing B, Edelman J, et al. Comparison of two yttrium-90 regimens in inflammatory and osteoarthropathies. *Ann Rheum Dis* 1992;51:262–265.

276. De Misa RF, Azana JM, Harto A, et al. Extracorporeal photochemotherapy in the treatment of severe psoriatic arthropathy. *Br J Dermatol* 1992;127: 448.

277. Fierlbeck G, Rassner G. Treatment of psoriasis and psoriatic arthritis with interferon gamma. *J Invest Dermatol* 1990;95(6 Suppl): 138S–141S.

278. Jorstad S, Bergh K, Iversen OJ, et al. Effects of cascade apheresis in patients with psoriasis and psoriatic arthropathy. *Blood Purif* 1998;16:37–42.

279. Cooley HM, Snowden JA, Grigg AP, et al. Outcome of rheumatoid arthritis and psoriasis following autologous stem cell transplantation for hematologic malignancy. *Arthritis Rheum* 1997; 40:1712–1715.

280. Lynfield YL, Ostroff G, Abraham J. Bacteria, skin sterilization and wound healing in psoriasis. *NY J Med* 1972;72:1247–1250.

281. Lambert JR, Wright V. Surgery in patients with psoriasis and arthritis. *Rheumatol Rehabil* 1979;18:35–37.

282. Belsky MR, Feldon P, Millender LH, et al. Hand involvement in psoriatic arthritis. *J Hand Surg* 1982;7:203–207.

283. Kononen M. Craniomandibular disorders in psoriatic arthritis. A radiographic and clinical study. *Proc Finn Dent Soc* 1987; 83(Suppl 8-10):1–45.

284. Mielants H, Veys EM. Enteropathic arthritis. In: Koopman WJ, ed. *Arthritis and allied conditions: a textbook of rheumatology*, 13th ed. Baltimore: Williams & Wilkins, 1996:1245–1263.

285. Mielants H, Veys EM, Cuvelier C, et al. Ileocolonoscopic findings in seronegative spondyloarthropathies. *Br J Rheumatol* 1988;27(Suppl II):95–105.

286. Simenon G, Van Gossum A, Adler M, et al. Macroscopic and microscopic gut lesions in seronegative spondylarthropathies. *J Rheumatol* 1990;17:1491–1494.

287. Leirisalo-Repo M, Turunen U, Stenman S, et al. High frequency of silent inflammatory bowel disease in spondylarthropathy. *Arthritis Rheum* 1994;37:23–31.

288. Altomonte L, Zoli A, Veneziani A, et al. Clinical silent inflam-

matory gut lesions in undifferentiated spondyloarthropathies. *Clin Rheumatol* 1994;13:565–570.

289. Lee YH, Ji JP, Sim JS, et al. Ileocolonoscopic and histological studies of Korean patients with ankylosing spondylitis. *Scand J Rheumatol* 1997;26:473–476.

290. Mayberry JF, Ballantyne KC, Hardcastle JD, et al. Epidemiological study of asymptomatic inflammatory bowel disease: the identification of cases during a screening programme for colorectal cancer. *Gut* 1989;30:481–483.

291. Gravallese EM, Kantrowitz FG. Arthritic manifestations of inflammatory bowel disease. *Am J Gastroenterol* 1988;83:703–709.

292. Orchard TR, Wordsworth BP, Jewell DP. Peripheral arthropathies in inflammatory bowel disease: their articular distribution and natural history. *Gut* 1998;42:387–391.

293. De Vlam K, De Vos M, Mielants H, et al. Spondyloarthropathy in inflammatory bowel disease: prevalence and HLA association. *J Rheumatol* 2000;27:2860–2865.

294. Mielants H, Veys EM. The gut in the spondyloarthropathies. *J Rheumatol* 1990;17:7–10.

295. Mielants H, Veys EM, Cuvelier C, et al. The evolution of spondylarthropathies in relation to gut histology. Part I: Clinical Aspects. *J Rheumatol* 1995;22:2266–2272.

296. Isdale A, Wright V. Seronegative arthritis and the bowel. *Baillieres Clin Rheumatol* 1989;3:285–301.

297. Dougados M, Van Der Linden J, Juhlin R, et al. The European Spondylarthropathy Study Group: The European Spondylarthropathy Study Group preliminary criteria for the classification of spondylarthropathy. *Arthritis Rheum* 1991;34:1218–1226.

298. Bardazzi G, Mannoni A, D'Albasio G, et al. Spondyloarthritis in patients with ulcerative colitis. *Ital J Gastroenterol* 1997;29:520–524.

299. Kennedy GL, Will R, Calin A. Sex ratio in the spondy-larthropathies and its relationship to phenotypic expression, mode of inheritance and age at onset. *J Rheumatol* 1993;20:1900–1904.

300. Edmonds L, Elswood J, Kennedy GL, et al. Primary ankylosing spondylitis in psoriatic and enteropathic spondylarthropathies: a controlled analysis. *J Rheumatol* 1991;19:696–698.

301. Schorr-Lesnick B, Brandt LJ. Selected rheumatologic and dermatologic manifestations of inflammatory bowel disease. *Am J Gastroenterol* 1988;83:216–223.

302. Rosenbaum T. Characterization of uveitis associated with spondyloarthritis. *J Rheumatol* 1989;16:792–796.

303. Banares AA, Jover JA, Fernandez-Gutiérrez B, et al. Bowel inflammation in anterior uveitis and spondylarthropathy. *J Rheumatol* 1995;22:1112–1117.

304. Greenstein AJ, Janowitz HD, Sachar DB. The extraintestinal complications of Crohn's disease and ulcerative colitis: a study of 700 patients. *Medicine* 1976;55:401–412.

305. Mielants H, Veys EM, Goethals K et al. Destructive hip lesions in seronegative spondylarthropathies. Relation to gut inflammation. *J Rheumatol* 1990;17:335–340.

306. Helliwell PS, Hickling P, Wright V. Do the radiological changes of classic ankylosing spondylitis differ from the changes found in the spondylitis associated with inflammatory bowel disease, psoriasis and reactive arthritis? *Ann Rheum Dis* 1998;57:135–140.

307. Nissila M, Lethinen K, Leirisalo-Repo M, et al. Sulphasalazine in the treatment of ankylosing spondylitis. *Arthritis Rheum* 1988;31:1111–1116.

308. Mielants H, Veys EM, Cuvelier C, et al. Course of gut inflammation in spondylarthropathies and therapeutic consequences. In: Veys EM, Mielants H, eds. *Ballieres Clin Rheumatol* 1996;10:147–164.

309. Baron TH, Truss CD, Elson CD. Low-dose oral MTX in refractory inflammatory bowel disease. *Dig Dis Sci* 1993;38:1551–1553.

SYSTEMIC LUPUS ERYTHEMATOSUS

MICHELLE PETRI

EPIDEMIOLOGY

Systemic lupus erythematosus (SLE) is predominantly a disease of women, with a ratio of 9:1, women to men. A recent study suggested that the incidence of SLE has increased threefold since the 1970s (1). In both the United States and the United Kingdom, SLE is more common in blacks (or blacks from the Caribbean) than in whites. It is estimated that as many as 500,000 people have been diagnosed with SLE in the United States.

Five- and 10-year survival has greatly improved in SLE. Among middle-class, privately insured SLE patients, survival rates are 97% at 5 years and 93% at 10 years. However, in the most recent American epidemiologic study, the 10-year survival rate in Rochester, Minnesota, was only about 80% (1). Inner-city academic centers in the United States generally report lower but still greatly improved 10-year survival rates. The major cause of death in SLE in developed countries is cardiovascular disease. Disability is common in SLE patients, either due to the disease itself (renal failure, stroke) or to complications of therapy, especially corticosteroids (osteoporotic fractures, avascular necrosis of bone).

PATHOPHYSIOLOGY/PATHOGENESIS

The pathogenesis of SLE is multifactorial. Apoptosis, or programmed cell death, appears to be a central factor in the development of lupus autoantibodies. Most of the self-antigens that become targets of autoantibody production are exposed on nuclear blebs during apoptosis (2). In murine models, mutations in proteins that control apoptosis are sufficient to cause SLE.

There is a complex genetic predisposition to human SLE, probably involving as many as 100 individual genes. Genes already identified as important in SLE diathesis include certain HLA DR and DQ alleles associated with individual autoantibody production; null complement alleles involved in both apoptosis and immune complex clearance; and Fc gamma receptors, also involved in immune complex clearance.

Hormonal factors are pivotal in both murine and human SLE. Most women with SLE do not become symptomatic until after puberty. Several sex hormones, including both estrogen and prolactin, can activate the immune system. Both case reports and cohort studies suggest that exposure to exogenous estrogen (either oral contraceptives or hormone replacement therapy) may predispose to SLE. A multicenter U.S. study, SELENA, is exploring whether SLE patients are more likely to flare if exposed to exogenous estrogen.

Environmental triggers are important in the onset of SLE. The classic environmental trigger, ultraviolet light, is now understood to induce apoptosis in keratinocytes. Either UV-B or UV-A wavelengths can induce SLE cutaneous flares. Drugs can also precipitate SLE. Sulfonamide antibiotics, such as Bactrim or Septra, are the most-well-known examples. Some over-the-counter alternative medicines, such as Echinacea (a cold remedy), have been associated with SLE as well. Some new anti–tumor necrosis factor therapies for rheumatoid arthritis, Enbrel and Remicade, have been associated both with the production of SLE autoantibodies and with true clinical lupus (although the latter occurs rarely). In several case-control studies, smoking has been incriminated as a risk factor for SLE. Finally, some infections, such as Epstein–Barr virus, have been strongly implicated in SLE, especially in children.

In established SLE, there is profound immune dysregulation. B cells are overactive, with both a hypergammaglobulinemia and production of autoantibodies. T-cell regulation has gone awry. Despite the hyperactivity against self, the SLE immune system is less effective in fighting infections, especially certain bacterial (salmonella, pneumococcal), and viral (herpes zoster, warts) infections. Routine vaccinations, such as influenza and pneumococcal vaccines, appear to be safe. The hepatitis B vaccine has been controversial because of case reports linking it to SLE, usually in children.

CLINICAL FEATURES

Signs

SLE is the prototypic autoimmune disease, as it can affect almost any organ system, and most patients have multisystem involvement (Table 13.1). The most recognized organ systems affected are cutaneous, musculoskeletal, and renal.

Cutaneous involvement is very frequent in SLE, eventually occurring in about 90% of patients. Most SLE rashes are photosensitive. The malar, or butterfly, rash, is a classic example. Discoid lesions occur predominantly on the face, but also in the ears and on the forearms. Mouth sores (aphthous ulcers) occur frequently in crops, can occur on the palate, and are often long-lasting; nasal sores are also seen. Raynaud phenomenon is frequent, but rarely severe. Alopecia is usually mild. More serious cutaneous involvement includes cutaneous vasculitis and digital gangrene.

Musculoskeletal involvement is usually polyarthralgias or polyarthritis, although myositis can also occur. The initial presentation usually mimics rheumatoid arthritis, with symmetric involvement of the small joints of the hands and wrists. Over time, unlike rheumatoid arthritis, lupus arthritis is rarely erosive, although reducible deformities (due to tendon and ligamentous laxity) do occur.

Renal lupus occurs in 50% of whites and probably as many as 75% of blacks with SLE. The classic findings on urinalysis include proteinuria, hematuria, and red blood cell (RBC) casts. The severe form, diffuse proliferative glomerulonephritis, can rapidly lead to renal failure if not controlled.

Hematologic manifestations of lupus are frequent and occasionally life-threatening. Anemia is frequent, but anemias of chronic disease and iron-deficiency anemia are actually more common than a Coombs-positive hemolytic ane-

mia. Leukopenia is common, but rarely severe (i.e., <2,000 cells/mm³). Lymphopenia is the rule, but some patients have neutropenia. Thrombocytopenia can be sudden and life-threatening, but more often a chronic mild thrombocytopenia is found. SLE patients frequently produce antiphospholipid antibodies (lupus anticoagulant, anticardiolipin, and anti-β2 glycoprotein I) that are associated with hypercoagulability and increased risk of venous thrombosis, arterial thrombosis (especially stroke), and pregnancy loss.

Lupus can affect any level of the neurologic system. Signs of neurologic lupus can include seizures, transient ischemic attacks, encephalopathy (including coma), cranial neuropathy, transverse myelitis, sensory or motor signs of mononeuritis multiplex or peripheral neuropathy, and entrapment neuropathy (most often carpal tunnel).

Bowel dysmotility can occur in SLE, with esophageal dysmotility, usually mild, being the most common. Severe gastrointestinal involvement, including mesenteric vasculitis, colitis, and protein-losing enteropathy, can occur, but rarely.

Constitutional signs of lupus include fever, weight loss, and lymphadenopathy.

Symptoms

The most frequent symptom of SLE is fatigue. Many SLE patients with chronic fatigue also have signs (tender points) and symptoms (sleep disturbance, migraine headaches, irritable bowel syndrome, dysesthesias, pain above and below the waist) associated with fibromyalgia (3).

Many SLE patients report subtle changes in cognitive function. Some of these patients may have small ischemic lesions on brain MRI ("unidentified bright objects," or "UBOs").

TABLE 13.1. SIGNS OF SYSTEMIC LUPUS ERYTHEMATOSUS

Organ System	Sign
Cutaneous	Malar rash, discoid rash, mouth/nasal sores, Raynaud phenomenon, cutaneous vasculitis, alopecia
Musculoskeletal	Polyarthritis, especially of small joints of hands and wrists, myositis
Renal	Proteinuria, hematuria, red blood cell casts, nephrotic syndrome, elevated creatinine
Cardiopulmonary	Pericarditis, pleurisy, pleural effusions, pneumonitis, pulmonary emboli, pulmonary hypertension, myocardial infarction
Hematologic	Anemia, leukopenia, thrombocytopenia, elevated sedimentation rate, lupus anticoagulant, anticardiolipin
Neurologic	Seizure, psychosis, stroke, encephalopathy, transverse myelitis, mononeuritis multiplex, peripheral neuropathy
Gastrointestinal	Esophageal dysmotility, intestinal vasculitis, protein-losing enteropathy
Constitutional	Fever, weight loss, lymphadenopathy

CLINICAL EVALUATION

Initial Evaluation

History and Physical Examination

Most SLE patients will eventually have a multisystem disease, making the diagnosis obvious to all. Early in the development of SLE there may be only nonspecific symptoms, such as fatigue and arthralgias, leading to a delay in diagnosis. The initial evaluation of a patient suspected of having lupus should include a complete history, including the chronology and evaluation of symptoms; a medication history (including exogenous estrogen, sulfonamide antibiotics, alternative medications); family history of autoimmune diseases; social history, including smoking; and a past medical history, including any thrombotic events or pregnancy losses that might suggest antiphospholipid antibody syndrome.

The physician should perform a complete physical examination, paying particular attention to characteristic organ system signs associated with SLE (Table 13.2). The physical examination, in addition to including vital signs, must be comprehensive, with special attention to each organ system detailed in Table 13.2.

Laboratory

Laboratory tests, especially routine laboratory tests, can be very helpful in making the diagnosis of SLE (Table 13.3). A positive ANA, however, does not mean that a patient has SLE. Most people with a positive ANA are normal: 10% to 15% of normal young women have a positive ANA. A patient in pain with a positive ANA is much more likely to have fibromyalgia (which occurs in 2% to 3% of the female population) than to have lupus.

Imaging

Imaging modalities that may be helpful in individual patients include chest x-ray, cardiac echocardiogram, pulmonary function tests, joint x-rays, and brain MRI.

TABLE 13.2. INITIAL EVALUATION FOR SYSTEMIC LUPUS ERYTHEMATOSUS

History of the present illness	Age at onset of symptoms and/or signs, chronology of symptoms/signs
Medications	Especially exogenous estrogen, sulfonamide antibiotics, alternative medications
Allergies	Allergy to sulfonamide antibiotics is common in SLE
Social habits	Smoking may be a risk factor for SLE; smokers are more likely to develop discoid lupus
Past medical history	Determine not just whether there is lupus in the family, but also whether there are other connective tissue diseases (such as rheumatoid arthritis) or localized autoimmune disorders (such as thyroid disease)
Review of Systems	
General health	Ask about fevers, weight loss
Skin	Ask about skin rashes, photosensitivity, alopecia
Eyes	Ask about eye dryness (Sjögren syndrome), uveitis, scleritis, and visual loss
Ears	Ask about discoid lesions in ear
Nose	Ask about nasal sores and dry, irritated nasal mucosa (Sjögren syndrome)
Mouth	Ask about mouth ulcers and dry mouth (Sjögren syndrome)
Endocrine	Ask about lymphadenopathy, thyroid disease, and diabetes
Chest	Ask about pleurisy, pleural effusions, and dyspnea
Cardiac	Ask about pericarditis and myocardial infarction
Gastrointestinal	Ask about difficulty swallowing, symptoms of colitis, abdominal pain
Renal	Ask if there have been laboratory tests showing abnormal urine findings
Gynecologic	Ask about pregnancy losses and severe preeclampsia
Extremities	Ask about ankle edema, history of thrombophlebitis, and Raynaud phenomenon
Neurologic	Ask about numbness, stroke, severe headaches, and weakness

SLE, systemic lupus erythematosus.

TABLE 13.3. LABORATORY TESTS HELPFUL IN THE EVALUATION OF SYSTEMIC LUPUS ERYTHEMATOSUS

Complete blood count	Look for anemia (check for retic count and direct Coombs' if the patient is anemic), leukopenia, thrombocytopenia
Differential	Look for lymphopenia
ESR	ESR is not specific for SLE but is often elevated
Creatinine	If elevated, look for renal lupus
Urinalysis	Look for proteinuria, hematuria, casts
RPR or VDRL	A false-positive test for syphilis can occur in SLE
Autoantibodies	A positive anti-ds DNA or anti-Sm is very specific for lupus. Other autoantibodies, like anti-RNP, anti-Ro, and anti-La can occur in other connective tissue diseases
Antiphospholipid antibodies	Both lupus anticoagulant and anticardiolipin antibody can occur in SLE
Complement	A low C3 and/or low C4, although not specific for lupus, are commonly found

ds DNA, double-stranded DNA; ESR, erythrocyte sedimentation rate; RPR, rapid plasma reagin; SLE, systemic lupus erythematosus; VDRL, Venereal Disease Research Laboratory.

Differential Diagnosis

The American College of Rheumatology has published a set of classification criteria for SLE, with four of 11 criteria required (Table 13.4) (4,5). It is important to emphasize that these are classification criteria for research studies and are not meant for diagnosis. However, they do serve to emphasize that the diagnosis of SLE is usually based on the presence of multisystem signs and that a positive ANA is neither necessary nor sufficient to diagnose SLE.

The differential diagnosis of SLE includes other connective tissue diseases—such as rheumatoid arthritis, Sjögren syndrome, scleroderma, and myositis—and other rheumatologic diseases, such as vasculitis and sarcoidosis. Drug-induced lupus can occur with procainamide, hydralazine, isoniazid, and minocycline. Infections that can mimic SLE

TABLE 13.4. REVISED AMERICAN COLLEGE OF RHEUMATOLOGY CLASSIFICATION CRITERIA FOR SYSTEMIC LUPUS ERYTHEMATOSUS

Malar rash	Fixed erythema, flat or raised, over the malar eminences, tending to spare the nasolabial folds
Discoid rash	Erythematous raised patches with adherent keratotic scaling and follicular plugging; atrophic scarring may occur in older persons
Photosensitivity	Skin rash as a result of unusual reaction to sunlight, by patient history or physician observation
Oral ulcers	Oral or nasopharyngeal ulceration, usually painless, observed by physician
Arthritis	Nonerosive arthritis involving two or more peripheral joints, characterized by tenderness, swelling, or effusion
Serositis	Pleuritis: convincing history of pleuritic pain or rub heard by a physician or evidence of pleural effusion *Or* Pericarditis: documented by electrocardiogram or rub or evidence of pericardial effusion
Renal disorder	Persistent proteinuria greater than 0.5 g/day or greater than 3+ if quantitation not performed *Or* Cellular casts: may be red cell, hemoglobin, granular, tubular, or mixed
Neurologic disorder	Seizures or psychosis in the absence of offending drugs or known metabolic derangements
Hematologic disorder	Hemolytic anemia with reticulocytosis; leukopenia less than 4000/mm^3 total on two or more occasions; lymphopenia less than 1500/mm^3 total on two or more occasions; or thrombocytopenia less than 100,000/mm^3 in the absence of offending drugs
Immunologic disorder	Antibody to native DNA in abnormal titer or antibody to Sm nuclear antigen; or positive finding of antiphospholipid antibodies based on (a) an abnormal serum level of IgG or IgM anticardiolipin antibodies, (b) a positive test result for lupus anticoagulant, or (c) a false-positive serologic test for syphilis
Antinuclear antibody	An abnormal titer of antinuclear antibody by immunofluorescence or an equivalent assay at any point in time and in the absence of drugs known to be associated with drug-induced lupus syndrome

Ig, immunoglobulin.

include bacterial endocarditis, Lyme disease, Epstein–Barr virus, hepatitis B and C, and parvovirus. Malignancy can cause a positive ANA, arthritis, and even vasculitis. Endocrine conditions, especially hypothyroidism, can mimic SLE, but other diseases, such as amyloidosis and acromegaly, should also be considered. Noninflammatory disorders, including depression and fibromyalgia, not only coexist with lupus, but can mimic symptoms of SLE.

Recurrent Flares

SLE may have several patterns over time. A few lucky patients may have a long period of quiescence, but most patients fall into two patterns—recurrent, unexpected exacerbations, or "flares," or chronic activity.

Laboratory

For many years it was thought that serologic tests, such as a rise in anti–double stranded (ds) DNA or a fall in C3 or C4, would predict a subsequent flare of SLE. Recent studies suggest, however, that most flares are not preceded by a rise in anti-ds DNA or fall in complement and must be diagnosed either on clinical grounds or by changes in routine laboratory tests (6).

The most useful screening tools for disease activity, in addition to the interval history and the physical examination, are the complete blood count, creatinine, and urinalysis.

Differential Diagnosis

A lupus patient who is febrile may have an infection or a lupus flare. Any lupus patient with a temperature of more than 101°F should be evaluated for an infection. In general, the best rule is to "think infection until proven otherwise."

PREVENTION AND THERAPY
Prevention
Nonpharmacologic

SLE patients should avoid known precipitants of SLE flares, such as ultraviolet light, and use sunblock. Most prevention efforts, however, are aimed at preventing complications of SLE and its treatment, especially atherosclerosis. SLE patients should invest in their future by maintaining their ideal body weight, exercising, stopping smoking, and eating a low-fat, low-cholesterol diet.

Pharmacologic
Atherosclerosis
Because all SLE patients are at high risk for atherosclerosis, it is worthwhile to check for traditional risk factors, includ-

ing hypertension, hyperlipidemia, elevated glucose, and elevated homocysteine. Patients with known atherosclerosis (either by history or by screening carotid duplex) should be treated aggressively. Patients with cardiovascular risk factors must be treated appropriately. ACE inhibitors are preferred for hypertension because they also reduce nephrosclerosis. B-vitamin supplementation can reduce homocysteine (7).

Osteoporosis
Limiting corticosteroid exposure is essential in preventing progression of osteoporosis. All SLE patients, unless they have calcium renal stones, should take calcium and vitamin D (800 IU daily). Screening bone mineral density is indicated, and if osteoporosis is present, bisphosphonate therapy should be considered (but not during pregnancy).

Surgical
Avascular Necrosis of Bone (Osteonecrosis)
A dreaded complication of high-dose corticosteroid therapy is avascular necrosis (AVN) of hips, knees, shoulders, or other joints. If detected early (usually by MRI scan), before joint destruction has occurred, its progression can often be stopped by a core decompression of bone.

Therapy
Nonpharmacologic

All SLE patients should be advised to have a healthy lifestyle in terms of rest; exercise; low-fat, low-cholesterol diet; no smoking; and maintenance of ideal body weight.

Pharmacologic
Cutaneous Lupus
The first step in treating photosensitive rashes is sun avoidance and use of sunblocks that block both UV-B and UV-A (Table 13.5). Topical steroids play a limited role; fluorinated topical steroids should not be used long term on the face because of the possibility of atrophy. The most important maintenance drug is the antimalarial drug hydroxychloroquine, usually at a dose of 400 mg daily in adults. Because it takes about a month to take effect, a bridging dose of prednisone is sometimes necessary. Retinopathy is very rare, but routine ophthalmology monitoring every 6 months is recommended. A dermatologist and/or a rheumatologist should treat severe cutaneous rashes, because steroid-sparing drugs (methotrexate, mycophenolate mofetil, or cyclophosphamide) may be needed.

Musculoskeletal Lupus
Lupus arthritis is initially treated with NSAIDs at antiinflammatory doses. The new class of NSAIDs, the COX-2-specific drugs (rofecoxib and celecoxib), which have greater gastrointestinal safety, do not have an antiplatelet effect and

TABLE 13.5. THERAPY OF SYSTEMIC LUPUS ERYTHEMATOSUS

Organ	Potential Approaches
Cutaneous	Sun avoidance, sun-block (UV-A and UV-B), hydroxychloroquine, topical steroids
Musculoskeletal	NSAIDs (antiinflammatory doses), hydroxychloroquine, low-dose prednisone
Renal	For diffuse proliferative glomerulonephritis: high-dose corticosteroids and i.v. cyclophosphamide
Cardiopulmonary	For pericarditis and pleurisy: NSAIDs if mild; corticosteroids if severe
Hematologic	For severe thrombocytopenia: i.v. methylprednisolone pulse therapy initially; i.v. immunoglobulin may be needed
Neurologic	For severe CNS–SLE: i.v. methylprednisolone pulse therapy initially; i.v. cyclophosphamide may be necessary

CNS–SLE, central nervous system–systemic lupus erythematosus; i.v., intravenous; NSAIDs, nonsteroidal anti-inflammatory drugs; UV, ultraviolet.

may reduce prostacyclin. For that reason, a patient with known hypercoagulability (such as antiphospholipid antibodies) might also need to take a baby aspirin (81 mg daily).

Hydroxychloroquine (400 mg daily in most adults) is a very useful drug for both polyarthralgias and polyarthritis. Severe polyarthritis may require prednisone, but if the maintenance dose cannot be kept at 7.5 mg or less, a steroid-sparing drug such as methotrexate, 7.5 mg weekly (with daily folic acid, 1 mg) should be considered. Patients with polyarthritis should be referred to a rheumatologist.

Renal Lupus

Proteinuria (1 g/day) and/or hematuria should lead to referral to a nephrologist and rheumatologist who work together to evaluate renal lupus. A renal biopsy can identify both the WHO class and the degree of activity and chronicity, which influences treatment choices. Diffuse proliferative glomerulonephritis is usually treated with high-dose corticosteroids initially (prednisone 40 to 60 mg daily, or IV methylprednisolone pulse therapy, 1,000 mg daily for 3 days), with the addition of monthly IV cyclophosphamide, 750 mg/m^2 body surface area. Mesna is given to avoid the complication of hemorrhagic cystitis. Other side effects of cyclophosphamide include cytopenias, infections, sterility, and malignancy. Lesser degrees of renal lupus, such as mesangial or focal proliferative glomerulonephritis, are often treated with less toxic immunosuppressive drugs, such as mycophenolate mofetil or azathioprine, in addition to prednisone. Attention should be paid to controlling hypertension, especially with ACE inhibitors to retard renal scarring.

Cardiopulmonary

Acute flares of pericarditis or pleurisy, if mild, can be treated with NSAIDs. Moderate to severe flares require corticosteroids.

The rheumatologist should manage severe cardiopulmonary lupus, often with a consulting cardiologist or pulmonologist.

Hematologic Lupus

Leukopenia may be tolerated, as long as there is not profound neutropenia with infections. G-CSF can cause SLE flares and should not be used unless life-threatening infection occurs. Thrombocytopenia is usually not associated with bleeding unless the platelet count is below 35,000/mm^3. Severe, life-threatening drops in the platelet count should lead to prompt hospitalization. Initial management is with IV methylprednisolone 1,000 mg daily for 3 days (followed by high-dose oral prednisone), with the addition of intravenous immunoglobulin if there is no response. Recalcitrant life-threatening thrombocytopenia may require splenectomy, although this should not be considered a curative procedure.

Antiphospholipid Antibody Syndrome

Some evidence suggests that SLE patients with antiphospholipid antibodies who take hydroxychloroquine have a reduced risk of thrombosis. Patients with antiphospholipid antibodies should avoid drugs, such as oral contraceptives, hormone replacement therapy, and raloxifene, which increase the risk of clotting.

Once a venous or arterial thrombosis has occurred, the current recommendation is high-intensity warfarin long term (8). To prevent pregnancy loss in a patient who has a history of miscarriage, prophylactic doses of heparin and a daily baby (81 mg) aspirin are recommended (9).

Pregnancy

Many studies have found an increase in lupus flares during pregnancy, likely mediated by higher estrogen and prolactin levels and a Th2 cytokine milieu. Therefore monthly visits with a rheumatologist are recommended.

SLE patients with a history of pregnancy loss need to be screened and treated for antiphospholipid antibodies. A second screening recommendation is to test for anti-Ro and anti-La, which are associated with congenital heart block. SLE pregnancies are considered high risk because of the increased frequency of preterm birth, preeclampsia, premature rupture of membranes, and intrauterine growth retardation.

Neurologic Lupus

Neurologic events in SLE patients require hospitalization and the consultation of rheumatology and neurology because of the wide differential diagnosis. A stroke, for example, could be due to CNS-SLE, antiphospholipid antibody syndrome, hypertension, atherosclerosis, infection, or even malignancy.

A severe presentation of CNS-SLE, such as encephalopathy, transverse myelitis, or stroke, will need to be treated urgently with IV pulse methylprednisolone and, on occasion, IV cyclophosphamide.

Corticosteroid Sparing

Much of the long-term morbidity of SLE is directly or indirectly due to reliance on corticosteroid therapy. Corticosteroid-related morbidity includes musculoskeletal damage (osteoporosis and avascular necrosis of bone), diabetes mellitus, hypertension, hyperlipidemia, and obesity (10). The role of the physician in the care of an SLE patient is not just to recognize and control manifestations of SLE, but also to judiciously introduce steroid-sparing approaches early in the disease course.

PATIENT EDUCATION AND SUPPORT

The Arthritis Foundation and Lupus Foundation of America are excellent sources of up-to-date educational materials for patients. Both organizations offer patient support groups, as well.

REFERENCES

1. Uramoto KM, Michet CJJ, Thumboo J, et al. Trends in the incidence and mortality of systemic lupus erythematosus, 1950–1992. *Arthritis Rheum* 1999;42:46–50.
2. Casciola-Rosen L, Rosen A, Petri M, et al. Surface blebs on apoptotic cells are sites of enhanced procoagulant activity: implications for coagulation events and antigenic spread in SLE. *Proc Natl Acad Sci USA* 1996;96:1624–1629.
3. Middleton GD, McFarlin JE, Lipsky PE. The prevalence and clinical impact of fibromyalgia in systemic lupus erythematosus. *Arthritis Rheum* 1994;37:1181–1188.
4. Tan EM, Cohen AS, Fries JF, et al. The 1982 revised criteria for the classification of systemic lupus erythematosus. *Arthritis Rheum* 1982;25:1271–1277.
5. Hochberg MC. Updating the American College of Rheumatology revised criteria for the classification of systemic lupus erythematosus [letter]. *Arthritis Rheum* 1997;40:1725.
6. Ho A, Magder L, Barr S, et al. Decreases in anti-double-stranded DNA levels are associated with concurrent flares in patients with systemic lupus erythematosus. *Arthritis Rheum* 2001;44: 2342–2349.
7. Petri M, Vu D, Omura A, et al. Effectiveness of B-vitamin therapy in reducing plasma total homocysteine in patients with systemic lupus [abstract]. *Arthritis Rheum* 1998;41(Suppl):S241.
8. Khamashta MA, Cuadrado MJ, Mujic F, et al. The management of thrombosis in the antiphospholipid antibody syndrome. *N Engl J Med* 1995;332:993–997.
9. Cowchock FS, Reece EA, Balaban D, et al. Repeated fetal losses associated with antiphospholipid antibodies: a collaborative randomized trial comparing prednisone with low-dose heparin treatment. *Am J Obstet Gynecol* 1992;166:1318–1323.
10. Zonana-Nacach A, Barr SG, Magder LS, et al. Damage in systemic lupus erythematosus and its association with corticosteroids. *Arthritis Rheum* 2000;43:1801–1808.

SYSTEMIC SCLEROSIS
AND RAYNAUD SYNDROME

THOMAS A. MEDSGER, JR.

Systemic sclerosis (SSc) is a chronic disorder of connective tissue characterized by inflammation, fibrosis, and degenerative changes in the blood vessels, skin, synovium, skeletal muscle, and certain internal organs, notably the gastrointestinal tract, lung, heart, and kidney. Although there is an early, often clinically unappreciated, inflammatory component, the hallmark of the disease is thickening of the skin (scleroderma) and other organs caused by excessive accumulation of connective tissue.

EPIDEMIOLOGY

SSc is divided into two major clinical variants, diffuse cutaneous (dc) and limited cutaneous (lc) disease, which are distinguished from one another primarily on the basis of the degree and extent of skin involvement. The term *overlap syndrome* is used when features commonly encountered in other connective-tissue diseases are also present. CREST syndrome (an acronym referring to the findings of *c*alcinosis, *R*aynaud phenomenon, *e*sophageal hypomotility, *s*clerodactyly, and *t*elangiectasias) is closely analogous to lcSSc (Table 14.1).

TABLE 14.1. CLASSIFICATION OF SYSTEMIC SCLEROSIS

A. *With diffuse cutaneous involvement:* symmetric widespread skin fibrosis affecting the distal and proximal extremities and often the trunk and face; tendency to rapid progression of skin changes and early apperance of internal organ involvement
B. *With limited cutaneous involvement:* symmetric restricted skin fibrosis affecting the distal extremities (often confined to the fingers) and face; prolonged delay in appearance of distinctive internal manifestations (e.g., pulmonary arterial hypertension); prominence of calcinosis and telangiectasias
C. *With "overlap":* having either diffuse or limited skin involvement and typical features of one or more of the other connective-tissue diseases

From Medsger TA Jr. Systemic sclerosis (scleroderma): clinical aspects. In: Koopman WJ, ed. *Arthritis and allied conditions: a textbook of rheumatology,* 14th ed. Philadelphia: Lippincott Williams & Wilkins, 2001:1590–1624, with permission.

SSc has been described in all races and is global in distribution. A U.S. community study detected nearly 20 new hospital-diagnosed cases per million population at risk annually (1). Overall, women are affected three times as often as men, and the female-to-male ratio is increased during the child-bearing years. No significant overall racial differences have been found. Systemic sclerosis usually begins in persons between 30 and 50 years of age. Onset during childhood and after age 80 has been reported but is uncommon. In black women, onset of disease occurs at a younger age, diffuse disease is more common, and survival is poor (2). Prevalence estimates for SSc have been in the range of 200 per million of population (3). Several environmental factors have been implicated as predisposing to or precipitating SSc, including occupational silica and organic solvent exposure (4).

An increased prevalence of familial SSc has been detected in three U.S. cohorts (5). Relatives of patients with SSc are often affected by other connective-tissue diseases, suggesting a heritable predisposition to this family of disorders. In multicase families, affected siblings shared HLA haplotypes, but the development of disease could not be entirely accounted for by HLA genes, suggesting that MHC complex genes are important, but not sufficient, for disease expression (6).

PATHOPHYSIOLOGY

The etiology of SSc is unknown. However, most investigators believe that the key players are endothelial cells, activated immune cells, and fibroblasts (Fig. 14.1). One frequently cited hypothesis suggests that the process is initiated by an immune attack on the endothelium, resulting in endothelial cell activation and/or injury. Subsequently, adjacent tissue fibroblasts are activated, resulting in subendothelial connective-tissue proliferation that leads to narrowing of the vascular lumen and Raynaud phenomenon. T cells are then selectively activated and populate affected areas such as the dermis (Fig. 14.2) and lung. These cells produce cytokines that stimulate resident fibroblasts to produce an excessive amount of procollagen, which is then converted extracellularly to mature colla-

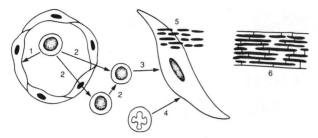

FIGURE 14.1. A simplified schematic of the pathophysiology of systemic sclerosis. Abnormalities include (*1*) endothelial cell damage/activation; (*2*) immune cell activation; (*3* and *4*) stimulation of fibroblasts by products of immune cells and mast cells; (*5*) overproduction of procollagen; and (*6*) excessive tissue deposition of mature collagen. (From Medsger TA Jr. Systemic sclerosis (scleroderma): clinical aspects. In: Koopman WJ, ed. *Arthritis and allied conditions: a textbook of rheumatology,* 14th ed. Philadelphia: Lippincott Williams & Wilkins, 2001:1590–1624, with permission.)

gen. Later in disease, especially dcSSc, the inflammatory process subsides and fibroblasts revert to a normal phenotype.

CLINICAL FEATURES

The important clinical manifestations of SSc are described in considerable detail in recent publications (7,8) and are summarized here.

Initial Symptoms

In most cases of lcSSc, the initial complaint is Raynaud phenomenon. In contrast, patients with dcSSc most often have generalized swelling of the hands, skin thickening, or arthritis as the first manifestation.

Distinguishing Diffuse from Limited Cutaneous Disease

Many demographic, clinical, and laboratory features help distinguish dc from lc disease (Table 14.2). Diffuse scleroderma is associated with palpable tendon friction rubs, arthritis with joint contractures, myopathy, serum antitopoisomerase I (anti-Scl 70) or anti-RNA polymerase antibodies, and earlier, more frequent occurrence of visceral disease affecting the heart and kidney. In contrast, lcSSc is characterized by calcinosis, telangiectasia, serum anticentromere antibodies, and occasional late development of pulmonary fibrosis, pulmonary arterial hypertension, or small bowel malabsorption. Overlap patients have convincing evidence of another connective-tissue disease, such as polymyositis (myositis, dermatomyositis rash) or systemic lupus erythematosus (leukopenia, glomerulonephritis, pleuropericarditis, typical rash). A common mistake is to prematurely classify a patient with new sclerodactyly alone as having limited cutaneous involvement. Close observation

over the next 3 to 6 months is necessary, since many such patients have rapid proximal evolution and obvious diffuse skin thickening during that interval.

Serum antinuclear antibody is found in more than 95% of SSc patients. The proportion of patients having one of seven SSc-associated autoantibodies is more than 85% (Fig. 14.3). Those with lcSSc most frequently have anticentromere or anti-Th antibody. Individuals with dcSSc have antitopoisomerase I or anti-RNA polymerase III antibody. Patients with SSc in overlap most often have anti-U1RNP, anti-PM-Scl, or anti-U3RNP antibodies.

Organ System Involvement

Skin

Initially, patients complain about tight, puffy fingers, especially on arising in the morning (*edematous phase*). Pitting or nonpitting edema of the fingers ("sausaging") and hands may occur. Edema may last indefinitely (e.g., fingers in lcSSc) or may be replaced gradually by thickening and tightening of the skin (*indurative phase*) during subsequent months. After several years, the dermis tends to soften somewhat and in some cases reverts to normal thickness or actually becomes thinner than normal (*atrophic phase*). At that time, the most striking finding is digital and facial telangiectasias, which consist of widely dilated capillary loops and distended venules.

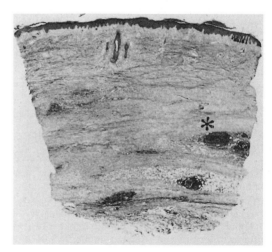

FIGURE 14.2. Photomicrograph of a skin punch biopsy from the dorsum of the forearm of a 53-year-old woman with diffuse cutaneous systemic sclerosis. Skin appendages are atrophic, the dermis is thickened with deposition of dense collagenous connective tissue, and there are prominent collections of small round cells (*asterisk*) that were identified as T-lymphocytes. (From Medsger TA Jr. Systemic sclerosis (scleroderma): clinical aspects. In: Koopman WJ, ed. *Arthritis and allied conditions: a textbook of rheumatology,* 14th ed. Philadelphia: Lippincott Williams & Wilkins, 2001:1590–1624, with permission.)

TABLE 14.2. COMPARISON OF CLINICAL AND LABORATORY FEATURES FOUND AT ANY TIME DURING THE COURSE OF SYSTEMIC SCLEROSIS (UNIVERSITY OF PITTSBURGH, 1989–1998)

	Diffuse Scleroderma (*n* = 534)	Limited Scleroderma (*n* = 543)	Overlap Syndrome (*n* = 128)
Demographic features			
Age at onset (<40)	38%	48%	63%
Race (nonwhite)	12%	6%	15%
Sex (female)	75%	86%	84%
Duration of symptoms at first visit (years)	3.8	11.3	6.9
Organ system involvement			
Skin thickening (maximum total skin score)	28.0	5.4	8.0
Telangiectasias	53%	70%	44%
Calcinosis	12%	32%	29%
Raynaud phenomenon	93%	96%	94%
Arthralgias or arthritis	93%	47%	81%
Tendon friction rubs	52%	4%	14%
Joint contractures	86%	29%	45%
Skeletal myopathy	10%	1%	57%
Esophageal hypomotility	60%	59%	52%
Pulmonary fibrosis	28%	31%	29%
Cardiac involvement	10%	5%	18%
Scleroderma renal crisis	16%	2%	5%
Laboratory data			
Antinuclear antibody positive (1:16+)	98%	98%	95%
Anticentromere antibody positive	3%	41%	7%
Anti-Scl 70 antibody positive	29%	16%	4%
Cumulative survival after first physician diagnosis			
5 years	80%	90%	93%
10 years	68%	78%	81%

From Medsger TA Jr. Systemic sclerosis (scleroderma): clinical aspects. In: Koopman WJ, ed. *Arthritis and allied conditions: a textbook of rheumatology*, 14th ed. Philadelphia: Lippincott Williams & Wilkins, 2001:1590–1624, with permission.

In dcSSc, skin thickening is typically the dominant feature (Fig. 14.4), whereas in lcSSc telangiectasias are more prominent (Fig. 14.5). The natural history of skin involvement in the two major variants of SSc is notably different (Fig. 14.6). In lcSSc, skin thickening is either absent or remains minimal over many years and bears no relation to visceral sequelae. In contrast, in dcSSc, early, rapid increase in skin thickness is the rule, reaching a peak after 1 to 2 years. Later in dcSSc, skin thickening typically improves.

In dcSSc, the skin overlying bony prominences, and especially over the proximal interphalangeal joints and elbows, becomes tightly stretched and is extremely vulnerable to trauma. These patients are often plagued by painful ulcerations at such sites and, less commonly, over the bony prominences about the shoulders and ankles.

Patients with lcSSc or late-stage dcSSc disease commonly develop intracutaneous and/or subcutaneous calcifications composed of hydroxyapatite. These palpable, yellow, rock-hard deposits occur chiefly in the digital pads and periarticular tissues, along the extensor surfaces of the forearms, in the olecranon bursae, prepatellar areas, and buttocks.

Peripheral Vascular System

Raynaud phenomenon occurs at some time during SSc in more than 95% of patients. Small areas of fingertip ischemic necrosis are frequent, often leaving pitted scars or ulcerations, but rarely gangrene. On microscopic examination, the capillary circulation is altered by the appearance of tortuous and dilated or "giant" loops, and in dcSSc, by a paucity of nailfold vessels or "dropout" (Fig. 14.7). Raynaud phenomenon is further discussed at the end of this chapter.

Joints and Tendons

Symmetric polyarthralgias and joint stiffness with or without gross synovitis of the fingers, wrists, knees, and ankles are frequent initial or early complaints in dcSSc. Some dcSSc patients have palpable tendon friction rubs (due to fibrinous tenosynovitis) over joint areas during motion. These rubs often antedate a rapid increase in skin thickness and are associated with active systemic disease, renal involvement, and reduced survival. Joint contractures, espe-

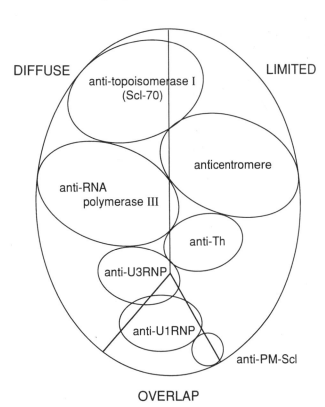

FIGURE 14.3. Classification of systemic sclerosis by clinical subsets and autoantibody types. (From Medsger TA Jr. Systemic sclerosis (scleroderma): clinical aspects. In: Koopman WJ, ed. *Arthritis and allied conditions: a textbook of rheumatology,* 14th ed. Philadelphia: Lippincott Williams & Wilkins, 2001:1590–1624, with permission.)

cially involving the hands, occur early in dcSSc and may be severe and disabling (Fig. 14.8).

Skeletal Muscle

Nonprogressive weakness and atrophy of skeletal muscle without inflammation result from disuse secondary to joint contractures or chronic disease in approximately 20% of patients. A minority of patients exhibit more pronounced proximal muscle weakness and both laboratory and clinical evidence typical of polymyositis.

Gastrointestinal Tract

Esophagus and Stomach

Esophageal dysfunction is the most common visceral manifestation of SSc and eventually develops in nearly 80% of patients. Lack of coordination of the normal propulsive peristalsis of the distal esophageal smooth muscle results in dysphagia when solids (meat, bread) become transiently "stuck" in the middle or lower esophagus (retrosternal location). Incomplete closure of the lower esophageal sphincter leads to gastroesophageal reflux with peptic esophagitis

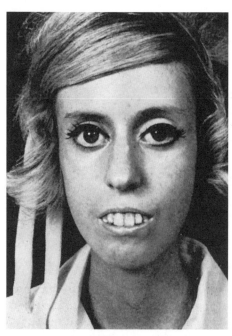

FIGURE 14.4. Face of a 19-year-old woman with diffuse cutaneous systemic sclerosis. Note loss of normal skin folds and retraction of lips. (From Medsger TA Jr. Systemic sclerosis (scleroderma): clinical aspects. In: Koopman WJ, ed. *Arthritis and allied conditions: a textbook of rheumatology,* 14th ed. Philadelphia: Lippincott Williams & Wilkins, 2001:1590–1624, with permission.)

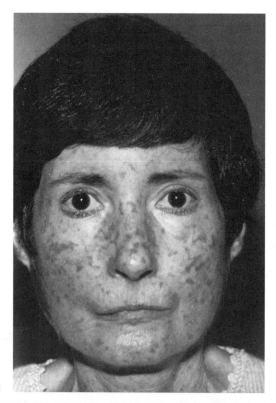

FIGURE 14.5. Face of a 45-year-old woman with limited cutaneous systemic sclerosis who had no skin thickening but had multiple telangiectasias. (From Medsger TA Jr. Systemic sclerosis (scleroderma): clinical aspects. In: Koopman WJ, ed. *Arthritis and allied conditions: a textbook of rheumatology,* 14th ed. Philadelphia: Lippincott Williams & Wilkins, 2001:1590–1624, with permission.)

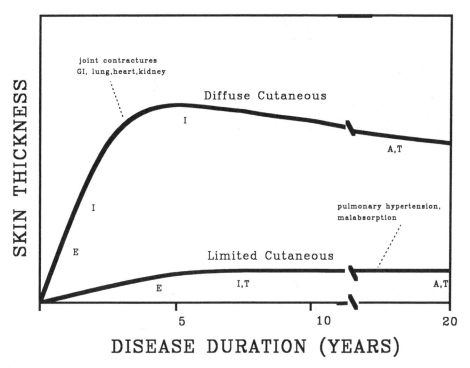

FIGURE 14.6. Natural history of skin thickness and timing of some serious complications during the course of systemic sclerosis with the two major disease variants. *E*, edema; *I*, induration; *A*, atrophy; *T*, telangiectasia. (From Medsger TA Jr. Systemic sclerosis (scleroderma): clinical aspects. In: Koopman WJ, ed. *Arthritis and allied conditions: a textbook of rheumatology,* 14th ed. Philadelphia: Lippincott Williams & Wilkins, 2001:1590–1624, with permission.)

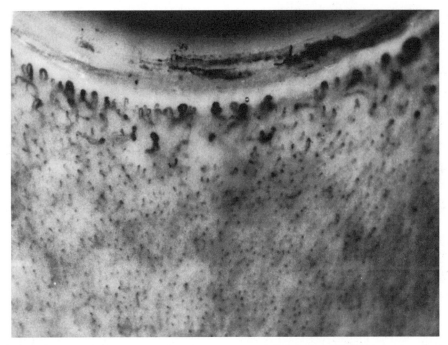

FIGURE 14.7. Nailfold capillary pattern of a patient with diffuse cutaneous systemic sclerosis (original magnification, ×18). Note extensive avascular area along the edge of the nailfold and grossly enlarged capillary loops. (From Maricq HR, LeRoy EC. Capillary blood flow in scleroderma. *Bibl Anat* 1973;11:352–358, with permission.)

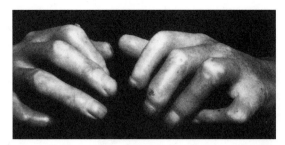

FIGURE 14.8. Proximal interphalangeal joint contractures in a patient with systemic sclerosis and diffuse scleroderma. (Reprinted from the *Clinical slide collection on the rheumatic diseases,* copyright 1991, 1995, 1997. Used by permission of the American College of Rheumatology.)

symptoms (heartburn). Distal esophageal stricture is likely to develop. Radiographic evidence of distal esophageal hypomotility with or without reflux has been found in three-fourths of SSc patients studied, including some who have no esophageal symptoms. Involvement of the stomach is uncommon, but heavy bleeding may result from an unusual condition termed *watermelon stomach,* which is the result of gastric antral vascular ectasia.

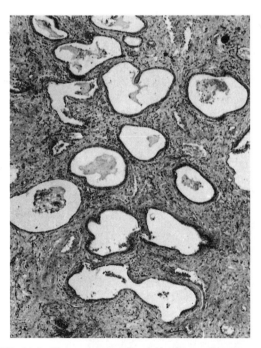

FIGURE 14.9. Photomicrograph of the lung of a 52-year-old woman with diffuse cutaneous systemic sclerosis who died as the result of respiratory insufficiency. Note the dramatic interstitial fibrosis and dilatation of air sacs (honeycomb lung). (From Medsger TA Jr. Systemic sclerosis (scleroderma): clinical aspects. In: Koopman WJ, ed. *Arthritis and allied conditions: a textbook of rheumatology,* 14th ed. Philadelphia: Lippincott Williams & Wilkins, 2001:1590–1624, with permission.)

Small Intestine

In a small proportion of patients, the illness is dominated by severe postprandial abdominal bloating and crampy abdominal pain. These symptoms are due to hypomotility and dilatation of the small intestine, and may result in a functional ileus (pseudoobstruction) with symptoms simulating mechanical obstruction. Profuse watery diarrhea, weight loss, and extreme wasting due to bacterial overgrowth and fat malabsorption can ensue despite adequate caloric intake, resulting in severe malnutrition. Radiographic findings of dilatation and hypomotility of the small intestine are uniformly present in such cases.

Colon and Rectum

Constipation, either alone or alternating with diarrhea, and rectal incontinence and prolapse may signal colonic and/or rectal involvement. Reduced anorectal capacity, motility, compliance, and sphincter pressure have been reported.

Lung

Pulmonary involvement occurs in more than 70% of patients and during the past 15 years has emerged as the most common SSc-related cause of death.

Interstitial Fibrosis

In more than one-third of patients with both dc and lcSSc, the chest radiograph shows interstitial thickening in a reticular pattern of linear, nodular, and lineonodular densities most pronounced in the lower lung fields. Dry bibasilar end-inspiratory "fibrotic" rales are frequently heard in these persons. A restrictive ventilatory defect, indicated by a reduction in forced vital capacity and decreased diffusing capacity, is most common. High-resolution computerized tomography (HRCT) is a more sensitive method for detecting interstitial lung disease and may identify a "ground-glass" appearance of inflammation (alveolitis) and/or "honeycombing" (fibrosis) (Fig. 14.9). Alveolitis also can be documented by either open-lung biopsy or bronchoalveolar lavage (BAL). Some patients with interstitial involvement develop slowly progressive respiratory failure over the course of 2 to 10 years, especially those with anti-topoisomerase I antibody. Secondary pulmonary hypertension often occurs in advanced cases.

"Intrinsic" Pulmonary Arterial Hypertension

This complication, without significant interstitial fibrosis, occurs predominantly in patients with lcSSc after 10 to 30 years. The rate of progression of dyspnea is alarmingly rapid, typically over 6 to 12 months. The pulmonic component of the second heart sound is accentuated, and ultimately, right-sided cardiac failure develops. The diffusing capacity is extremely low, consistent with impaired gas exchange across thickened small pulmonary blood vessels. Diagnosis is confirmed by echocardiogram or by right heart catheterization. The prognosis is poor.

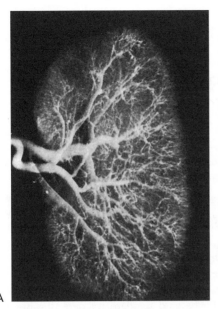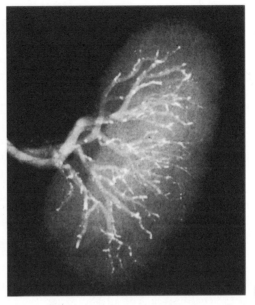

FIGURE 14.10. Roentgenograms of the kidneys, injected post mortem, of two patients with diffuse cutaneous systemic sclerosis. **A:** Kidney of a man who died of cardiac disease without clinical evidence of renal involvement. Filling of the interlobular and small cortical vessels is normal. **B:** Kidney of a man who developed "scleroderma renal crisis" with malignant hypertension and renal failure. There is irregular narrowing of the interlobular vessels and little filling of smaller vessels supplying the renal cortex. (From Medsger TA Jr. Systemic sclerosis (scleroderma): clinical aspects. In: Koopman WJ, ed. *Arthritis and allied conditions: a textbook of rheumatology,* 14th ed. Philadelphia: Lippincott Williams & Wilkins, 2001:1590–1624, with permission.)

Heart

Cardiac involvement may be classified as primary or secondary. Primary disease consists of pericarditis with or without effusion, left ventricular or biventricular congestive failure, or a serious supraventricular or ventricular arrhythmia. Acute symptomatic pericarditis is unusual, and cardiac tamponade is rare. Left-sided congestive failure secondary to myocardial fibrosis occurs in fewer than 5% of dcSSc patients. Myocarditis is rare and is associated with polymyositis. Cardiac arrhythmias include complete heart block and other electrocardiographic abnormalities.

Kidney

Clinically evident renal involvement is restricted almost exclusively to persons with dcSSc, especially those with rapidly progressive skin thickening of less than 5 years' duration. Twenty percent of patients with dcSSc develop a dramatic complication termed *scleroderma renal crisis,* with the abrupt onset of accelerated hypertension, followed promptly by oliguric renal failure. The presenting symptoms are varied and include headache and visual blurring from hypertensive retinopathy, seizures, and acute dyspnea due to sudden left ventricular failure. Within several days or weeks, microscopic hematuria and low-grade proteinuria are noted, along with rapidly increasing serum creatinine,

and finally, oliguria or anuria. Microangiopathic hemolytic anemia with thrombocytopenia is a frequent concomitant. A bland vasculopathy with subintimal hyperplasia and fibrinoid necrosis affecting the interlobular and small cortical arterioles is found (Fig. 14.10).

Sjögren Syndrome

Dry eyes and dry mouth are frequent complaints. Only a few affected persons have serum anti-SSA/Ro and/or anti-SSB/La antibodies. As in primary Sjögren syndrome, vasculitis involving the skin (palpable purpura and leg ulcers) and peripheral nervous system (sensory neuropathy and mononeuritis multiplex) may occur.

Thyroid Gland

Hypothyroidism, often clinically unrecognized, occurs in one-fourth of patients with SSc.

DISEASE COURSE

The natural history of SSc is extremely variable (Fig. 14.6). In addition to a poor prognosis if visceral involvement occurs, many patients with dcSSc experience steadily increasing sclerosis of the fingers and hands, as well as tenosynovitis and arthritis, leading to deforming joint contractures. Rapid progression of skin thickness is associated with the development of internal organ problems, including involvement of the gastrointestinal tract, lung, heart, and kidney. Thus, although extensive skin thickening per se does not influence prognosis, the associated visceral disease is clearly life-threatening. After maximal skin thickening has developed in dcSSc, slow but definite regression of cutaneous sclerosis ensues and in some cases is remarkable (9). The classic pattern of improvement is that the most recently affected areas (usually the anterior chest and abdomen) are the first to improve. Late cutaneous (and visceral) flares in dcSSc do occur and resemble the initial skin manifestations, but they are unusual (<10% of patients) (10).

Patients with lcSSc have a relatively favorable prognosis. Their life span is significantly longer than that of patients with dcSSc, in part because they rarely, if ever, develop myocardial or renal disease. For all SSc patients combined, most authors agree that male sex, older age, and involvement of the kidney, heart, and lung adversely affect outcome. The cumulative survival rates in our patients first evaluated during 1989–1998 are 86% at 5 years and 74% at 10 years after first physician diagnosis (from Table 14.2).

CLINICAL EVALUATION

If active SSc is suspected, regardless of when in the course of disease, certain clinical and laboratory evaluations are useful (Table 14.3). The important point to remember is that careful history and physical examination provide the most information.

Cutaneous involvement is best assessed by physical examination. A validated, reliable scoring system (modified Rodnan skin scoring method) has been developed that is of great assistance in assessing the degree and extent of skin thickening and in following cutaneous changes over time (especially important in dcSSc) (11). Skin biopsy is not as useful as the physical examination for the diagnosis of SSc.

The gold standard for detecting distal esophageal hypomotility is the cine esophagram, performed in the sitting and supine position. Esophagogastroduodenoscopy is less reliable in assessing esophageal muscular contraction but is superior for identifying erosive esophagitis. Small intestinal SSc

---

TABLE 14.3. USEFUL CLINICAL FINDINGS AND LABORATORY STUDIES TO PERFORM IN EVALUATION OF SYSTEMIC SCLEROSIS PATIENTS

Organ System	History	Physical Examination	Laboratory Studies
General	Fatigue	Weight	Hematocrit, ESR
Skin	Pruritis	Increasing skin thickness	
Peripheral vascular	Raynaud phenomenon	Digital tip pitting scars, ulcers, gangrene	
Joints/tendons	Duration of morning stiffness, carpal tunnel symptoms	Arthritis/tenosynovitis, palpable tendon friction rubs, Tinel sign, reduced finger-to-palm distance	Radiographs (joint erosions, paraarticular bone loss)
Muscle	Proximal weakness	Proximal muscle weakness	CK, EMG, muscle biopsy
GI tract	Distal dysphagia, heartburn, postprandial distention, watery diarrhea, rectal incontinence, weight loss	Abdominal distention, hypertympany, lax rectal sphincter	Cine esophagram, esophageal manometry, small bowel series, hydrogren breath test, total fecal fat excretion
Lung	Dyspnea, pleurisy	Bibasilar rales, pleural friction rub, increased P_2	Chest radiograph, PFTs (including DLCO), HRCT of lung, BAL, right heart catherization, echocardiogram
Heart	Dyspnea, orthopnea, PND, palpitations, syncope, pericardial pain	Pericardial rub, S3 gallop	Chest radiograph, ECG, echocardiogram with estimation of LVEF; thallium perfusion test; left heart catheterization
Kidney	Dyspnea, severe headache, visual blurring	Severe hypertension, hypertensive retinopathy	Urinalysis, serum creatinine; 24-hour urine for creatinine clearance and protein; hematocrit and reticulocyte count; platelet count

BAL, bronchoalveolar lavage; CK, creatine kinase; DLCO, diffusing capacity for carbon monoxide; ECG, electrocardiogram; EMG, electromyogram; ESR, erythrocyte sedimentation rate; GI, gastrointestinal; HRCT, high-resolution computerized tomography; LVEF, left ventricular ejection fraction; PFTs, pulmonary function tests; PND, paroxysmal nocturnal dyspnea.

involvement should not be considered unless the small bowel series shows characteristic hypomotility and dilatation.

Although many SSc patients have mild hypertension and increased serum creatinine and/or proteinuria, scleroderma renal crisis is a distinct and dramatic complication that occurs very rapidly (over the course of several weeks) and should be considered one of the true rheumatic disease emergencies.

TREATMENT

Considering the proposed pathophysiology, a number of potential sites of intervention can be considered (Fig. 14.1).

Pharmacologic

In the past, no drug or combination of drugs has proved of value in adequately controlled prospective trials. Because of their potential toxicity, including possibly precipitating acute renal failure (12), corticosteroids are typically restricted to patients with inflammatory myopathy or symptomatic serositis inadequately controlled with nonsteroidal antiinflammatory drugs (NSAIDs). D-Penicillamine, which has both immunomodulating and antifibrotic potential, was shown in two retrospective U.S. studies of early diffuse disease to result in striking improvement in skin thickening, reduced frequency of subsequent renal involvement, and increased survival (13,14). However, this therapy remains controversial (15). Immunosuppressive measures seem justified in patients with early, rapidly progressive, life-threatening, and/or disabling diffuse disease, but to date, there is no general agreement about their effectiveness. Agents designed to protect injured endothelial cells and to prevent platelet aggregation and subsequent release of platelet-derived growth factors, such as dipyridamole and aspirin, have not altered disease progression.

Supporting Measures

Proper treatment of individual organ system complications of SSc may prolong survival and enhance quality of life (Table 14.4).

Raynaud Phenomenon

Commonsense self-management includes avoiding undue cold exposure, dressing warmly, and abstaining from tobacco use. Vasodilating drugs, such as the calcium channel blocker nifedipine and the angiotensin converting enzyme receptor blocking agent losartan, have proved useful. Digital sympathectomy and microvascular reconstruction for affected larger vessels in selected patients can be successful.

Calcinosis

Reliable medical treatment to eradicate or prevent calcinosis is not available. Surgical excision of large calcinotic masses may be helpful.

Joints and Muscles

Articular complaints may be treated with NSAIDs, with careful attention to their potential to aggravate gastroesophageal reflux and to reduce renal blood flow. A vigorous twice-daily range-of-motion exercise program can maintain or improve joint range of motion.

Surgical fusion of severely flexed proximal interphalangeal joints may reduce skin breakdown and infection. Active polymyositis with proximal muscle weakness should be

---

TABLE 14.4. SUPPORTING MEASURES USEFUL IN SYSTEMIC SCLEROSIS

Problem	Management
Raynaud phenomenon	Commonsense measures, vasodilators
Digital ischemia	Digital sympathectomy, microvascular reconstruction
Calcinosis	Surgical excision
Arthralgias/arthritis	NSAIDs, range of motion exercise program
PIP joint contractures	Surgical fusion
Polymyositis	Low-dose corticosteroids ± immunosuppressive drug
Distal dysphagia	Prokinetic drug
Esophageal reflux	Commonsense measures, H_2 blockers, proton pump inhibitors
Esophageal stricture	Dilatation
"Watermelon stomach"	Laser coagulation
Malabsorption/bacterial overgrowth	Prokinetic drugs, rotating antibiotics, hyperalimentation
Alveolitis	Cyclophosphamide, oxygen, transplantation
Pulmonary hypertension	Vasodilators (prostacyclin analogs), transplantation
"Renal crisis"	ACE inhibitors, dialysis, transplantation

ACE, angiotensin converting enzyme; NSAIDs, nonsteroidal anti-inflammatory drugs; PIP, proximal interphalangeal.

treated with moderate doses of corticosteroids (prednisone 15 to 20 mg/day) alone or combined with another immunosuppressive agent such as methotrexate or azathioprine.

Gastrointestinal Tract

Metoclopramide and erythromycin act as prokinetic drugs. Nifedipine is capable of relaxing intestinal smooth muscle tone and thus may aggravate esophageal symptoms. Reflux esophagitis can be minimized by appropriate commonsense measures and the use of H_2 blocking drugs or proton pump inhibitors (e.g., omeprazole). Esophageal stricture requires periodic endoscopic dilatation. Bleeding telangiectasias and the ectatic superficial vessels of "watermelon stomach" can be treated with sclerotherapy and laser coagulation, respectively. Transient improvement in steatorrhea and other signs of intestinal malabsorption may follow rotating, 2-week courses of broad-spectrum antibiotics. In advanced circumstances, one must resort to parenteral hyperalimentation, but the mortality from infection is high in such patients. Rectal sphincter surgery is difficult because of the lax tissues involved, and results are frequently unsatisfactory.

Lung

If pulmonary involvement is present, prophylactic influenza and *Pneumococcus pneumoniae* vaccinations should be given. In persons with alveolitis, corticosteroids with immunosuppressive drugs (particularly cyclophosphamide) may be efficacious. When there is resting or exercise-precipitated hypoxia, supplemental oxygen should be administered. In "intrinsic" pulmonary arterial hypertension, both intermittent and continuous intravenous prostacyclin analogs have resulted in improvement and the endothelin–1 antagonist bosentan has been approved for use. Anticoagulation is often prescribed. Heart–lung or single lung transplantation is an option for either type of end-stage lung disease.

Heart

Symptomatic pericarditis should be treated with NSAIDs or corticosteroids. If myocarditis is identified clinically or by endomyocardial biopsy, high-dose glucocorticoid therapy should be tried. The typical progressive left ventricular failure caused by myocardial fibrosis is unaffected by any therapy and is uniformly fatal, unless some correctable non-sclerodermatous problem is also present. Digitalis toxicity is frequent, and diuretics are the mainstay of therapy. Serious arrhythmias are treated in a standard fashion.

Kidney

The most important aspect of therapy for renal crisis is prompt detection. Patients with early dcSSc are advised to have their blood pressure taken every 2 weeks and to report a rise of systolic pressure of 30 mmHg or greater. The angiotensin-converting enzyme (ACE) inhibitors are the drugs of choice (16), but early aggressive therapy with other potent antihypertensive agents can be successful. Some patients require dialysis, but most maintained on ACE inhibitors can discontinue dialysis after 3 to 24 months. Numerous successful renal transplants have now been reported.

RAYNAUD SYNDROME

Raynaud phenomenon is defined as paroxysmal vasospasm in response to cold exposure or emotional stress, leading to pallor and cyanosis of the digits, which also become cold, numb, and painful. Typical episodes last from 5 to 20 minutes. During rewarming, reactive hyperemia is common. The toes are often affected. Less frequently involved sites include the tip of the nose, earlobes, and tongue. Raynaud phenomenon is relatively common, occurring in up to 20% of female and 13% of male adults in the general population (17).

Many patients with bilateral Raynaud phenomenon but no obvious symptoms or signs of underlying connective tissue disease are referred to internists or rheumatologists for evaluation. Some of these individuals will develop a connective tissue disorder within the first several years of the onset of Raynaud phenomenon (18). After 2 years, few patients (less than 5%) do so, and they almost all ultimately have lcSSc (19). The two most important clinical clues predicting the later appearance of a connective-tissue disorder in patients with Raynaud phenomenon only are nailfold capillary microscopic abnormalities (20) (Fig. 14.6) and a positive antinuclear antibody test (21,22).

A variety of other causes of Raynaud phenomenon should be considered. They fall into several categories, as noted in Table 14.5. Blood elements that may reduce blood flow velocity in otherwise normal vessels include paraproteins and cryoglobulins, cold agglutinins, and an excess of

TABLE 14.5. CONDITIONS ASSOCIATED WITH RAYNAUD SYNDROME

(I) *Connective-tissue diseases:* SSc, SLE, PM/DM, mixed connective-tissue disease, Sjögren syndrome
(II) *Hyperviscosity:* polycythemia, cryoglobulinemia, paraproteinemia, cold agglutinins
(III) *Drugs:* β-blockers, ergotamine, methysergide, bleomycin, cisplatin, nicotine, estrogen/progesterone, pseudoephedrine
(IV) *Environmental agents:* vibrating tools, polyvinyl chloride, heavy metals (arsenic, lead)
(V) *Large blood vessel disease:* atherosclerosis, Buerger disease, vasculitis, costoclavicular compression syndrome (cervical rib)
(VI) *Others:* hypothyroidism

PM/DM, polymyositis/dermatomyositis; SLE, systemic lupus erythematosus; SSc, systemic sclerosis.

red blood cells (polycythemia). Drug-induced spasm of otherwise normal arterioles can be due to beta blockers, ergot-containing compounds, and cisplatin. Bleomycin may affect both vascular structure and function, leading to Raynaud phenomenon, scleroderma-like skin changes, and pulmonary fibrosis. Structural damage to small arteries and arterioles may result from cold (frostbite) or vibration injury (e.g., chain saw operators' "vibration white finger"). Large and medium-sized arteries are the target of thoracic outlet syndrome (extrinsic compression due to cervical rib) or intrinsic disorders leading to vascular narrowing such as Takayasu disease, giant cell arteritis, or atherosclerosis. Most frequently, the latter disorders are unilateral and/or unidigital, a helpful diagnostic point. Finally, profound hypothyroidism, with its severe cold sensitivity, may be associated with very cool, slightly dusky, puffy digits, but these changes are persistent rather than episodic. Other conditions that must be differentiated from Raynaud phenomenon include reflex sympathetic dystrophy, acrocyanosis, and erythromelalgia.

Patients with Raynaud phenomenon have a persistently reduced digital pad temperature in the basal state and subnormal capillary blood flow in the fingers in both warm and cool environments (23). Reduction in finger systolic blood pressure (24), unaltered by blockade of the sympathetic nervous system (25), has been observed.

The treatment of Raynaud phenomenon has been discussed earlier.

REFERENCES

1. Steen V, Oddis CV, Conte CG, et al. Incidence of systemic sclerosis: a twenty year study of hospital diagnosed cases in Allegheny County, PA, 1963–1982. *Arthritis Rheum* 1997;40:441–445.
2. Laing TJ, Gillespie BW, Toth MB, et al. Racial differences in scleroderma among women in Michigan. *Arthritis Rheum* 1997;40:734–742.
3. Lawrence RV, Helmick CG, Arnett FC, et al. Estimates of the prevalence of arthritis and selected musculoskeletal disorders in the United States. *Arthritis Rheum* 1998;41:778–799.
4. Silman H, Hochberg MC. Occupational and environmental influences on scleroderma. *Rheum Dis Clin North Am* 1996;22:737–749.
5. Aguilar MB, Cho M, Reveille JD, et al. Prevalences of familial systemic sclerosis and other autoimmune diseases in three U.S. Cohorts. *Arthritis Rheum* 1999;42:S186.
6. Mandios N, Dunckley H, Chivers T, et al. Immunogenetic analysis of 5 families with multicase occurrence of scleroderma and/or related variants. *J Rheumatol* 1995;22:85–92.
7. Medsger TA Jr. Systemic sclerosis (scleroderma): clinical aspects. In: Koopman WJ, ed. *Arthritis and allied conditions: a textbook of rheumatology,* 14th ed. Philadelphia: Lippincott Williams & Wilkins, 2001:1590–1624.
8. Medsger TA Jr, Steen VD. Classification, prognosis. In: Clements PJ, Furst DE, eds. *Systemic sclerosis.* Baltimore: Williams & Wilkins, 1996:51–64.
9. Black C, Dieppe PK, Huskisson T, et al. Regressive systemic sclerosis. *Ann Rheum Dis* 1986;45:384–388.
10. Steen V, Medsger TA Jr. Skin flares in systemic sclerosis with diffuse scleroderma (dcSSc). *Arthritis Rheum* 2000;43:S319.
11. Clements PJ, Lachenbruch PA, Ng SW, et al. Skin score. A semiquantitative measure of cutaneous involvement that improves prediction of prognosis in systemic sclerosis. *Arthritis Rheum* 1990;33:1256–1263.
12. Steen VD, Medsger TA Jr. Case-control study of corticosteroids and other drugs that either precipitate or protect from the development of scleroderma renal crisis. *Arthritis Rheum* 1998;42:1613–1619.
13. Steen VD, Medsger TA Jr, Rodnan GP. D-penicillamine therapy in progressive systemic sclerosis (scleroderma). *Ann Intern Med* 1982;97:652–658.
14. Jimenez SA, Andrews RP, Myers AR. Treatment of rapidly progressive scleroderma (PSS) with D-penicillamine: a prospective study. In: Black CM, Myers AR, eds. *Systemic sclerosis (scleroderma): current topics in rheumatology.* New York: Gower Medical Publishing, 1985:387–393.
15. Clements PJ, Furst DE, Wong W-K, et al. High-dose versus low dose D-penicillamine in early diffuse systemic sclerosis: analysis of a two-year, double-blind, randomized, controlled clinical trial. *Arthritis Rheum* 1999;42:1194–1203.
16. Steen VD, Costantino JP, Shapiro AP, et al. Outcome of renal crisis in systemic sclerosis: relation to availability of angiotensin converting enzyme (ACE) inhibitors. *Ann Intern Med* 1990;113:352–357.
17. Maricq HR, Carpentier PH, Weinrich MC, et al. Geographic variation in the prevalence of Raynaud's phenomenon: Charleston, SC, USA, vs Tarentaise, Savoie, France. *J Rheumatol* 1993;20:70–76.
18. Sheiner NM, Small P. Isolated Raynaud's phenomenon: a benign disorder. *Ann Allergy* 1987;58:114–117.
19. Gerbracht DD, Steen VD, Ziegler GL, et al. Evolution of primary Raynaud's phenomenon (Raynaud's disease) to connective tissue disease. *Arthritis Rheum* 1985;28:87–92.
20. Fitzgerald O, Hess EV, O'Connor GT, et al. Prospective study of the evolution of Raynaud's phenomenon. *Am J Med* 1988;84:718–726.
21. Okano Y, Medsger TA Jr. Antibody to Th ribonucleoprotein (nucleolar 7–2 RNA protein particle) in patients with systemic sclerosis (scleroderma). *Arthritis Rheum* 1990;33:1822–1828.
22. Kallenberg CGM, Wouda AA, Hoet MH, et al. Development of connective tissue disease in patients presenting with Raynaud's phenomenon: a six-year follow-up with emphasis on the predictive value of antinuclear antibodies as detected by immunoblotting. *Ann Rheum Dis* 1988;47:634–641.
23. Coffman JD, Cohen AS. Total and capillary fingertip blood flow in Raynaud's phenomenon. *N Engl J Med* 1971;285:259–263.
24. Maricq HR, Diat F, Weinrich MC, et al. Digital pressure responses to cooling in patients with suspected early vs. definite scleroderma (systemic sclerosis) vs. primary Raynaud's phenomenon. *J. Rheumatol* 1994;21:1472–1476.
25. Hendriksen O, Kristensen JK. Reduced systolic blood pressure in fingers of patients with generalized scleroderma (acrosclerosis). *Acta Derm Venereol (Stockh)* 1981;61:531–534.

INFLAMMATORY MYOPATHIES: POLYMYOSITIS, DERMATOMYOSITIS, AND RELATED CONDITIONS

FREDERICK W. MILLER

Diseases characterized by acquired muscle inflammation are designated *inflammatory myopathies*. This term encompasses a large number of disorders that include viral, fungal, and parasitic infections of muscle, toxic myopathies, and other causes of muscle damage (Table 15.1). When the appropriate clinical, laboratory, and pathologic studies eliminate known causes of muscle inflammation, however, a diagnosis of idiopathic inflammatory myopathy (IIM) can be made (1).

The most common forms of IIM are polymyositis (PM), in which patients have inflammation of multiple muscles, and dermatomyositis (DM), in which inflammatory changes occur in the skin as well as muscles. Yet the IIM themselves are a heterogeneous group of rare syndromes that differ considerably in their clinical presentations, pathologic findings, disease courses, and prognoses (2). This heterogeneity has delayed progress in the field and certainly reflects multiple etiologies and pathogeneses that result in a final common path of muscle inflammation (2,3).

Mononuclear cell infiltration in muscle and frequent immune abnormalities, including autoantibodies, in patients with IIM, have resulted in most of these disorders being thought of as autoimmune diseases. This has also been the basis for the major therapies for IIM aimed at decreasing inflammation in organs that may be affected (4).

DIFFERENTIAL DIAGNOSIS AND CRITERIA

Because the differential diagnosis of muscle complaints is large, many disorders must be considered in their evaluation (Table 15.2). The first priority is to define the patient's primary problems. Questions should focus upon (a) the exact nature and location of weakness, myalgias, or other muscle symptoms; (b) any exacerbating or ameliorating factors; (c) the time frame and tempo of the progression of symptoms; and (d) the development of any associated nonmuscular symptoms, such as fatigue, rashes, breathing or swallowing difficulties, or arthralgias. Next, one needs to consider the possible causes for these problems. Has the individual been exposed to any myotoxins, licit or illicit drugs, botanical or other over-the-counter preparations that could result in myopathy, or had any unusual exposure, infections, or travel? Do any symptoms or findings suggest thyroid disease? Does a family history of a similar disorder suggest a dystrophy or inherited myopathy?

Muscle weakness needs to be distinguished from fatigability or pain that might limit function. The distribution of muscle tenderness or atrophy should be noted. Involvement of other muscles—including the heart, oropharynx, gastrointestinal tract, or ocular and respiratory muscles, as well as any other abnormalities—should be documented. Rashes should be evaluated and in some cases biopsied. Although molecular genetic studies have identified genes responsible for many dystrophies, metabolic, and mitochondrial myopathies, some patients continue to defy diagnostic evaluations and remain enigmas. These individuals need to be fully educated about the limitations of our understanding of muscle disease and the risks and benefits of possible empiric therapy.

Criteria to define the IIM syndromes and distinguish them from other myopathies were proposed more than 20 years ago (5). Although in need of reassessment, given recent findings regarding the role of autoantibodies and magnetic resonance imaging (MRI) in the diagnosis of myositis (6), they remain useful today. They include muscle weakness, elevation of muscle enzymes, EMG and muscle biopsy findings, or rashes consistent with IIM (Table 15.3). In unclear cases, additional clues that can assist in making the diagnosis of IIM include the presence of antinuclear or myositis-specific autoantibodies (7,8), a family history of autoimmune disease, inflammatory changes in muscles on MRI (9,10), or a clinical response to immunosuppressive therapy (11) (Table 15.4).

TABLE 15.1. INFLAMMATORY MYOPATHIES

Infectious myopathies
  Bacterial
    Staphylococcus
    Streptococcus
    Clostridia
    Borrelia
    Mycoplasma pneumoniae
    Serratia marcescens
    Citrobacter freundii
    Salmonella
  Viral
    Influenza
    Adenovirus
    Epstein–Barr virus
    Coxsackievirus
    Echovirus
    Hepatitis B
    Hepatitis C
    HIV
    Human T-cell leukemia (HTLV-1)
  Fungal
    Candida
    Coccidioidomycosis
  Protozoal
    Toxoplasmosis
    Sarcocystis
    Trypanosomiasis
    Microsporidia, increasingly described in AIDS
    Malaria
  Cestode infections
    Cysticercosis
    Echinococcosis
  Nematode infections
    Trichinosis
    Toxocariasis
Toxic myopathies
  Adulterated rapeseed oil (toxic oil syndrome)
  Cimetidine
  Cocaine–heroin
  D-penicillamine
  Ethanol
  L-tryptophan (eosinophilia myalgia syndrome)
Myositis associated with graft-versus-host disease
Myositis ossificans
Myositis associated with the vasculitides
Idiopathic inflammatory myopathies (see Tables 15.6 and 15.8)

AIDS, acquired immunodeficiency syndrome; HIV, human immunodeficiency virus.
From Miller FW. Inflammatory myopathies: polymyositis, dermatomyositis, and related conditions. In: Koopman WJ, ed. *Arthritis and allied conditions: a textbook of rheumatology,* 14th ed. Philadelphia: Lippincott Williams & Wilkins, 2001:1562–1589, with permission.

TABLE 15.2. A DIFFERENTIAL DIAGNOSIS OF MUSCLE WEAKNESS/PAIN

Inflammatory myopathies (see Table 15.1)
Noninflammatory myopathies
  Congenital—nemaline rod, centronuclear, central core
  Mitochondrial—with genetic defects
  Metabolic—acid maltase deficiency, McArdle's phosphofructokinase deficiency, carnitine and carnitine palmityltransferase deficiency, uremia
  Endocrine—hypo- and hyperthyroidism, acromegaly, diabetes, Cushing's, Addison's, hypo- and hyperparathyroidism, hypocalcemia, hypokalemia
  Toxic—from many drugs, including ethanol, corticosteroids, cocaine, colchicine, clofibrate, chloroquine, lovastatin, emetine, ipecac, zidovudine (AZT)
  Nutritional—vitamin E deficiency, malabsorption syndromes
Malignant hyperthermia
Muscular dystrophies
  Duchenne
  Becker
  Fascioscapulohumeral
  Limb-girdle
  Emery–Dreifuss
  Distal
  Oculopharyngeal
Myotonia
Neuropathies
  Denervating conditions
    Spinal muscular atrophy
    Amyotrophic lateral sclerosis
  Proximal neuropathies
    Guillain–Barré syndrome
    Autoimmune polyneuropathy
    Diabetic plexopathy
    Acute intermittent porphyria
Neuromuscular junction disorders
  Eaton–Lambert syndrome
  Myasthenia gravis
Overuse syndromes
Periodic paralyses
Paraneoplastic syndromes
  Carcinomatous neuropathy
  Cachexia
  Myonecrosis
Rhabdomyolysis
Rheumatic syndromes
  Giant cell arteritis/polymyalgia rheumatica
  Wegener granulomatosus
  Polyarteritis nodosa
  Fibromyalgia syndromes
Tendonitis–fasciitis syndromes
Trauma

From Miller FW. Inflammatory myopathies: polymyositis, dermatomyositis, and related conditions. In: Koopman WJ, ed. *Arthritis and allied conditions: a textbook of rheumatology,* 14th ed. Philadelphia: Lippincott Williams & Wilkins, 2001:1562–1589, with permission.

Regarding the recently defined entity of inclusion-body myositis (IBM), a diagnosis is usually possible based on the finding of IIM criteria in the context of slowly progressive proximal and distal weakness, serum creatine kinase (CK) levels of less than 12 times the upper limits of normal, and characteristic rimmed vacuoles by light microscopic evaluation of stained sections of frozen muscle specimens (12,13).

The association of cancer with myositis remains controversial. Yet, in view of data from population-based studies (14) and many other clinical series and anecdotes, most investigators consider a patient to have cancer-associated myositis if both diagnoses are made within 2 years of each other.

TABLE 15.3. CRITERIA FOR THE DIAGNOSIS OF IDIOPATHIC INFLAMMATORY MYOPATHY (IIM)[a]

1. Symmetric weakness, usually progressive, of the limb-girdle muscles
2. Muscle biopsy evidence of myositis
   Necrosis of type I and type II muscle fibers
   Phagocytosis
   Degeneration and regeneration of myofibers with variation in myofiber size
   Endomysial, perimysial, perivascular, or interstitial mononuclear cells
3. Elevation of serum levels of muscle-associated enzymes
   Creatine kinase
   Aldolase
   Lactate dehydrogenase
   Transaminases (ALT/SGPT and AST/SGOT)
4. Electromyographic triad of myopathy
   Short, small, low-amplitude polyphasic motor unit potentials
   Fibrillation potentials, even at rest
   Bizarre high-frequency repetitive discharges
5. Characteristic rashes of dermatomyositis
   Heliotrope rash—a lilac discoloration of the eyelids and periorbital area
   Gottron papules—scaly erythematous eruptions over the metacarpophalangeal and
      interphalangeal joints, or over other extensor surfaces (knees, elbows, and medial
      malleoli)
   Gottron sign—erythema in the distribution of Gottron papules but without papules

[a]In patients in whom all known causes of myopathy have been excluded.
Definite IIM = 4 of the above criteria 1–4; or 4 of the above (including the rash) for dermatomyositis.
Probable IIM = 3 of the above criteria 1–4; or 3 of the above (including the rash) for dermatomyositis.
Possible IIM = 2 of the above criteria 1–4; or 2 of the above (including the rash) for dermatomyositis.
ALT/SGPT, alanine aminotransferase/serum glutamic-pyruvic transaminase; AST/SGOT, aspartate
aminotransferase/serum glutamic–oxaloacetic transaminase.
Modified from Bohan A, Peter JB. Polymyositis and dermatomyositis (parts 1 and 2). *N Engl J Med*
1975;292:344–347, 403–407.

TABLE 15.4. USEFUL DISCRIMINATORS FOR MYOSITIS IN CONFUSING CASES OF MYOPATHY

Features Leading Toward Myositis	Features Leading Away from Myositis
Family history of autoimmune disease	Family history of a similar syndrome as the patient's signs/symptoms
Symmetric, chronic, proximal > distal weakness[a]	Weakness related to exercise, eating or fasting, or of the face
Muscle atrophy after chronic symptoms	Muscle atrophy early or hypertrophy ever
Absence of neuropathy by exam or EMG/NCV[a]	Presence of neuropathy
Lack of fasciculations and little muscle cramping	Fasciculations or prominent muscle cramping
Gottron[a], Heliotrope[a], V sign, shawl-sign rashes, linear extensor erythema, cuticular overgrowth, or vasculitis	No rash or vasculitis
Features of CTD—fevers, arthritis, ILD, Raynaud, etc.	No CTD symptoms
CK, AST, ALT, LD, aldolase levels 2–100× normal[a]	Enzymes <2× normal range, or >100× normal
Positive ANA, MSA, or ENA	Negative autoantibodies
Muscle biopsy evidence of myofiber degeneration–regeneration with inflammation[a], strong alkaline phosphatase staining of the interstitium[a]	Myofiber vacuoles, ragged red fibers, parasites—neither inflammation nor alkaline phosphatase staining in the interstitium
MRI—spotty bright symmetric areas in muscle by STIR	MRI normal or only shows atrophy
Clinical response to immunosuppressives	No clinical response to immunosuppressives

[a]Accepted criteria for the diagnosis of idiopathic inflammatory myopathy (IIM) per Table 15.3. CTD,
connective-tissue disease; ILD, interstitial lung disease; ANA, antinuclear antibody; MSA, myositis-
specific autoantibody; ENA, antibody to extractable nuclear antigens (Ro, La, RNP, etc.); STIR, short
tau inversion repeat.
ALT, alanine aminotransferase; AST, aspartate aminotransferase; CK, creatine kinase; EMG,
electromyogram; LD, lactate dehydrogenase; MRI, magnetic resonance imaging; NCV, nerve
conduction velocity.
From Miller FW. Inflammatory myopathies: polymyositis, dermatomyositis, and related conditions. In:
Koopman WJ, ed. *Arthritis and allied conditions: a textbook of rheumatology,* 14th ed. Philadelphia:
Lippincott Williams & Wilkins, 2001:1562–1589, with permission.

CLINICAL CHARACTERISTICS AND THEIR EVALUATION

Most patients present with acute or subacute onset of proximal weakness. This is usually manifested by complaints of hip muscle weakness, which may include increasing difficulty getting up from a chair or climbing stairs. The shoulder muscles often become symptomatic later, resulting in difficulty combing or styling the hair or getting objects from high shelves. The physical examination should be focused on the evaluation of muscle strength using standard manual muscle strength testing, noting how a patient arises from a squatting or sitting position, how rapidly he or she can dress or undress, walk times, and what he or she can do compared with a previous point in time (15). A simple, easily scored activities-of-daily-living questionnaire is often useful (16).

Because the IIM are systemic connective-tissue diseases, other organ systems can be involved with inflammation or other pathologic processes (Table 15.5). The location and nature of arthritis, skin rashes, and subcutaneous tenderness, vasomotor instability, and pulmonary, cardiac, and gastrointestinal abnormalities should all be documented (Figs. 15.1 and 15.2), and consideration should be given for further evaluation of any positive findings by radiologic studies, electrocardiography, biopsy, or other laboratory testing (Table 15.6). None of the many skin lesions that have been described in DM patients (17,18) is pathognomonic except Gottron papules. These are palpable lesions overlying the extensor surfaces of the hand joints, elbows, knees, or malleoli with an erythematous base. Other rashes characteristic for DM include the purplish discoloration around the eyes, known as the heliotrope rash (Fig. 15.1) and Gottron sign, scaling erythema without papules in the same distribution as Gottron papules. Other common rashes include linear extensor erythema, periungual vasculitic changes and cuticular overgrowth, photosensitive erythroderma, accentuated erythema in the V of the neck (V sign), and a drying and cracking of the skin over the lateral and palmar surfaces of the fingers, known as *mechanic's hands.*

TABLE 15.5. SYSTEMIC MANIFESTATIONS OF THE IDIOPATHIC INFLAMMATORY MYOPATHIES

General
 Fatigue
 Fevers
 Weight loss
 Voice changes—nasal speech, hoarseness
 Raynaud phenomenon and other vasomotor instability
Musculoskeletal system
 Muscle weakness—proximal > distal, upper and lower limbs, neck muscles, rare facial weakness
 Unexpected falling
 Myalgia
 Muscle tenderness
 Muscle atrophy
 Contractures
 Arthralgias
 Arthritis
 Deforming arthropathy[a]
Respiratory system
 Dyspnea at rest and on exertion
 Dry cough
 Wheezing/rales/rhonchi
 Atelectasis
 Interstitial lung disease
 Pneumonia secondary to immunosuppression and poor clearing of secretions
 Pneumothorax[a]
 Pneumomediastinum[a]
 Cricopharyngeal obstruction[a]
Cardiac system
 Myocarditis
 Arrhythmias
 Congestive failure

Pericarditis[a]
Gastrointestinal system
 Dysarthria—poor tongue propulsions
 Dysphagia—upper and lower esophagus
 Odynophagia
 Nasal regurgitation
 Reflux esophagitis
 Poorly coordinated peristalsis
 Constipation/diarrhea
 Ulcerations (particularly in juvenile dermatomyositis)
 Pneumatosis intestinalis[a]
Skin
 Dermatomyositis-specific rashes—Gottron's papules, Gottron sign, heliotrope
  Less specific rashes—diffuse rashes, erythroderma, V sign, shawl sign, mechanic's hands, linear extensor erythema, acrosclerosis
  Poikiloderma vasculare atrophicans
  Photosensitivity
 Mucin deposition
 Panniculitis
 Scleredema
 Calcifications
 Vasculitis and ulceration
 Periungual capillary changes
 Cuticular overgrowth
 Alopecia[a]
 Purpura[a]
Renal
 Membranous nephropathy[a]
 Insufficiency from myoglobinuria[a]

[a]Rare manifestations.
From Miller FW. Inflammatory myopathies: polymyositis, dermatomyositis, and related conditions. In: Koopman WJ, ed. *Arthritis and allied conditions: a textbook of rheumatology,* 14th ed. Philadelphia: Lippincott Williams & Wilkins, 2001:1562–1589, with permission.

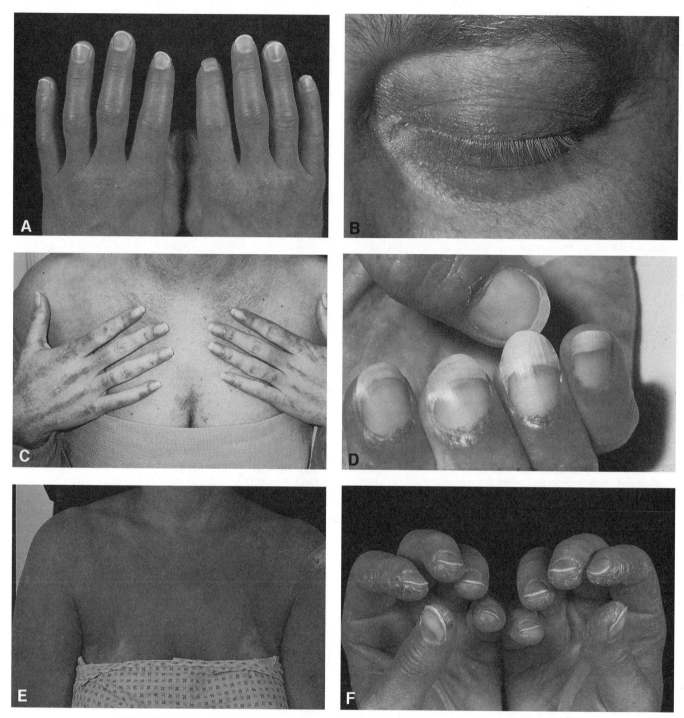

FIGURE 15.1. Skin changes seen in dermatomyositis. **A:** Gottron papules are scaly papules overlying the extensor surfaces of the hands (over the metacarpophalangeal and proximal interphalangeal joints in this case), elbows, knees, or malleoli. This patient also has sclerodactyly and arthritis of the metacarpophalangeal and proximal interphalangeal joints. **B:** The heliotrope rash is a purplish discoloration around the eyes, especially on the upper lids. **C:** Linear extensor erythema overlies the extensor surface of the hands beyond the usual location of Gottron papules or sign. **D:** Periungual vasculitic changes and cuticular overgrowth. **E:** Photosensitive diffuse erythroderma with accentuated erythema in the V of the neck (V sign) in a patient with cancer-associated dermatomyositis. **F:** Drying and cracking of the skin over the lateral and palmar surfaces of the fingers, known as "mechanic's hands," is seen frequently in patients with autoantibodies to aminoacyl-tRNA synthetases (the antisynthetase syndrome). (From Miller FW. Inflammatory myopathies: polymyositis, dermatomyositis, and related conditions. In: Koopman WJ, ed. *Arthritis and allied conditions: a textbook of rheumatology,* 14th ed. Philadelphia: Lippincott Williams & Wilkins, 2001:1562–1589, with permission.). See Color Plate 1.

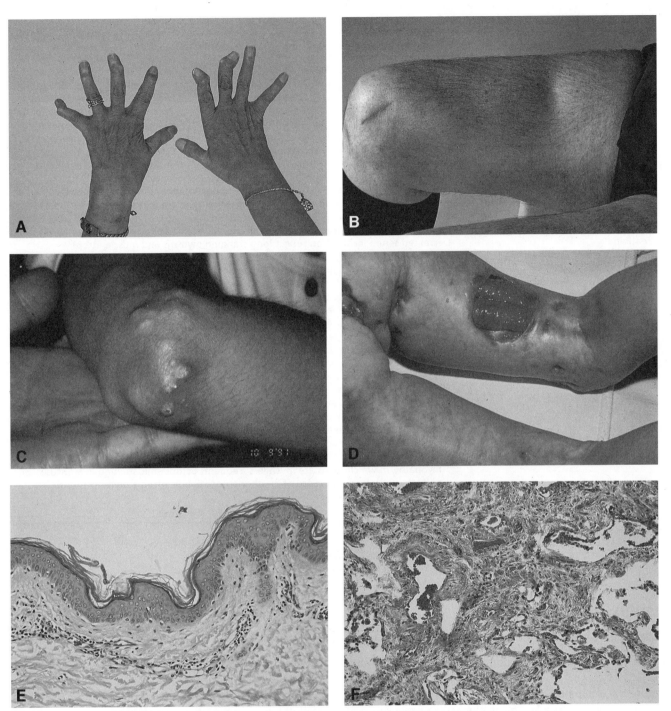

FIGURE 15.2. Manifestations of idiopathic inflammatory myopathy. **A:** A deforming arthropathy is occasionally seen in polymyositis patients as a manifestation of the antisynthetase syndrome as seen in this patient with anti-Jo-1 autoantibodies. **B:** Irregular and asymmetric muscle atrophy, often in the anterior thigh muscles, is often seen in patients with inclusion-body myositis. **C:** Extensive calcifications over the elbow in a child with juvenile dermatomyositis (courtesy of Dr. Robert Rennebohm). **D:** Severe vasculitis with erosions into muscle in a patient with dermatomyositis (courtesy of Dr. Robert Rennebohm). **E:** Biopsy from affected skin demonstrating surface scaling, vacuolization, and subcutaneous perivascular mononuclear cells characteristic, but not diagnostic, of dermatomyositis (hematoxylin and eosin) (courtesy of Dr. Lori A. Love). **F:** Lung biopsy from a patient with antisynthetase syndrome and interstitial lung disease demonstrating destruction of the normal architecture and extensive replacement by inflammatory cells and fibrotic tissue (hematoxylin and eosin) (courtesy of Dr. Lori A. Love). (From Miller FW. Inflammatory myopathies: polymyositis, dermatomyositis, and related conditions. In: Koopman WJ, ed. *Arthritis and allied conditions: a textbook of rheumatology,* 14th ed. Philadelphia: Lippincott Williams & Wilkins, 2001:1562–1589, with permission.) See Color Plate 2.

TABLE 15.6. LABORATORY ABNORMALITIES IN MYOSITIS PATIENTS

Laboratory Test	Comments
Muscle-associated enzymes	CK, AST, ALT, LD, aldolase—generally useful to assess the presence and degree of myositis, but may not always correlate with disease activity. May be normal in 5% to 10% of IIM patients at myositis onset and may become normal later despite active disease because of loss of muscle mass or circulating inhibitors of enzyme activity. Elevations may predate clinical flares of disease by weeks to months, and, conversely, decreases may precede clinical responses to therapy by a similar time period. Levels also relate to muscle mass, so are higher in men than in women and higher in blacks than in whites. Elevation of transaminases often results in the misdiagnosis of non-A non-B hepatitis in myositis patients.
CK MB fraction	A correlate of disease activity and a common source of misdiagnosis of myocardial infarction. Probably arises from myoblasts rather than from cardiac muscle in most myositis patients.
Creatinuria	Increased urinary exretion of creatine indicates muscle damage.
Creatinine	Decreased serum levels often reflect long-standing myositis and muscle atrophy.
Myoglobin serum/urine	May correlate with muscle strength better than muscle enzymes and may predict clinical relapse. Because of diurnal variation, myoglobin levels should be measured at the same time of day.
Heme + urine without red blood cells	Usually indicates myoglobinuria.
White blood cell and platelet counts	Elevated values sometimes seen with active myositis.
Hypergammaglobulinemia	Seen in about 10% of IIM patients in whom the level correlates with myositis activity. Elevated IgE can be seen in juvenile myositis.
Hypo- or agammaglobulinemia	A rare finding except in echovirus-associated cases of juvenile dermatomyositis.
Monoclonal gammopathy	Rare but sometimes seen in cancer-associated myositis.
IgA deficiency	Increased frequency in some series of myositis patients.
ESR	Elevated in less than half of IIM patients. Does not correlate with disease activity.
C-reactive protein	Normal in most IIM patients. Elevation often indicative of bacterial infection.
↑ Factor VIII related antigen	Elevated in active juvenile dermatomyositis and correlates with disease activity, but elevation occurs in only a subset of patients.
↑ Neopterin	Correlates with disease activity in many juvenile dermatomyositis patients.
ANA present	Seen in 60% to 90% of IIM patients and a good discriminator of IIM from other forms of myopathy, in which ANAs are much less frequent. Cytoplasmic staining in a diffuse pattern suggests the presence of another autoantibody, often a myositis-specific autoantibody.
Other autoantibodies	See Table 15.7.

ANA, antinuclear autoantibody; CK, creatine kinase; ESR, erythrocyte sedimentation rate; Ig, immunoglobulin; LD, lactate dehydrogenase.
Modified from Rider LG, Miller FW. Laboratory evaluation of the inflammatory myopathies. *Clin Diag Lab Immunol* 1995;2:1–9.

LABORATORY FINDINGS

Clinical Chemistry

The laboratory plays an important role in evaluating the IIM (19,20), and many abnormalities may be detected in routine screening blood tests (Table 15.6). One of the primary laboratory clues to a myopathy is the presence in the serum of elevated levels of enzymes originating from the cytoplasm of the muscle cell (sarcoplasm). The most frequently measured enzyme is CK, because of its high sensitivity, muscle specificity, and relatively good correlation with disease activity and muscle strength. Nonetheless, in IIM patients lactate dehydrogenase, SGOT/aspartate aminotransferase, SGPT/alanine aminotransferase, and aldolase serum levels all tend to correlate with CK levels (19). At the onset of illness, serum CK levels may be elevated as much as 10 to 100 times the upper limit of normal. The serum levels of CK and other muscle-derived enzymes are generally useful in following myositis activity and responses to therapy, although the magnitude of elevation does not always correlate with global disease activity, especially in DM and children. Therefore CK levels alone can never substitute for a thorough evaluation of the patient, which includes functional assessment. The lack of correlation of CK levels with disease activity is partly due to the 3- to 8-week delay between normalization of CK and improvement in muscle strength, and the 5- to 6-week lag between elevation of CKs and clinical relapse (21).

The presence of a normal CK level in the face of active disease, demonstrated by muscle weakness and accompanied by inflammation on muscle biopsy or MRI, may be related to suppression of CK by corticosteroids, the presence of serum inhibitors of CK enzyme activity, racial differences not taken into account by the testing laboratory, or extensive muscle atrophy due to chronic disease. Also, patients with systemic lupus erythematosus (SLE), rheumatoid arthritis, and other connective-tissue diseases tend to have abnormally low CK levels (19). Thus a normal CK level in these patients may indicate active myositis. Most of the elevation of serum CK levels in IIM is due to increases in the MM isoenzyme fraction, which is released from skeletal muscle. Elevation of the MB isoenzyme, found primarily in myocardium, may also occur not only as a result of myocarditis but also as an indicator of skeletal muscle regeneration (19).

Abnormalities of nonspecific markers of inflammation, such as leukocytosis, elevated platelet counts, high C-reactive protein, and erythrocyte sedimentation rates may be found in myositis patients. These are generally not useful in assessing IIM activity, but usually reflect coexisting processes. Twenty-four-hour urinary creatine excretion, which reflects muscle mass and damage, is elevated in many patients with muscle diseases. Abnormally low serum creatinine levels may result from the loss of muscle mass and should alert the clinician to the presence of chronic myositis.

Immunology

Immunologic abnormalities are sometimes the first clue that a patient has IIM. The most frequent abnormalities are hypergammaglobulinemia or the presence of an autoantibody. Antinuclear autoantibodies (ANAs) are the most common autoantibodies. The ANA usually displays a speckled pattern, although any other pattern can also be present. Other immune abnormalities, however, may be present, including hypogammaglobulinemia, hypergammaglobulinemia, monoclonal gammopathy, cryoglobulinemia, and a variety of autoantibodies, some of which are specific for myositis (Tables 15.6 and 15.7).

Electromyography and Other Tests

Electromyography (EMG) and nerve conduction velocity (NCV) measurements are often performed to distinguish neuropathies from myopathies. They also can add to the probability that the patient has an inflammatory myopathy when characteristic abnormalities are present (Table 15.3). Radiographs, electrocardiograms, and other laboratory studies should be based upon the nature of the symptoms and findings, and concern for the presence of cancer, which may be associated with IIM.

Muscle Biopsy

Although physicians may be reluctant to perform a muscle biopsy in what would appear to be straightforward cases of myositis, a biopsy should be included early in evaluating most patients. The biopsy may reveal an unexpected disease, sometimes with important therapeutic, prognostic, or reproductive implications (Fig. 15.3).

TABLE 15.7. A SEROLOGIC CLASSIFICATION OF THE INFLAMMATORY MYOPATHIES

Serologic Category	Associations and Comments
Myositis-specific autoantibodies[a]	
Antisynthetase[b]	High frequency of symmetric nonerosive arthritis, interstitial lung disease, fever, mechanic's hands, Raynaud phenomenon; often occurs as an acute, severe myositis with onset in the spring, moderate response to therapy, myositis flare with tapering of therapy; seen in 20% to 25% of all myositis cases
Antisignal recognition particle	Cardiac involvement with frequent palpitations and myalgias; very acute onset of severe polymyositis in the fall; most often in black women; poor response to therapy; seen in <5% of myositis patients
Anti-Mi-2	Classic dermatomyositis with V sign, shawl sign, and cuticular overgrowth; good response to therapy; seen in 5% to 10% of myositis patients
Anti-Mas[c]	Polymyositis following alcoholic rhabdomyolysis
Anti-Fer[c]	Seen in <1% of myositis patients
Anti-KJ[c]	Polymyositis interstitial lung disease, Raynaud phenomenon
None of the above (MSA negative)	A heterogeneous group of patients
Myositis-associated autoantibodies[b]	
Anti-PM-Scl	Scleroderma/myositis overlap syndromes
Anti-Ku[c]	Scleroderma/myositis overlap syndromes
Anti-U1RNP[c]	Myositis overlap syndromes
Anti-U2RNP[c]	Scleroderma/myositis overlap syndromes
Anti-U5RNP[c]	Myositis overlap syndromes

[a]Myositis-specific autoantibodies are only seen in myositis patients; myositis-associated autoantibodies are seen in myositis patients and those with other autoimmune disorders.
[b]Includes patients with anti-Jo-1 autoantibodies (directed against histidyl-tRNA synthetase) and those with autoantibodies to threoryl-(PL-7), alanyl-(PL-12), isoleucyl-(OJ), and glycyl-(EJ) tRNA synthetases.
[c]Possibly distinct entities for which less substantiating data exist than do for the other categories.
Modified from Miller FW. Classification and prognosis of inflammatory muscle disease. *Rheum Dis Clin North Am* 1994;20:811–826.

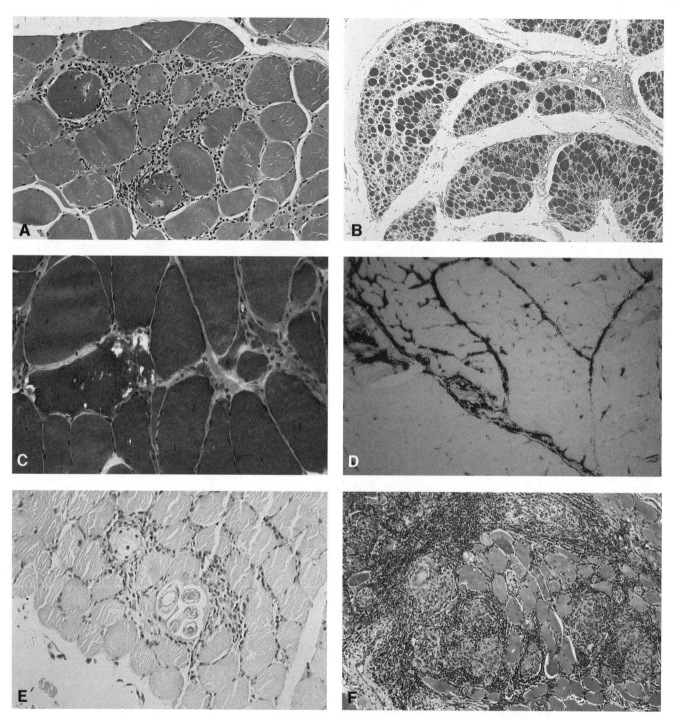

FIGURE 15.3. Histopathology of inflammatory myopathies. **A–B:** Muscle biopsies from polymyositis patients tend to show focal endomysial infiltration by mononuclear cells (**A,** hematoxylin and eosin stain), while those from dermatomyositis patients show more perivascular and interstitial inflammation with perifascicular myofiber atrophy (**B,** modified trichrome stain). **C:** Transverse fresh-frozen section of muscle from a patient with inclusion-body myositis displaying purplish granular material lining the multiple vacuoles in several myofibers and the presence of angulated myofibers (modified trichrome stain). **D:** Strong alkaline phosphatase staining of the interstitium is common in idiopathic inflammatory myopathy and can help distinguish this condition from other myopathies even in the absence of inflammation. **E:** Trichinosis parasites in a myofiber surrounded by mononuclear inflammatory cells in a patient originally misdiagnosed with polymyositis (courtesy Dr. Lori A. Love). **F:** Intensely inflammatory granulomatous myositis is characterized by the presence of granulomata and endomysial inflammation in this patient with sarcoidosis (hematoxylin and eosin stain). (From Miller FW. Inflammatory myopathies: polymyositis, dermatomyositis, and related conditions. In: Koopman WJ, ed. *Arthritis and allied conditions: a textbook of rheumatology,* 14th ed. Philadelphia: Lippincott Williams & Wilkins, 2001: 1562–1589, with permission.) See Color Plate 3.

Nonetheless, the biopsy may not always be diagnostic. Inflammation in typical myositis may be missed because of its spotty nature or as a result of therapy. Conversely, muscle inflammation can be present in some dystrophies, especially fascioscapulohumeral dystrophy, and toxic myopathies. MRI can detect muscle inflammation and damage and may improve the yield of biopsy diagnosis by directing the site of biopsy. When a muscle cell dies a secondary inflammatory process may occur. What distinguishes the IIM, however, is that the inflammation is primary and chronic. Chronic inflammatory cells, mononuclear cells that are predominantly lymphocytes, may be found not only in direct contact with a dying myocyte (endomysial), but between unaffected cells and fascicles (perimysial), or in the adjacent interstitial tissue. Predominance of neutrophils or perineural inflammation usually points to a process other than IIM, whereas predominant plasma cells, eosinophils, or granulomata in an otherwise typical myositis suggest the type of IIM present (Fig. 15.3F).

Irregular red-rimmed inclusions on trichrome stain can identify IBM, the most common form of IIM in those more than 50 years of age (Fig. 15.3C). Strong activity of the alkaline phosphatase stain in the interstitium suggests an IIM even if inflammation is not prominent (Fig. 15.3D). The finding of prominent glycogen (by PAS stain), fat (by oil red O stain), abnormal mitochondria (the ragged red fiber on hematoxylin and eosin stain), or other inclusions should move the clinician away from the diagnosis of IIM toward that of other syndromes.

Imaging Studies

Radiographic studies are useful in screening for and assessing gastrointestinal, cardiac, and pulmonary disease; erosive arthropathy; or calcifications (Fig. 15.4). Interest is increasing in using computed tomography (CT), ultrasound, MRI, and a related technique called magnetic resonance spectroscopy to assess muscle disease because these techniques are noninvasive and can sample larger volumes of muscle than EMG and muscle biopsy. Most investigators agree that MRI is superior to CT or ultrasound scanning because of the added information it provides (Fig. 15.5). Studies suggest that a combination of the T1-weighted image and the STIR (short tau inversion repeat) or other fat-suppressed image should be employed to assess muscle disease in IIM (9,10). Multiple cross sections of the thighs are usually useful views, but the location to be evaluated should depend on the signs and symptoms of the individual. Despite the expense of MRI, it may be a cost-effective adjunct for diagnosing and assessing selected patients. Active exercise can cause muscle changes that result in transient elevations in serum CK levels and inflammatory changes on MRI. Therefore patients should rest for at least an hour before these studies (22).

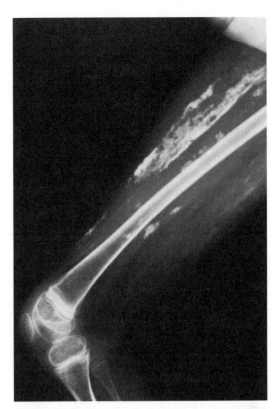

FIGURE 15.4. Subcutaneous and perimuscular calcifications in a patient with juvenile dermatomyositis. (From Miller FW. Inflammatory myopathies: polymyositis, dermatomyositis, and related conditions. In: Koopman WJ, ed. *Arthritis and allied conditions: a textbook of rheumatology,* 14th ed. Philadelphia: Lippincott Williams & Wilkins, 2001:1562–1589, with permission.)

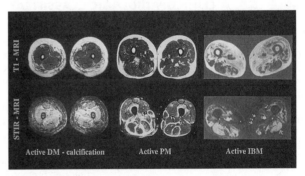

FIGURE 15.5. Magnetic resonance imaging (MRI) of the thighs is a useful modality to quantitate and distinguish IIM disease activity (muscle inflammation) from disease damage (muscle atrophy and fibrosis). The MRIs from three patients with both disease activity and damage are shown: dermatomyositis with subcutaneous calcifications (which appear black) on the left, polymyositis in the middle, and inclusion-body myositis on the right. The T1-weighted MRIs **(top)** define anatomic details and show disease damage represented by severe muscle atrophy and replacement of muscle by fat. The STIR (short tau inversion recovery)-MRIs **(bottom)** help quantitate inflammation demonstrated by bright areas in muscle (active myositis), subcutaneous tissue (panniculitis), and skin (active dermatitis). (Courtesy of Dr. Elizabeth Adams. From Miller FW. Inflammatory myopathies: polymyositis, dermatomyositis, and related conditions. In: Koopman WJ, ed. *Arthritis and allied conditions: a textbook of rheumatology,* 14th ed. Philadelphia: Lippincott Williams & Wilkins, 2001:1562–1589, with permission.)

CLASSIFICATION

Although the simplest differentiation of these syndromes is into PM, DM, and IBM (23), this approach does not capture all the useful information that divisions into the more specific forms can generate (24). Two major classification systems have proved the most useful to date in terms of research and patient care: serologic (Table 15.7) and clinicopathologic (Table 15.8) divisions.

Clinicopathologic Groups

Primary PM differs from primary DM in clinical presentation, histopathology (1), the number and distribution of both circulating and muscle-infiltrating CD4+ and CD8+ T cells and B cells, and responses to therapy (25). Some physicians believe that a distinct entity known as DM without myositis (dermatomyositis sine myositis) exists (26); however, it remains unclear whether this is a separate entity or simply at one end of a continuum in myositis severity. MRI and spectroscopy, as well as histopathologic studies (27), suggest that there are abnormalities in the muscles of some patients who exhibit typical dermatomyositis rash but do not have clinical evidence of muscle weakness.

Overlap myositis syndromes refer to the occurrence of myositis in association with criteria for other connective tissue disorders such as systemic sclerosis, SLE, or Sjögren syndrome. These overlap diseases tend to be characterized by a higher frequency of Raynaud, arthritis (28), higher frequencies and titers of autoantibodies (28), and less severe myositis with a better response to therapy (25), compared with other forms of myositis.

Juvenile myositis is being recognized as an increasingly heterogeneous group of disorders, and there may be fewer differences from the adult forms of myositis than previously believed (29,30). Nonetheless, juvenile DM patients have more frequent vasculitic complications and calcifications (Fig. 15.6), and a better response to therapy than that seen in most adult myositis patients (31).

Cases of myositis developing in association with malignancy, responding to simple resection of the cancer, and returning to herald the recurrence of the cancer, anecdotally supported a cancer-associated form of myositis. Although this has been a controversial area, there appears to be an increased risk of a variety of cancers with certain forms of IIM. A recent population survey has demonstrated a significantly increased risk of cancer in patients with either PM or DM, with most, but not all cancers, developing within 2 years of the onset of IIM (14). Although many forms of cancer have been associated with myositis in case series, gastric and ovarian cancers may be overrepresented (32,33).

The association of myositis with cancer in population studies raises the difficult question of how to address cancer

TABLE 15.8. A CLINICOPATHOLOGIC CLASSIFICATION OF THE INFLAMMATORY MYOPATHIES[a]

Clinicopathologic Category	Associations and Comments
Primary idiopathic polymyositis	A diagnosis of exclusion—defined by the absence of all below[b]
Primary idiopathic dermatomyositis	Heliotrope rash, Gottron papules or sign is present, but other rashes may coexist; myositis may be clinically silent (dermatomyositis sine myositis)
Myositis associated with another connective-tissue disease	Mild myositis, good response to therapy; rheumatoid arthritis, systemic sclerosis, and systemic lupus erythematosus most common as overlaps
Juvenile myositis	More frequent calcifications and gastrointestinal vasculitis than seen in adults; may be more heterogeneous than previously thought
Myositis associated with malignancy	Myositis onset often within 2 years of cancer; ovarian cancer may be overrepresented
Inclusion body myositis	Occurs mainly in older white men with insidious onset and progression; poor response to therapy; rimmed inclusions in myocytes
Granulomatous myositis	Granulomas prominent and frequent in muscle biopsy; can be seen in sarcoidosis
Eosinophilic myositis	Eosinophils prominent in muscle; can be a part of hypereosinophilic syndrome or eosinophilic fasciitis
Vasculitic myositis	Vasculitis prominent in muscle; can be part of other vasculitides, including polyarteritis nodosa
Orbital or ocular myositis	Involvement of extraocular muscles only; often diagnosed by computerized tomography or magnetic resonance imaging
Focal or nodular myositis[c]	Focal involvement of one or more limbs; can progress to polymyositis, remain isolated, or resolve
Myositis ossificans[c]	Occurs as a local limited phenomenon or more generalized excessive proliferation of connective tissue and replacement by bone

[a]Categories are not mutually exclusive.
[b]In a patient meeting criteria for definite or probable myositis (5)
[c]Possibly distinct entities for which less substantiating data exist than for the other categories.
Modified from Miller FW. Classification and prognosis of inflammatory muscle disease. *Rheum Dis Clin North Am* 1994;20:811–826.

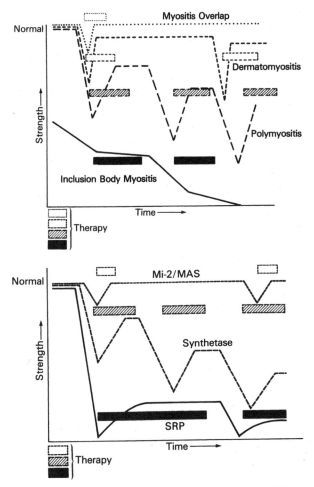

FIGURE 15.6. Generalized myositis courses differ in different idiopathic inflammatory myopathy clinical **(top)** and serologic **(bottom)** subgroups. (From Koopman WJ, ed. *Arthritis and allied conditions: a textbook of rheumatology,* 14th ed. Philadelphia: Lippincott Williams & Wilkins, 2001:1562–1589, with permission.)

screening in the individual IIM patient. A careful history, physical examination, and routine laboratory screening, with rigorous follow-up of any abnormalities suspicious of cancer, is preferable to a nondirected series of radiologic or invasive studies (1). Increased vigilance for cancer is warranted in myositis patients more than 50 years of age, in those with other risk factors for cancer, in IIM patients without autoantibodies, and in those with severe or unresponsive skin rashes, erythroderma, or vasculitis (34). Because of the heightened concern about ovarian cancer, most women with DM, including those with normal pelvic examinations and pap smears, should undergo testing with CA-125 and ovarian ultrasound evaluations.

IBM is perhaps the most underdiagnosed form of IIM. The inclusion-body myopathy syndromes consist of two major groups of disorders: (a) inflammatory conditions in which activated lymphocytes infiltrating normal muscle are seen in muscle biopsies, making these entities a form

of IIM (these are referred to as the IBM syndromes), and (b) noninflammatory disorders (the noninflammatory inclusion-body myopathy syndromes). Both the inflammatory and noninflammatory forms can be either sporadic or familial. A continuing confusion in the field relates to the unfortunate use by workers in this area of a similar abbreviation—IBM—to represent both types of these disorders. Because inclusion-body myopathy and Alzheimer disease share slowly progressive target organ damage that affects older individuals, and accumulate some of the same proteins in pathologic lesions, it is tempting to speculate that a similar process is at work in both of these diseases. IBM differs clinically, pathologically, serologically, and prognostically from all the other forms of IIM. Whenever an elderly white man presents with a slowly progressive, often asymmetric proximal and distal weakness, unexpected falling, quadriceps atrophy, few serologic abnormalities or extraskeletal manifestations, serum CK levels of less than 12 times the upper limits of normal, and a poor response to corticosteroids, the diagnosis of IBM should be strongly considered (28).

Eosinophilic, granulomatous, and vasculitic myositis have distinctive muscle pathology features (35); however, because they are extremely rare, little is known about them. Another unusual inflammatory myopathy is termed *ocular* or *orbital myositis* and involves chronic inflammation of structures within the orbit. Individuals with this form of IIM usually present with unilateral periorbital pain that is often made worse with eye movement, as well as proptosis, diplopia, and swelling of the eyelid (36).

Syndromes defined by local areas of pain, swelling, or weakness but that on biopsy show the typical features of IIM have been called *focal, nodular,* or *focal nodular myositis.* These disorders probably represent a number of diseases with heterogeneous etiologies and pathogeneses inasmuch as they can progress to systemic polymyositis, remain chronically focal, or resolve spontaneously. MRI is a particularly useful modality for the diagnosis and follow-up evaluation of these conditions (37).

Serologic Groups

The past decade has seen an explosion of immunologic studies that has redefined our thinking about the IIM. This is largely the result of identifying particular autoantibodies only in myositis patients, the myositis-specific autoantibodies (MSAs), which define relatively homogeneous groups of patients with similar signs and symptoms, immunogenetics, disease course, and prognoses. Other autoantibodies that are frequently, but not exclusively, found in myositis patients, the myositis-associated autoantibodies, have also been identified recently. Thus a new serologic classification of the inflammatory myopathies using the myositis-specific and myositis-associated autoantibodies has been proposed (Table 15.7).

Possible Environmental Triggers for Idiopathic Inflammatory Myopathy

Anecdotal reports of the clustering in onset of myositis cases have suggested strong environmental influences in the development of IIM. Additionally, a metaanalysis of all published pedigrees of familial myositis demonstrated that the differences in the time of onset of myositis (median 1.1 years) were significantly less than the differences in age at myositis onset (median, 7.5 years) in the affected family members (38,39). These data are consistent with the hypothesis that genetically susceptible family members shared common environmental exposures within a short time frame that may have triggered IIM in that family. Yet a growing number of noninfectious agents are being investigated as possible triggers of disease as well (40) (Table 15.9). Although there may be a temporal association between the putative environmental exposure and the myositis, the pathophysiologic mechanisms involved in the evolution of the inflammation and a cause–effect relationship with the exposure are often unclear (41).

TABLE 15.9. POSSIBLE ENVIRONMENTAL TRIGGERS FOR IIM

Infections	Gemfibrozil
Viruses	Tiopronin
Hepatitis B	Foods
Hepatitis C	L-tryptophan
Human immunodeficiency virus (HIV)	Adulterated rapeseed oil
	Ciguatera toxin
HTLV-1	Biologics
Echovirus	Human growth hormone therapy
Coxsackievirus	Interleukin-2 therapy
Parasites	Vaccines
Lyme	Medical devices
Toxoplasmosis	Silicone implants
Bacteria	Collagen implants
Staph/streptococcus	Occupational exposures
Noninfectious agents	Silica
Drugs	Polyvinyl chloride
D-penicillamine	Dyes and organic solvents
Cimetidine	Ultraviolet light

HTLV-I, human T cell lymphotrophic virus type I.
From Miller FW. Inflammatory myopathies: polymyositis, dermatomyositis, and related conditions. In: Koopman WJ, ed. *Arthritis and allied conditions: a textbook of rheumatology,* 14th ed. Philadelphia: Lippincott Williams & Wilkins, 2001:1562–1589, with permission.

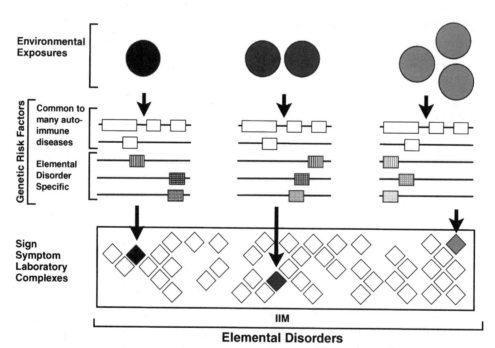

FIGURE 15.7. Possible mechanisms by which IIM subgroups (elemental disorders) may arise. The elemental disorder hypothesis posits that each autoimmune disease, as currently classified, is a heterogeneous collection of clinical signs, symptoms, and laboratory findings composed of many elemental disorders. Elemental disorders are recognized clinically by selected cardinal signs, symptoms, and laboratory findings, and are defined by the minimal necessary and sufficient environmental exposures and genes that need to be present in individuals to induce a common pathology that results in the given sign–symptom–lab complex. The environmental risk factors in this hypothetical construct could be single exposures or multiple sequential or concomitant exposures. The genetic risk factors for autoimmunity would consist of two forms: those that are common to many autoimmune diseases and those that are specific for a given elemental disorder. (From Miller FW. Inflammatory myopathies: polymyositis, dermatomyositis, and related conditions. In: Koopman WJ, ed. *Arthritis and allied conditions: a textbook of rheumatology,* 14th ed. Philadelphia: Lippincott Williams & Wilkins, 2001:1562–1589, with permission.)

Etiology

Although the causes of the IIM are by definition unknown, evidence suggests that they likely result from one or more environmental stimuli acting on genetically susceptible individuals to induce chronic immune activation and subsequent myositis. Gene–environment interactions may lead to different pathophysiologic processes that result in unique syndromes, each of which may be distinguished by a distinct matrix of signs, symptoms, or laboratory abnormalities, which all share myositis. Each of these syndromes has been referred to as an elemental disorder (39,41) and has been defined by the minimal necessary and sufficient environmental exposures and genes that result in the pathology that leads to a given sign–symptom complex (Fig. 15.7). The heterogeneity of the myositis syndromes suggests that they, like most autoimmune diseases, are composed of many elemental disorders.

Many lines of indirect evidence suggest that cellular immune activation is responsible for the pathologic effects seen in myositis (Table 15.10). Evaluation of biopsy specimens by immunologic techniques suggests a role for both cellular and humoral immune systems in muscle damage as well as differences among some of the clinical groups that may point to different pathogenic mechanisms (42). In DM, B cells and CD4+ cells predominate in muscle, whereas in both PM and IBM, individual myocytes that appear otherwise normal are invaded mainly by CD8+ T cells. Analyses of the T-cell receptors utilized by myocyte-infiltrating cells suggest that dermatomyositis patients have more polyclonal T-cell receptor patterns, whereas polymyositis and IBM patients exhibit more oligoclonal T-cell receptor patterns, suggesting an antigen-driven pathogenesis.

Considerable evidence, beyond the frequent occurrence of autoantibodies, indicates that abnormalities of the humoral arm of the immune system exist in IIM patients (Table 15.10). Early damage and loss of capillaries in DM before the development of muscle weakness suggest that a vasculopathy may be the primary event responsible for the later muscle damage.

PROGNOSIS

The IIM are serious and sometimes life-threatening diseases. Survival of myositis patients has been increasing dur-

---

TABLE 15.10. IMMUNOLOGIC ABNORMALITIES IN THE IDIOPATHIC INFLAMMATORY MYOPATHIES

Cellular abnormalities
  Activated mononuclear cells in muscle
  Restricted T-cell receptor expression in muscle
  Common motifs found in putative T-cell receptor antigen-binding regions in muscle of some
    clinical and serologic groups
  Altered expression of activation markers on myocytes
  Elevated levels of soluble CD8, IL-2 receptors, and cytokines in serum
  Altered peripheral mononuclear cell immunophenotypes
  Altered peripheral mononuclear cell trafficking to muscle
  Decreased autologous mixed lymphocyte and mitogenic responses
  Proliferative responses of peripheral lymphocytes to autologous muscle
Humoral abnormalities
  Autoantibodies

Myositis-specific	Antisynthetases [directed against histidyl-(Jo-1), alanyl-, glycyl-, threonyl-, and isoleucyl-tRNA synthetases]
	Anti-MI-2
	Antisignal recognition particle (SRP) and others
Not specific to myositis	Antinuclear antibodies
	Rheumatoid factor
	Antimuscle
	Antithyroid
	Anti-nRNP
	Anti-Ro/La
	Anti-PM-ScL
	Anti-Ku and others

  Immunoglobulin and complement deposition in muscle
  Hypergammaglobulinemia, hypogammaglobulinemia, and agammaglobulinemia
  Monoclonal gammopathies
  Circulating immune complexes

From Miller FW. Inflammatory myopathies: polymyositis, dermatomyositis, and related conditions. In: Koopman WJ, ed. *Arthritis and allied conditions: a textbook of rheumatology,* 14th ed. Philadelphia: Lippincott Williams & Wilkins, 2001:1562–1589, with permission.

TABLE 15.11. POOR PROGNOSTIC FACTORS IN THE INFLAMMATORY MYOPATHIES

Based on demographics
   Black (versus white) race
   Old (versus young)
   Female (versus male) gender
Based on sign-symptom complex
   Severe myositis
   Dysphagia
   Pulmonary involvement
   Cardiac involvement
   Delay to diagnosis and therapy
   Normal creatine kinase
Based on clinicopathologic group
   Polymyositis (versus dermatomyositis)
   Cancer-associated myositis
   Adult (versus juvenile myositis)
   Inclusion body myositis
Based on serologic group
   Antisynthetase autoantibodies
   Antisignal recognition particle autoantibodies

Modified from Miller FW. Classification and prognosis of inflammatory disease. *Rheum Dis Clin North Am* 1994;20:811–826.

ing the past few decades, from 50% before the introduction of corticosteroid therapy to 5-year survival rates of 65% in 1947–1968 and approximately 80% more recently (43,44). This improvement is probably the result of many factors, including better general medical care, earlier diagnosis, and improved treatment of the myositis syndromes. The rarity and heterogeneity of myositis has limited the collection of such data, yet a number of studies have attempted to define prognostic factors in the IIM (Table 15.11).

Studies imply that poor prognostic factors include the following: polymyositis as opposed to dermatomyositis, older age, associated malignancy, cardiopulmonary disease, severe weakness, longer duration of weakness before diagnosis, fever, dysphagia, IBM, or antisynthetase or antisignal recognition particle autoantibodies (24,25). Some serologic findings predict a more benign myositis course. These include anti-Mi-2, anti-PM-Scl, and anti-U1RNP autoantibodies (4,8).

MANAGEMENT

General Considerations

Therapy must be individualized, taking into account prognostic factors, severity of disease, and risk factors for the adverse events associated with each therapeutic agent. It is more difficult to assess disease severity, especially in chronic cases, than is often appreciated. This is because of the absence of generally accepted validated tools to assess and distinguish myositis disease activity (defined as inflammatory changes that may respond to immunosuppressive therapy) from disease damage (defined as irreversible changes that result from prior disease activity). Also, there are few validated tools to assess any of the extramuscular manifestations of IIM, and there is a lack of a "gold standard" for disease activity (45).

The past decade has seen a shift from the traditional approach of stepped therapy—in which a structured series of first-line, second-line, and third-line agents is prescribed in rigid chronological order as disease severity increases—to more individualized, and often more aggressive, forms of therapy that take into account the risk profile for poor prognostic outcomes.

Rehabilitation

The goal of all therapy is to optimize the functional levels of patients and, if possible, to return them to normal. In this regard, physical and occupational therapy remain underutilized. Graded rehabilitation that takes into account the stage and severity of the patient's myositis is the best approach (46). Although bed rest is often necessary during periods of severe disease, passive range-of-motion exercises and stretching should be initiated early, especially in very debilitated, hospitalized patients, to prevent the formation of contractures. As the degree of myositis decreases, patients should increase their activity through stages: active-assisted range of motion, followed by isometric, then isotonic, and, finally, aerobic exercise.

Therapeutic Approaches for Myositis

Corticosteroids remain the primary therapy for the IIM and should be initiated as early as possible in nearly all patients. Factors important in determining corticosteroid responses are an adequate initial dose (in most cases at least 1 mg/kg/day), continuation of prednisone until or after the serum CK becomes normal, and a slow rate of prednisone tapering (47). The roles of pulse corticosteroids and alternate-day therapy as treatment remain unclear. Those individuals with poor prognostic factors should be considered for more aggressive therapy, using corticosteroids with an added cytotoxic agent from the beginning of their disease.

The clinical and serologic groups differ in the rapidity of myositis onset, severity of disease, responses to therapy, and clinical course (Fig. 15.6). The treatment of IBM remains controversial, and most patients with IBM do not respond to therapy as well as patients in the other clinical groups. Some patients with IBM, however, may benefit from corticosteroid and cytotoxic therapy in terms of slowing the rate of progression of disease (48,49). Although most patients have at least a partial response to corticosteroids, some do not respond adequately, many more experience disease activity increases during steroid tapering, and most eventually suffer from the toxicities of corticosteroids. Little is known about optimal therapy in corticosteroid-resistant patients. Oral methotrexate, at doses of 7.5 to 25 mg/week, and azathioprine, at 50 to 150 mg/day, are the major therapeutic options for corticosteroid-resistant patients (25). A combination of methotrexate and azathioprine leads to improvement in some patients who have had inadequate responses to either agent given alone (50). Intravenous gammaglobulin (IVIg), cyclophosphamide, cyclosporine A, FK506, chlorambucil, high-dose intravenous methotrexate with leucovorin rescue, or other combinations of cytotoxics may be beneficial in some patients and warrant further evaluation. A double-blind, placebo-controlled trial has shown that intravenous gammaglobulin at least transiently increases strength and decreases CK, rash, and muscle inflammation in some DM patients (51). Nonetheless, the long-term efficacy and safety, usefulness in other IIM groups, and cost-effectiveness of intravenous gammaglobulin have been questioned. Novel therapies using biologic antiinflammatory agents and autologous stem cell transplants are now under study and may represent important advances in the treatment of myositis in the future.

The treatment of IBM is controversial. Retrospective reviews of corticosteroid and cytotoxic therapy, a prospective open trial of intravenous gammaglobulin, and a randomized trial of combination oral methotrexate–azathioprine versus high-dose methotrexate with leucovorin rescue, all suggest that the rate of deterioration may be decreased or stabilized and strength improved in IBM patients with evidence of active myositis.

Many organ systems may be affected in IIM and cause significant morbidity and mortality. General symptoms of fatigue, fever, and weight loss often respond to corticosteroid or cytotoxic therapy for the underlying myositis. Raynaud phenomenon may respond to avoidance of the cold or calcium channel blockers. The rash of dermatomyositis may be a very troublesome problem for the patient and may persist long after the myositis has resolved. In addition to avoidance of sun and photosensitizers, topical sunscreens and steroids may be helpful, but often hydroxychloroquine or methotrexate is required. Some authors have used quinacrine successfully, and isotretinoin, despite teratogenic concerns, may be useful in treating IIM rashes (4). Subcutaneous calcifications, more common in children than in adults, can be very troubling. No treatment, other than therapy for the underlying myositis, has improved the calcifications. Pulmonary fibrosis is a worrisome complication in IIM patients, and some patients do not improve with any therapy. Yet methotrexate, pulse corticosteroids, and cyclophosphamide are often tried in an attempt to treat this cause of great morbidity and mortality. The role of pulmonary transplantation in pulmonary dysfunction associated with systemic autoimmune disease remains unclear, but anecdotal reports suggest successful outcomes in some patients. Symptomatic cardiac disease should be treated with diuretics or digitalis to resolve heart failure, antiarrhythmics as needed, and corticosteroids and cytotoxics if evidence of myocarditis is present. Some patients have such severe dysphagia and are at such risk of aspiration that tube feedings are necessary. Reflux esophagitis is common and should be treated by the usual approaches of elevating the head of the bed, prescribing antacids, or H_2-receptor antagonists. Cricopharyngeal dysfunction can be the cause of significant dysphagia and odynophagia and may improve with myotomy.

REFERENCES

1. Plotz PH, Dalakas M, Leff RL, et al. Current concepts in the idiopathic inflammatory myopathies: polymyositis, dermatomyositis, and related disorders. *Ann Intern Med* 1989;111: 143–157.
2. Targoff IN. Dermatomyositis and polymyositis. *Curr Prob Dermatol* 1991;3:131–180.
3. Plotz PH, Rider LG, Targoff IN, et al. Myositis: immunologic contributions to understanding cause, pathogenesis, and therapy. *Ann Int Med* 1995;122:715–724.
4. Oddis CV. Therapy of inflammatory myopathy. *Rheum Dis Clin North Am* 1994;20:899–918.
5. Bohan A, Peter JB, Bowman RL, et al. Computer-assisted analysis of 153 patients with polymyositis and dermatomyositis. *Medicine (Baltimore)* 1977;56:255–286.
6. Targoff IN, Miller FW, Medsger TAJ, et al. Classification criteria for the idiopathic inflammatory myopathies. *Curr Opin Rheumatol* 1997;9:527–535.
7. Miller FW. Myositis-specific autoantibodies. Touchstones for understanding the inflammatory myopathies (clinical conference). *JAMA* 1993;270:1846–1849.
8. Targoff IN. Immune manifestations of inflammatory muscle disease. *Rheum Dis Clin North Am* 1994;20:857–880.
9. Fraser DD, Frank JA, Dalakas M, et al. Magnetic resonance imaging in the idiopathic inflammatory myopathies. *J Rheumatol* 1991;18:1693–1700.
10. Park JH, Olsen NJ, King L Jr, et al. Use of magnetic resonance imaging and P-31 magnetic resonance spectroscopy to detect and quantify muscle dysfunction in the amyopathic and myopathic variants of dermatomyositis. *Arthritis Rheum* 1995;38:68–77.
11. Love LA, Miller FW. Understanding the idiopathic inflammatory myopathies. *Contemp Internal Med* 1995;7:29–43.
12. Lotz BP, Engel AG, Nishino H, et al. Inclusion body myositis. Observations in 40 patients. *Brain* 1989;112:727–747.
13. Griggs RC, Askanas V, DiMauro S, et al. Inclusion body myositis and myopathies. *Ann Neurol* 1995;38:705–713.
14. Sigurgeirsson B, Lindelöf B, Edhag O, et al. Risk of cancer in patients with dermatomyositis or polymyositis: a population-based study. *N Engl J Med* 1992;326:363–367.
15. Moxley RT. Evaluation of neuromuscular function in inflammatory myopathy. *Rheum Dis Clin North Am* 1994;20:827–843.
16. Kagen LJ. Inflammatory muscle disease. Management. In: Klippel JH, Dieppe PA, eds. *Rheumatology.* St Louis: CV Mosby, 1994:14.1–14.4.
17. Franks AG. Important cutaneous markers of dermatomyositis. *J Musculoskelet Med* 1988;5:39–63.
18. Kasteler JS, Callen JP. Scalp involvement in dermatomyositis: often overlooked or misdiagnosed. *JAMA* 1994;272:1939–1941.
19. Rider LG, Miller FW. Laboratory evaluation of the inflammatory myopathies. *Clin Diagn Lab Immunol* 1995;2:1–9.
20. Bohlmeyer TJ, Wu AH, Perryman MB. Evaluation of laboratory tests as a guide to diagnosis and therapy of myositis. *Rheum Dis Clin North Am* 1994;20:845–856.

21. Kroll M, Otis J, Kagen L. Serum enzyme, myoglobin and muscle strength relationships in polymyositis and dermatomyositis. *J Rheumatol* 1986;13:349–355.

22. Summers RM, Brune AM, Choyke PL, et al. Juvenile idiopathic inflammatory myopathy: exercise-induced changes in muscle at short inversion time inversion-recovery MR imaging. *Radiology* 1998;209:191–196.

23. Dalakas MC. Polymyositis, dermatomyositis and inclusion-body myositis. *N Engl J Med* 1991;325:1487–1498.

24. Miller FW. Classification and prognosis of inflammatory muscle disease. *Rheum Dis Clin North Am* 1994;20:811–826.

25. Joffe MM, Love LA, Leff RL, et al. Drug therapy of the idiopathic inflammatory myopathies: predictors of response to prednisone, azathioprine, and methotrexate and a comparison of their efficacy. *Am J Med* 1993;94:379–387.

26. Euwer RL, Sontheimer RD. Amyopathic dermatomyositis (dermatomyositis sine myositis): presentation of six new cases and review of the literature. *J Am Acad Dermatol* 1991;24:959–966.

27. Emslie-Smith AM, Engel AG. Microvascular changes in early and advanced dermatomyositis: a quantitative study. *Ann Neurol* 1990;27:343–356.

28. Love LA, Leff RL, Fraser DD, et al. A new approach to the classification of idiopathic inflammatory myopathy: myositis-specific autoantibodies define useful homogeneous patient groups. *Medicine* 1991;70:360–374.

29. Rider LG, Miller FW, Targoff IN, et al. A broadened spectrum of juvenile myositis: myositis-specific autoantibodies in children. *Arthritis Rheum* 1994;37:1534–1538.

30. Rider LG, Miller FW. Classification and treatment of the juvenile idiopathic inflammatory myopathies. *Rheum Dis Clin North Am* 1997;23:619–655.

31. Pachman LM, Miller FW. Idiopathic inflammatory myopathies: dermatomyositis, polymyositis and related disorders. In: Frank MM, Austin KF, Claman HN, eds. *Samter's immunologic diseases.* Boston: Little, Brown, 1995:791–803.

32. Sakon M, Monden M, Fujimoto Y, et al. Gastric carcinoma associated with dermatomyositis. *Acta Chir Scand* 1989;155:365–366.

33. Whitmore SE, Rosenshein NB, Provost TT. Ovarian cancer in patients with dermatomyositis. *Medicine (Baltimore)* 1994;73:153–160.

34. Basset-Seguin N, Roujeau JC, Gherardi R, et al. Prognostic factors and predictive signs of malignancy in adult dermatomyositis: a study of 32 cases. *Arch Dermatol* 1990;126:633–637.

35. Engel AG, Franzini-Armstrong C. *Myology,* 2nd ed. New York: McGraw-Hill, 1994;1–1937.

36. Scott IU, Siatkowski RM. Idiopathic orbital myositis. *Curr Opin Rheumatol* 1997;9:504–512.

37. Moreno-Lugris C, Gonzalez-Gay MA, Sanchez-Andrade A, et al. Magnetic resonance imaging: a useful technique in the diagnosis and follow up of focal myositis. *Ann Rheum Dis* 1996;55:856.

38. Rider LG, Gurley RC, Pandey JP, et al. Clinical, serologic, and immunogenetic features of familial idiopathic inflammatory myopathy. *Arthritis Rheum* 1998;41:710–719.

39. Shamim E, Miller FW. Familial autoimmunity and the idiopathic inflammatory myopathies. *Curr Rheumatol Rep* 2000;2:201–211.

40. Love LA, Miller FW. Noninfectious environmental agents associated with myopathies. *Curr Opin Rheum* 1993;5:712–718.

41. Miller FW. Genetics of environmentally associated rheumatic disease. In: Kaufman LD, Varga J, eds. *Rheumatic diseases and the environment.* London: Arnold Publishers, 1999:33–45.

42. Engel AG, Arahata K. Mononuclear cells in myopathies: quantitation of functionally distinct subsets, recognition of antigen-specific cell-mediated cytotoxicity in some diseases, and implications for the pathogenesis of the different inflammatory myopathies. *Hum Pathol* 1986;17:704–721.

43. Medsger TA, Robinson H, Masi AT. Factors affecting survivorship in polymyositis. *Arthritis Rheum* 1971;14:249–258.

44. Hochberg MC, Feldman D, Stevens MB. Adult onset polymyositis/dermatomyositis: an analysis of clinical and laboratory features and survival in 76 patients with a review of the literature. *Semin Arthritis Rheum* 1986;15:168–178.

45. Rider LG. Assessment of disease activity and its sequelae in children and adults with myositis. *Curr Opin Rheumatol* 1996;8:495–506.

46. Hicks JE. Rehabilitation of patients with myositis. In: Klippel JH, Dieppe PA, eds. *Rheumatology.* St Louis: CV Mosby, 1994;15.4–15.6.

47. Oddis CV. Therapy for myositis. *Curr Opin Rheumatol* 1993;5:742–748.

48. Cohen MR, Sulaiman AR, Garancis JC, et al. Clinical heterogeneity and treatment response in inclusion body myositis. *Arthritis Rheum* 1989;32:734–740.

49. Leff RL, Miller FW, Hicks J, et al. The treatment of inclusion body myositis: a retrospective review and a randomized, prospective trial of immunosuppressive therapy. *Medicine (Baltimore)* 1993;72:225–235.

50. Villalba L, Hicks JE, Adams EM, et al. Treatment of refractory myositis: a randomized crossover study of two new cytotoxic regimens. *Arthritis Rheum* 1998;41:392–399.

51. Dalakas MC, Illa I, Dambrosia JM, et al. A controlled trial of high-dose intravenous immune globulin infusions as treatment for dermatomyositis. *N Engl J Med* 1993;329:1993–2000.

52. Sokoloff MC, Goldberg LS, Pearson CM. Treatment of corticosteroid-resistant polymyositis with methotrexate. *Lancet* 1971;1:14–16.

VASCULITIS

KENNETH E. SACK

The term *vasculitis* literally means "inflammation of blood vessels." It refers to a host of conditions with multiple causes and, depending on the size of the involved vessels, multiple consequences. The various forms of vasculitis are usually classified by the size of the affected vessel, but they might just as well be categorized by their etiology or histopathologic findings. Additionally, a given type of vasculitis may affect vessels of varying sizes, and similar histopathologic findings may occur in a variety of vasculitides, irrespective of their cause.

Although certain clinical features can suggest vasculitis, biopsy of the affected tissue is necessary to confirm the diagnosis. Awareness of this fact becomes paramount when one is contemplating use of potentially toxic therapy. Furthermore, the histopathologic finding of inflammation in a vessel wall does not necessarily indicate the cause of the vascular damage. And an angiogram showing vascular irregularities, aneurysms, and stenoses is not necessarily diagnostic of vasculitis (Table 16.1).

One should keep these caveats in mind as clinical descriptions of several stereotypic vasculitis syndromes are presented.

TABLE 16.1. ANGIOGRAPHIC MIMICKERS OF VASCULITIS

Amyloidosis
Atrial myxoma
Cold exposure
Drug abuse
Dye injection
Ehlers–Danlos syndrome
Fibromuscular dysplasia
Hypertension
Infection
Migraine
Moyamoya
Neurofibromatosis
Neoplasia
Pseudoxanthoma elasticum
Radiation exposure
Reperfusion of normal vessels
Thrombotic thrombocytopenic purpura
Trauma

VASCULITIS AFFECTING PREDOMINANTLY SMALL VESSELS

Hypersensitivity Vasculitis

Epidemiology

Hypersensitivity vasculitis represents an immune response to an exogenous substance, most often a drug; it primarily affects arterioles and venules. Precise data on its incidence are lacking, but its prevalence is approximately 3 to 6/100,000. Both genders and all ethnic groups are equally susceptible.

Pathophysiology/Pathogenesis

The finding of various antigens (e.g., infectious agents), immunoglobulins, and complement components by immunofluorescent study of early cutaneous lesions suggests that immune complexes mediate this condition.

Clinical Features

Palpable purpura (Fig. 16.1), the characteristic feature of hypersensitivity vasculitis, typically appears rapidly, with lesions ranging from 3 to 6 mm and occasionally up to 1 cm in diameter. Some lesions become confluent and form plaques. Although the vasculitis is usually limited to the skin, arthralgias or arthritis, and constitutional symptoms such as fever, malaise, or fatigue may occur.

Clinical Evaluation

Laboratory abnormalities are nonspecific and include leukocytosis, thrombocytosis, eosinophilia, elevated erythrocyte sedimentation rate (ESR), and reduced serum complement. Microhematuria may occur, but renal failure is uncommon. Biopsy of a skin lesion typically shows leukocytoclastic vasculitis (i.e., neutrophils and nuclear fragments in and around the walls of arterioles and venules), accompanied occasionally by eosinophils. Rarely, lymphocytes predominate.

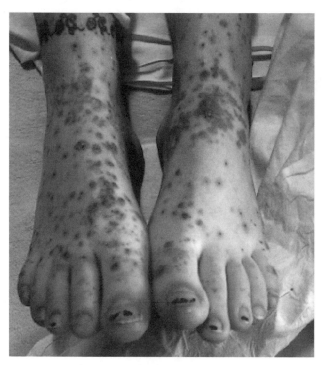

FIGURE 16.1. Palpable purpura in a young woman (courtesy Dr. Jonathan Graf). See Color Plate 4.

Differential diagnosis includes other vasculitides that affect small vessels. These are Henoch–Schönlein purpura, cryoglobulinemia, Wegener granulomatosis, Churg–Strauss syndrome, autoimmune diseases (e.g., systemic lupus erythematosus, rheumatoid arthritis, Sjögren syndrome), infection, malignancy, coagulopathies, and atheromatous emboli.

Treatment

Hypersensitivity vasculitis usually remits after removing the offending agent, but temporary use of corticosteroids may become necessary.

Henoch–Schönlein Purpura

Epidemiology

Henoch–Schönlein purpura (HSP) is the most common form of childhood vasculitis, striking approximately 10/100,000 children per year. It typically affects males less than 20 years of age, with a peak incidence at about age 5.

Pathophysiology/Pathogenesis

HSP is probably an immune-complex-mediated disease; the complexes—whether from the patient's serum or affected tissues—invariably contain immunoglobulin A (IgA). The cause is unknown, but infection and exposure to drugs are common triggers.

Clinical Features

Purpura, arthritis, abdominal pain, gastrointestinal (GI) hemorrhage, and glomerulonephritis characterize HSP. The skin lesions appear in gravity-dependent areas such as the buttocks and legs, and consist of purpura or petechiae occurring within erythematous maculopapules or in areas of urticaria. Cramping abdominal pain, with or without occult GI bleeding, ordinarily follows but sometimes precedes the skin lesions. The joint pain is short-lived, usually involves the knees and ankles, and is accompanied by periarticular swelling. Angioedema is common, affecting the face and extremities, and occasionally the scrotum.

Severe intestinal hemorrhage is rare; other GI complications include ileocolic intussusception, infarction or perforation of bowel, pancreatitis, and hydrops of the gallbladder. Renal manifestations develop in about 20% of the patients and range from transient microscopic hematuria to those of rapidly progressive glomerulonephritis. In most cases, however, renal function ultimately returns to normal.

Involvement of other organs in HSP may include scrotal swelling and hemorrhage, testicular pain, headache, seizures, intracerebral hemorrhage or infarction, subarachnoid hemorrhage, and pulmonary hemorrhage.

Laboratory Evaluation

Mild anemia is common and results from chronic inflammation, GI blood loss, or both. Hematuria and proteinuria characteristically signal glomerulonephritis. Histopathologic examination of a purpuric skin lesion typically shows leukocytoclastic vasculitis. Renal histopathology ranges from mild proliferation of mesangial cells to crescentic glomerulonephritis. Deposition of IgA in an involved organ (e.g., skin, kidney, or intestine), or an elevation in serum IgA levels occurs frequently and is virtually specific for HSP.

Treatment

Because full recovery is the rule, supportive care usually suffices. In patients with evidence of aggressive glomerulonephritis, treatment with corticosteroids, immunosuppressive drugs, and anticoagulants has yielded variable results.

Wegener Granulomatosis

Epidemiology

Wegener granulomatosis (WG) is a relatively rare granulomatous vasculitis affecting primarily the upper respiratory tract, lung parenchyma, and kidneys. The disease typically appears in whites in their fourth or fifth decades and is slightly more common in men.

Pathogenesis

The triggering event in WG is unknown, but patients with active disease typically have antibodies directed against cytoplasmic components of neutrophils (ANCAs), more specifically, antiserine proteinase 3. When inflammatory mediators prime the neutrophil, serine proteinase 3 (PR-3) translocates to the cell surface, where it can interact with ANCAs. The activated neutrophil is then able to interact with endothelial cells and induce vasculitis. T-lymphocytes directed against PR-3 may also participate in this process.

Clinical Features

Most patients have evidence of respiratory and kidney disease. Acute or chronic sinusitis, nasal ulceration or obstruction, and necrosis of nasal cartilage (occasionally causing saddle-nose deformity) are common, but oral ulcers, gingival hypertrophy, scleritis, orbital pseudotumor, inflammation of the external and internal ear, and subglottic tracheal stenosis may also occur. Cough, chest pain, dyspnea, and hemoptysis indicate lower respiratory tract disease. Additional manifestations sometimes include myalgias, arthralgias and arthritis, purpuric or ulcerative skin lesions, peripheral neuropathy, cerebral infarction, GI ulceration, and cardiac ischemia. Rarely, WG presents with localized organ involvement (e.g., lower genitourinary tract, breast). Renal involvement ranges from mild glomerulonephritis to rapidly progressive renal failure. Occasionally, the disease remains localized to the upper respiratory tract ("limited WG").

Laboratory Evaluation

In addition to the nonspecific markers that typify chronic inflammation, hematuria, pyuria, and proteinuria signify renal involvement. Nodular, often cavitary, infiltrates in the middle and lower lung fields are characteristic radiographic findings. Most patients with active systemic disease have anti PR-3 antibodies that produce a cytoplasmic pattern on immunofluorescent staining of ethanol-fixed neutrophils (c-ANCA). A smaller percentage has the more nonspecific antimyeloperoxidase antibodies, yielding a perinuclear staining pattern (p-ANCA). The diagnosis is reasonably certain if the patient has characteristic symptoms and signs together with a positive test for c-ANCA. Nevertheless, diagnostic confirmation requires histopathologic evidence of tissue necrosis and granuloma formation. In patients with abnormal chest x-rays, lung biopsy can help establish the diagnosis while ruling out an infectious process. Renal

histopathologic findings are nonspecific and usually show a crescentic glomerulonephritis with varying amounts of fibrinoid necrosis.

Treatment

Systemic corticosteroids temporarily alleviate some of the inflammatory manifestations but do not affect long-term survival. Cytotoxic drugs, however, particularly cyclophosphamide, dramatically improve the prognosis. Initial therapy for active disease typically consists of prednisone 1 mg/kg/day plus cyclophosphamide 2 mg/kg/day. Rapid tapering and eventual discontinuation of prednisone are usually possible after disease manifestations abate. A maintenance dose of cyclophosphamide between 1 and 1.5 mg/kg/day usually allows the peripheral WBC count to remain at a safe level (>3,000/mm³). Although azathioprine is not effective for inducing a remission, it may be an acceptable substitute for cyclophosphamide once the disease is quiescent. Methotrexate is sometimes effective in patients who cannot tolerate cyclophosphamide. Trimethoprim/sulfa may also suppress disease activity, especially in patients with limited WG.

Churg–Strauss Syndrome

Churg–Strauss syndrome (CSS), also termed *allergic granulomatosis* and *angiitis,* is a rare disorder, usually affecting middle-aged men. It consists of asthma, peripheral eosinophilia, and an accompanying vasculitis of various organ systems.

Pathogenesis

The cause is unknown, but the increased serum levels of IgE and peripheral eosinophilia in untreated patients suggest an allergic component. Most patients have ANCAs, which may play a role in injuring vessel walls.

Clinical Features

Patients typically have a long-standing history of allergic rhinitis, frequently with nasal polyposis. Asthma ordinarily begins in middle age and gradually increases in severity. A dramatic remission in the asthma often heralds the onset of systemic vasculitis that may affect lungs, heart, peripheral nerves, gastrointestinal tract, skin, or kidneys. Arthralgias and arthritis occur in up to half of the patients. Severe renal disease is uncommon.

Laboratory Evaluation

Peripheral eosinophilia, often greater than 10,000/mm³, is the rule. Many patients also have pANCAs, usually with antimyeloperoxidase activity. Chest radiographs typically show migratory or transitory pulmonary infiltrates. Biopsy of affected tissues shows granulomatous or nongranulomatous vasculitis along with extravascular necrotizing granulomas. The predominant renal lesion is a focal segmental glomerulonephritis.

Treatment

Prednisone in a dose of 40 to 60 mg/day induces a favorable response in most patients. When such treatment fails, the addition of azathioprine or cyclophosphamide is usually effective. Most patients do well, with a 50-year survival of greater than 50%.

OTHER SMALL-VESSEL VASCULITIDES

Behçet Disease

Behçet disease is an inflammatory disorder characterized by recurrent oral aphthous ulcers, genital ulcers, uveitis, and skin lesions. Cases tend to cluster around the ancient "Silk Route," which extends from eastern Asia to the Mediterranean basin. The disease is most common in Turkey (100 to 400 cases 100,000 population). Its prevalence in Middle and Far Eastern countries ranges from 10 to 20 cases per 100,000, and in Western countries, it occurs in less than one out of every 100,000 people.

The cause is unknown. Nevertheless, hyperfunction of neutrophils, altered immune responses, hypercoagulability, and injury to small vessels are common findings. Additionally, involvement of the vasa vasorum may lead to damage of large vessels.

Behçet disease typically begins in the third or fourth decade of life. Oral ulceration is usually the first symptom and may precede other manifestations by years. Cutaneous and mucosal lesions are self-limited, but uveitis may recur and cause blindness. Less frequently, the disease affects the gastrointestinal tract, central nervous system, and large blood vessels. Erythema nodosum is common in female patients, while chronic progressive central nervous system disease occurs more frequently in males.

Diagnosis rests primarily on clinical findings. Pathergy—the occurrence of a 2-mm or larger erythematous nodule or pustule 48 hours after pricking the skin with a sterile 20-G needle—is a relatively specific phenomenon. However, it occurs infrequently in non-Mediterranean populations and may be seen in patients with Sweet syndrome (a neutrophilic dermatosis) and in those with pyoderma gangrenosum.

Treatment is largely symptomatic, consisting mainly of nonsteroidal antiinflammatory drugs and topical application of steroids, antihistamines, or antibiotics. Recalcitrant disease or involvement of vital organs may require the use of colchicine, sulfasalazine, oral corticosteroids, or immuno-

suppressive agents. Prognosis depends primarily on the extent of organ involvement and the rapidity of treatment.

Microscopic Polyangiitis

Microscopic polyangiitis is a disease of unknown cause affecting arterioles, capillaries, and venules. It is slightly more common in men and typically begins at about 50 years of age. Although glomerulonephritis, with or without pulmonary hemorrhage, is the predominant manifestation, diffuse pulmonary infiltrates, gastrointestinal pain or bleeding, arthralgias or arthritis, peripheral neuropathy, and purpuric skin lesions may also occur. Laboratory findings are nonspecific, but two-thirds of the patients have serum perinuclear–antineutrophil cytoplasmic antibodies (pANCA), directed predominantly against myeloperoxidase. Renal biopsy typically shows focal pauciimmune segmental necrotizing glomerulonephritis with crescents. Treatment with corticosteroids induces a clinical remission in some patients, but many others require the addition of an immunosuppressive agent such as cyclophosphamide or azathioprine.

Cryoglobulinemic Vasculitis

Cryoglobulins are immunoglobulins that precipitate at cold temperatures and dissolve as the temperature rises. Vasculitis occurs when cryoglobulins deposit in the walls of arterioles, capillaries, and venules. Purpura, arthralgias, and glomerulonephritis are common manifestations, although virtually any organ may be affected. Cryoglobulinemia accompanies a variety of illnesses, the most frequent being infection with hepatitis C virus. Many patients also have a reduction in serum complement level. Treating the underlying cause of cryoglobulinemia sometimes alleviates symptoms, but often the vasculitis requires addition of nonsteroidal antiinflammatory drugs, colchicine, corticosteroids, or immunosuppressive agents. When the concentration of cryoglobulins is high, plasmapheresis may be beneficial.

Miscellaneous Conditions

Small-vessel vasculitis may accompany a variety of infectious, neoplastic, and autoimmune diseases. Treating the underlying condition often alleviates the vasculitis.

VASCULITIS AFFECTING PREDOMINANTLY MEDIUM-SIZED VESSELS

Polyarteritis Nodosa

Epidemiology

Polyarteritis nodosa (PAN) is a necrotizing vasculitis involving predominantly peripheral nerves, intestinal tract, kidneys, skin, and joints. It is a rare disorder, affecting less than one out of 100,000 people per year. Middle-aged adults of all racial groups are the usual targets.

Pathophysiology/Pathogenesis

The vasculitis likely results from complexes of immunoglobulin and antigen (e.g., viral) that deposit in the vessel wall, activate the complement cascade, and attract neutrophils. CD4+ lymphocytes and ANCAs may also play a role.

Clinical Features

Patients may present with constitutional symptoms (e.g., malaise, fever, and weight loss), myalgias or arthralgias, or evidence of ischemia of major organs. Typical manifestations include mononeuritis multiplex, cutaneous lesions [e.g., livedo reticularis (Fig. 16.2), papulopetechial eruptions, digital gangrene], hypertension, renal insufficiency, abdominal pain, gastrointestinal bleeding, coronary insufficiency, and orchitis. Symptoms referable to the central nervous system are uncommon and usually appear several years after the onset of the disease. Occasionally, PAN affects a single organ system without evidence of systemic disease.

Laboratory Evaluation

Signs of chronic inflammation (e.g., anemia, leukocytosis, elevated ESR), or abnormal liver function tests may be the only laboratory abnormalities. Many patients, however,

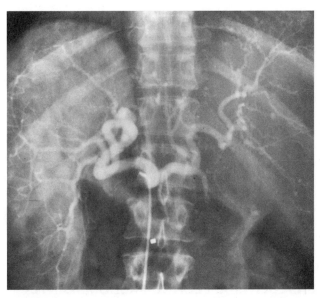

FIGURE 16.3. Visceral angiogram showing stenoses, dilatations, and small aneurysms in small and medium-sized arteries (courtesy Dr. Kenneth Fye).

have hematuria, proteinuria, an elevated serum creatinine level, and evidence of infection with hepatitis B virus. ANCAs, usually directed against myeloperoxidase, occur in a small percentage of cases. Characteristic angiographic abnormalities include microaneurysms, occlusions, and irregularities of visceral arteries (Fig. 16.3). Diagnostic confirmation requires evidence of necrotizing vasculitis of medium-sized arteries (e.g., 0.5 to 1 mm in diameter). Common biopsy sites are skin, muscle, or sural nerve.

Treatment

The prognosis is poor, especially in patients with proteinuria of more than 1g/day, renal insufficiency, cardiomyopathy, gastrointestinal involvement, or central nervous system disease. Use of corticosteroids usually causes substantial improvement, but additional treatment with cytotoxic drugs is often necessary. Azathioprine in doses of 2 to 2.5 mg/kg/day is frequently effective and well tolerated. When organ-threatening disease is present, cyclophosphamide is required. The usual oral regimen of 2 mg/kg/day may cause hemorrhagic cystitis or bladder malignancy. Intravenous injections of 1 g/m²/month are safer, but their efficacy is unproven. Studies in France have shown impressive survival in patients with hepatitis B–related PAN who receive plasmapheresis and antiviral agents (vidarabine or IFNα-2b) without other immunosuppressive treatment.

Kawasaki Disease

Kawasaki disease (KD), formerly known as mucocutaneous lymph node syndrome, is an acute systemic vasculitis pre-

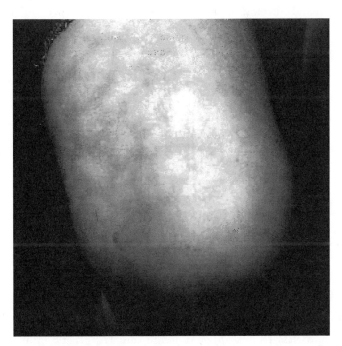

FIGURE 16.2. Livedo reticularis (courtesy Dr. Jonathan Graf). See Color Plate 5.

dominantly affecting Asian, black, and white children, in descending order. Its acute, self-limited nature, seasonal incidence, geographic clustering, and predilection for children suggest an infectious etiology. Typical manifestations include high fevers, conjunctival injection, fissuring or crusting of the lips, strawberry tongue, oropharyngeal erythema, cervical adenopathy, erythema of the palms and soles, and eventual desquamation of the skin of the hands and feet. Although KD also affects the lungs, kidneys, gastrointestinal tract, and nervous system, its most dreaded complication is that of coronary arteritis. Such involvement can lead to the formation of aneurysms and subsequent stenosis or atherosclerosis of affected vessels. Treatment with aspirin and intravenous immunoglobulin has greatly reduced the long-term morbidity of this disease.

VASCULITIS AFFECTING PREDOMINANTLY LARGE VESSELS

Giant Cell Arteritis

Epidemiology

Giant cell arteritis (GCA) characteristically affects the large and medium-sized extracranial arteries of the head and neck. It occurs almost exclusively in whites more than 50 years of age, and for unknown reasons is more common in northern than in southern regions of the United States and Europe.

Pathophysiology/Pathogenesis

Patients with GCA share a common sequence of amino acids in the antigen-binding cleft of an HLA-DR molecule, possibly setting the stage for a specific immune response to an exogenous, endogenous, or altered self-antigen in the vessel wall. T cells are likely the prime mediators of the vascular injury.

Clinical Manifestations

Fever (often exceeding 39°C), malaise, and weight loss are common and may be the only manifestations of GCA. As many as 40% of patients have aching and stiffness in the neck, shoulders, or pelvic girdle—characteristic symptoms of polymyalgia rheumatica. Inflammation and narrowing of cranial vessels may cause headache, tenderness over the temporal artery, loss of vision (usually abrupt), jaw "claudication" (i.e., pain in the muscles of mastication during chewing), or gangrene of the scalp or tongue. In patients with visual impairment, initial funduscopic examination may be normal or show signs of ischemic optic neuropathy. Inflammation of the aortic arch and its branches occurs in 10% to 15% of patients and may cause reduced blood pressure in one or both upper extremities, arm claudication, focal cerebral ischemia, or aneurysm of the affected aorta. Involvement of skin, peripheral nerves, kidneys, heart, lungs, or intracranial vessels is rare.

Laboratory Evaluation

In most cases, the ESR and C-reactive protein (CRP) are markedly elevated. Rarely, they are in the normal range. Many patients also have increased levels of hepatic enzymes. Histopathologic examination of an affected temporal artery shows mononuclear and giant cells in the media, thickening of the intima, and fragmentation of the internal elastic lamina. Because involvement of the artery is patchy, obtaining a specimen at least 4 to 5 cm in length is essential. In addition, the yield of a positive biopsy increases in patients with symptoms or signs referable to cranial vessels.

Treatment

GCA is a medical emergency. Early treatment with 0.5 to 1 mg/kg/d corticosteroids is critical in preventing irreversible loss of vision. Such treatment for up to 1 week will not affect the findings on temporal artery biopsy. After symptoms subside and the ESR (or CRP) returns to normal, steroids may be tapered slowly to a maintenance range of 10 to 20 mg/day. Return of symptoms or a rise in ESR usually necessitates an increase in steroid dosage. In the rare patient who requires prolonged treatment with high-dose steroids, addition of an immunosuppressive agent such as methotrexate may become necessary. Although most clinicians terminate treatment after 2 years, studies have shown active disease on temporal artery biopsy after 9 years of steroid therapy. Consequently, managing patients with GCA demands relentless vigilance.

Takayasu Arteritis

Epidemiology

Takayasu arteritis (TA) affects predominantly the aorta and its primary branches, usually in women of reproductive age. Although once considered a disease of Asians, TA is now known to occur in all ethnic groups. Its estimated incidence in the United States is 2.6 cases per million persons per year.

Pathogenesis/Pathophysiology

The frequent association of circulating immune complexes and autoantibodies with TA suggests that disordered humoral immunity plays a causative role. T-lymphocytes that recognize heat shock proteins probably contribute to the vascular damage as well. Despite the fact that familial clustering occasionally occurs and that certain class I HLA antigens accompany TA, genetic influences appear weak.

Clinical Manifestations

Nonspecific symptoms (e.g., malaise, fever, weight loss, myalgias, arthralgias, headache) are common and can occur at any time during the course of the illness. More characteristic, however, is evidence of vascular insufficiency of an organ or extremity such as limb claudication, postural dizziness, visual disturbances, arterial bruits, or reduced or absent pulses. Systemic hypertension—consequent to aortic or renal artery stenosis—is common but may be overlooked if blood pressure readings are not obtained in both arms. Mild to moderate pulmonary hypertension also is common but is not often clinically apparent. Congestive heart failure occurs more frequently in children than in adults and results from systemic hypertension, valvular regurgitation, myocarditis, or coronary artery disease. A variety of retinal vascular lesions may appear, but the usual funduscopic findings are those of hypertensive retinopathy. Skin manifestations include palpable purpura, erythema nodosum, and pyoderma gangrenosum.

Laboratory Evaluation

An elevated ESR typifies active disease, but a normal ESR does not preclude ongoing vascular inflammation. Chest radiographs may show widening or irregularities of the aorta, evidence of pulmonary hypertension, or notching of the ribs. Invasive or magnetic resonance angiography shows characteristic stenosis or aneurysm in the aorta or its major branches.

Treatment

Glucocorticoids are the mainstay of treatment. Dose adjustments are made according to the patient's symptoms and ESR, but predicting active disease is often difficult. Methotrexate is usually effective in allowing a reduction in steroid dosage. Controlling blood pressure is critical in preventing morbidity and mortality from congestive heart failure and cerebrovascular accidents. When medications fail to control hypertension, angioplasty—with or without stenting—of a stenosed renal artery may yield lasting benefit.

Mimickers of Vasculitis

Any form of vascular damage can produce the same signs and symptoms as those of true vasculitis (Table 16.1). That damage can result from ischemic processes, neoplasia, infection, drug effects, exposure to cold, congenital or inherited abnormalities, and ailments such as sarcoidosis and Moyamoya disease. Thus digital ischemia or unexplained organ failure could represent atheromatous emboli or cardiac myxoma just as well as polyarteritis nodosa. Consequently, maintaining an ongoing awareness of the numerous mimickers of vasculitis can help streamline diagnostic testing and avoid the inappropriate use of toxic medications.

BIBLIOGRAPHY

Bradley DJ, Glode MP. Kawasaki disease. *West J Med* 1998;168: 23–29.

Cohen MD, Conn DL. Approach to the patient with suspected vasculitis. *Bull Rheum Dis* 1999;48:1–4.

Ball GV, Gay RM Jr. Vasculitis. In: Koopman WJ, ed. *Arthritis and allied conditions: a textbook of rheuamtology*, 14th ed. Philadelphia: Lippincott Williams & Wilkins, 2001:1655–1695.

Jennette JC, Falk RJ. Small-vessel vasculitis. *N Engl J Med,* 1997; 337:1512–1523.

Kerr GS, Hallahan CW, Giordano J, et al. Takayasu arteritis. *Ann Intern Med* 1994;120:919–929.

Lhote F, Guillevin L. Polyarteritis nodosa, microscopic polyangiitis, and Churg-Strauss syndrome: clinical aspects and treatment. *Rheum Dis Clin North Am* 1995;21:911–947.

Lie JT. Histopathologic specificity of systemic vasculitis. *Rheum Dis Clin North Am* 1995;21:883–909.

Martinez-Taboada VM, Blanco R, Garcia-Fuentes M, et al. Clinical features and outcome of 95 patients with hypersensitivity vasculitis. *Am J Med* 1997;102:186–191.

Nordborg E, Nordborg C, Malmvall B, et al. Giant cell arteritis. *Rheum Dis Clin North Am* 1995;21:1013–1026.

Sack KE. Mimickers of vasculitis In: Koopman WJ, ed. *Arthritis and allied conditions: a textbook of rheumatology*, 14th ed. Philadelphia: Lippincott Williams & Wilkins, 2001:1711–1735.

POLYMYALGIA RHEUMATICA AND TEMPORAL ARTERITIS

RAMESH KUMAR

POLYMYALGIA RHEUMATICA

Polymyalgia rheumatica is a descriptive term introduced by Barber in 1957. It is characterized by pain and stiffness in the muscles of the neck, shoulders, and pelvic girdle of at least 4 weeks' duration (Table 17.1), elevated erythrocyte sedimentation rate (ESR), and prompt response to corticosteroid therapy. The diagnosis should be made only if other diseases—such as rheumatoid arthritis, myositis, infection, and malignancy—have been excluded.

Epidemiology

Polymyalgia rheumatica is a relatively common syndrome in the elderly white population and is more common than temporal arteritis. In a study from Olmstead County, Minnesota, the annual incidence of polymyalgia rheumatica was 53.7 cases/100,000 persons 50 years of age or older. This rate compares with an annual incidence of 28.6/100,000 in Göteborg, Sweden.

Polymyalgia rheumatica rarely affects those under 50 years of age and becomes more common with increasing age. Most patients are more than 60 years of age, with the mean age of onset being approximately 70 years. Women are affected twice as often as men. Polymyalgia rheumatica, like temporal arteritis, largely affects white individuals and is uncommon in blacks, Hispanics, Asians, and Native Americans. Whites in the southern United States appear to be less frequently affected than those in northern areas.

Etiology and Pathogenesis

The cause and pathogenesis of polymyalgia rheumatica is unknown, and there is no evidence of an infectious agent or toxin. The clues are presumably provided by epidemiology of the disease, yet the association of polymyalgia rheumatica with aging is without clear explanation. Up to 15% of the patients with polymyalgia rheumatica also have giant cell arteritis.

Familial aggregation and increased incidence in patients of northern European background suggest a genetic predisposition, and an association with HLA-DR4 has been reported. The immune system is implicated in the pathogenesis, but no persistent immune defects or characteristic antibodies have been identified.

Clinical Features

Onset

In most instances, symptoms have been present for weeks or months before the diagnosis is established. In one series, the mean was 6.2 months. Infrequently, the onset may be so acute that patients can tell the exact date and hour of their first symptoms, although typically it is more insidious.

Constitutional Symptoms

Patients with polymyalgia rheumatica frequently display systemic symptoms such as low-grade fever, malaise, weight loss, and anorexia. Although these constitutional symptoms may mimic the symptoms of a malignancy, there is no

TABLE 17.1. CLINICAL FEATURES OF POLYMYALGIA RHEUMATICA

Pain in the muscles of the shoulder girdle, pelvic girdle, and neck (commonly bilateral and symmetric, of at least 4 weeks duration)
Stiffness after rest
Elevation of the erythrocyte sedimentation rate (≥40 mm/hr)
Frequent constitutional features, including anemia, weight loss, fever, and general malaise
Prompt clinical response to corticosteroid treatment

From Weyard CM, Govonzy JJ. Polymyalgia rheumatica and giant cell arteritis. In: Koopman WJ, ed. *Arthritis and allied conditions: a textbook of rheumatology,* 14th ed. Philadelphia: Lippincott Williams & Wilkins, 2001:1784–1798, with permission.

direct association of polymyalgia rheumatica with neoplastic disease.

Proximal Myalgia

Polymyalgia rheumatica is usually characterized by chronic symmetric, profound proximal muscle aching and stiffness. The symptoms are most prominent in the neck, shoulders, and pelvic girdle, but distal muscle may also be involved. Aching and stiffness are worse in the morning and may be severe and incapacitating. Unlike patients with rheumatoid arthritis, in whom symptoms arise from small joints and cause difficulty performing tasks such as buttoning clothes, patients with polymyalgia rheumatica localize their symptoms to the proximal muscles and joints and complain of difficulty in performing such activities as getting out of bed, rising from a chair, climbing stairs, cleaning windows, or combing their hair. In one-third of the patients, aching and stiffness are so severe that self-care becomes difficult.

Despite these distressing clinical symptoms, objective findings are rare. On physical examination proximal muscles may be tender, and with longer duration of illness muscle atrophy may occur because of disuse of muscles. Contractures may develop, but only after long-standing disease. Muscle strength is often difficult to evaluate because pain is present. If the patient can disregard the pain, strength should be normal unless disuse atrophy has occurred.

Joints

Most patients have clinical manifestations of synovitis. The syndrome's original description excluded synovitis as a feature, with moderate effusions occasionally seen in knees and other joints. When present, the synovitis is often transient, relatively mild, and likely present either at disease onset or with rapid tapering of the glucocorticoid dose.

Temporal Arteritis

A detailed discussion of temporal arteritis and its relationship to polymyalgia rheumatica can be found in the following section, "Temporal Arteritis." The precise incidence of temporal arteritis in polymyalgia rheumatica is a subject of controversy. Polymyalgia rheumatica has been noted in 40% to 60% of patients with temporal arteritis. Conversely, temporal arteritis occurs in patients with polymyalgia rheumatica roughly 15% of the time.

Laboratory Studies

An elevated ESR is the characteristic lab finding of polymyalgia rheumatica. It is usually in excess of 50 mm/hour and may exceed 100 mm/hour. Although the ESR provides a useful means of monitoring treatment, some elevation of ESR might occur in otherwise healthy elderly people. Polymyalgia rheumatica may infrequently occur with normal or only mildly elevated ESR.

Normocytic and normochromic anemias can occur and may be the presenting symptom. Other findings reflecting the systemic inflammatory process, such as thrombocytosis, increased gamma globulins, and elevated acute-phase reactants are common, but they are no more helpful than the ESR in the assessment of disease activity.

Liver-associated enzyme abnormalities may be seen in up to one-third of the patients; an increased alkaline phosphatase level is most common. Renal function, urinalysis, serum creatine kinase levels, the ANA, and the RF are negative or normal. Radiographs are consistent with the expected changes seen in this age group. Synovial fluid is typically inflammatory, with leukocyte count varying from 1,000 to 20,000 cells/mm^3 with 40% to 50% polymorphonuclear leukocytes. Culture and crystal examinations are negative.

Differential Diagnosis

The diagnosis of polymyalgia rheumatica remains based on clinical presentation, and despite well-recognized laboratory abnormalities, no pathognomonic laboratory test exists. The differential diagnosis (Table 17.2) in an elderly patient with muscle pain, stiffness, and a raised ESR is wide because the prodromal phase of several conditions can mimic it. Nonspecific clinical features and the frequent absence of physical signs make diagnosis difficult. Frequently, the diagnosis is made after an exhaustive search for other diagnostic possibilities has proved fruitless.

TABLE 17.2. DIFFERENTIAL DIAGNOSIS OF POLYMYALGIA RHEUMATICA

Arthropathies
  Rheumatoid arthritis
  Fibromyalgia
  Other inflammatory joint diseases in elderly
  Degenerative joint disease
  Shoulder disorder
  Inflammatory muscle disease
  Malignant diseases
  Infection
  Hypothyroidism
  Depression

Adapted from Weyard C, Govonzy J. Polymyalgia rheumatica and giant cell arteritis In: Koopman WJ, ed. *Arthritis and allied conditions: a textbook of rheumatology,* 14th ed. Philadelphia: Lippincott Williams & Wilkins, 2001:1784–1798.

Rheumatoid Arthritis

It is often difficult to distinguish polymyalgia rheumatica from the early onset of rheumatoid arthritis. Both conditions have constitutional symptoms and morning stiffness surpassing joint manifestations of synovitis. Features that support the diagnosis of polymyalgia rheumatica are absence of rheumatoid factor, absence of peripheral joint involvement, lack of joint damage, and absence of erosive disease during follow-up.

Moreover, a prompt response to corticosteroid in the dose of 10 to 20 mg daily is typical for polymyalgia rheumatica. Although response to the corticosteroids is not a reliable distinguishing feature, an insufficient or incomplete response to corticosteroid therapy should prompt the physician to rethink the diagnosis of polymyalgia rheumatica.

Other Inflammatory Diseases

Inflammatory myopathies that may present with muscle pain usually have predominant muscle weakness with elevated creatine kinase and electromyographic evidence of myositis. Osteoarthritis of shoulders and hips can mimic a polymyalgia syndrome with radiographic studies and laboratory tests assisting in the correct diagnosis. Difficulties in diagnosis may arise in case of bilateral capsulitis of the shoulders. The full range of passive motion of the shoulder joints in polymyalgia rheumatica should distinguish these cases. Diffuse myalgia is not infrequent in patients with infectious diseases; however, postviral syndromes usually do not persist for 2 months. Generally, patients with polymyalgia rheumatica do not have spiking fevers and chills, and the presence of these features should always prompt an evaluation for underlying infectious diseases.

Malignant Disease

A hidden malignancy can mimic the symptoms of polymyalgia rheumatica but the prompt response to corticosteroids does not occur in malignancies. At present, no evidence suggests that neoplastic syndromes are more common in patients with polymyalgia rheumatica than in other people. Deterioration in health or an incomplete and delayed clinical response to corticosteroid should be taken seriously and alert the physician to reevaluate the patient and search for an occult neoplasm.

Other Diagnoses

Other diseases, such as the fibromyalgia syndrome, hypothyroidism, and depression, should also be considered in differential diagnosis. Although a normal ESR is present in all of them, they can be distinguished with the presence of tender points in fibromyalgia and an elevated thyroid-stimulating hormone in hypothyroidism.

Management

The therapeutic goal in polymyalgia rheumatica is to alleviate stiffness and constitutional features. Corticosteroids are the drug of choice, and NSAIDs may be used when symptoms are mild. The recommendation on initial dose of prednisone will vary according to the level of suspicion or presence of underlying giant cell arteritis.

For patients with polymyalgia rheumatica, the current recommendation is to initiate treatment with 15 to 20 mg of prednisone per day. Although most patients are significantly better within 24 hours, a few may take 48 to 72 hours to respond completely. The dose should be tapered according to the clinical response and the ESR. Complete normalization of the ESR is helpful, but it may take several weeks. Generally, the daily dose of prednisone can be decreased by 2.5 mg every 2 weeks until a dose of 10 mg/day is reached. Further tapering by 1-mg decrements every 4 weeks is recommended while following the clinical features and ESR. Optimally, prednisone should be tapered and discontinued as quickly as possible. When patients cannot tolerate the outlined dose reduction program and relapse occurs, the dose of prednisone must be increased to the previous dose to recapture control of the disease activity.

If there is no evidence of recurrence, prednisone is tapered slowly until discontinued. Patients with polymyalgia rheumatica should be monitored for 6 to 12 months after discontinuation of corticosteroids. Although corticosteroids relieve the symptoms of polymyalgia rheumatica, no evidence suggests that they shorten the duration of the disease. Therapy should continue for those with continued symptoms on tapering. Typically, treatment is required for 6 to 24 months. Because of the known complications of chronic corticosteroid treatment, osteoporosis and corticosteroid-induced glucose tolerance must be addressed with each patient.

Some patients can be effectively managed with NSAIDs. These agents can be tried in those with milder disease or in patients with multiple co-morbid risks, such as with hypertension, diabetes mellitus, and ischemic heart disease. As with other diseases, no individual NSAID is necessarily more effective than another, and selection should be based upon tolerability and safety for the patient. NSAID may be added to the corticosteroid therapy to facilitate steroid tapering. The clinician must remember the toxicity of NSAIDs, particularly given the age of these patients and duration of therapy.

Other than medication, reassurance and treatment should be part of the treatment plan of polymyalgia rheumatica. This can be achieved by educating patients about the disease's self-limiting chronic course. If diagnosis and treatment occur promptly, then the prognosis is excellent. Attention to side effects from corticosteroids and NSAIDs should be given in view of their morbidity in this age group.

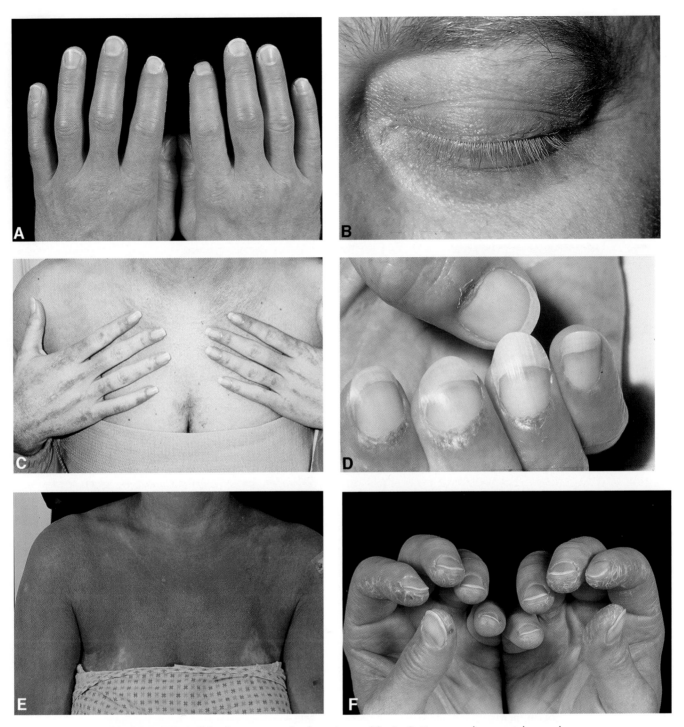

COLOR PLATE 1. Skin changes seen in dermatomyositis. **A:** Gottron papules are scaly papules overlying the extensor surfaces of the hands (over the metacarpophalangeal and proximal interphalangeal joints in this case), elbows, knees, or malleoli. This patient also has sclerodactyly and arthritis of the metacarpophalangeal and proximal interphalangeal joints. **B:** The heliotrope rash is a purplish discoloration around the eyes, especially on the upper lids. **C:** Linear extensor erythema overlies the extensor surface of the hands beyond the usual location of Gottron papules or sign. **D:** Periungual vasculitic changes and cuticular overgrowth. **E:** Photosensitive diffuse erythroderma with accentuated erythema in the V of the neck (V sign) in a patient with cancer-associated dermatomyositis. **F:** Drying and cracking of the skin over the lateral and palmar surfaces of the fingers, known as "mechanic's hands," is seen frequently in patients with autoantibodies to aminoacyl-tRNA synthetases (the antisynthetase syndrome). (From Miller FW. Inflammatory myopathies: polymyositis, dermatomyositis, and related conditions. In: Koopman WJ, ed. *Arthritis and allied conditions: a textbook of rheumatology,* 14th ed. Philadelphia: Lippincott Williams & Wilkins, 2001:1562–1589, with permission.) See Figure 15.1 on page 186.

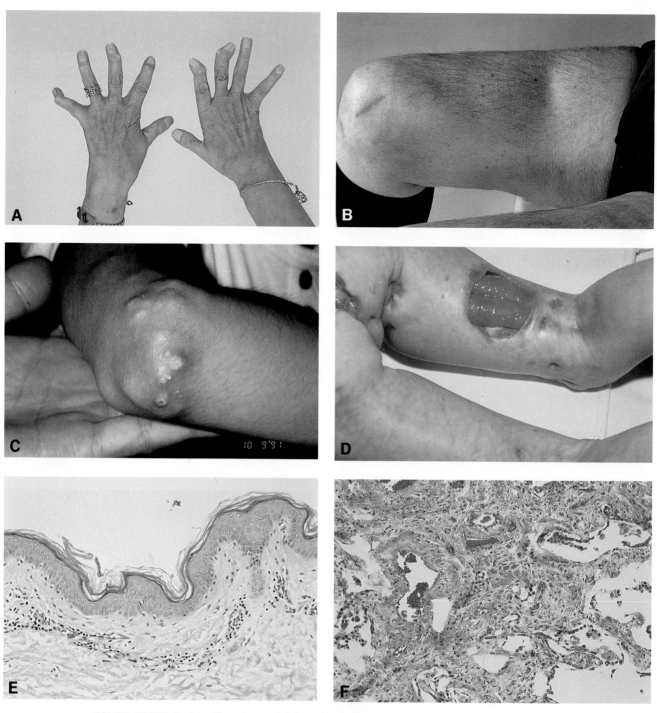

COLOR PLATE 2. Manifestations of idiopathic inflammatory myopathy. **A:** A deforming arthropathy is occasionally seen in polymyositis patients as a manifestation of the antisynthetase syndrome as seen in this patient with anti-Jo-1 autoantibodies. **B:** Irregular and asymmetric muscle atrophy, often in the anterior thigh muscles, is often seen in patients with inclusion-body myositis. **C:** Extensive calcifications over the elbow in a child with juvenile dermatomyositis (courtesy of Dr. Robert Rennebohm). **D:** Severe vasculitis with erosions into muscle in a patient with dermatomyositis (courtesy of Dr. Robert Rennebohm). **E:** Biopsy from affected skin demonstrating surface scaling, vacuolization, and subcutaneous perivascular mononuclear cells characteristic, but not diagnostic, of dermatomyositis (hematoxylin and eosin) (courtesy of Dr. Lori A. Love). **F:** Lung biopsy from a patient with antisynthetase syndrome and interstitial lung disease demonstrating destruction of the normal architecture and extensive replacement by inflammatory cells and fibrotic tissue (hematoxylin and eosin) (courtesy of Dr. Lori A. Love.) (From Miller FW. Inflammatory myopathies: polymyositis, dermatomyositis, and related conditions. In: Koopman WJ, ed. *Arthritis and allied conditions: a textbook of rheumatology,* 14th ed. Philadelphia: Lippincott Williams & Wilkins, 2001:1562–1589, with permission.) See Figure 15.2 on page 187.

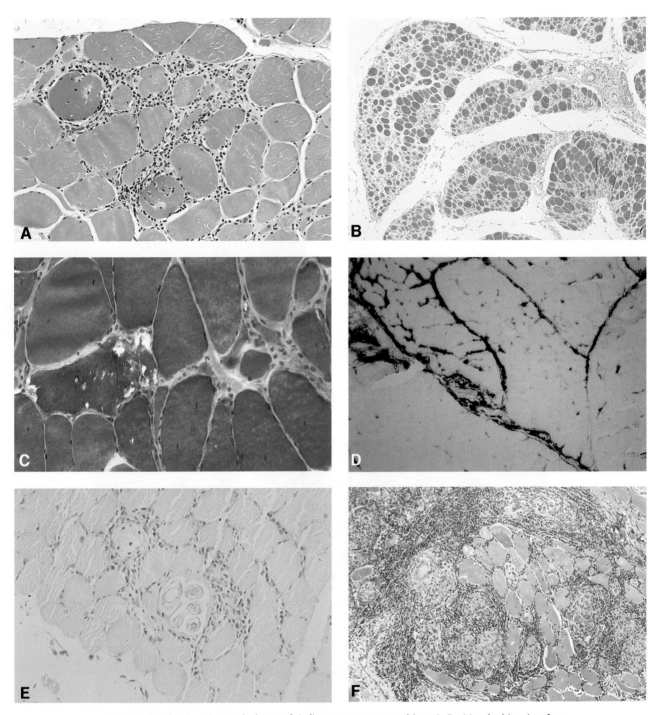

COLOR PLATE 3. Histopathology of inflammatory myopathies. **A–B:** Muscle biopsies from polymyositis patients tend to show focal endomysial infiltration by mononuclear cells (**A**, hematoxylin and eosin stain), whereas those from dermatomyositis patients show more perivascular and interstitial inflammation with perifascicular myofiber atrophy (**B**, modified trichrome stain). **C:** Transverse fresh-frozen section of muscle from a patient with inclusion-body myositis displaying purplish granular material lining the multiple vacuoles in several myofibers and the presence of angulated myofibers (modified trichrome stain). **D:** Strong alkaline phosphatase staining of the interstitium is common in idiopathic inflammatory myopathy and can help distinguish this condition from other myopathies even in the absence of inflammation. **E:** Trichinosis parasites in a myofiber surrounded by mononuclear inflammatory cells in a patient originally misdiagnosed with polymyositis (courtesy Dr. Lori A. Love). **F:** Intensely inflammatory granulomatous myositis is characterized by the presence of granulomata and endomysial inflammation in this patient with sarcoidosis (hematoxylin and eosin stain). (From Miller FW. Inflammatory myopathies: polymyositis, dermatomyositis, and related conditions. In: Koopman WJ, ed. *Arthritis and allied conditions: a textbook of rheumatology,* 14th ed. Philadelphia: Lippincott Williams & Wilkins, 2001:1562–1589, with permission.) See Figure 15.3 on page 190.

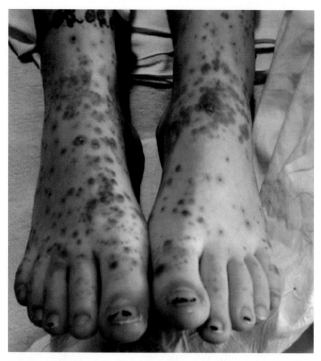

COLOR PLATE 4. Palpable purpura in a young woman (courtesy Dr. Jonathan Graf). See Figure 16.1 on page 200.

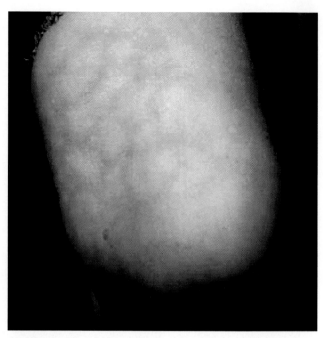

COLOR PLATE 5. Livedo reticularis (courtesy Dr. Jonathan Graf). See Figure 16.2 on page 203.

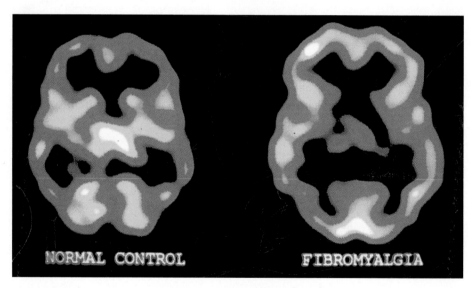

COLOR PLATE 6. Single photon emission computerized tomography of the brain in a normal individual and one with fibromyalgia. There is decreased regional cerebral flow to the thalamus and caudate nuclei in the fibromyalgia patient. [Modified from Alarcón GS. *WMN Health Pri Care (Orth Ed.)* 1999; 2:11–22.] See Figure 20.3 on page 231.

TEMPORAL ARTERITIS

Temporal arteritis, also referred to as giant cell or cranial arteritis, predominantly affects medium and large-sized cranial arteries. Although the term *temporal arteritis* appears to have existed in the late nineteenth century, it was not until 1932 that Horton et al. established the term *giant cell arteritis.*

Temporal arteritis occurs almost exclusively in those more than 50 years of age. There is a wide range of symptoms, with most patients having clinical findings related to involved arteritis. The American College of Rheumatology developed the criteria for classifying vasculitides to distinguish seven vasculitic syndromes. These criteria are useful for differentiating the various vasculitic diseases (Table 17.3).

Epidemiology

Giant cell arteritis is the most frequent vasculitis in North America and Western Europe. The prevalence is highest in Scandinavian whites and lowest in Hispanics, blacks, and Asians. In a study from Minnesota, a population of largely northern European descent had an incidence of 17 per 100,000 persons, with the prevalence rate averaging 223 per 100,000 in those older than 50 years. This rate compares with the annual incidence of 18.3 per 100,000 in Göteborg, Sweden.

Temporal arteritis is rare in people less than 50 years of age, with the incidence increasing with age, and it is more common among women than among men.

Pathology

The diagnosis of temporal arteritis is made when typical histologic changes are noted. The arteritis is histologically a panarteritis with giant cell granuloma formation often in close proximity to a disrupted internal elastic lamina. Large and medium-sized arteries are affected, the involvement is patchy, and "skip lesions" often occur. The frequency of skip lesions necessitates an adequate sample size on temporal artery biopsy.

TABLE 17.3. AMERICAN COLLEGE OF RHEUMATOLOGY 1990, CRITERIA FOR THE CLASSIFICATION OF GIANT CELL ARTERITIS

1. Age at disease onset ≥50 years
2. Headache of new onset or new type
3. Tenderness or decreased pulsation of temporal artery
4. Elevated erythrocyte sedimentation rate (≥50 mm/hr)
5. Histologic changes of arteritis (either granulomatous lesions, usually with multinucleated giant cell, or diffuse mononuclear cell infiltration)

From Hunder GG, Bloch DA, Michel BA, et al. The American College of Rheumatology 1990 criteria for the classification of giant cell arteritis. *Arthritis Rheum* 1990;33:1122–1228, with permission.

Multinucleated giant cells are not always present and, although characteristic, are not required to establish the diagnosis. If present, multinucleated giant cells are often close to a fragmented internal elastic lamina and the giant cells may be localized circumferentially along the degenerated elastic membrane. Careful examination of the area of arteritis enhances the likelihood of finding giant cells.

In 90% of the patients, morphologic changes occur in extracranial medium-sized branches of the aorta. Superficial temporal, vertebral, ophthalmic, and posterior ciliary arteries were involved most frequently. In 10% to 15% of patients, inflammatory changes are found in large elastic arteries, including the aorta and its major branches.

Etiology and Pathogenesis

The course of giant cell arteritis is unknown, and pathogenesis is poorly understood. The similarity of incidence rates in different geographic regions and different ethnic or racial groups is highly suggestive of the contribution of genetic elements to disease pathogenesis. The location of the inflammatory reaction around the fragmented internal elastic lamina suggests that giant cell arteritis may result from an autoimmune reaction to elastin or other macromolecules, although this remains unproven. The inflammatory infiltrate is primarily macrophages, and CD4+ T-lymphocytes of the Th1 type, with approximately 25% being activated T cells. Recent reports show that most temporal arteritis and polymyalgia rheumatica patients express the HLA-DR4 allele (50% to 60%). These patients have a common sequence motif of amino acids, which can be mapped to the antigen-binding site of the HLA-DR molecule, suggesting that the selective binding of a disease-inducing antigen by the HLA-DR molecule is a crucial event in the pathogenesis.

Clinical Features

Temporal arteritis occurs almost exclusively in individuals older than 50 years. Seventy percent to 80% of patients are female, with the mean age at onset about 70 years. Temporal arteritis can involve a spectrum of arteries causing a wide spectrum of symptoms.

The onset of symptoms may be acute or insidious, with most patients having constitutional symptoms, such as malaise, anorexia, weight loss, low-grade fever, fatigue, and depression. Occasionally, fever of unknown origin with spiking temperatures and chills can be the dominant features of giant cell arteritis. The vast majority of patients (80% to 90%) have clinical findings related to involvement with extracranial branches of the proximal aorta, although it is now recognized that the disease has a more widespread arterial lesion. The varied spectrum of symptoms can be classified according to anatomic vascular distribution (Table 17.4).

TABLE 17.4. CLINICAL FEATURES OF GIANT CELL ARTERITIS

Symptoms Directly Related to Vascular Involvement
  Frequent
    Headaches
    Abnormalities of temporal arteritis
  Common
    Ocular symptoms
    Jaw claudication
  Infrequent
    Tongue claudication
    Respiratory symptoms
    Vision loss
    Limb claudication
    Circulatory insufficiency of central nervous system
    Peripheral neuropathic syndromes
    Aortic arch syndrome
Symptoms Related to Systemic Illness
  Frequent
    Laboratory evidence for acute-phase response (elevated
      erythrocyte sedimentation rate, anemia, elevated
      C-reactive protein)
  Common
    Malaise, fever, anorexia, weight loss, night sweats,
      polymyalgia rheumatica
  Infrequent
    Arthralgias/arthritis

From Weyard CM, Govonzy JJ. Polymyalgia rheumatica and giant cell arteritis. In: Koopman WJ, ed. *Arthritis and allied conditions: a textbook of rheumatology*, 14th ed. Philadelphia: Lippincott Williams & Wilkins, 2001:1784–1798, with permission.

Symptoms Related to External Carotid Artery Branches

Headache is the most common symptom and occurs in 70% to 80% of patients. It usually begins early in the course of the disease and may be the presenting symptom. The headache is usually severe and the patient describes throbbing, sharp, or dull pain that often is localized to one area of the head. Tenderness of the scalp, particularly in the temporal region, when wearing glasses, combing the hair, or touching the pillow with the head at night is a frequent complaint. Physical findings of significance are thickened vessels, with tenderness, nodularity, induration, and absent or reduced pulses.

Jaw claudication, when present, is highly suggestive of the syndrome. It is usually due to reduced blood flow in the extracranial branches of the aorta supplying the masseter and temporalis muscle. About 50% of the patients complain of pain in the jaw or tongue, induced by chewing or prolonged talking. *Temporomandibular joint pain* may occur due to the involvement of the temporal artery. *Ear pain* may occur secondary to involvement of the posterior auricular branch.

Symptoms Related to Internal Carotid Artery

Giant cell arteritis causes *visual symptoms* in 25% to 30% of all cases. The spectrum of ocular manifestation includes diplopia, amaurosis fugax, scotoma, ptosis, and partial or complete blindness. Sudden blindness is a well-recognized and feared complication. It can be the presenting symptom and is abrupt and painless, and it is most commonly due to ischemic optic neuritis. Anatomic lesions that produce ischemic optic neuritis in these patients result from arteritis involving the posterior ciliary branches of the ophthalmic arteries, resulting in ischemia of the optic nerve. Blindness due to retinal artery involvement appears to be a relatively uncommon cause of blindness.

Blurring of vision, transient visual loss (amaurosis fugax), scotoma, and ophthalmoplegia due to ischemia of extraocular muscles may also be manifestations of giant cell arteritis. Visual blurring and/or amaurosis fugax can occur as waning signs for months before sudden blindness develops.

Neurologic symptoms can infrequently occur and are due to narrowing and occlusion of the internal carotid and vertebrobasilar arteries, resulting in transient ischemic attacks, seizures, and cerebral dysfunction. The involvement of the intracranial arteries is unusual, since these vessels lack an internal elastic lamina.

Symptoms Related to Large Artery Involvement

Although cranial involvement is the most frequently recognized and characteristic presentation of temporal arteritis, the process not only is limited to cranial vessels, but also can involve large arteries in 10% to 15% of patients. It may present as *aortic arch syndrome,* a serious complication of the disease, producing upper-extremity claudication, decreased or absent peripheral pulses, paresthesias, and Raynaud phenomenon. Vascular bruits can be heard over the carotid, subclavian, and axillary arteries.

Although *abdominal aortic* involvement is rare, it can produce symptoms secondary to aortic aneurysms or as claudication of extremities when involving the distal aorta, iliac, or femoral vessels. Despite involvement of both large and medium-sized arteries, pulmonary artery involvement is unusual. Because small artery involvement is uncommon, skin manifestations are rare.

Symptoms Related to Polymyalgia Rheumatica

Patients with giant cell arteritis with or without polymyalgia rheumatica usually have similar systemic symptoms, such as malaise, fatigue, fever, weight loss, depression, and arthralgia. However, it is still difficult to predict which patient with polymyalgia rheumatica will have temporal arteritis. Some physicians recommend treating all patients with polymyalgia rheumatica as if they had giant cell arteritis. However, this approach involves unnecessary treatment of a large group of patients with high-dose steroids. Because temporal artery biopsy is a relatively benign procedure, this should be done in all patients with polymyalgia rheumatica who also display classic signs or symptoms of giant cell arteritis.

Laboratory Studies

As in polymyalgia rheumatica, the ESR is the most consistently abnormal laboratory test, and it is usually higher in temporal arteritis than in the other vasculitides. It is almost always more than 50 mm/hr and is commonly more than 100 mm/hr. On rare occasion, it may be normal. Although in the appropriate clinical setting the ESR is a sensitive indicator of temporal arteritis, its specificity is very low. Indeed, other diseases, particularly infections and multiple myeloma, can give systemic symptoms with associated ESR of more than 100 mm/hr.

A mild to moderate normochromic or hypochromic anemia and elevated platelet counts are common. Acute-phase serum proteins, such as c-reactive, are frequently increased. Additional laboratory results include increased hepatic enzymes in 20% to 30% of patients and elevated levels of factor VIII and interleukin-6.

Diagnostic Studies

Temporal arteritis should be suspected in a patient who is more than 50 years of age and develops a new type of headache, jaw claudication, fever, or polymyalgia rheumatica. Careful physical examination may reveal a thickened or tender temporal artery. An abnormal segment should be biopsied to confirm the diagnosis. Temporal arteritis is characterized by patchy or segmental arterial involvement, and the diagnosis can be missed if the biopsy specimen does not include one of the patchy infiltrates. Therefore arterial segments of several centimeters should be removed and should be sliced like salami at 1- to 2-mm intervals and examined histologically at multiple levels. If the first side is negative, consideration should be given to biopsying the other temporal artery. Most of the positive biopsies show mural lymphocytes, macrophages, giant cells, and a disrupted lamina. A properly performed biopsy will define the need for therapy in about 90% of cases.

Differential Diagnosis

A vasculitic infiltration of temporal arteries is sometimes found in other vasculitides; however, the histopathologic and clinical features are sufficiently distinct. In patients with *polyarteritis nodosa,* however, these arteries are rarely abnormal on examination, and clinical features are distinct from it. *Takayasu arteritis* and temporal arteritis are pathologically similar, but the clinical findings and age at onset may help to distinguish them.

Management

Currently, high-dose corticosteroids remain the treatment of choice. Usually, the dose ranges from 40 to 60 mg prednisone per day. If clinical response is inadequate, higher doses are necessary. Patients with visual symptoms should be started on intravenous methyl prednisone. Failure to initiate appropriate therapy can result in blindness. Corticosteroids usually are dramatically effective in suppressing systemic symptoms of temporal arteritis within 72 hours after initiation of therapy. Localized manifestations of arteritis, such as headache, scalp tenderness, and jaw or tongue claudication, slowly improve over a longer period of time. The dose of 40 to 60 mg prednisone should be continued until clinical evidence of the inflammatory process, including symptoms and laboratory evidence of inflammation, has subsided; then the corticosteroid dose can be reduced gradually. A good rule of thumb is to start tapering 1 month after clinical and laboratory parameters, particularly ESR, have normalized. Excessively rapid tapering may result in a relapse. Frequently, doses of 15 to 25 mg or more must be given for several months before further dose reduction can be attempted. Alternate-day therapy is usually insufficient to control disease activity. Most patients with temporal arteritis had a disease course of less than 2 years. Discontinuation of corticosteroids should be tried 2 years after initial diagnosis, and careful clinical monitoring is needed for 6 to 12 years after withdrawal from corticosteroids. Every effort should be made to limit side effects of corticosteroids, such as osteoporosis (calcium supplementation and vitamin D therapy). If patients do not achieve clinical remission or are not able to be tapered to low doses of corticosteroids, immunosuppressive agents should be considered. Azathioprine has shown a modest corticosteroid-sparing effect. Studies with methotrexate have not been shown to have beneficial effects.

In conclusion, when temporal arteritis is strongly suspected there should be no delay in starting therapy. as the artery biopsy will still show inflammatory changes for several days after corticosteroids have been started and the result is unlikely to alter the therapeutic decision. If the temporal (or other) artery biopsy shows no arteritis but suspicion of disease is strong, corticosteroids should be started.

Summary

The classic clinical presentation of temporal arteritis is a combination of constitutional features associated with marked acute-phase reaction and symptoms related to the inflammation of extracranial branches of proximal aorta. If treated promptly, mortality is low and feared consequences, such as permanent vision loss and cerebral malperfusion, can be prevented. Histologic confirmation should be sought in clinically suspected cases because the treatment of choice, high doses of corticosteroids given over several months, can cause serious side effects.

BIBLIOGRAPHY

Cohen MD, Ginsburg WW. Polymyalgia rheumatica. *Rheum Dis Clin North Am* 1990;16:325–338.

De Silva M, Hazleman BL. Azathioprine in giant cell arteritis/ polymyalgia rheumatica: a double blind study. *Ann Rheum Dis* 1986;45:136–138.

Evan JM, O'Fallon WM, Hunder GG. Increased incidence of aortic aneurysm and dissection in giant cell (temporal) arteritis: a population based study. *Ann Intern Med* 1995;122:502–507.

Healy LA. On epidemiology of polymyalgia rheumatica and temporal arteritis. *J Rheumatol* 1993;20:1639–1640.

Horton BT, Magath TB, Brown GE. An undescribed form of arteritis of the temporal vessels. *Proc Staff Meet Mayo Clin* 1932;7:700.

Mourat AG, Hazelmon BL. PMR. *J Rheumatol* 1974;1:190–202.

Weyard CM, Govonzy JJ. Polymyalgia rheumatica and giant cell arteritis In: Koopman WJ, ed. *Arthritis and allied conditions: a textbook of rheumatology,* 14th ed. Philadelphia: Lippincott Williams & Wilkins, 2001:1784–1798.

18

UNCLASSIFIED OR UNDIFFERENTIATED CONNECTIVE TISSUE DISEASE

GRACIELA S. ALARCÓN

Despite significant gains in the understanding of the immunopathogenesis of the different connective tissue diseases (CTDs), their etiology remains elusive. The diagnosis of the different CTDs is thus a matter of clinical judgment as patients present with constellations of symptoms, physical findings, and laboratory features that permit their recognition (1–6). Often, however, patients present with manifestations of more than one different CTD or with manifestations that defeat classification (7–10). The term *overlap* is used in this chapter for the first group of patients, whereas the terms *unclassified* or *undifferentiated* are used for the second group. The term *mixed* (M) *CTD* is reserved for patients with a defined overlap syndrome (see later) (10–12). As our understanding of the etiopathogenesis of the CTDs improves, more precise labels will certainly be used.

The term *atypical* (A) *CTD* has arisen from the consensus reached by nonphysicians working with silicone breast implant patients (13). The "legal" definition of ACTD is such that almost any individual presenting some (subjective, for the most part) neuropsychologic or musculoskeletal manifestation may be diagnosed with this "entity." The rheumatologic community has not validated the existence of such a disorder; thus ACTD will not be discussed.

Table 18.1 summarizes the terminology/nomenclature used in this chapter.

THE OVERLAP SYNDROMES

The following overlap syndromes have been described in the literature: rhupus, or the overlap between rheumatoid arthritis and lupus (8,14–18); sclerodermatomyositis (or scleromyositis), or the overlap between scleroderma and myositis (7,19–22); and MCTD, or the overlap between poly/dermatomyositis, scleroderma, systemic lupus erythematosus (SLE), and rheumatoid arthritis (RA), in the presence of anti-U1-RNP antibodies and HLA-DR4 (10,11,23). Other "overlaps" are considered subsets of defined CTDs rather than overlaps; such is the case for patients with SLE or RA who also have myositis or vasculitis, as well as for patients with SLE who have clinical and laboratory features of the antiphospholipid antibody syndrome (APS). Other patients with a defined CTD present overlapping manifestations with non-CTD disorders; such is the case of patients with luposclerosis, as the overlapping clinical syndrome of SLE and multiple sclerosis has been called (24,25). Finally, patients with primary APS may also present with manifestations of multiple sclerosis (26). Table 18.2 summarizes these different conditions by categories.

The first three overlap syndromes will now be described in some detail.

Rhupus

Arthralgias and arthritis are rather common in patients with SLE; however, in some patients with SLE, the most prominent clinical manifestation is that of a symmetric polyarthritis. These patients may or may not have a positive rheumatoid factor (RF). Likewise, patients with RA may present some extraarticular features and a positive antinuclear antibody (ANA) test that may suggest the diagnosis of

TABLE 18.1. TERMINOLOGY/NOMENCLATURE

ACR	American College of Rheumatology
CTD	connective tissue disease
Defined CTD	Clear-cut diagnosis of systemic lupus erythematosus, rheumatoid arthritis, polydermatomyositis, or scleroderma
Overlap syndrome	Presence of two defined CTDs (see Table 18.2)
Undifferentiated CTD	Patients with clinical features of CTDs who do not meet criteria for a defined CTD
Mixed CTD	A particular form of overlap syndrome (see Table 18.2)
Atypical CTD	Term used in the silicone breast implant litigation (not sanctioned by the ACR)

SLE. The term *rhupus,* however, is reserved for those patients who clearly meet criteria for both SLE and RA and who present characteristic clinical features of both disorders (8,14–18,27). These patients usually have a seropositive, erosive, symmetric polyarthritis, which antedates the onset of unequivocal clinical features of SLE (14–18,27). They also present autoantibodies characteristic of both disorders; these include IgM-RF, ANA, anti-DNA, and in about half the patients, antibodies to Ro (27). Some of the extraarticular features these patients present may be related to the presence of rheumatoid nodules rather than to SLE; this distinction may have therapeutic implications.

Rhupus patients should be distinguished from those SLE patients who develop deforming nonerosive arthropathy that resembles that occurring in patients with recurrent rheumatic fever (Jaccoud arthropathy) (16,28–30). These patients present with (initially) correctable subluxation of the MCP joints with ulnar deviation as well as swan neck and boutonniere finger and Z-thumb deformities. These abnormalities appear to be the result of ligamentous laxity and compression of hand musculature rather than the result of pannus (16,28). The magnitude of the previously described features was the basis for the development of an index to aid in the diagnosis of Jaccoud arthropathy (16,31). Van Vugt et al. have developed an algorithm to classify the deforming hand arthropathy of lupus patients (16). Figure 18.1 presents a revision of this algorithm.

The frequency of rhupus at the population level is unknown, since most cases have been recognized at tertiary care centers; this probably reflects the degree of awareness about this condition rather than its true frequency. It is also unclear whether the coexistence of SLE and RA is the result of the random association of these disorders (8) or the result of genetic predisposition for both, as postulated by Brand et al. (27).

TABLE 18.2. OVERLAP CONNECTIVE TISSUE DISEASES AND RELATED SYNDROMES

Recognized overlap CTDs
  SLE/RA: rhupus
  Myositis/scleroderma: sclerodermatomyositis or scleromyositis
  Myositis/scleroderma/RA/SLE: MCTD
Subsets within defined CTDs
  SLE/myositis
  RA/myositis
  SLE/APS
  RA/vasculitis
  SLE/vasculitis
Overlap CTD and a nonrheumatic disorder
  SLE/multiple sclerosis
Overlap CTD-like and a nonrheumatic disorder
  APS/Multiple sclerosis

APS, antiphospholipid antibody syndrome; CTD, connective tissue disease; MCTD, mixed CTD; RA, rheumatoid arthritis; SLE, systemic lupus erythematosus.

From the practical point of view, rhupus patients should be treated according to their clinical manifestations (and their severity), utilizing compounds proven to be effective in both RA and SLE. Thus antimalarials may be needed to prevent SLE flares, but methotrexate or leflunomide may be needed to prevent joint damage. Until the etiopathogenesis of both SLE and RA are defined, it is unclear whether anti-TNF therapies found to be beneficial in patients with RA but possibly detrimental in patients with SLE should or could be used in these patients. (See chapter 10.)

Sclerodermatomyositis or Scleromyositis

Patients with sclerodermatomyositis or scleromyositis show scleroderma and poly/dermatomyositis with variable cutaneous, muscular, and organ system manifestations (7,19,21). Although this overlap syndrome was originally described in adults, pediatric cases have been reported (19). Skin changes occur characteristically over the span of years and are described as not being very severe (no digital ulcerations, no trunk or face involvement, absence of prominent telangiectasia); "mechanic's" hands have been described (19). My own experience with this rare disorder, however, is quite different. The patients (children and adults) I have followed have had severe and generalized skin involvement with the consequent occurrence of flexion contractures. Pulmonary, gastrointestinal, and renal involvement, as the one described in scleroderma, is characteristically mild, but severe megacolon and restrictive lung function have been described (20).

Patients with sclerodermatomyositis usually exhibit high ANA titers in a homogenous pattern, which correspond to the presence of the PM-Scl antigen (a nucleolar antigenic complex of 11 to 16 polypeptides). Anti-U1-RNP antibodies are characteristically absent. From the immunogenetic point of view, patients with sclerodermatomyositis are either HLA-DR3 homozygous or HLA-DR3/DR4 heterozygous. They are thus quite different from patients with MCTD (19).

The frequency of this disorder is largely unknown. As with rhupus, most publications on sclerodermatomyositis come from tertiary care facilities. Thus population-based figures are unavailable.

The treatment of these patients should be aimed at controlling the inflammatory process in muscles and other tissues involved. Muscle inflammation is usually mild and steroid responsive. The inability to taper corticosteroids rapidly may lead to the successive use of "sparing" agents; methotrexate is the most common compound utilized with this purpose, but intravenous immunoglobulin G has also been used (32). The prognosis of patients with this overlap syndrome depends on the degree of organ system involvement, whether or not manifestations respond to corticosteroids, and whether or not other complications supervene (19,20,33).

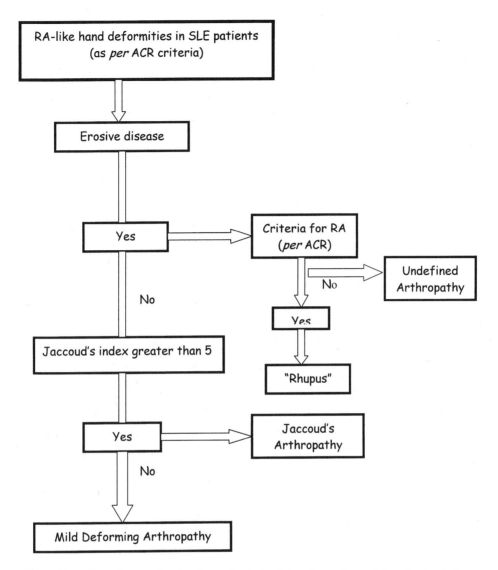

FIGURE 18.1. Flow diagram for the diagnosis of the deforming arthropathies of systemic lupus erythematosus (*SLE*). *ACR*, American College of Rheumatology; *RA*, rheumatoid arthritis. (Modified from Van Vugt RM, Derksen RH, Kater L, et al. Deforming arthropathy of lupus and rhupus hands in systemic lupus erythematosus. *Ann Rheum Dis* 1998;57:540–544.)

Mixed Connective Tissue Disease

The first description of MCTD dates back to 1972, when Sharp described 25 patients with overlapping clinical manifestations of RA, SLE, myositis, and scleroderma occurring predominantly in adult women. Similar cases have been described in children and older adults. Patients with MCTD also exhibit extremely high titers of antibodies to ENA (extractable nuclear antigen) (10,11), later identified as antibodies to U1-RNP (10,34,35) and HLA-DR4 positivity (23,36). Since then, to date, this syndrome has been at the center of discussion, with some rheumatologists favoring its recognition and others not (23,35–38). Some argue that patients with MCTD, including the ones originally described by Sharp, tend to evolve into one of the more defined CTDs, such as SLE, myositis, or scleroderma (12), and should not be considered to have a defined syndrome. Others, however, propose that patients with anti-U1-RNP antibodies but no clear-cut manifestations of MCTD represent early or undefined MCTD and that as time goes on they show the full-blown MCTD syndrome (23). So the presence of antibodies to U1-RNP, although characteristic of MCTD, is not, in the absence of other clinical features, sufficient to make this diagnosis. The fact that some patients evolve into a more defined CTD has been postulated to have genetic basis. Patients who start as MCTD and who are HLA-DR3 or HLA-DR5 evolve into SLE or scleroderma, whereas those who are HLA-DR4 remain as MCTD (23,27,36). Table 18.3 shows the distinct clinical features of MCTD: Raynaud phenomenon, sclerodactyly, sausage digits, lymphoadenopathy, malar rash, myositis, pulmonary involvement, esophageal dysmotility, symmetric polyarthritis (in a RA-like distribution), and serositis. Organ system involvement, particularly gastrointestinal and pulmonary, occurs with variable frequency, but renal and central nervous system involvement are conspicuously absent. Raynaud phenomenon severe enough to produce severe digital ischemia and necrosis, sausage digits, swollen hands, polyarthritis, and rash are the more common presenting manifestations of MCTD (10,12,23,39). Sharp and subsequently other investigators (39) have proposed criteria for the diagnosis of MCTD. They include, in addition to the clinical manifestations described, the presence of antibodies to ENA (anti-U1-RNP) at very high titers (in the millions), in the absence of anti-Sm antibodies. A pathogenic role for anti-U1-RNP antibodies has not been determined to date (39). It is quite possible (and, in fact, has been proposed) that these antibodies modify the clinical expression of a CTD (39). Treatment in patients with MCTD is directed at the clinical manifestations present and at the prevention of structural damage in affected organs, using standard pharmacologic compounds commonly used in the more defined CTDs, such as corticosteroids, methotrexate, and other immunosuppressive drugs. The prognosis in patients with MCTD is variable. Patients who evolve into a defined CTD adopt the clinical course and outcome of the new entity, whereas those who remain as an overlap may develop prominent digital ischemic/necrotic events as well as pulmonary hypertension or significant gastroesophageal reflux.

THE UNCLASSIFIED OR UNDIFFERENTIATED CONNECTIVE TISSUE DISEASES

There is no consensus on how to diagnose these patients. Some authors consider these patients to be the preamble of MCTD; some, of lupus (prelupus, latent lupus, incomplete lupus) (40,41); others, including our group, of an ANA-positive fibromyalgia-like syndrome (see chapter 20) (42). Still others prefer to refer to these patients as having "unclassified" or "undifferentiated" CTD, only to indicate that these patients often evolve into a defined CTD (43). Indeed, a large effort by rheumatologists at different U.S. academic centers took place between 1982 and 1995 (44,45). This study involved the largest cohort of "unclassified" patients with disease manifestations of up to 12 months' duration, and followed these patients over time. The aim was to identify among these patients the predictors of a given outcome. Three subgroups of patients were recognized within this cohort of unclassified patients: (a) those with isolated Raynaud phenomenon, (b) those with unexplained polyarthritis (patients not quite meeting criteria for the diagnosis of RA), and (c) those with truly undefined manifestations (as shown in Table 18.4). It can be argued that not all patients entering the undefined category would have been included as such to date; indeed, some of these patients probably could have been considered as having an ANA-positive, fibromyalgia-like syndrome, as described by our group several years ago (42) (see chapter 20). This multicentric group constituted also a second cohort of patients with well-defined CTDs that served as a comparison for the unclassified patients.

Patients in this study were followed longitudinally in an effort to determine the patients' final diagnosis. Yearly visits were done during the first 5 years; an additional visit was conducted at 10 years. The protocol required only an update interval history, a physical examination, and a core of laboratory tests. Any other laboratory test or more sophisticated

TABLE 18.3. CLINICAL AND LABORATORY FEATURES OF MIXED CONNECTIVE TISSUE DISEASE

Major
  Swollen fingers and/or hands
  Raynaud phenomenon
  Esophageal dysmotility
  Sclerodactyly
  Myositis
  Serositis
  Pulmonary involvement
  Anti-U1-RNP antibodies
  Negative anti-Sm antibodies
Minor
  Arthritis
  Alopecia
  Myositis
  Trigeminal neuropathy
  Cytopenias

TABLE 18.4. CLINICAL FEATURES OF PATIENTS WITH UNCLASSIFIED OR UNDIFFERENTIATED CONNECTIVE TISSUE DISEASE

Arthralgias/arthritis
Myalgias
Rashes
Sicca
Pericarditis/pleuritis
Pulmonary involvement
Peripheral neuropathy
Elevated acute phase reactant(s)
Positive serologic test for syphilis

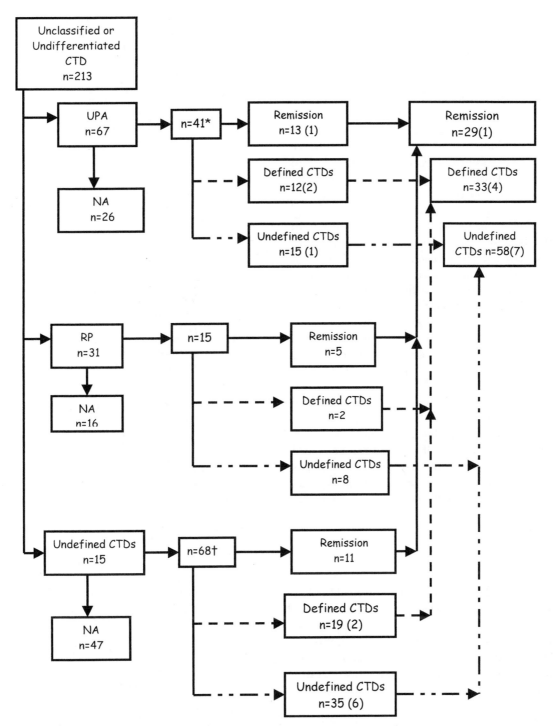

FIGURE 18.2. Ten-year follow-up diagnoses of patients with unclassified or undifferentiated connective tissue disease (*CTD*). *NA*, not available; *RP*, Raynaud phenomenon; *UPA*, unexplained polyarthritis. The *asterisk* indicates that one patient in this group developed psoriatic arthritis. The *dagger* indicates that one patient in this group each developed psoriatic arthritis, sarcoidosis, and myasthenia gravis. (Modified from Alarcón GS. Unclassified or undifferentiated connective tissue disease. In: Woolf AD, ed. *Bailliere's BEST practice and research: clinical rheumatology.* London: Harcourt Ltd., 2000:125–137.)

ancillary procedure required the presence of clinical manifestations that could justify ordering or performing them (44,45). The results of this study are worth discussing. First, the overwhelming majority of patients entering the study as defined CTDs kept the same diagnosis later. This contrasts with less than 50% for those with undifferentiated disease (46–50) that kept the same diagnosis. Among those with unclassified diseases, there were some differences, depending on the subgroup within this cohort at enrollment. Of those who started as "unexplained polyarthritis," about one-third remained undifferentiated, one-third went into remission, and the other third evolved into a defined CTD (47). In contrast, of those patients who entered the cohort as "isolated Raynaud phenomenon" or as undefined manifestations of a CTD, about one-half remained as undifferentiated. Patients with Raynaud phenomenon were more likely to go into remission, whereas those with undefined manifestations were more likely to evolve into a defined CTD (47). Figure 18.2 summarizes the initial and final diagnoses of patients from this undifferentiated CTD cohort.

The examination of socioeconomic–demographic and clinical parameters for predictors of a given outcome among patients from the entire undifferentiated cohort provided some interesting data. Young African American patients with alopecia, serosis, discoid lupus, positive ANAs, and anti-Smith antibodies were more likely to evolve into SLE (50). Those with small hand joints involvement were more likely to evolve into RA (46). Of course it can be argued that in both cases patients could have been diagnosed as having SLE and RA, respectively, but following the strict guidelines established a priori they could not, since they did not meet criteria for either disorder.

SUMMARY

More than a precise diagnosis, the generalist should follow patients with manifestations suggestive but not diagnostic of a CTD with a very open mind and be ready to diagnose and treat a CTD if clear-cut manifestations evolve. Patients should be treated according to their clinical manifestations, trying to minimize the impact of the disorder as well as that of the therapies utilized.

REFERENCES

1. Tan EM, Cohen AS, Fries JF, et al. The 1982 revised criteria for the classification of systemic lupus erythematosus. *Arthritis Rheum* 1982;25:1271–1277.
2. Subcommittee for Scleroderma Criteria of the American Rheumatism Association Diagnostic and Therapeutic Criteria Committee. Preliminary criteria for the classification of systemic sclerosis (scleroderma). *Arthritis Rheum* 1980;23:581–590.
3. Bohan A, Peter JB. Polymyositis and dermatomyositis (first of two parts). *N Engl J Med* 1975;292:344–347.
4. Bohan A, Peter JB. Polymyositis and dermatomyositis (second of two parts). *N Engl J Med* 1975;292:403–407.
5. A Committee of the American Rheumatism Association. Revision of diagnostic criteria for rheumatoid arthritis. *Arthritis Rheum* 1959;2:16–20.
6. Arnett FC, Edworthy SM, Bloch DA, et al. The American Rheumatism Association 1987 revised criteria for the classification of rheumatoid arthritis. *Arthritis Rheum* 1988;31:315–324.
7. Guiziou C, Lebreton C, Kaplan G, et al. Sclerodermatomyositis. Apropos of 13 cases [Les sclérodermatomyosites. A propos de 13 observations]. *Rev Rheumat Maladies Ostéo-Articulaires* 1987;54:457–461.
8. Panush RS, Edwards L, Longley S, et al. "Rhupus" syndrome. *Arch Intern Med* 1999;148:1633–1636.
9. Vincent FM, van Houzen RN. Trigeminal sensory neuropathy and bilateral carpal tunnel syndrome: the initial manifestation of mixed connective tissue disease. *J Neurol Neurosurg Psychiatry* 1980;43:458–460.
10. Sharp GC, Irvin WS, May CM, et al. Association of antibodies to ribonucleoprotein and Sm antigens with mixed connective tissue disease, systemic lupus erythematosus, and other rheumatic diseases. *N Engl J Med* 1976;295:1149–1154.
11. Sharp GC, Irvin WS, Tan EM, et al. Mixed connective tissue disease—an apparently distinct rheumatic disease syndrome associated with a specific antibody to an extractable nuclear antigen (ENA). *Am J Med* 1972;52:148–159.
12. Nimelstein SH, Brody S, McShane D, et al. Mixed connective tissue disease: a subsequent evaluation of the original 25 patients. *Medicine* 1980;59:239–248.
13. Blackburn WD Jr, Everson MP. Silicone-associated rheumatic disease: an unsupported myth. *Plastic Reconstruc Surg* 1997;99:1362–1367.
14. Venegoni C, Chevallard M, Mele G, et al. The coexistence of rheumatoid arthritis and systemic lupus erythematosus. *Clin Rheumatol* 1987;6:439–445.
15. Cohen MG, Webb J. Concurrence of rheumatoid arthritis and systemic lupus erythematosus: report of 11 cases. *Ann Rheum Dis* 1987;46:853–858.
16. Van Vugt RM, Derksen RH, Kater L, et al. Deforming arthropathy of lupus and rhupus hands in systemic lupus erythematosus. *Ann Rheum Dis* 1998;57:540–544.
17. Fischman AS, Abeles M, Zanetti M, et al. The coexistence of rheumatoid arthritis and systemic lupus erythematosus: a review of the literature. *J Rheumatol* 1981;8:405–415.
18. Jawad ASM, Habib S. The definition for coexistent rheumatoid arthritis and systemic lupus erythematosus. *Lupus* 1995;4:166–168.
19. Garcia-Patos V, Bartralot R, Fonollosa V, et al. Childhood sclerodermatomyositis: report of a case with the anti-PM/Scl antibody and mechanic's hands. *Br J Dermatol* 1996;135:613–616.
20. Srinivas V. Sclerodermatomyositis with megacolon, small-bowel involvement and impaired lung function. *Proc R Soc Med* 1976;69:263–264.
21. Mimori T. Scleroderma-polymyositis overlap syndrome. *Int J Dermatol* 1987;26:419–425.
22. Blaszczyk M, Jablonska S, Szymanska-Jagiello W, et al. Childhood scleromyositis: an overlap syndrome associated with PM-Scl antibody. *Pediatr Dermatol* 1991;8:1–8.
23. Smolen JS, Steiner G. Mixed connective tissue disease: to be or not to be? *Arthritis Rheum* 1998;41:768–777.
24. Bonnet F, Mercie P, Hocke C, et al. Devic's neuromyelitis optica during pregnancy in a patient with systemic lupus. *Lupus* 1999;8:244–247.
25. Van der Kaaden AJ, Kamphuis DJ, Nossent JC, et al. Long-standing isolated cerebral systemic lupus erythematosus in an 8-

year-old: resemblance with multiple sclerosis. *Clin Neurol Neurosurg* 1993;95:241–244.

26. Cuadrado MJ, Khamashta MA, Ballesteros A, et al. Can neurologic manifestations of Hughes (antiphospholipid) syndrome be multiple sclerosis? Analysis of 27 patients and review of the literature. *Medicine* 2000;79:57–68.

27. Brand CA, Rowley MJ, Tait BD, et al. Coexistent rheumatoid arthritis and systemic lupus erythematosus: clinical, serological, and phenotypic features. *Ann Rheum Dis* 1992;51:173–176.

28. Bywaters EGL. The relation between heart and joint disease (type Jaccoud's). *Br Heart J* 1950;12:101–131.

29. Reilly PA, Evison G, McHugh NJ, et al. Arthropathy of hands and feet in systemic lupus erythematosus. *J Rheumatol* 1990; 17:777–784.

30. Alarcón-Segovia D, Abud-Mendoza C, Diaz-Jouanen E, et al. Deforming arthropathy of the hands in systemic lupus erythematosus. *J Rheumatol* 1988;15:65–69.

31. Spronk PE, ter Borg EJ, Kallenberg CGM. Jaccoud arthropathy: a clinical subset with an increased C-reactive protein response? *Ann Rheum Dis* 1992;51:358–361.

32. Bodemer C, Teillac D, Le Bourgeois M, et al. Efficacy of intravenous immunoglobulin in sclerodermatomyositis. *Br J Dermatol* 1990;123:545–546.

33. Orihara T, Yanase S, Furuya T. A case of sclerodermatomyositis with cutaneous amyloidosis. *Br J Dermatol* 1985;112:213–219.

34. Burdt MA, Hoffman RW, Deutscher SL, et al. Long-term outcome in mixed connective tissue disease: longitudinal clinical and serologic findings. *Lupus* 1999;42:899–909.

35. Piirainen HI. Patients with arthritis and anti-U1-RNP antibodies: a 10-year follow-up. *Br J Rheumatol* 1990;29:345–348.

36. Gendi NS, Welsh KI, van Venrooij WJ, et al. HLA type as a predictor of mixed connective tissue disease differentiation: ten-year clinical and immunogenetic followup of 46 patients. *Arthritis Rheum* 1995;38:259–266.

37. Grant KD, Adams LE, Hess EV. Mixed connective tissue disease: a subset with sequential clinical and laboratory features. *J Rheumatol* 1981;8:587–598.

38. Mukerji B, Hardin JG. Undifferentiated, overlapping and mixed connective tissue diseases. *Am J Med Sci* 1993;305:114–119.

39. Maddison PJ. Mixed connective tissue disease: overlap syndromes. In: Woolf AD, ed. *Bailliere's BEST practice and research: clinical rheumatology.* London: Harcourt Ltd, 2000:111–124.

40. Ganczarczyk L, Urowitz MB, Gladman DD. Latent lupus. *J Rheumatol* 1989;16:475–478.

41. Greer JM, Panush RS. Incomplete lupus erythematosus. *Arch Intern Med* 1989;149:2473–2476.

42. Calvo-Alén J, Bastian HM, Mikhail I, et al. Identification of patient subsets among those presumptively diagnosed with, referred and/or followed up for systemic lupus erythematosus at a large tertiary care center. *Arthritis Rheum* 1995;38:1475–1484.

43. Alarcón GS. Unclassified or undifferentiated connective tissue disease. In: Woolf AD, ed. *Bailliere's BEST practice and research: clinical rheumatology.* London: Harcourt Ltd., 2000:125–137.

44. Clegg DO, Williams HJ, Singer JZ, et al. Early undifferentiated connective tissue disease. II. The frequency of circulating antinuclear antibodies in patients with early rheumatic diseases. *J Rheumatol* 1991;18:1340–1353.

45. Alarcón GS, Williams GV, Singer JZ, et al. Early undifferentiated connective tissue disease. I. Early clinical manifestation in a large cohort of patients with undifferentiated connective tissue diseases compared with cohorts of well established connective tissue disease. *J Rheumatol* 1991;18:1332–1339.

46. Alarcón GS, Willkens RF, Ward JR, et al. Early undifferentiated connective tissue disease. IV. Musculoskeletal manifestations in a large cohort of patients with undifferentiated connective tissue diseases compared with cohorts of patients with well-established connective tissue diseases: follow-up analyses in patients with unexplained polyarthritis and patients with rheumatoid arthritis at baseline. *Arthritis Rheum* 1996;39:403–414.

47. Williams HJ, Alarcón GS, Joks R, et al. Early undifferentiated connective tissue disease (CTD). VI. An inception cohort after ten years: disease remissions and changes in diagnosis in well-established and undifferentiated CTD. *J Rheumatol* 1999;26: 816–825.

48. Williams HJ, Alarcón GS, Neuner R, et al. Early undifferentiated connective tissue disease V. An inception cohort five years later: disease remissions and changes in diagnosis in well established and undifferentiated connective tissue diseases. *J Rheumatol* 1998;25:261–268.

49. Bulpitt KJ, Clements PJ, Lachenbruch PA, et al. Early undifferentiated connective tissue disease: III. Outcome and prognostic indicators in early scleroderma (Systemic sclerosis). *Ann Intern Med* 1993;118:602–609.

50. Calvo-Alén J, Alarcón GS, Burgard SL, et al. Systemic lupus erythematosus: predictors of its occurrence among a cohort of patients with early undifferentiated connective tissue disease: multivariate analyses and identification of risk factors. *J Rheumatol* 1996;23:469–475.

RHEUMATIC FEVER, SJÖGREN SYNDROME, AND RELAPSING POLYCHONDRITIS

YUSUF YAZICI
ALLAN GIBOFSKY

RHEUMATIC FEVER

Acute rheumatic fever (RF) is a delayed, nonsuppurative sequela of a pharyngeal infection with a group A streptococcus. Following the initial streptococcal pharyngitis, there is a latent period of 2 to 3 weeks. The onset of disease is usually characterized by one of three classic ways: (a) migratory arthritis predominantly involving large joints, (b) clinical and laboratory signs of carditis and valvulitis, and (c) involvement of the central nervous system, manifesting itself as Sydenham chorea.

Epidemiology

The incidence of RF actually began to decline before the introduction of antibiotics. The introduction of antibiotics rapidly accelerated this decline, and by 1980 the incidence ranged from 0.23 to 1.88 patients per 100,000, primarily in children and teenagers. Only a few M serotypes (types 5,14,18,24) have been identified with outbreaks of RF, suggesting that certain strains of group A streptococci may be more "rheumatogenic" than others (1).

Pathogenesis

Epidemiologic and immunologic evidence indirectly implicates the group A streptococcus in the initiation of the disease process: (a) outbreaks of RF closely follow epidemics of either streptococcal sore throats or scarlet fever, (b) adequate treatment of a documented streptococcal pharyngitis markedly reduces the incidence of subsequent RF, (c) appropriate antimicrobial prophylaxis prevents the recurrences of disease in known patients with RF, (d) the vast majority of RF patients have elevated antibody (streptolysin "O," hyaluronidase, and streptokinase) titers to streptococcal antigens.

An intriguing and as yet unexplained observation has been the invariable association of RF only with streptococcal pharyngitis. Although there are many outbreaks of

impetigo, RF almost never occurs following infection with these strains. Many hypotheses have been advanced to explain the occurrence of RF and exact genesis of rheumatic carditis and other clinical manifestations. The most acceptable has been that the disease represents a damaging immune response on the part of the host to an antecedent group A streptococcal infection involving microbial antigens cross-reacting with target organs.

Clinical Features

The clinical presentation of RF is quite variable and the lack of a single pathognomonic feature has resulted in the development of the revised Jones criteria (Table 19.1). All patients should have evidence of a preceding streptococcal infection and the presence of two major or one major and two minor manifestations. These criteria were established only as guidelines and were not intended to be "etched in stone." Manifestations of RF (Table 19.2) that are not clearly expressed pose a dilemma because of the importance of identifying a first rheumatic attack clearly in order to establish the need for prophylaxis of recurrences.

In the classic, untreated case, the arthritis of RF affects several joints in quick succession, each for a short time. The terms *migrating* or *migratory* are often used to describe the arthritis. The various locations usually overlap in time. Classically, each joint is maximally inflamed only for a few days, or a week at most. In routine practice, however, many patients with arthralgias or arthritis are treated empirically with antiinflammatory medications with subsequent resolution of the arthritis, not having an opportunity to "migrate" to other joints. Involvement of only a single large joint is common, with one or both knees involved in 76% of the cases (2). Analysis of the synovial fluid generally reveals a sterile, inflammatory fluid.

Carditis can manifest in a variety of signs and symptoms, including organic heart murmurs, cardiomegaly, congestive

TABLE 19.1. REVISED JONES CRITERIA FOR DIAGNOSIS OF ACUTE RHEUMATIC FEVER

Major Criteria	Minor Criteria
Carditis	Fever
Polyarthritis	Arthralgias
Chorea	Previous RF or rheumatic heart disease
Erythema marginatum	
Subcutaneous nodules	

Laboratory Findings
Elevated acute-phase reactants (ESR, C-reactive protein)
Prolonged P-R interval

Supporting Evidence of Preceding Streptococcal Infection
1. Increased ASO or other streptococcal antibodies
2. Positive throat culture for Group A–hemolytic streptococci
3. Recent scarlet fever

ASO, antistreptolysin O; ESR, erythrocyte sedimentation rate.
From Jones Criteria Update 1992. Guidelines for diagnosis of rheumatic fever. *JAMA* 1992;268:2069–2070.

heart failure, or pericarditis. Congestive heart failure is the most life-threatening clinical syndrome of RF. Even though earlier reports put the rate of carditis at presentation at 65% (3), when Doppler sonography was employed in the clinical evaluation, 91% had carditis, indicating that with more sensitive measurements, almost all patients with RF have signs of acute carditis (4).

Rheumatic heart disease is the most severe sequela of RF. Usually occurring 10 to 20 years after the original attack, it is the major cause of acquired valvular disease in the world. The mitral valve is mainly involved, and mitral stenosis is a classic rheumatic heart disease finding and can manifest as a combination of mitral insufficiency and stenosis, due to severe calcification of the mitral valve. Valvular damage manifesting as organic murmurs later in life is likely to occur in 50% of patients with RF, particularly if they present with evidence of carditis at initial diagnosis.

Sydenham chorea is a neurologic disorder, consisting of abrupt, purposeless, nonrhythmic involuntary movements, muscular weakness, and emotional disturbances. Involuntary movements disappear during sleep and may be suppressible at the beginning. They are commonly more marked on one side and are occasionally completely unilateral. The neurologic examination fails to reveal sensory losses or pyramidal tract involvement. Chorea may follow streptococcal infections after a latent period, which is longer, on the average, than the latent period of other rheumatic manifestations.

Subcutaneous nodules of RF are firm and painless. The overlying skin is not inflamed and can usually be moved over the nodules. Nodules rarely present for more than a month. They are located over bony surfaces or prominences, and the elbows are most frequently involved. They appear only after the first few weeks of illness.

Erythema marginatum (EM) is an evanescent, nonpruritic skin rash, pink or faintly red, usually affecting the trunk, sometimes the proximal parts or the limbs, but not the face. Lesions extend centrifugally, whereas the skin in the center returns gradually to normal, hence the name *erythema marginatum*. The individual lesions may appear and disappear in a matter of hours, usually to return. EM usually occurs in the early phase of the disease.

Laboratory Findings

The diagnosis of RF cannot be established readily by laboratory tests. Nevertheless, such tests may be helpful in two ways: first, in demonstrating that an antecedent streptococcal infection has occurred, and second, in documenting the presence or persistence of an inflammatory process.

Throat cultures are usually negative, but an attempt should be made to isolate the organism. Three throat cul-

TABLE 19.2. PHYSICAL SIGNS AND SYMPTOMS OF RHEUMATIC FEVER

Signs and Symptoms	Prevalence (%)
Carditis	90.1
Arthritis	67.8
Epistaxis	5.7
Chorea	3.4
Pericarditis	3.4
Nodules	3.4
Erythema marginatum	2.3

tures should be done during the first 24 hours, before administering antibiotics. Streptococcal antibodies are more useful because (a) they reach a peak titer at about the time of onset of RF, (b) they indicate true infection rather than transient carriage, and (c) any significant recent streptococcal infection can be detected by performing several tests for different antibodies. The antibody tests are directed against extracellular products, including antistreptolysin O, anti-DNAse B, antihyaluronidase, anti-NADase, and anti-streptokinase. Antistreptolysin O has been the most widely used test and is generally available in hospitals in the United States. Antistreptolysin O titers may vary with age, season, and geography. Streptococcal antibodies, when increased, support, but do not prove, the diagnosis of RF, nor are they a measure of disease activity.

Acute-phase reactants are elevated during RF but may be normal during episodes of pure chorea or persistent EM. If either the C-reactive protein or ESR remain normal a few weeks after discontinuing antirheumatic therapy, the attack may be considered ended unless chorea appears.

Clinical Course and Treatment

The mainstay of treatment of RF has always been antiinflammatory agents, most commonly aspirin. Dramatic improvement in symptoms is usually seen after the initiation of therapy. Usually, 80 to 100 mg/kg/day in children and 4 to 8 g/day in adults are required for an effect to be seen. Duration of antiinflammatory therapy can vary but needs to be maintained until all symptoms are absent and laboratory values are normal. If severe carditis is present, steroid therapy, usually at the dose of 2 mg/kg/day, can be started for the first 1 to 2 weeks. Depending on the clinical improvement, the dosage can then be tapered over the next 2 weeks and aspirin can be added during the last week.

Whether or not signs of pharyngitis are present at the time of diagnosis, antibiotic therapy with penicillin should be started and maintained at least for 10 days, in doses recommended for the eradication of streptococcal pharyngitis. In addition, family members should be cultured and treated for streptococcal infection, if positive.

Antibiotic prophylaxis with penicillin should be started immediately following resolution of the acute episode. The optimal regimen consists of oral penicillin VK 250,000 twice a day or parenteral penicillin G, 1.2 million units IM, every 4 weeks. Some data suggest that every-3-week injections may be more effective at preventing recurrences (5). If the patient is allergic to penicillin, erythromycin 250 mg per day can be substituted. The endpoint of prophylaxis is unclear. Most believe it should continue at least until the patient is a young adult, which is usually 10 years from an acute attack with no recurrence. Individuals with documented evidence of rheumatic heart disease should be on continuous prophylaxis indefinitely since RF recurrences can occur even in the fifth or sixth decade.

Despite its disappearance in many areas of the world, RF continues to be a serious problem in geographic areas inhabited by two-thirds of the population. The importance of early diagnosis and therapy cannot be overemphasized.

SJÖGREN SYNDROME

Epidemiology

Sjögren syndrome (SS) is a slowly progressive, inflammatory autoimmune disease affecting primarily the exocrine glands. It affects mostly females, with a female-to-male ratio of 9:1. The peak incidence is in the fourth and fifth decades of life, but SS can occur in any age group. Studies looking at the prevalence of SS estimate the rate at approximately 3% (6).

Clinical Features

Most patients run a slow and benign course, and may require many years to develop the full syndrome. Most common clinical findings are mucosal dryness manifested in keratoconjuctivitis sicca (KS), xerostomia, xerotrachea, and vaginal dryness (Table 19.3). Major salivary gland enlargement and atrophic gastritis are also seen.

Diminished tear production leads to destruction of corneal and bulbar conjunctival epithelium, leading to symptoms of keratoconjunctivitis sicca, pericorneal injection, irregularity of corneal image, and lacrimal gland enlargement. Patients usually complain of a sandy, scratchy, burning sensation in their eyes.

Xerostomia, dry mouth, stems from the decreased production of saliva by the salivary glands. Patients complain of difficulty swallowing, changes in taste, and increased dental carries. Parotid or major salivary gland enlargement is seen in 60% of primary SS patients, usually starting unilaterally but progressing to bilateral enlargement with continued disease activity. Dryness may affect other mucosal surfaces, including but not limited to vaginal, bronchial, and dermal surfaces and pancreatic secretions.

About 50% of primary SS patients experience arthritis that usually does not lead to erosive changes.

TABLE 19.3. SIGNS AND SYMPTOMS OF SJÖGREN SYNDROME (SS)

SS Manifestations	Percentage
Xerophthalmia	47
Xerostomia	42
Parotid gland enlargement	24
Dyspareunia	5
Arthralgias/arthritis	28
Raynaud phenomenon	21
Kidney involvement	1.5
Lung involvement	1.5
Fever/fatigue	10

The most common skin manifestation is Raynaud phenomenon, which is seen in 30% of patients. Primary SS patients may present with swollen hands, like the scleroderma patients, but do not progress to digital ulcers. Purpura and annular erythema also may be noted.

Dysphagia, nausea, and epigastric pain are common symptoms. Gastric mucosa biopsies can show chronic atrophic gastritis and lymphocyte infiltrates, similar to salivary gland biopsies. Although acute or chronic pancreatitis has been rarely reported, subclinical involvement occurs in close to 25% of patients, manifesting as hyperamylasemia. SS has an established relationship to chronic liver disease. Patients can present with hepatomegaly and antimitochondrial antibodies, and have elevated liver function tests. In primary biliary cirrhosis, there is an increased occurrence of secondary SS (Table 19.4).

Ten percent of SS patients have overt kidney disease, presenting with hypokalemia and renal tubular acidosis. Some cases of membranous or membranoproliferative glomerulonephritis in SS have been described.

Vasculitis presents as purpura, recurrent urticaria, and mononeuritis multiplex and skin ulcerations.

Patients with primary SS have a 40-fold increase in relative risk of developing lymphoma (7). Immunohistologic studies show that these are usually of B-cell origin. Pseudolymphoma, a tumorlike collection of lymphoid cells not meeting criteria for malignancy, sometimes makes interpretation of biopsies very difficult and should be considered in a patient with lymphadenopathy, organomegaly, or salivary gland enlargement.

Pathogenesis

The manifestations of SS result from lymphocyte infiltration of glandular and nonglandular organs. Lymphocytic infiltration of the lacrimal glands and salivary glands interferes with the production of tears and saliva, respectively. Lymphocytic infiltration of other organs, such as the lungs and gastrointestinal tract, results in a variety of major organ manifestations. The lymphocytes are predominantly CD4+ helper T cells. B cells account for 20% of the lymphocytes and are responsible for increased immunoglobulin production.

TABLE 19.4. DISEASES ASSOCIATED WITH SECONDARY SJÖGREN SYNDROME

Rheumatoid arthritis
Systemic lupus erythematosus
Scleroderma
Mixed connective-tissue disease
Primary biliary cirrhosis
Vasculitis
Myositis
Chronic active hepatitis
Thyroiditis
Mixed cryoglobulinemia

Clinical Investigations

Laboratory tests reveal mild anemia, high ESR, but a normal CRP. Hypergammaglobulinemia is a common finding. Autoantibodies usually found are rheumatoid factor, antinuclear antibodies, and organ-specific antibodies as thyroglobulin thyroid microsomal, mitochondrial, and salivary duct antibodies. Antibodies to Ro (SS-A), and La (SS-B) occur frequently (Table 19.5).

The Schirmer test is used to evaluate tear production. Strips of filter paper are placed beneath the inferior lid, and after 5 minutes, the wetting length of the paper is measured. Less than 5 mm after 5 minutes is a sign of decreased secretion. Rose Bengal staining of the corneum is used to diagnose KS. Rose Bengal stains the damaged or devitalized epithelium of the cornea and conjunctiva, and slit lamp examination reveals keratitis. Sialometry (measuring salivary flow rates) and sialography (radiologically assessing anatomic changes in the salivary duct system) may also be utilized to evaluate salivary gland involvement in SS.

The cornerstone for the diagnosis of SS is the minor salivary gland biopsy. Microscopic examination reveals lymphocytic replacement of the salivary epithelium and epimyoepithelial islands made of keratin-containing epithelial cells.

Treatment

The key to treatment in SS is to prevent manifestations of underproduction of tears and saliva (8). Artificial teardrops should be used as often as needed to lubricate the eyes. Soft contact lenses may be used to protect the cornea, but these lenses themselves require wetting. Drugs that can have anticholinergic effects (tricyclic antidepressants, antispasmodics, anti-Parkinsonian agents, and phenothiazines) should be avoided.

No single method is best for the treatment of xerostomia. Salivary flow stimulation by sugar-free, flavored lozenges and chewing gum have been used. Oral hygiene is very important because of the predisposition to dental caries. Pilocarpine hydrochloride may be used to stimulate salivary production in severe cases, with the side effects of sweating and flushing. For severe extraglandular disease (interstitial pneumonitis, glomerulonephritis, vasculitis), systemic steroids (1 mg/kg/day prednisone) and immunosuppressive agents can be used (9).

TABLE 19.5. AUTOANTIBODY FINDINGS IN SJÖGREN SYNDROME (SS)

Autoantibody	Percentage
Rheumatoid factor	80–95
Antinuclear antibody (ANA)	90
Anti-SS-A antibody	70–90
Anti-SS-B antibody	40–50

TABLE 19.6. DEMOGRAPHICS OF RELAPSING POLYCHONDRITIS

Age at onset	40–50 years
Female:male	1:1
Racial distribution	Equal in all races

RELAPSING POLYCHONDRITIS

Epidemiology

Relapsing polychondritis (RP) is a rare, multisystem disorder that can be life-threatening, debilitating, and difficult to diagnose (10). An estimate from Rochester, Minnesota, puts the incidence of RP at 3.5 cases per million. Peak onset is usually at 40 to 50 years of age, but can also be seen in children and the elderly. It is equally frequent among all ethnic groups and in both sexes (Table 19.6). The estimated 5-year survival is 74% in one series, and life expectancy is reduced. About 30% of the cases are associated with other autoimmune disorders (Table 19.7). Disease manifestations can vary, depending on the age and sex of the patients, with young females having more nasal and subglottic chondritis.

Pathogenesis

The cause and pathogenesis of RP is unknown. Evidence of cell-mediated immune response, serum antibodies to type II collagen found during acute attacks in some patients (11,12), an association with HLA-DR4 antigen (13) points toward an autoimmune cause. Further genotyping has not shown a significant subtype to be increased. Generally good response to steroids and the frequent association with other autoimmune disease also support the hypothesis that RP is immunologically mediated.

TABLE 19.7. CONDITIONS ASSOCIATED WITH RELAPSING POLYCHONDRITIS

Systemic vasculitic syndromes
Rheumatoid arthritis
Systemic lupus erythematosus
Sjögren syndrome
Ankylosing spondylitis
Mixed cryoglobulinemia
Reiter syndrome
Psoriatic arthritis
Inflammatory bowel disease
Behçet syndrome
Myelodysplastic syndromes
Hodgkin disease
Primary biliary cirrhosis
Diabetes mellitus
Thymoma
Panniculitis
Retroperitoneal fibrosis

There is no pathognomonic biopsy finding for RP. Specimens of inflamed cartilage may show distinctive features. Loss of basophilic staining of the cartilage matrix, with perichondral inflammation at the cartilage–soft-tissue interface, perivascular mononuclear, and polymorphonuclear cell infiltrates may be seen (14).

Clinical Features

RP can present in many different ways (Table 19.8), but the classic clinical presentation is acute unilateral or bilateral auricular chondritis. It is a manifestation of the disease in more than 85% of patients. It typically spares the lobe, affecting only the pinna, because the lobe lacks cartilage. Unilateral or bilateral redness, warmth, and swelling usually last days to weeks and resolve with or without treatment. After repeated attacks, the pinna loses its firmness and may become soft and deformed. The external auditory canal may be involved, leading to narrowing. Both a conductive and sensorineural pattern of hearing loss may be seen, the latter presumed to be due to vasculitis of the internal auditory artery. Nasal chondritis may lead to collapse and saddle deformity.

Laryngotracheal or bronchial chondritis is the most life-threatening complication of RP (15). Symptoms include sore throat, hoarseness, cough, stridor, choking, and dyspnea. An anatomic narrowing is identified in 20% of patients. Strictures usually form in the subglottic area and may cause increased susceptibility to infections. The reported mortality rate from respiratory complications ranges from 10% to 50%.

Seronegative, asymmetric, oligo-, or polyarticular joint involvement can be seen. This is nondeforming and nonerosive. Most commonly involved joints are the ankles, wrists, and proximal interphalangeal and metacarpophalangeal joints. Because RP can be associated with other connective-tissue diseases, patients may have symptoms of arthritis stemming form the associated disorder.

Cardiac involvement includes aneurysms of the thoracic and abdominal aorta, aortitis causing thinning of the media and leading to the dilatation of the root of the aorta, and

TABLE 19.8. CLINICAL MANIFESTATIONS OF RELAPSING POLYCHONDRITIS

Clinical Manifestations	Presenting (%)	Cumulative (%)
Auricular chondritis	39	85
Nasal cartilage changes	24	54
Laryngotracheal symptoms	26	48
Arthritis	36	52
Ocular symptoms	19	51
Hearing loss	9	30
Systemic vasculitis	3	10
Cutaneous symptoms	7	28

leakage of aortic valves. Also, aortic and mitral valves can be sites of inflammation and may develop incompetence.

About 50% of patients have ocular symptoms during the course of their disease. Episcleritis, local or diffuse, and scleritis can occur at onset or anytime during the course of the disease.

Skin manifestations are variable, ranging from palpable purpura to urticaria and livedo reticularis.

Clinical Evaluation

Clinical presentation alone is enough to diagnose RP, but because it may be seen with many other diseases, the presentation may be confusing and may take time to establish the diagnosis. No pathognomonic laboratory abnormalities are associated with RP. During attacks, acute-phase reactants (ESR, CRP) are elevated. Thrombocytosis, leukocytosis, and anemia may occur. Autoantibodies and hypocomplementemia are found when RP occurs with another connective-tissue disease.

Because of the potential for serious airway involvement, patients should be evaluated for laryngotracheal disease. Computed tomography (CT) can show wall thickening by edema or granulation tissue in the trachea. Renal status should also be determined to exclude any glomerulonephritis.

Differential diagnosis includes acute infections of the ear and trauma, and although sparing of the ear lobe is characteristic, a biopsy may be required for diagnosis. Nasal damage can be part of local infections from fungi, tuberculosis, syphilis or granulomatous lesions as Wegener granulomatosis, and lymphomatoid granulomatosis. All the systemic vasculitides should also be considered and ruled out.

Treatment

For mild cases, presenting with mild auricular and/or nasal chondritis or arthritis, nonsteroidal antiinflammatory drugs and low-dose prednisone are used initially. For severe cases with laryngotracheal or ocular symptoms, inner ear inflammation, vasculitis, or severe auricular/nasal chondritis, prednisone at a dose of 1 mg/kg is indicated. Depending on the response of the patient, the prednisone may be tapered. If relapses occur, patients may require standing doses of prednisone. Anecdotal reports of dapsone, colchicine, and immunosuppressive drugs (azathioprine, cyclophosphamide, cyclosporine, chlorambucil) and plasmapheresis exist in the literature but no clinical trials had been done to determine the ideal treatment regimen. Treatment is monitored by clinical response.

Laryngotracheal involvement may require special treatment options. If airway damage has occurred, tracheostomy may be required to treat a symptomatic subglottic stenosis. For diffuse airway disease with flaccid collapse, treatment options are limited. Nasal continuous positive airway pressure may be tried to keep the airway open. Surgical correction can be attempted when the disease is no longer active.

REFERENCES

1. Markowitz M. Rheumatic fever: recent outbreaks of an old disease. *Conn Med* 1987;51:229–233.
2. Gibofsky A, Zabriskie JB. Rheumatic fever: etiology, diagnosis, and treatment. In: Koopman WJ, ed. *Arthritis and allied conditions: a textbook of rheumatology,* 13th ed. Baltimore: Williams & Wilkins, 1997:1581–1594.
3. Bland EF, Jones TD. Rheumatic fever and rheumatic heart disease: a twenty-year report on 1,000 patients followed since childhood. *Circulation* 1951;4:836–843.
4. Veasy LG, Wiedmeier SE, Orsmond GS, et al. Resurgence of acute rheumatic fever in the intermountain area of the United States. *N Engl J Med* 1987;316:421–427.
5. Lue HC, Wu MH, Hsieh KH, et al. Rheumatic fever recurrences: controlled study of 3 week versus 4 week benzathine penicillin prevention programs. *J Pediatr* 1986, 108:299–304.
6. Drosos AA, Andonopoulos AP, Costopoulos JS, et al. Prevalence of primary Sjögren's syndrome in an elderly population. *Br J Rheumatol* 1988;27:123–127.
7. Yazici Y, Kagen L. Malignancy and rheumatic diseases. *UpToDate* 1999;7:2.
8. Tzioufas AG, Moutsopoulos HM. Sjögren's syndrome. In: Klippel JH, Dieppe PA, eds. *Rheumatology.* St Louis: CV Mosby, 1998;7:32:1–12.
9. Fox RI, Tornwall J, Michelson P. Current issues in the diagnosis and treatment of Sjögren's syndrome. *Curr Opin Rheumatol* 1999;11:364–371.
10. Luthra HS. Relapsing polychondritis. In: Klippel JH, Dieppe PA, eds. *Rheumatology.* St Louis: CV Mosby, 1998:5;27:1–4.
11. Foidart JM, Abe S, Martin GR, et al. Antibodies to type II collagen in relapsing polychondritis. *N Engl J Med* 1978;299:1203–1207.
12. Terato K, Shimozuru Y, Katayama K, et al. Specificities to antibodies to type II collagen in rheumatoid arthritis. *Arthritis Rheum* 1990;33:1493–1500.
13. Lang B, Rothenfusser A, Lanchbury JS, et al. Susceptibility to relapsing polychondritis is associated with HLA-DR4. *Arthritis Rheum* 1993; 36: 660–664.
14. Trentham DE. Relapsing polychondritis. In: McCarty DJ, Koopman WJ, eds. *Arthritis and allied conditions: a textbook of rheumatology,* 12th ed. Philadelphia: Lea & Febiger, 1993:1369–1375.
15. Trentham DE, Le CH. Relapsing polychondritis. *Ann Intern Med* 1998;129:114–122.

FIBROMYALGIA

GRACIELA S. ALARCÓN

Fibromyalgia (FM) is a chronic musculoskeletal disorder characterized by generalized pain and tenderness at specific anatomic sites, called *tender points* (1). Patients with FM commonly have other clinical manifestations, including fatigue, altered sleep, headache, and irritable bowel syndrome. Although the condition had been recognized for decades under other names (*nonarticular rheumatism, psychogenic rheumatism,* and *fibrositis*), it was not until 1990 that the American College of Rheumatology (ACR) defined criteria for the classification of these patients and FM was "officially" accepted (2). Despite this endorsement, not all clinicians accept the mere existence of FM as an entity. Some think that patients with FM are only the result of the medicalization of otherwise unrelated symptoms; others consider this a defined disease. An intermediate and practical approach, and one our group favors, is that of considering these patients as having a painful musculoskeletal syndrome. The increased acceptance of FM among clinicians has resulted in lobbying efforts by interest groups to secure funding for research into the nature of this disorder. Research in FM is now being conducted at different academic centers and the field is advancing rapidly.

In the past, we have recognized that FM can occur in isolation or in the setting of another musculoskeletal or rheumatic disorder (primary versus secondary FM) (1,2). In fact, the overwhelming clinical manifestations in some patients with rheumatoid arthritis (RA) or systemic lupus erythematosus (SLE) are those of FM, and not the ones we typically attribute to either RA or SLE. These FM symptoms are, by and large, unresponsive to therapies commonly used for the treatment of the underlying condition. The ACR does not favor the distinction between primary and secondary FM (2). Our research group decided, however, to limit studies on FM to those patients with no other rheumatic or musculoskeletal condition. We feel this is the only way to tease out the mechanisms involved in the pathogenesis of pain in these patients.

The ACR defines FM as present if patients have evidence of widespread pain and at least 11 tender points (2). Widespread pain is defined as pain present above and below the waist, at both sides of the body, and in the axial skeleton. (This includes not only the upper and lower back, but also the anterior chest wall.) Some patients also have peripheral pain, which patients may refer to as "joint pain" (3). In addition to widespread pain, patients with FM must have pain or tenderness in response to relatively minor levels of pressure stimulation in 11 of 18 anatomic sites (tender points). In the research setting these points are ascertained using a calibrated dolorimeter; a point is considered positive if the patient reports pain at a pressure of 4 kg/cm^2 or less; in the clinical setting these points are ascertained exerting comparable pressure with the thumb. In our experience normal individuals have a mean threshold for pain above 5 kg/cm^2 and it is not uncommon that they do not report pain even at higher levels of pressure (1,4,5). In contrast, patients with FM report pain at pressure of around 2 kg/cm^2. It should be added that these criteria were developed for research purposes. In the clinical setting it is unnecessary for patients to have exactly 11 tender points. Most patients seeking care have in fact more, rather than fewer, tender points (2). These tender points are listed and illustrated in Fig. 20.1. The most important practical issues regarding FM will now be discussed.

CLINICAL MANIFESTATIONS
Musculoskeletal Manifestations

In addition to generalized pain and tender points, patients with FM often complain of diffuse arthralgias and myalgias as well as of subjective but not objective evidence of joint swelling, particularly in the small joints of the hands and feet (3). Some patients also complain of morning stiffness lasting from minutes to hours; others exhibit joint hypermobility (6). It is unclear whether this is a predisposing factor to the occurrence of FM or an associated clinical finding (see Fig. 20.2. A model of abnormal pain perception).

Other Clinical Manifestations

As already noted, patients with FM may experience numerous other clinical manifestations. In fact, these other manifestations may be the ones that bring these patients to seek medical help. Symptoms referred to all organ systems have been described. In some cases these other manifestations,

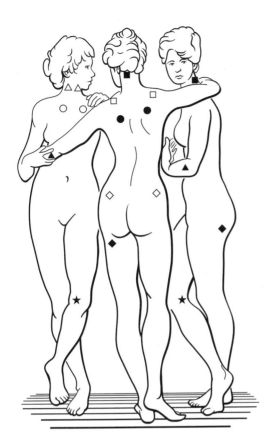

FIGURE 20.1. Localization of tender points in patients with fibromyalgia. *Solid squares,* occiput: suboccipital muscle insertions; *open triangles,* low cervical: anterior aspects of the intertransverse spaces at C5–C7; *open circles,* second rib: second costochondral junctions; *open diamonds,* gluteal: upper outer quadrants of buttocks; *stars,* knee: medial fat pad proximal to the joint line; *open squares,* trapezius: midpoint of the upper border; *solid circles,* supraspinatus: above the medial border of the scapular spine; *solid triangles,* lateral epicondyle: 2 cm distal to the epicondyles; *solid diamonds,* greater trochanter: posterior to the trochanteric prominence. [Modified from Alarcón GS. *Wmn Health Pri Care (Orth Ed)* 1999;2:11–22.]

rather than pain, may be the predominant ones. A discussion of some of these manifestations follows.

Fatigue

Patients with FM often complain of some degree of fatigue; rarely, however, is fatigue so intense as to be the factor determining incapacitation, unlike the situation of patients with chronic fatigue syndrome (CFS) (4,7–9). In turn, patients with CFS may experience arthralgias and myalgias, and may exhibit some tender points. Rarely, the patients may meet criteria for both disorders. Like pain, fatigue is a subjective manifestation, which can only be quantified by self-report.

Sleep Disturbances

Patients with FM, regardless of the intensity of their pain, usually complain of poor sleep; they may have difficulty falling asleep or may wake up throughout the night. As a result, they awake in the morning unrefreshed and tired. Some investigators have postulated that the musculoskeletal pain in FM results from sleep deprivation. Sleep studies conducted in patients with FM have indeed shown abnormal recordings during deep sleep. This pattern, called "non–rapid eye movement anomaly," is characterized by a relative fast frequency (alpha waves) superimposed in a slower delta frequency (10–12). Similar findings have been obtained in normal individuals subjected to sleep deprivation; these abnormalities are neither specific nor sensitive for FM. Another abnormality, sleep apnea, described in some patients with FM, primarily overweight men, can be considered a marker for this disorder. However, only a careful assessment of sleep (including the spouse or bed partner) may uncover the presence and severity of sleep apnea.

Other Manifestations

Table 20.1 lists other clinical manifestations described in FM patients. These patients may be under the care of different physicians for their various symptoms. Often these patients are subjected to extensive, expensive, and even invasive tests and procedures, in order to rule out more serious or different disorders. Imaging and nuclear medicine studies, endoscopies, and exploratory surgeries are, unfortunately, not uncommonly performed. Patients usually present to each new provider carrying their multiple imaging studies and medical records, seeking one more opinion to either confirm or rule out the diagnosis of FM (or associated disorder) (5). Table 20.1 lists procedures and tests commonly obtained in patients with FM.

Rheumatologists see patients with possible FM in consultation in different situations. One scenario is that of patients with FM who have failed numerous treatments and who come seeking a cure for their ailment. A second scenario is that of patients who want to legitimize their diagnosis for legal purposes (e.g., workman's compensation or disability determination) (13,14). Still others are patients with different musculoskeletal disorders who had been diagnosed as having FM but whose diagnoses have been overlooked. Examples include spinal stenosis, peripheral neuropathies, systemic vasculitis, myositis, and polymyalgia rheumatica, among others. A fourth scenario is that of patients who have been diagnosed as having "refractory RA" and have received multiple medications but have significant joint complaints (pain primarily). If patients are obese, the differentiation between puffy or fatty hands and true arthritis may not be readily evident to the nonrheumatologist. Lastly, other patients have been diagnosed as having SLE or have been referred for evaluation of possible SLE. They present FM-like manifestations and a positive test for antinuclear antibodies (ANA). They may also have subjective but not objective clinical manifestations that render the diagnosis of SLE plausible, until the history is examined more critically (15). For example, patients may present after having had oral/nasal ulcers, photosensitivity, and photosensitive

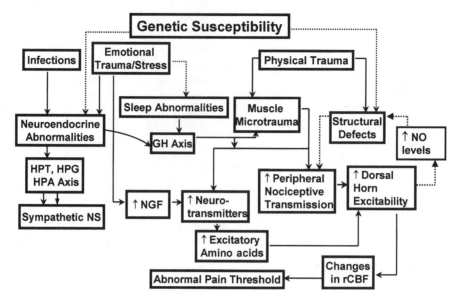

FIGURE 20.2. Model of abnormal pain perception in fibromyalgia. *Broken lines* are proposed mechanisms; *solid lines* are defined mechanisms. *HPT,* hypothalamic–pituitary–thyroid axis; *HPG,* hypothalamic–pituitary–gonadal axis; *HPA,* hypothalamic–pituitary–adrenal axis; *GH,* growth hormone axis; *NGF,* nerve growth factor; *NS,* nervous system; *NO,* nitric oxyde; *rCBF,* regional cerebral blood flow. (Modified from Weigent DA, Bradley LA, Blalock JE, et al. *Am J Med Sci* 1998;315:405–412.)

rashes. Similarly, they may complain of Raynaud-like manifestations, alopecia, chest pain (which worsens in inspiration), and of course arthralgias and myalgias. A positive ANA in this setting reinforces the diagnosis of SLE and, unfortunately, may prompt the initiation of potentially toxic pharmacologic compounds. These patients may be considered to have "pre-lupus" or "latent lupus" (16,17). Although it is never possible to be sure whether such patients may eventually develop SLE, it is preferable to wait until objective evidence of SLE becomes evident (16–18) and to not alarm these patients unduly.

EPIDEMIOLOGY

Fibromyalgia is a condition affecting preferentially middle-aged white women; men, children of either gender, and older adults can be affected, however (1,19). FM has been recognized primarily in the middle and upper socioeconomic strata. Whether this reflects only access to health care or true differences in the incidence and prevalence of the disorder among disadvantaged populations remains to be determined. In our center, as in others of North America, there is a white predominance among FM patients.

The true incidence and prevalence of FM is unknown. Population-based studies are difficult to interpret; issues such as the criteria used to diagnose FM, whether primary and secondary cases are included, the method used to ascertain them, and the demographic characteristics of the population that is being surveyed need to be considered. Studies from North America and Europe, imperfect as they may be, reveal overall prevalence rates of between 1% and 5%, but figures as high as 13% have been reported. These population-based studies confirm the gender distribution (predominantly female) of the FM syndrome. In the clinical setting, the frequency of FM depends, to a certain extent, on the degree of awareness about this condition. Figures of between 2% and 4% have been reported in the primary care setting. In rheumatology clinics, the frequency of FM fluctuates between 3% and 20%. These figures probably reflect the rheumatologists' interest in FM and the level of awareness about this condition among community physicians and the public at large (1,20).

ETIOPATHOGENESIS

Like many other rheumatic disorders, the etiopathogenesis of FM is probably multifactorial (21). Susceptible individuals may develop FM as a result of the interaction of peripheral and central factors. Familial aggregation of FM does not of itself prove genetic susceptibility; in fact, it can be argued that familial aggregation only reflects learned behavior among the offspring of adult FM patients. However, the familial pattern of FM (affecting primarily the female gender) suggests an autosomal dominant transmission (22). Animal data indeed suggest that genetic factors may influence pain sensitivity and pain modulation; human data are just emerging (22,23).

TABLE 20.1. SYMPTOMS, DIAGNOSTIC TESTS/PROCEDURES AND DIAGNOSES IN FIBROMYALGIA PATIENTS SEEKING HEALTH CARE

Specialist	Reasons for Consultation	Potential Tests/Procedures	Possible Diagnoses[a]
Internist	Malaise, fatigue, weakness	Various	Various
Cardiologist	Palpitations, chest pain, syncope, hypotension	ECG, exercise test, echocardiogram, conventional and MR angiograms, cardiac catheterization, tilt table evaluation	Mitral valve prolapse Atypical angina Dysautonomia
Pulmonologist	Dyspnea, snoring	Pulmonary function tests, arterial blood gases, polysomnogram	Asthma Sleep apnea
Gastroenterologist	Dysphagia, dyspepsia, abdominal pain, bloating, constipation, diarrhea	Upper and lower GI tract endoscopies, radiographs and/or biopsies, abdominal CT and/or ultrasound, abdominal angiogram	Noncardiac chest pain Irritable bowel syndrome Gastroesophageal reflux
Endocrinologist	Weakness, faintness	Fasting blood sugars, serum hormone levels	Hypoglycemia
Rheumatologist	Myalgias, arthralgias, Raynaud phenomenon, weakness, neck and/or back pain, fatigue	Serologic tests, electrophysiologic studies	"Latent", "Variant" or "Pre-lupus" Costochondritis Polymyalgia rheumatica "Undifferentiated" CTD
Dermatologist	Pruritus, hives, skin rashes, "photosensitivity"	Skin biopsies	Dermatitis
Allergist	"Allergies"	Skin tests, suppression tests	Allergies Multiple chemical sensitivities
Neurologist	Dizziness, dysesthesias, vertigo, headache, syncope, seizures	CT scans and/or MRIs, MR angiograms, electrophysiologic studies, lumbar puncture, biopsies	Migraine, restless leg syndrome, dysautonomia, anxiety
Gynecologist	Polyuria, dysuria, dyspareunia, "vaginitis," pelvic pain	Cystoscopies, colposcopies	UTI, cystitis, vaginitis, endometriosis
Otorhinolaryngologist	Tinnitus, cough, headache, hoarseness, snoring, vertigo, dizziness	Audiograms, CT scans or MRIs, polysomnogram	Rhinitis, sinusitis, Menière, sleep apnea
Orthopedist	Neck and/or back pain	Radiographs, MRIs, and/or CT scans	"Arthritis"
Neurosurgeon	Headache, neck and/or back pain, dysesthesias	CT scans and/or MRIs, electrophysiologic studies	Spinal stenosis, radiculopathy
Ophthalmologist	Dry eyes, blurred vision, double vision	Shirmer test, fluorescein test	Sicca syndrome
Psychiatrist	Anxiety, depression, insomnia, decreased memory, sexual and/or physical abuse	MMPI, neurocognitive evaluation, other psychologic tests	Anxiety, depression, abuse (sexual and/or physical)
Dentist	Dry mouth	Salivary gland biopsy	Sicca syndrome

[a]Some of these diagnoses represent true associations. Others, unfortunately, are given to patients in an effort to explain their symptoms, but lack organic basis.
CT, computerized tomography; CTD, connective-tissue disease; ECG, electrocardiograms; GI, gastrointestinal; MMPI, Minnesota Multiphasic Personality Inventory; MR, magnetic resonance; MRI, MR imaging; UTI, urinary tract infection.
Modified from Alarcón GS. *Wmn Health Pri Care* (Orth Ed) 1999;2:11–22.

Peripheral Factors

Patients with FM describe their pain as being "muscular." It is therefore logical that investigators targeted their efforts to study the muscle tissue in these patients; for the most part, these investigations have failed to reveal abnormalities consistently either at the tender points or elsewhere until recently. It is conceivable that initially muscle microtrauma may occur, pain persists despite apparent healing, and no further abnormalities are found either histologically, immunohistochemically, or electrophysiologically. An alternative explanation is that healing is slow to occur due to altered growth hormone (GH) production (needed for muscle repair); in turn, these altered levels of GH result from disturbed sleep (sleep modulates the GH axis). However, magnetic resonance (MR) imaging of tender points and muscles has failed to demonstrate structural abnormalities of muscles. Studies of ^{31}P MR spectroscopy, however, suggest alterations of the oxidative capacity of muscle tissue at rest (24), and ultrastructural studies demonstrate increased DNA repair in muscle fibers of patients with FM relative to control subjects (25).

Central Factors

Given the initial inconsistency and relative paucity of peripheral abnormalities in patients with FM, efforts have been directed at the elucidation of the central mechanisms that may be responsible for the musculoskeletal pain these patients present. Of course there are those who consider FM patients to have pain with no organic basis and dismiss them as a nuance to the medical system. In support of their assertion is the well-recognized fact that patients with FM who are cared for at tertiary-level facilities usually exhibit a significant degree of psychopathology (26–29). The fact that we do not understand the nature of this disorder (and why pain occurs) does not give us permission to consider the pain these patients report unreal, which unfortunately is a pervasive attitude among physicians when confronted with unexplained events. We and others have shown that many individuals meet criteria for the diagnosis of FM as per ACR criteria but who do not seek medical care for their symptoms (we have called them "FM nonpatients" to distinguish them from the ones seeking care at our center or elsewhere) (30–32). These nonpatients experience levels of pain threshold nearly comparable to those of the patients but tend to have a smaller cumulative number of psychiatric diagnoses, using the Diagnostic Interview Schedule. In other words, what prompts FM subjects to seek medical care is not pain per se, but the degree of psychologic disturbance they have. Furthermore, over a 30-month follow-up period, ten of our 40 nonpatients became patients; that is, they sought medical care for their symptoms. Features that distinguished these "new" patients from those who remained as nonpatients were, in addition to the number of psychiatric diagnoses, work-related stress and higher use of prescription medications (31,33).

Different groups of investigators are pursuing important areas of research trying to determine the factors responsible for the pain of FM. The following should be considered: sleep disturbances (described), neuroendocrine abnormalities, neuropeptide abnormalities, and abnormalities in functional brain activity.

Neuroendocrine Abnormalities

Abnormalities of the hypothalamic–pituitary–adrenal (HPA) axis are now well recognized in patients with FM. It has now clearly been shown that patients with FM exhibit a reduced 24-hour excretion of free cortisol. In addition, patients with FM respond with an exaggerated excretion of ACTH but a blunted cortisol response to the administration of corticotrophin-releasing hormone. The infusion of ACTH is followed, however, by a normal cortisol response. Abnormalities of the autonomic nervous system (e.g., response to orthostatic stress), which have been well documented in patients with FM, may be related to an altered HPA axis and abnormal sympathoadrenal responses (34–37). There is also a reciprocal interaction between the HPA axis and brain limbic system structures. These interactions may explain the high levels of aversiveness that characterizes the pain of FM (38).

Neuroendocrine abnormalities in FM go beyond the HPA axis, the sympathoadrenal responses, and limbic system structures; they include the HP-thyroid, the HP-gonadal (G), and the GH axis. The study of the hypothalamic–pituitary–gonadal (HPG) axis, including pain perception and stimulation during the different phases of the menstrual cycle, for example, may provide insights into the predominant female distribution of FM or explain the variability of symptoms patients usually describe in conjunction with the occurrence of menses. Sleep abnormalities may disturb the secretion of GH, necessary for muscle homeostasis. This disturbance, in turn, may contribute to poor healing when muscle microtrauma occurs and to the perpetuation of nociception (1).

Neuropeptide Abnormalities

Our group and others have demonstrated that patients with FM exhibit a number of different abnormalities in neuropeptides, suggesting that indeed pain in FM involves abnormalities in pain modulation. Serum and cerebrospinal fluid (CSF) levels of different neuropeptides have been described (39–43). Abnormalities that have been consistently found include low serum levels of serotonin and its metabolite, 5-hydroxyindolacetic (5-HIAA), and high CSF levels of substance P. Of interest, our group has shown elevated levels of substance P in the group of nonpatients, supporting the notion that these subjects experience a disorder similar to that of the FM subjects who seek medical care, yet the former seem to manage their symptoms without obtaining such help (4). Investigations in patients with CFS should provide further evidence that these two syndromes are different, clinically and pathogenically. Other neuropeptides found to be abnormal in patients with FM include nerve growth factor, dynorphin A, and calcitonin-related gene peptide. These neuropeptides could contribute to increased excitability of dorsal horn neurons after injury. This increased excitability results in increased neural input (which is mediated by neurons with N-methyl-D-aspartase, or NMDA, receptors). By this process (which is called *central sensitization*), the receptive area of nociception experiences an enlargement in quantity (increased peripheral perceptive field) and quality (responsive to all kinds of stimulation). Studies of pain perception conducted in our laboratory support this increased pain sensitivity in both patients and nonpatients with FM. This increase in nociceptive transmission may result in functional alterations of brain structures involved in pain modulation. It has also been proposed that the hyperexcitability of the NMDA receptors may lead to increased synthesis of nitric oxide (NO), which in turn contributes to maintaining abnormal muscle tissue and leads to increased nociception, and to a vicious cycle that is difficult to interrupt. Our group has indeed shown that serum NO levels are increased in patients with FM (44).

Abnormalities in Functional Brain Activity

Our group was the first to demonstrate that patients with FM have abnormalities in the functional activity of specific brain structures (thalamus and caudate nucleus). These studies, now replicated by other investigators, further support the contribution of central mechanisms to the pathogenesis of pain in FM (39). Initially, we studied a small group of women with FM by single photon emission computerized tomography (SPECT) and found decreased regional cerebral blood flow (rCBF) to these brain structures, particularly in patients whose manifestations started insidiously (Fig. 20.3) (45,46). These abnormalities were found in the resting state. We are now examining rCBF after painful stimulation. Such stimulation is followed in normal individuals by activation not only of the contralateral thalamus but also of the anterior cingulate (AC) cortex, the primary and secondary somatosensory (SS) cortices, and the insula. In contrast, our FM patients have shown bilateral activation of the SS cortices and of the right AC cortex. The level of painful stimulation utilized in these studies was tailored to the patients' own threshold levels of pain. Thus, by and large, patients received lower levels of painful stimulation than the controls (4). These data should be considered preliminary but are described here to emphasize the basis for these patients' main symptom—that is, musculoskeletal pain.

Before leaving this section we should state clearly that our group is not recommending the inclusion of either imaging brain studies (particularly SPECT) or the study of serum and CSF levels of neuropeptides in all FM patients. As useful as these studies have been, and continue to be, in clarifying the nature of this mysterious condition, their diagnostic properties (sensitivity; specificity; and negative, positive, and overall predictive value) have not been determined, and their risk and cost make them currently unjustifiable.

Precipitating Factors

In some patients FM evolves in an insidious manner. It is impossible to determine precisely when symptoms really started. Other patients, however, can time the onset of their symptoms to a traumatic event (physical or emotional), or to a well-defined infectious process. In fact, these postinfectious cases were called in the past "reactive FM" [comparing them to other postinfectious rheumatic disorders (reactive arthritis)] (47), but this term is no longer used. With regard to trauma, the nature of the trauma does not really matter (severity of injury or even if the event was predominantly physical, but perceived as emotional by the patient) (48,49). Numerous infectious processes have been described as capable of precipitating FM. They include infections with the human immunodeficiency virus, hepatitis C virus, Coxsackie virus, and Parvovirus B19 (50–52). Infections with *Borrelia burgdorferi* (Lyme disease) have also been recognized as capable of precipitating FM. It should be noted that, unfortunately, many cases of post-Lyme FM are erroneously

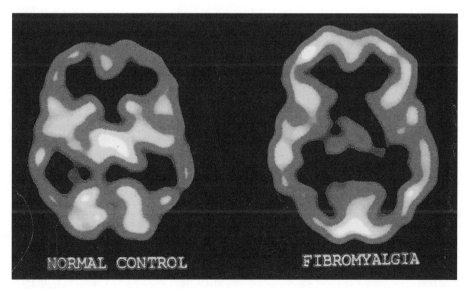

FIGURE 20.3. Single photon emission computerized tomography of the brain in a normal individual and one with fibromyalgia. There is decreased regional cerebral flow to the thalamus and caudate nuclei in the fibromyalgia patient. [Modified from Alarcón GS. *Wmn Health Pri Care (Orth Ed)* 1999; 2:11–22.] See Color Plate 6.

diagnosed as chronic Lyme disease and patients are subjected to costly, unnecessary, and lengthy treatments. (See chapters 27–30.)

Conclusions

Although we do not completely understand all the mechanisms involved in the musculoskeletal pain patients with FM have, we have made significant strides toward understanding them. Drawing from our studies and those of other investigators, we have put together a testable pain model. The contributions of peripheral and central factors to the pathogenesis of pain in FM are shown in Fig. 20.4, which is an iteration of the model our group has published before (21). This model should be modified as we and others confirm or discard the different dotted lines (mechanisms postulated but not demonstrated) that may have an important role in this disorder.

♦ Fibromyalgia is an organic, not a psychiatric, disorder. The misperception that fibromyalgia may be an affective disorder arose from the fact that the patients seen in tertiary care centers (patients included in most clinical trials and studies) often have psychiatric illness. However, they are not typical of all persons with fibromyalgia

---

♦ Official criteria for the classification of fibromyalgia include: widespread and persistent musculoskeletal pain and the presence of soft tissue tender points in at least 11 of 18 defined anatomic sites called "tender points'. However, these criteria were developed for research (not clinical) purposes. In clinical practice, there is no reason to require a specific number of tender points for diagnosis (but most patients have more rather than less points).

♦ The following findings help support a diagnosis of fibromyalgia: fatigue; difficulty sleeping; arthralgias; headache, chest, abdominal, pelvic, or perineal pain; weakness; and dysesthesias.

♦ Why patients with fibromyalgia experience chronic pain remains unknown, although evidence points to aberrations in CNS processing of stimuli. Abnormalities of the neuroendocrine system, sleep disturbances, altered cerebral blood flow to the thalamus and caudate nucleus, altered neuropeptide serum and CSF levels and changes in pain perception are frequently seen in these patients.

♦ Although the etiology of fibromyalgia is unknown, several triggers have been identified: bacterial (i.e., *Borrelia burgdorferi*) or viral (i.e., Parvovirus) infection, physical or emotional trauma, and sleep deprivation. However, in some patients, onset is insidious, and no trigger can be found.

♦ Managing fibromyalgia is challenging. A combination of pharmacologic and nonpharmacologic options is recommended. Nonpharmacologic options recommended. Nonpharmacologic options include low-impact exercise (such as aquatics, which are well tolerated) and a structured day with defined periods of sleep.

♦ Antidepressants may alleviate the symptoms of fibromyalgia if patients can tolerate their side effects. NSAIDs and corticosteroids can be used if a patient has a localized area of pain in addition to the more typical manifestations of fibromyalgia. NSAIDs may also be used sparingly for their analgesic effects. Narcotic analgesics should be avoided if at all possible

---

FIGURE 20.4. Important practical issues in fibromyalgia. [Modified from Alarcón GS. *Wmn Health Pri Care (Orth Ed)* 1999; 2:11–22.]

TREATMENT GUIDELINES

Given that we are just beginning to understand this disorder, it should not come as a surprise that we lack effective therapies or the data to support many of the ones that are advocated. Primary care physicians (PCPs) have the tremendous responsibility of steering patients away from unproved (and often risky) treatments. Patients with FM need first to believe that we, their health care providers, acknowledge that their pain is real and causes suffering (53). Second, we need to establish realistic goals from the outset. Third, we need to emphasize to our patients that pharmacologic compounds constitute only one element in their overall treatment plan. Other elements include a balance between exercise and rest; a diet aimed at achieving or maintaining an ideal body weight; avoidance of alcohol, caffeine, nicotine, and recreational drugs; and modification of abnormal sleep behaviors/habits.

Patients with FM are so often overweight and deconditioned that they have to start an exercise program very gradually. Aquatic exercises rather than land exercises are better tolerated; unfortunately, year-round aquatic programs exist only in urban areas and are not accessible to all patients. If these facilities exist, however, patients should be strongly advised to enter aquatic exercise programs under proper supervision. Low-impact aerobics are an alternative for patients lacking aquatic facilities. As with pharmacologic compounds, the data in favor of including an exercise program, weight control, and adequate sleep and health behaviors in the management of patients with FM are scarce. In many cases, the only evidence in favor of their use is the overall favorable influence these measures have on health. Data, however, are being generated for both pharmacologic and nonpharmacologic treatment modalities in FM (54–57).

Unfortunately, many patients with FM present to rheumatologists with a (sometimes very large) sac or box, which includes current and past medications (in addition to a binder with medical records and a stack of radiographs and imaging studies). Once patients have reached this level of polypharmacy, it is extremely difficult to simplify their therapeutic regimen. Moreover, the rationale for the use of some compounds is virtually lacking. That is the case, for example, for nonsteroidal antiinflammatory drugs (NSAIDs) usually detailed to generalists and specialists alike as the panacea for "arthritis" and prescribed quite often to FM patients. Other than their possible central effect (purely analgesic), there is no reason to use them; more often than not, however, they are used (despite their potential side effects and/or cost) (1). Narcotic analgesics (of different strength and quality) are, unfortunately, also commonly used, even in children and young adults. It is my experience that once FM patients start this type of analgesic, they rarely discontinue them. Muscle relaxants are also commonly used for a prolonged time. NSAIDs, narcotic analgesics, and muscle relaxants, if used, need to be prescribed judiciously, and for limited time periods (e.g., during exacerbation of background pain or after trauma in patients with joint hypermobility). This should be discussed with the patient from the outset (1,5). As our understanding of FM improves, our therapies will become more rational; for now, our patients need to understand that FM per se does not produce physical deformities and that despite pain, a relatively normal life, including work, family, and recreational activities, is possible. We are available to help them periodically, but the day-to-day management of their symptoms rests entirely in their hands.

Pharmacologic compounds found to be beneficial in patients with FM include the tricyclic antidepressants (TCAs) as well as the selective serotonin reuptake inhibitors, or SSRIs, independent of whether patients are depressed (58). These drugs probably exert their effect by ameliorating the patients' level of psychologic distress, modulating their abnormal pain perception, inducing sleep, and modifying their fatigue. Among the TCAs, amitriptyline is the most commonly used (59,60). The starting dose varies between 10 and 25 mg/day and can be escalated to 50 to 75 mg/day. In terms of the SSRIs, the most commonly used is fluoxetine; the most frequent dose is 20 mg/day, but higher doses have been used. Other SSRIs—including citalopram, sertraline hydrochloride, and venlafaxine—have also been used. Anxiolytics and other psychopharmaceuticals should be restricted to patients with clear-cut indications for their use (concomitant psychopathology). A compound not available in North America, S-adenosylmethiomine (SAMe), is a methyl donor, which appears to exert an antiinflammatory, antidepressant, and analgesic effect. Convincing case-controlled efficacy data for this compound are, however, lacking.

Other Treatment Modalities

The role of liniments and other topical preparations (substance P antagonists, such as capsaicin) in the treatment of FM is probably limited to those circumstances in which there is definite added local pathology to a region/area of the musculoskeletal system (e.g., a shoulder, elbow, trochanteric or anserine bursa). In the past, rheumatologists frequently injected several tender points with corticosteroids and anesthetics every so often. Some patients indeed reported these injections to be beneficial. This effect probably relates to the use of steroids and their systemic absorption, rather than to their local effect. These soft-tissue injections are probably justified when there is convincing evidence of local pathology as noted earlier. The rationality for performing periodic soft-tissue injections in all other FM patients is nonexistent, other than perhaps "needling" these patients, in much the same way as is done with acupuncture, now a recognized alternative treatment for FM (61). The role of soft-tissue massages, hypnotherapy, relaxation, and spinal manipulations for the treatment of FM is undetermined for now.

Recently, claims have appeared on the Internet of the successful treatment of FM with decompressive surgery of the craniocervical junction (62). This surgery is based on the reported possible association of FM with Chiari malformation (protrusion of the tonsils below the level of the foramen magnum). Although we recognize that patients with cervical spinal stenosis may exhibit some FM-like manifestations, searching for this association should be done only if clinical manifestations indicative of canal stenosis and compressive myelopathy, but not otherwise (63). Unfortunately, the Internet has favored the dissemination of unfiltered information capable of directly reaching many more patients than with methods used in the past. PCPs should be properly informed so that patients receive adequate counseling and unnecessary and risky surgical procedures are avoided.

IMPACT OF FIBROMYALGIA

Although FM patients do not develop obvious physical deformities or impairments, this disorder can impact several domains of their lives (pain, iatrogenesis, employment, and financial and family stability) (64). Patients who remain employed, physically active, and trim; take few medications; and have adequate coping skills and a supportive family tend to do better than those who are physically inactive, unemployed, overweight, and already taking many medications.

REFERENCES

1. Bradley LA, Alarcón GS. Fibromyalgia. In: Koopman WJ, ed. *Arthritis and allied conditions: a textbook of rheumatology,* 14th ed. Philadelphia: Lippincott Williams & Wilkins, 2001:1811–1844.
2. Wolfe F, Smythe HA, Yunus MB, et al. The American College of Rheumatology 1990 criteria for the classification of fibromyalgia. Report of the Multicenter Criteria Committee. *Arthritis Rheum* 1990;33:160–172.
3. Reilly PA, Littlejohn GO. Peripheral arthralgic presentation of fibrositis/fibromyalgia syndrome. *J Rheumatol* 1992;19:281–283.
4. Bradley LA, McKendree-Smith NL, Alarcón GS. Pain complaints in patients with fibromyalgia versus chronic fatigue syndrome. *Cur Rev Pain* 2000;4:148–157.
5. Alarcón GS. Fibromyalgia: dispelling diagnostic and treatment myths. Is this common condition organic or affective? *Wmn Health Pri Care (Ortho Ed)* 1999;2:775–783.
6. Acasuso-Diaz M, Collantes-Estevez E. Joint hypermobility in patients with fibromyalgia syndrome. *Arthritis Care Res* 1998;11:39–42.
7. Evengard B, Nilsson CG, Lindh G, et al. Chronic fatigue syndrome differs from fibromyalgia: no evidence for elevated substance P levels in cerebrospinal fluid of patients with chronic fatigue syndrome. *Pain* 1998;78:153–155.
8. Demitrack MA. Chronic fatigue syndrome and fibromyalgia: dilemmas in diagnosis and clinical management. *Psychiatr Clin North Am* 1999;21:671–692.
9. Buchwald D. Fibromyalgia and chronic fatigue syndrome: similarities and differences. *Rheum Dis Clin North Am* 1996;22:219–243.
10. Drewes AM. Pain and sleep disturbances with special reference to fibromyalgia and rheumatoid arthritis. *Br Soc Rheumatol* 1999;38:1035–1038.
11. Harding SM. Sleep in fibromyalgia patients: subjective and objective findings. *Am J Med Sci* 1998;315:367–376.
12. Moldofsky H, Saskin P, Lue FA. Sleep and symptoms in fibrositis syndrome after a febrile illness. *J Rheumatol* 1988;15:1701–1704.
13. Anonymous. Does fibromyalgia qualify as a work-related illness or injury? *J Occup Med* 1992;34:968.
14. Bennett RM. Fibromyalgia and the disability dilemma: a new era in understanding a complex, multidimensional pain syndrome. *Arthritis Rheum* 1996;39:1627–1634.
15. Calvo-Alén J, Bastian HM, Mikhail I, et al. Identification of patient subsets among those presumptively diagnosed with, referred and/or followed up for systemic lupus erythematosus at a large tertiary care center. *Arthritis Rheum* 1995;38:1475–1484.
16. Greer JM, Panush RS. Incomplete lupus erythematosus. *Arch Intern Med* 1989;149:2473–2476.
17. Panush RS, Schur PH. Is it lupus? *Bull Rheum Dis* 1997;46:3–8.
18. Bastian HM, Alarcón GS. A response on the positive ANA in an asymptomatic young woman (letter). *J Clin Rheumatol* 1998;4:169–170.
19. Buskila D. Fibromyalgia in children—lessons from assessing nonarticular tenderness. *J Rheumatol* 1997;24:2017–2019.
20. White KP, Speechley M, Harth M, et al. Fibromyalgia in rheumatology practice: a survey of Canadian rheumatologists. *J Rheumatol* 1995;22:722–726.
21. Weigent DA, Bradley LA, Blalock JE, et al. Current concepts in the pathophysiology of abnormal pain perception in fibromyalgia. *Am J Med Sci* 1998;315:405–412.
22. Yunus MB, Khan MA, Rawlings KK, et al. Genetic linkage analysis of multicase families with fibromyalgia. *J Rheumatol* 1999;26:408–412.
23. Offenbaecher M, Bondy B, DeJonge S, et al. Possible association of fibromyalgia with a polymorphism in the serotonin transporter gene regulatory region. *Arthritis Rheum* 1999;42:2482–2488.
24. Olsen NJ, Park JH. Skeletal muscle abnormalities in patients with fibromyalgia. *Am J Med Sci* 1998;315:351–358.
25. Salemi S, Kaeser L, Bradley LA, et al. Expression of opioid receptor variants in skin and muscle tissues of fibromyalgia patients. *Arthritis Rheum* 2000;43:S173[Abstract].
26. Hudson JI, Goldenberg DL, Pope HGJ, et al. Comorbidity of fibromyalgia with medical and psychiatric disorders. *Am J Med* 1992;92:363–367.
27. Hawley DJ, Wolfe F, Cathey MA. Pain, functional disability, and psychological status: a 120-month study of severity in fibromyalgia. *J Rheumatol* 1988;15:1551–1556.
28. Ashles TA, Yunus MB, Riley SD, et al. Psychological factors associated with primary fibromyalgia syndrome. *Arthritis Rheum* 1984;27:1101–1106.
29. Bennett RM. Emerging concepts in the neurobiology of chronic pain. *Mayo Clin Proc* 1999;74:385–398.
30. Forseth KO, Gran JT. The occurrence of fibromyalgia-like syndromes in a general female population. *Clin Rheumatol* 1993;12:23–27.
31. Aaron LA, Bradley LA, Alarcón GS, et al. Psychiatric diagnoses in patients with fibromyalgia are related to health care-seeking behavior rather than to illness. *Arthritis Rheum* 1996;39:436–445.
32. Jacobsen S, Bredkjaer SR. The prevalence of fibromyalgia and widespread chronic musculoskeletal pain in the general population [letter; comment]. *Scand J Rheumatol* 1992;21:261–263.

33. Bradley LA, Alarcón GS, Triana M, et al. Health care seeking behavior in fibromyalgia: associations with pain thresholds, symptom severity, and psychiatric morbidity. *J Musculoskel Pain* 1994;2:79–87.
34. Crofford LJ. Neuroendocrine abnormalities in fibromyalgia and related disorders. *Am J Med Sci* 1998;315:359–366.
35. Crofford LJ, Pillemer SR, Kalogeras KT, et al. Hypothalamic–pituitary–adrenal axis perturbations in patients with fibromyalgia. *Arthritis Rheum* 1994;37:1583–1592.
36. Martinez-Lavín M, Hermosillo AG, Mendoza C, et al. Orthostatic sympathetic derangement in subjects with fibromyalgia. *J Rheumatol* 1997;24:714–718.
37. Russell IJ. Neurohormonal aspects of fibromyalgia syndrome. *Rheum Dis Clin North Am* 1989;15:149–168.
38. Alberts KR, Bradley LA, Alarcón GS, et al. Anticipation of acute pain and high arousal feedback in women with fibromyalgia, high pain anxiety, and high negative affectivity evokes increased pain and anterior cingulate cortex activity without nociception. *Arthritis Rheum* 2000;43:S173[Abstract].
39. Johansson G, Risberg J, Rosenhall U, et al. Cerebral dysfunction in fibromyalgia: evidence from regional cerebral blood flow measurements, otoneurological tests and cerebrospinal fluid analysis. *Acta Psychiatr Scand* 1995;91:86–94.
40. Bennett RM. Fibromyalgia syndrome: new insights into causes. High substance P, low serotonin contribute to pain magnification. *J Musculoskel Med* 1999;16:S13–S19.
41. Giovengo SL, Russell IJ, Larson AA. Increased concentrations of nerve growth factor in cerebrospinal fluid of patients with fibromyalgia. *J Rheumatol* 1999;26:1564–1569.
42. Russell IJ. Advances in fibromyalgia: possible role for central neurochemicals. *Am J Med Sci* 1998;315:377–384.
43. Russell IJ, Orr MD, Littman B, et al. Elevated cerebrospinal fluid levels of substance P in patients with the fibromyalgia syndrome. *Arthritis Rheum* 1994;37:1593–1601.
44. Bradley LA, Weigent DA, Sotolongo A, et al. Blood serum levels of nitric oxide (NO) are elevated in women with fibromyalgia (FM): possible contributions to central and peripheral sensitization. *Arthritis Rheum* 2000;43:S173[Abstract].
45. Mountz JM, Bradley LA, Modell JG, et al. Fibromyalgia in women: abnormalities of regional cerebral blood flow in the thalamus and the caudate nucleus are associated with low pain threshold levels. *Arthritis Rheum* 1995;38:926–938.
46. Mountz JM, Bradley LA, Alarcón GS. Abnormal functional activity of the central nervous system in fibromyalgia syndrome. *Am J Med Sci* 1998;315:385–396.
47. Greenfield S, Fitzcharles MA, Esdaile JM. Reactive fibromyalgia syndrome. *Arthritis Rheum* 1992;35:678–681.
48. Buskila D, Neumann L, Vaisberg G, et al. Increased rates of fibromyalgia following cervical spine injury: a controlled study of 161 cases of traumatic injury. *Arthritis Rheum* 1997;40:446–452.
49. Aaron LA, Bradley LA, Alarcón GS, et al. Perceived physical and emotional trauma as precipitating events in fibromyalgia: associations with health care seeking and disability status but not pain severity. *Arthritis Rheum* 1997;40:453–460.
50. Goldenberg D. Fibromyalgia and its relation to chronic fatigue syndrome, viral illness, and immune abnormalities. *J Rheumatol* 1989;16:91–93.
51. Buskila D, Gladman D, Langevitz P, et al. Fibromyalgia in human immunodeficiency virus infection. *J Rheumatol* 1990;17:1202–1206.
52. Berg AM, Naides SJ, Simms RW. Established fibromyalgia and parvovirus B19 infection. *J Rheumatol* 1993;20:1941–1943.
53. Bendtsen L, Norregaard J, Jensen R, et al. Evidence of qualitatively altered nociception in patients with fibromyalgia. *Arthritis Rheum* 1997;40:98–102.
54. Bennett RM. Multidisciplinary group programs to treat fibromyalgia patients. *Rheum Dis Clin North Am* 1996;22:351–367.
55. Bennett RM, Campbell S, Burckhardt C, et al. Balanced approach provides small but significant gains: a multidisciplinary approach to fibromyalgia management. *J Musculoskelet Med* 1991;8:21–32.
56. Russell IJ. Nonpharmacologic care, NSAIDs, and tricyclics are mainstays. Fibromyalgia syndrome: formulating a strategy for relief. *J Musculoskelet Med* 1998;15:4–21.
57. Alarcón GS, Bradley LA. Advances in the treatment of fibromyalgia: current status and future directions. *Am J Med Sci* 1998;315:397–404.
58. Goldenberg D, Mayskiy M, Mossey C, et al. A randomized double-blind crossover trial of fluoxetine and amitriptyline in the treatment of fibromyalgia. *Arthritis Rheum* 1996;39:1852–1859.
59. Carette S, Bell MJ, Reynolds WJ, et al. Comparison of amitriptyline, cyclobenzaprine, and placebo in the treatment of fibromyalgia: a randomized, double-blind clinical trial. *Arthritis Rheum* 1994;37:32–40.
60. Carette S, McCain GA, Bell DA, et al. Evaluation of amitriptyline in primary fibrositis: a double-blind, placebo-controlled study. *Arthritis Rheum* 1986;29:655–659.
61. NIH Consensus Development Panel on Acupuncture. Acupuncture. *JAMA* 1999;280:1518–1524.
62. Hoh D. Spine, skull surgery may help many with CFIDS, FMS: Chiari malformation or cervical stenosis may be common in CFIDS and fibromyalgia. *CFIDS Chronicle* 1999;10–12.
63. Milhorat TH, Chou MW, Trinidad EM, et al. Chiari I malformation redefined: clinical and radiographic findings for 364 symptomatic patients. *Neurosurgery* 1999;44:1005–1017.
64. Henriksson CM. Long-term effects of fibromyalgia on everyday life. A study of 56 patients. *Scand J Rheumatol* 1994;23:36–41.

PREGNANCY AND RHEUMATIC DISEASES

MICHAEL D. LOCKSHIN

In order of frequency during pregnancy, the rheumatic diagnoses of pregnant women are systemic lupus erythematosus (SLE), antiphospholipid antibody, rheumatoid arthritis scleroderma, juvenile chronic arthritis, dermatomyositis, spondyloarthropathy, Takayasu arteritis, polyarteritis nodosa, Wegener granulomatosis, and relapsing polychondritis. Table 21.1 lists pregnancy-related maternal and fetal complications for the common rheumatic illnesses. The complications should be understood in the context of normal changes during pregnancy.

NORMAL PREGNANCY

Blood volume and cardiac output increase by 45% during pregnancy. The glomerular filtration rate increases by 50%: a normal creatinine clearance in late pregnancy is 150 mL/min. Estradiol increases 100-fold and estriol, 1,000-fold in pregnancy. Progesterone and prolactin excretion also rise by orders of magnitude. Because, in vitro, estrogens upregulate and androgens down-regulate T-cell responses and immunoglobulin synthesis, in pregnancy cell-mediated immunity, leukocyte chemotaxis and adhesion, and immune responses to specific microbial antigens are depressed. In normal pregnancy total C3, C4, and CH50 complement levels are usually unchanged or raised, but low-grade classic pathway activation is normal in pregnant women. Thrombocytopenia is common in uncomplicated late pregnancy (1). Table 21.2 outlines the potential effects on rheumatic illness of the normal physiologic changes of pregnancy.

Antirheumatic Drug Therapy During Pregnancy

Drug metabolism increases during pregnancy, necessitating dose adjustments for some medications, such as anticonvulsants. Nonsteroidal antiinflammatory drugs may rarely injure fetal kidneys or induce premature closure of the ductus arteriosus. Prednisone and methylprednisolone are inactivated by placental enzymes and do not reach the fetus; flu-

orinated corticosteroids (dexamethasone and betamethasone) are not inactivated and should be used only to treat the fetus. There is no published experience verifying safety of "pulse" bolus corticosteroid in pregnancy. Hydroxychloroquine is probably safe (2). Azathioprine, widely used in renal transplant patients, is relatively safe, but fetal cytopenias and malformations have occurred. Cyclosporine is fetotoxic at maternal toxic doses. Cyclophosphamide, methotrexate, and leflunomide are contraindicated in early pregnancy because of their teratogenic and abortifacient properties (3). Table 21.3 provides guidelines to commonly used antirheumatic drugs (4).

Fertility, Oral Contraception, Paternity

Patients with SLE, antiphospholipid antibody syndrome, or spondyloarthropathy have normal fertility, and those with rheumatoid arthritis and scleroderma probably have slight reductions in fertility. Oral contraceptives have only small effect, if any, on SLE incidence or activity (5). Paternal rheumatic illness does not affect the child.

SPECIFIC RHEUMATIC DISEASES

Systemic Lupus Erythematosus

Whether pregnancy induces lupus flare remains controversial; flares, if they do occur, are generally mild (6). Diagnosing flare during pregnancy is difficult because pregnancy-induced thrombocytopenia, preeclamptic proteinuria, and erythemas all resemble SLE flare.

Maternal Complications

Approximately one in four SLE patients develops thrombocytopenia during pregnancy. Causes include antiphospholipid antibody (asymptomatic, occurs before 15 weeks, does not fall lower than 50×10^9/L, remits after delivery, recurs with subsequent pregnancies); preeclampsia (after 25 weeks, worsens as pregnancy progresses, is associated with deteriorating maternal and fetal health, remits after delivery); HELLP

TABLE 21.1. COMMON RHEUMATIC ILLNESSES AND THEIR MAJOR PREGNANCY COMPLICATIONS

Disease	Maternal Complications	Fetal Complications	Comments
SLE	Flare, worsening renal function, low platelets	Prematurity, neonatal lupus	Anti-SSA/Ro, anti-SSB/La, antiphospholipid antibody common; renal flare, preeclampsia hard to distinguish
APS	Phlebitis, stroke postpartum	IUGR, prematurity, death	Some patients have SLE
MCTD	Similar to SLE	Similar to SLE	Manage like SLE
UCTD	Similar to SLE	Similar to SLE	Manage like SLE
RA	Remission during pregnancy, flare after	None	Patient positioning difficult
Sjögren syndrome	Similar to RA	Neonatal lupus	Anti-SSA/Ro, anti-SSB/La antibody common
JRA	Worsening during pregnancy	Insufficient data	Patient positioning difficult
Scleroderma	Fluid volume a problem	Prematurity	Renal crisis life-threatening, hard to distinguish from preeclampsia
AS, Reiter disease	Worsens during, better after pregnancy	Probably none	Hip involvement common
Psoriatic arthritis	Improves during pregnancy, worsens after	Probably none	
Dermatomyositis	Respiratory insufficiency	Probably none	Maternal strength a problem
Takayasu arteritis	Cardiac failure, hypertension hard to measure	Probably none	Hypertension hard to measure
Polyarteritis nodosa	Hypertension	Insufficient data	Very few cases known, high maternal morbidity
Wegener granulomatosis	Worsens	Insufficient data	Very few cases known
Relapsing polychondritis	No change	Insufficient data	Normal delivery usual
Ehlers–Danlos syndrome	Uterine rupture	May be affected	—
Marfan syndrome	Aortic dissection	May be affected	—
Total hip replacement	Loosens	Insufficient data	Antibiotic coverage for delivery; positioning for vaginal delivery

APS, antiphospholipid antibody syndrome; SLE, systemic lupus erythematosus; aSSB/La, antibodies to Sjögren syndrome B; aSSA/Ro, antibodies to Sjögren's syndrome A; IUGR, intrauterine growth retardation; JRA, juvenile rheumatoid arthritis; MCTD, mixed connective-tissue disease; RA, rheumatoid arthritis; UCTD, undifferentiated connective tissue disease.
From Lockshin MD. Pregnancy and rheumatic diseases. In: Koopman WJ, ed. *Arthritis and allied conditions: a textbook of rheumatology,* Philadelphia: Lippincott Williams & Wilkins, 2001:1799–1808, with permission.

syndrome (*h*emolysis, *e*levated *l*iver enzymes, *l*ow *p*latelet count, resembles severe preeclampsia with liver failure; benign thrombocytopenia of late pregnancy (average 130×10^9/L, asymptomatic, remits after delivery); idiopathic thrombocytopenic purpura (ITP) (severe, abrupt in onset); and lupus-related (reflects disease activity). Severe *anemia* (hematocrit <25%) due to chronic illness or to hemolysis indicates a need to use corticosteroid or erythropoietin for protection of the fetus, even if the mother tolerates the anemia well.

Clinical signs of active SLE, rising anti-dsDNA antibody, and erythrocyte casts favor a diagnosis of lupus *nephritis* as opposed to *preeclampsia*. Rapid worsening over days suggests preeclampsia. Normal complement in the face of progressive renal disease is most consistent with preeclampsia.

Fetal Complications

Active SLE, in the absence of maternal fever, severe anemia, uremia, hypertension, or preeclampsia, does not compromise pregnancy. Maternal IgG (and hence autoantibody) is transmitted to the fetus; nonetheless, infants born of SLE mothers with IgG-induced thrombocytopenia usually have normal platelet counts. Other autoantibodies appear in fetal blood but, except for anti-SSA/Ro and anti-SSB/La, they cause no symptoms.

Mothers with anti-SSA/Ro and anti-SSB/La antibodies, whether or not they have a clinical diagnosis of SLE, are at risk to deliver a child with neonatal lupus. The syndrome of *neonatal lupus* includes photosensitive rash, thrombocytopenia, hepatitis, and hemolytic anemia, all of which are transient, and congenital complete heart block, which is not (7). Congenital heart block is first diagnosable *in utero* by fetal electrocardiography, ultrasound, or cardiac rate monitoring between 18 and 25 weeks' gestation (average, 23 weeks). Among SLE patients with anti-SSA/Ro antibody, the risk that a liveborn child will have neonatal lupus rash is 25% and for congenital complete heart block, less than 3%. However, the risk of recurrent congenital heart block is 18% and that of *recurrent* neonatal lupus rash is 25%. Dexamethasone and plasmapheresis of the mother have been used

TABLE 21.2. COMMON PREGNANCY CHANGES THAT MAY INFLUENCE THE INTERPRETATION OR MANAGEMENT OF RHEUMATIC ILLNESS

Normal Pregnancy Change	Effect on Rheumatic Disease
Cardiovascular	
Increased intravascular volume	May cause heart failure, hypertension
Hematologic	
Hemodilutional anemia	Mimics disease exacerbation
Increased platelet activation	May worsen disease-induced thrombocytopenia
Increased fibrinogen	Suggests inflammation
Increased factor VIII, IX, X	Suggests vasculitis; lowers prothrombin time, thromboplastin time
Immunologic	
Immune complexes present	Mimics disease exacerbation
Increased complement	Modifies interpretation of disease-induced hypocomplementemia
Complement activation	Mimics disease exacerbation
Endocrine	
Increased cortisol	Induces remission during pregnancy? Decrease postpartum results in flare?
Increased estrogen	Worsens systemic lupus erythematosus?
Renal	
Inreased clearance	If clearance does not increase, fluid overload occurs
Proteinuria/hypertension	Preeclampsia versus disease exacerbation may be hard to distinguish
Joints	
Ligament loosening	Joint effusions mimic active arthritis; C1–2 subluxation may worsen in rheumatoid arthritis

From Lockshin MD. Pregnancy and rheumatic diseases. In: Koopman WJ, ed. *Arthritis and allied conditions: a textbook of rheumatology,* 14th ed. Philadelphia: Lippincott Williams & Wilkins, 2001:1799–1808, with permission.

to treat fetal incomplete heart block, myocarditis, heart failure, and *hydrops fetalis* (8). Even with a pacemaker, cardiac failure and sudden death may occur before 5 years of age.

Antiphospholipid Antibody Syndrome

Patients with antiphospholipid antibody syndrome and anticardiolipin antibody have a high frequency of midpregnancy intrauterine growth restriction or fetal death. High titer and IgG isotype suggest poor prognosis and are the only antibody characteristics that predict pregnancy outcome. Maternal history of prior fetal death markedly increases the risk of new fetal death. Low-titer IgM and IgG anticardiolipin antibody are not associated with poor fetal outcome, nor is an isolated positive test for syphilis. Fetal loss is not specific for the antiphospholipid antibody syndrome, since protein C, protein S, and antithrombin III deficiencies and Factor V_{Leiden} and prothrombin mutations also predispose to fetal death (9,10). Risk for stroke and thrombophlebitis is increased postpartum, especially after discontinuation of anticoagulant therapy.

Fetal monitoring after 15 weeks shows, in sequence, slowed fetal growth, nonreactive fetal heart rate pattern, spontaneous bradycardia, diminished fetal motion, decreased amniotic fluid, reduced placental size, and if delivery is not accomplished, fetal death. Untreated women with secondary antiphospholipid antibody syndrome, anticardiolipin antibody of 80 GPL units/mL or more, and

prior fetal deaths have fetal survival rates as low as 20%. With treatment, fetal survival rates of more than 80% are possible.

Monitoring of antiphospholipid antibody pregnancies consists of ultrasound evaluation of fetal growth rate and placental volume and appearance (11). Spontaneous fetal sinus bradycardia indicates a need to deliver. Table 21.4 lists guidelines for monitoring pregnancy. Table 21.5 gives treatment recommendations for antiphospholipid antibody pregnancy. Low-dose aspirin (81 mg/day) plus subcutaneous heparin, 5,000 to 12,000 units twice daily, begun after ultrasonographic confirmation of a viable pregnancy results in more than 80% live (not necessarily term) births (12,13). Low-molecular-weight heparin has been used successfully. Warfarin is teratogenic. Anticoagulation should continue postpartum for up to 3 months. Aspirin (if used during pregnancy) should also continue for at least 3 months. Although absolute points at which anticoagulation might end have not been established, recent data suggest that aspirin should continue indefinitely.

Sjögren Syndrome

Management of pregnancy of patients with secondary Sjögren syndrome is that of the accompanying connective-tissue disease. Patients with primary Sjögren syndrome have increased risks of fetal loss and of neonatal lupus in their offspring (14).

TABLE 21.3. DRUGS COMMONLY USED IN RHEUMATIC DISEASES

Drug	FDA Risk Category[a]	Safety	Comments
Aspirin[b]	C/D[c]	Variable, depends on dose and time of use	May be protective against fetal death in antiphospholipid antibody syndrome; may cause maternal and fetal bleeding if administered near term; high dose, uncertain safety
Naproxen, ibuprofen, ketoprofen, nabumetone and similar drugs[b]	B/D[c]	Variable, depends on dose and time of use	Experience largely accumulated through treatment of headache or dysmenorrhea; no major teratogenicity noted; use at term not advised
Ketorolac[b]	C	Causes dystocia and neonatal death in animals	Insufficient human experience
Indomethacin[b]	B/D[c]	Variable, depends on dose and time of use	Rare cases of fetal pulmonary hypertension if used at term
Celecoxib, rofecoxib	C	Double doses cause malformations in rabbits	Little available human experience
Prednisone	B	Generally safe	Trivial passage across placenta; safe in lactation, but may suppress milk production
Methylprednisolone	B	Probably safe	Similar to prednisone, but fewer data available
Dexamethasone, betamethasone	C	Probably safe in late pregnancy	Important transfer across placenta; used to induce fetal lung maturation
Hydroxychloroquine	Unclassified	Questionable safety	Small published experience indicating safety
Azathioprine	D	Safety uncertain	Large experience with renal transplant patients indicates no immediate danger to offspring if maternal dose is <2 mg/kg/d; rare reports of congenital anomalies, including immunodeficiency
Cyclosporine	C	Probably safe	Little experience, none suggesting high fetal risk
Cyclophosphamide, methotrexate, chlorambucil	D	Dangerous	Abortifacient, teratogenic
Leflunomide	X	Dangerous	Abortifacient, teratogenic, no data available
Heparin	B	Appears to be safe	Anticoagulant of choice; usually given subcutaneously twice daily; dose control essential for safety; causes osteoporosis
Low-molecular-weight heparin	B	Appears to be safe	No American controlled trials
Warfarin	X	Teratogenic and possibly fetotoxic	Fetal warfarin syndrome when given in first trimester; may cause CNS defects in second and third trimesters; risk of severe neonatal hemorrhage when given near term
Infliximab	C	No animal studies	No human studies
Etanercept	B	Animal tests without problems	No human studies
Intravenous immunoglobulin	C	No animal tests	Human experience suggests no problems

[a]Food and Drug Administration (FDA) pregnancy risk classification. A, controlled trials show no risk in humans; B, animal studies show no risk, no definitive studies in humans; C, animal studies show risk *or* no studies in humans *or* no information; D, positive evidence of risk, risk:benefit ratio may be acceptable in some circumstances; X, fetal risk, risk:benefit ratio always unacceptable.
[b]All inhibitors of prostaglandin synthesis activity may inhibit labor and prolong gestation. There is also a risk of *in utero* closure of the ductus arteriosus, particularly when used after the thirty-fourth gestational week.
[c]Risk category D when used near delivery.
Adapted from Lockshin MD. Pregnancy and rheumatic diseases. In: Koopman WJ, *Arthritis and allied conditions: a textbook of rheumatology,* 14th ed. Philadelphia: Lippincott Williams & Wilkins, 2001: 1799–1808.

TABLE 21.4. MONITORING OF THE PREGNANT RHEUMATIC DISEASE PATIENT

Recommended Frequency	Monitoring Test
First visit	Complete blood count, including platelets
	Urinalysis
	Creatinine clearance
	Anticardiolipin antibody
	Lupus anticoagulant
	Anti-SSA/Ro and anti-SSB/La antibodies
	Anti-dsDNA antibody (SLE patients)
	Complement (C3 and C4 or CH_{50}) (SLE patients)
Monthly	Platelet count[b]
Each trimester	Creatinine clearance[b]
	24-hr urine protein if screening urinalysis abnormal[b]
	Anticardiolipin antibody
	Complement[b]
	Anti-dsDNA antibody[b]
Weekly (last trimester, mothers with antiphospholipid antibody)	Antenatal fetal heart rate testing ("nonstress test"), periodic biophysical profile[c]
Between 18 and 25 weeks (mothers with anti-SSA/Ro and anti-SSB/La antibodies)	Fetal echocardiogram, ?fetal electrocardiogram

[a]The erythrocyte sedimentation rate is often abnormal in uncomplicated pregnancy.
[b]More frequently if abnormal.
[c]Measure of fetal size, activity, and domestic fluid volume.
dsDNA, double-stranded DNA; SLE, systemic lupus erythematosus.
From Lockshin MD. Pregnancy and rheumatic diseases. In: Koopman WJ, ed. *Arthritis and allied conditions: a textbook of rheumatology,* Philadelphia: Lippincott Williams & Wilkins, 2001:1799–1808, with permission.

Rheumatoid Arthritis

Patients with established rheumatoid arthritis frequently experience lessening of illness during pregnancy, probably because of maternal-fetal HLA-DQ and -DR disparity (15). Flare of rheumatoid arthritis often follows delivery.

Pregnancy is usually uneventful in rheumatoid patients. Rheumatoid joints may become unstable in late pregnancy as physiologic joint loosening occurs and as the patient's weight distribution changes. Because anticardiolipin and anti-SSA/Ro and anti-SSB/La antibodies are rarely present in rheumatoid patients, high-risk pregnancy monitoring is not generally necessary. Gold, hydroxychloroquine, cyclosporine, and azathioprine have been used during pregnancy without apparent effect on the fetus, but experience is limited and they are not recommended. Cyclophosphamide, methotrexate, and leflunomide are contraindicated. Etanercept, infliximab, and other biologics have unknown effects in pregnancy and should not be used. Low-dose prednisone is the safest option for treating active disease.

Before delivery the team managing the patient must take special care to identify the patient's disabilities to prepare for labor. Points for special emphasis are hip, knee, and neck arthritis. If intubation is planned, an anesthesiologist familiar with temporomandibular arthritis and rheumatoid cervical spine disease should be available.

Scleroderma

Problems in patients with scleroderma derive from nondistensible vascular beds and from preexisting renal, cardiac, and pulmonary insufficiency. Gastroesophageal reflux, common during pregnancy even in women with normal esophageal motility, can be disabling. Treatment is standard: small meals, elevating the head of the bed, histamine-2 blockers and proton pump inhibitors but not the prostaglandin E_1 analog, misoprostol. Maternal preeclampsia, congestive heart failure, pulmonary hypertension, pulmonary insufficiency, and renal insufficiency may occur. Renal scleroderma may be indistinguishable from preeclampsia and may justify termination of pregnancy (16). Angiotensin-converting enzyme inhibitors are relatively contraindicated in pregnancy, unless renal hypertensive crisis occurs. Patients with severe atonic small bowel disease can carry a pregnancy to term with the use of parenteral nutritional support. Prematurity or intrauterine growth restriction constitutes the greatest risk to the infant.

Spondyloarthropathy

Most patients with ankylosing spondylitis experience either no change or modest worsening of complaints during pregnancy; those who worsen return to baseline postpartum

TABLE 21.5. TREATMENT RECOMMENDATIONS FOR PREGNANT WOMEN WITH ANTIPHOSPHOLIPID ANTIBODY

Patient Characteristic	Recommendation
High-titer IgG or IgM aPL antibody[a]	
Primipara	Consider aspirin, 81 mg/d, or no therapy initially; if modest ($>50 \times 10^9$/L) thrombocytopenia occurs, add aspirin[b]
Multipara, most recent pregnancy liveborn	Consider aspirin, 81 mg/d, or no therapy initially; if modest ($>50 \times 10^9$/L) thrombocytopenia occurs, add aspirin[b]
Multipara, most recent pregnancy failure <15 weeks (1 loss)	Aspirin
Multipara, most recent pregnancy failure ≥15 weeks without other explanation, or >1 loss	Aspirin while trying to conceive; add heparin, 5,000 U b.i.d. at confirmation of fetal heartbeat, continue for duration of pregnancy
Low-titer IgG or IgM aPL antibody	
Primipara	No therapy
Multipara, no prior fetal loss	No therapy
Multipara, most recent pregnancy failure <15 weeks (1 loss)	Aspirin
Multipara, most recent pregnancy failure ≥15 weeks without other explanation, or >1 loss	Aspirin while trying to conceive; add heparin, 5,000 U b.i.d. at confirmation of fetal heartbeat, continue for duration of pregnancy
Multipara, most recent pregnancy failure ≥15 weeks without other explanation	Aspirin while trying to conceive; add heparin, 5,000 U b.i.d. at confirmation of fetal heartbeat, continue for duration of pregnancy
Multipara, prior preeclampsia, IUGR, hypertension or renal disease	Aspirin, beginning after first trimester
Normal aPL antibody	
Primipara	No therapy
Multipara, prior preeclampsia, IUGR, hypertension, or renal disease	Aspirin, beginning after first trimester
Multipara, all others	No therapy indicated by antiphospholipid antibody

[a]At our institution normal IgG <16 GPL U/mL; low positive, 16–40; high positive, >40; normal, IgM <8 MPL U/mL; low positive, 8–40; high positive, >40.
[b]For thrombocytopenia <50 × 10^9/L, consider intravenous immunoglobulin and/or prednisone.
aPL, antiphospholipid antibody; Ig, immunoglobulin; IUGR, intrauterine growth retardation.
From Lockshin MD. Pregnancy and rheumatic diseases. In: Koopman WJ, ed. *Arthritis and allied conditions: a textbook of rheumatology,* 14th ed. Philadelphia: Lippincott Williams & Wilkins, 2001:1799–1808, with permission.

(17). Patients with psoriatic arthritis may improve during pregnancy. Most patients have no unusual problems with pregnancy.

Vasculitis

Patients with *Takayasu arteritis* may do well, but renovascular occlusive disease (and preeclampsia), pulmonary hypertension, and cardiac insufficiency are important potential problems (18). Pregnancy associated with *polyarteritis nodosa* (PAN) is rare. Onset of PAN during pregnancy results in high maternal morbidity. Maternal and fetal outcome for patients in clinical remission is good. Pregnancies in patients with *leukocytoclastic vasculitis* are uneventful. Some pregnant patients with *Wegener granulomatosis* experience exacerbation and even death, but others do well (19). *Erythema nodosum* may be triggered by pregnancy (*erythema nodosum gravidarum*), but it does not harm the fetus. The course of *relapsing polychondritis* does not change during pregnancy, and full-term pregnancy is probable (20).

Dermatomyositis

Muscle fatigue and respiratory impairment are the greatest dangers for the pregnant patient with inflammatory myositis. Pulmonary fibrosis may compromise maternal respiratory reserve, especially in late pregnancy. Muscle strength and pulmonary function must be repeatedly monitored during pregnancy and delivery. The risk to the fetus is that of the mother's therapy and of the complications she suffers during pregnancy.

PREGNANCY MANAGEMENT

Table 21.4 lists monitoring recommendations for rheumatic disease patients.

Decisions regarding timing and route of delivery are dictated by the status of the fetus but may be influenced by maternal illness and its complications. There is little information about the use of tocolytics or stimulators of labor in rheumatic disease pregnancy. At delivery, "stress" corticosteroid doses (usually 100 mg hydrocortisone every 8 hours from onset of labor until 24 hours after delivery) are administered to patients currently or recently taking corticosteroids. Asymptomatic bacteremia occurs during vaginal delivery in 3.6% of deliveries.

REFERENCES

1. Crowther MA, Kelton, JG, Ginsberg J, et al. Thrombocytopenia in pregnancy: diagnosis, pathogenesis and management. *Blood Rev* 1996;10:8–16.
2. Parke AL. Antimalarial drugs in pregnancy. *Scand J Rheumatol* 1998;(Suppl 107):125–127.
3. Bermas BL, Hill JA. Effects of immunosuppressive drugs during pregnancy. *Arthritis Rheum* 1995;38:722–732.
4. Koren G, Pastuszak A, Ito S. Drugs in pregnancy. *N Engl J Med* 1998;338:1128–1137.
5. Petri M, Robinson C. Oral contraceptives and systemic lupus erythematosus. *Arthritis Rheum* 1997;40:797–803.
6. Ruiz-Irastorza G, Lima F, Alves J, et al. Increased rate of lupus flare during pregnancy and the puerperium: a prospective study of 78 pregnancies. *Br J Rheumatol* 1996;35:133–138.
7. Buyon JP, Hiebert R, Copel J, et al. Autoimmune-associated congenital heart block: demographics, mortality, morbidity and recurrence rates obtained from a national neonatal lupus registry. *J Am Coll Cardiol* 1998;31:1658–1666.
8. Rosenthal, D, Druzin M, Chin C, et al. A new therapeutic approach to the fetus with congenital complete heart block: preemptive targeted therapy with dexamethasone. *Obstet Gynecol* 1998;92:689–691.
9. Kupferminc MJ, Eldor A, Steinman N, et al. Increased frequency of genetic thrombophilia in women with complications of pregnancy. *N Engl J Med* 1999;340:9–13.
10. Lima F, Khamashta MA, Buchanan NM, et al. A study of sixty pregnancies in patients with antiphospholipid syndrome. *Clin Exp Rheumatol* 1996;14:131–136.
11. Adams D, Druzin ML, Edersheim T, et al. Antepartum testing—systemic lupus erythematosus and associated serologic abnormalities. *Am J Reprod Immunol* 1992;28:159–164.
12. Kutteh WH, Ermel LD. A clinical trial for the treatment of aPL associated recurrent pregnancy loss with lower dose heparin and aspirin. *Am J Reprod Immunol* 1996;35:402–407.
13. Rai R, Cohen H, Dave M, et al. Randomized controlled trial of aspirin and aspirin plus heparin in pregnant women with recurrent miscarriage associated with phospholipid antibodies (or antiphospholipid antibodies). *Br Med J* 1997;314:253–257.
14. Julkunen H, Kaaja R, Kurki P, et al. Fetal outcome in women with primary Sjögren's syndrome: a retrospective case-control study. *Clin Exp Rheumatol* 1995;13:65–71.
15. Nelson JL, Hughes KA, Smith AG, et al. Maternal–fetal disparity in HLA class ll alloantigens and the pregnancy-induced amelioration of rheumatoid arthritis. *N Engl J Med* 1993;329:466–471.
16. Steen VD, Medsger TA, Jr. Fertility and pregnancy outcome in women with systemic sclerosis. *Arthritis Rheum* 1999;42:763–768.
17. Gran JT, Ostensen M. Spondylarthritides in females. *Baillieres Clin Rheumatol* 1998;12:695–715.
18. Bassa A, Desai DK, Moodley J. Takayasu's disease and pregnancy: three case studies and a review of the literature. *S Afr Med J* 1995;85:107–112.
19. Luisiri P, Lance NJ, Curran JJ. Wegener's granulomatosis in pregnancy. *Arthritis Rheum* 1997;40:1354–1360.
20. Papo T, Wechsler B, Bletry O, et al. Pregnancy in relapsing polychondritis: twenty–five pregnancies in eleven patients. *Arthritis Rheum* 1997;40:1245–1249.

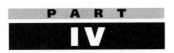

PART

IV

OSTEOARTHRITIS AND METABOLIC BONE AND JOINT DISEASE

22

OSTEOARTHRITIS

CARLOS J. LOZADA
ROY D. ALTMAN

Osteoarthritis (OA) is the most common articular disease worldwide. It is probably the oldest documented human disease and occurs in some form in all mammals. Age is its most notable risk factor. OA affects more than 20 million individuals in the United States alone (1). This high prevalence entails significant costs to society. It has been estimated that the economic impact of OA is 30 times greater than that of rheumatoid arthritis (RA) (2). Direct costs include items such as physician visits, medications, and surgical intervention but are perhaps not as significant as indirect costs, such as time lost from work or the isolation and inability to perform self-care of an elderly patient with OA. As the population of developed nations ages over the next decades, the need for better understanding and better therapeutic alternatives for OA will continue to grow (1).

With significant improvement in our understanding of the etiopathogenesis of OA, there have been changes in the conceptual approach to management, providing new emphasis on potential preventive measures and a more comprehensive approach to treatment (3). Guidelines for the management of OA at specific sites have been developed and reported (4,5). Guidelines for the conduct of clinical trials in OA have also been developed (6). OA is no longer considered a "degenerative" or "wear-and-tear" arthritis, but rather involves dynamic biomechanical, biochemical, and cellular processes (7). Indeed, the joint damage that occurs in OA is at least in part through active remodeling involving all the joint structures (8).

The development of a therapeutic program needs to consider that OA differs in symptoms, signs, and function when in different joints, implying different therapeutic options. As with any disease, the most effective therapeutic program is prevention. Several factors may predispose to the development of OA, such as trauma, infection, and obesity. Specific preventive measures can be directed at altering these risk factors.

Presently, therapy is directed at relieving pain, the most common symptom that causes the patient to seek assistance. Symptom-modifying agents may be directed at short-term-benefit (e.g., nonsteroidal antiinflammatory drugs, NSAIDs) or longer-term-benefit (e.g., intraarticular depocorticosteroids or hyaluronate). Unlike rheumatoid arthritis (RA), no proven structure-modifying (disease-modifying) agents presently exist. These medications would prevent, arrest, or reverse the process of OA.

There has also been an effort to subject therapies that have been generally considered "alternative" to appropriate clinical trials as symptom-modifying or structure-modifying (9,10).

EPIDEMIOLOGY

Osteoarthritis can be defined epidemiologically (using radiographic criteria) or clinically (radiographs plus clinical symptoms/signs) (11–13). Using radiographic criteria, 30% of individuals between the ages of 45 and 65 are affected, and more than 80% are affected by their eighth decade of life. However, most of these individuals are asymptomatic.

Prevalence of disease increases with age in both men and women. It appears to be greater among men under 45 years of age. In adults more than 55 years of age, women have a higher prevalence than men, with an increasing gap as the patients get older (14,15). In addition to age, risk factors include genetics, obesity, trauma, and others (Table 22.1).

Although OA is common worldwide, there appear to be some ethnic differences. For example, OA of the hip appears to be less common in South African blacks, east Indians, and Native Americans than in white populations (16). Genetics can be determinant in certain types of OA. Distal interphalangeal joint (DIP) OA is 10 times more likely to present in women than in men (17). Mothers and

TABLE 22.1. RISK FACTORS FOR OSTEOARTHRITIS

Age
Female sex
Obesity
Trauma
Genetic factors

sisters of women with DIP OA are two to three times more likely to be affected by it (18). Human leukocyte antigen (HLA)-A1 and HLA-B8 are associated with an increased incidence of OA (19). Certain genetic articular cartilage defects have been described as well, such as a point mutation in the cDNA for type II collagen (20,21).

Obesity in women has been linked to OA of the knees (22,23) and is probably a risk factor in both the knee and hip joints in both sexes. The mechanisms for this have not been clearly elucidated and may include increase in body mass, altered biomechanics of gait, genetic predisposition, and altered metabolism (24). Less clear still is the reason for the linkage of weight and OA of non–weight-bearing joints such as the sternoclavicular joints and the DIPs (25).

The relationship between OA and osteoporosis is unclear. There is some epidemiologic evidence for an inverse relationship between OA and osteoporosis (26). Perhaps the less dense periarticular bone in osteoporosis stresses cartilage to a lesser extent than normal bone.

PATHOLOGY/PATHOGENESIS

Initially thought of as a disease only of articular cartilage, OA involves the entire joint, including subchondral bone. There is also increasing appreciation of the role of inflammation in OA with expression of cytokines and metalloproteinases in synovium and cartilage. Therefore the term *degenerative joint disease* is no longer appropriate when referring to OA (27).

Grossly, cartilage is initially affected. Ulcerations within cartilage are seen. This damage eventually leads to cartilage loss and eburnation. There is subchondral bone formation, and eventually bony osteophytes are seen. Disease progression is characteristically slow, over several years or decades. Histologically, the earliest changes are also seen in cartilage. Proteoglycan staining is diminished and irregularity appears on the articular surface with clefts and eventual erosions.

The etiopathogenesis of OA has been divided into three stages (28). In stage 1 proteolytic breakdown of cartilage matrix occurs. Chondrocyte metabolism is affected, leading to increased production of enzymes such as metalloproteinases (e.g., collagenase and stromelysin) that destroy the cartilage matrix. Chondrocytes also produce inhibitors of proteolysis such as tissue inhibitors of metalloproteinases (TIMP) 1 and 2 but in amounts insufficient to counteract the proteolytic effect. Stage 2 involves fibrillation and erosion of the surface of the cartilage with subsequent release of proteoglycan and collagen fragments into the synovial fluid. Finally, in stage 3, these breakdown products of cartilage induce a chronic inflammatory response in the synovium. There is synovial macrophage production of cytokines such as interleukin-1 (IL-1) and tumor necrosis factor (TNF)α, and of metalloproteinases. These can diffuse back into the cartilage, where they can directly destroy tissue or stimulate chondrocytes to produce more metalloproteinases. Other pro-inflammatory molecules, such as nitric oxide (NO), an inorganic free radical, may also have a role.

Eventually these events alter joint architecture, and bone overgrowth occurs in an attempt to stabilize the joint. As the joint architecture is changed and further mechanical and inflammatory insults occur on the articular surfaces, the disease can progress unabated.

CLINICAL FEATURES

Pain is most often the reason a patient with OA seeks the help of a physician (29). It is unclear why only 40% of patients with severe radiographic OA [Kellgren and Lawrence grade III and IV (30)] have pain (31). Even when present, the origin of the pain is often not clear, as pain in OA has many potential causes (32). Damage to *articular cartilage* is the hallmark of osteoarthritis, yet articular cartilage does not generate a pain response, since it lacks nerve endings (33,34). *Menisci,* similarly, do not contain nerves, except away from compressive forces on their outer third, and cannot directly account for pain. It makes evolutionary sense that compressive or shear forces on cartilage would not elicit pain, as pain would make locomotion burdensome. Nevertheless, *articular cartilage, menisci,* and even *synovial fluid* can indirectly cause pain in OA. These are among the many possible etiologies of pain in OA, which include stretching of the joint capsule, increased vascular pressure in subchondral bone, surrounding muscle spasm, release of inflammatory cells in the synovium, and others (35) (Table 22.2). The *synovium* contains nerve fibers. These include A-β large myelinated mechanoreceptors, A-δ small myelinated nociceptors, and C-small nonmyelinated nociceptors. The nociceptors can release both substance P and calcitonin gene-related peptide (CGRP). Substance P stimulates both the pain response and inflammation (36). The *subchondral bone* is directly related to pain in OA by virtue of nociceptors such as substance P and CGRP (37). When subchondral ischemia or increased arterial pressures occur, these peptides are released from the nerve endings in bone (38). The pain of ischemic bone is aching and deep-seated—so-called bone angina. Pain recurs with bone repair and remodeling. In OA, subchondral cysts and sclerosis are the eventual radiographic evidence that localized avascular necrosis has taken place. The presence of crystals such as calcium pyrophosphate dehydrate (CPPD) can aggravate inflammation and pain (39).

Pain can be difficult to localize to an area within the joint. A thorough history and physical examination may help direct effective symptomatic therapy by revealing, and hence allowing the physician to address, the origin of the pain. Joint pain is also related to the individuals' perception of that pain and to the individual's unique ethnic, cultural, and personal circumstances. Pain tends to be more severe in

TABLE 22.2. PAIN IN OSTEOARTHRITIS

Structure	Mechanism
Cartilage	"Char" fragments, crystal release, enzyme release, stimulation of inflammatory mediators, stress on subchondral bone, joint instability
Menisci	Tearing or degeneration, stretching at their insertion to the capsule
Synovium	Increase in fluid volume that can carry cartilage products and inflammatory cells, infiltration with inflammatory cells
Subchondral bone	Ischemia and increased vascular pressure, repair of infarcted bone
Osteophytes	Periosteal elevation, neural impingement
Joint capsule	Stretch from joint distention, stress at insertion to periosteum and bone
Ligaments	Stretch at insertion to periosteum and bone
Bursae	Inflammation, with or without calcification
Muscle	Spasm, nocturnal myoclonus, contractures
Central nervous system	Psychologic stress, sleep deprivation

From Lozada CJ, Altman RD. Management of osteoarthritis. In: Koopman WJ, ed. *Arthritis and allied conditions: a textbook of rheumatology,* 14th ed. Philadelphia: Lippincott Williams & Wilkins, 2001:2246–2263, with permission.

TABLE 22.3. COMMON SITES OF INVOLVEMENT IN OSTEOARTHRITIS

Cervical spine
First carpometacarpal (CMC) joint
Distal interphalangeal joints (DIPs)
Proximal interphalangeal joints (PIPs)
  Lumbar spine
    Hips
    Knees
First metatarsophalangeal (MTP) joint

evenings, on weekends, and early in the workweek (40). Pain is complicated by the presence of dysthymia, other forms of depression, cyclothymia, and secondary gains. Psychologic intervention may be needed in the evaluation of the overlying psychologic influences on the pain response.

Initially, in symptomatic patients with OA, pain occurs during activity, relieved by rest and responsive to simple analgesia. There is short-duration morning stiffness in the joint(s), commonly lasting less than half an hour. Stiffness at times of rest or "gelling" may develop. As the disease progresses, joints may become unstable. The patient may complain of his knees "locking" or "giving way." Pain becomes more prominent, even at times of rest, and may respond less optimally to medications. Joints most commonly involved are predominantly weight-bearing, including the knees, hips, cervical and lumbosacral spine, and feet (Table 22.3). Hand joints commonly affected include the first carpometacarpal joints, distal interphalangeal joints (DIP), and proximal interphalangeal (PIP) joints.

Physical examination findings are limited to the affected joints. On inspection there may be bony enlargement and malalignment, depending on disease severity. Heberden and/or Bouchard nodes can be present. These usually develop slowly over time, although certain patients may have rapid growth with gelatinous cysts appearing before the node itself.

An effusion may be present, but there is usually no erythema or significant warmth over the joint. There is pain on active or passive range of motion of the affected joints. Crepitus (a grating sensation upon joint motion) is characteristic on range-of-motion testing of larger joints such as the knees. There can be periarticular muscle atrophy secondary to disuse. Limitation of joint motion may be present in more advanced cases.

A particular presentation in younger adults with patellar pain is chondromalacia patellae. In chondromalacia, there is damage to the patellar cartilage, and pain is most notable when walking uphill or upstairs. It is also present characteristically with marked knee flexion, as may be present when sitting in a movie theater.

Symptomatic hip OA is usually insidious in onset. Diminished internal rotation, a limp, and groin pain can be prominent features. Complaints of pain in the buttocks, sciatic region, or even knee are not uncommon. Pain in the lateral aspect of the thigh around the greater trochanter of the femur most often represents trochanteric bursitis and not OA pain. The pain is usually reproducible on palpation of the affected area.

Severe OA of the lumbar spine can result in spinal stenosis. Symptoms of pseudoclaudication occur with intermittent or constant pain in the legs worsened by exercise and relieved by sitting down. Diffuse idiopathic skeletal hyperostosis (DISH) is characterized by flowing ossification along the anterolateral aspect of the vertebral bodies, particularly the anterior longitudinal ligament. There is no associated disc space narrowing or anterior vertebral body squaring.

Erosive OA is a particular presentation in which there is prominent DIP or PIP involvement. There are inflammatory flares, resulting in joint erosion, deformity, and ankylosis.

There are also multiple causes of secondary OA, including trauma, rheumatoid arthritis, Paget disease, infectious arthritides, gout, hemophilia, acromegaly, neuropathic or Charcot joints, metabolic disorders, and congenital disorders.

LABORATORY AND RADIOGRAPHIC FINDINGS

There are no *laboratory abnormalities* specific for OA. Acute-phase reactants such as the erythrocyte sedimenta-

TABLE 22.4. RADIOLOGIC FEATURES OF OSTEOARTHRITIS

Joint space narrowing
Osteophyte formation
Subchondral sclerosis
Subchondral cysts

tion rate (ESR) are not elevated. Synovial fluid analysis usually indicates a leukocyte cell count of less than 2,000/mm³, with a mononuclear predominance.

Radiographic findings that are most indicative of OA are bony spurs at the joint margins known as osteophytes (Table 22.4). Other findings include asymmetric joint space narrowing, subchondral sclerosis, and subchondral cyst formation. The severity of the radiographic findings often fails to correlate with symptoms.

DIFFERENTIAL DIAGNOSIS

The diagnosis of OA can usually be made on clinical grounds. History and physical examination findings are usually sufficient. Radiographic findings can confirm the initial impression. Laboratory values are typically within the normal range. The initial goal is to differentiate OA from the other arthritides, such as rheumatoid arthritis (RA).

RA usually affects predominantly wrists, metacarpophalangeal (MCP), and proximal interphalangeal joints (PIP). Unlike OA, it rarely, if ever, involves the DIPs and lumbosacral spine. RA is typically associated with prominent morning stiffness of more than 1 hour, and radiographic findings are those of bone erosion (periarticular osteopenia; marginal erosions of bone) rather than bone formation. Laboratory findings in RA correlate with systemic inflammation and commonly include elevated acute-phase reactants (ESR, C-reactive protein). Eighty percent of patients eventually have a positive serum rheumatoid factor. Joint fluid with a polymorphonuclear cell predominance and substantially elevated white blood cell (WBC) count further differentiates the two diseases.

Secondary forms of OA must be considered in individuals with chondrocalcinosis, joint trauma, metabolic bone disorders, hypermobility syndromes, and neuropathic diseases. Spondyloarthropathies (e.g., Reiter syndrome, ankylosing spondylitis, and psoriatic arthritis) with sacroiliac and lumbosacral spine involvement can be differentiated by clinical history and characteristic radiographic findings.

MANAGEMENT OF OSTEOARTHRITIS

The management of OA includes preventive and therapeutic (nonpharmacologic and pharmacologic) components.

Preventive Therapy

Although many of the presently established risk factors, such as age and genetics, cannot be modified, some can be altered. The single most important factor emerging from epidemiologic trials that can be altered is obesity. Obesity in women has been linked to OA of the knees (41,42) and is probably a risk factor in both the hip and knee joints in both sexes (43). A link between weight and OA of the hands has been proposed as well (44,45). The mechanisms have not been clearly elaborated and may include increase in body mass, altered biodynamics of gait (46), genetic predisposition (genetically obese mice get more OA), and/or altered metabolism (e.g., estrogens).

Metabolic correlates of OA have been investigated as well. Data from 1,003 women between the ages of 45 and 64 from the Chingford population study have suggested that, even after adjustment for age and body mass index, hypertension, hypercholesterolemia, and elevated blood glucose may be associated with unilateral and bilateral OA of the knee (47). The Baltimore Longitudinal Study of Aging cohort did not show these relationships when adjustments for age and obesity were made (48).

Weight loss should be a goal in obese patients, as modest weight loss has been accompanied by a decrease in symptomatology (49), and perhaps reduced radiographic progression. Other studies have shown that a reduction in percent body fat rather than weight may be significant in reducing pain from OA of the knee (50).

The role of occupational trauma in OA is not always clear. However, occupations involving considerable bending seem to be related to OA of the knees. Changes in certain repetitive motions, severe trauma, and bending may be indicated. Weakness of the quadriceps muscles relative to body weight has been listed as a possible risk factor for OA of the knees (51).

Symptomatic Therapy of OA

An individualized therapeutic program should be designed once the causes of pain have been assessed. The most effective symptomatic therapy combines several approaches and may be more effective if multidisciplinary (e.g., the rheumatologist, physiatrist, orthopedist, physical therapist, occupational therapist, psychologist, psychiatrist, nurse/nurse coordinator, dietician, and social worker).

The physician-directed therapeutic program should include a combination of physical measures, medicinal measures, psychologic approaches, and surgical interventions.

Physical Measures

A variety of physical modalities are of value for the relief of pain, reducing stiffness, and limiting muscle spasm. These include strengthening the paraarticular structures to provide improved joint support. Physical measures make up an integral part of any successful therapeutic program for OA. Physical measures may be subdivided into exercise, supportive devices, alterations in activities of daily living, and thermal modalities (Table 22.5).

Exercise is the most commonly employed physical measure and is most effectively employed after some pain relief has been obtained. In patients with OA, exercise programs have been linked to reduced pain and improved function (52,53). Although professional guidance will be required in some patients, in most instances, exercises can be performed by the patient after minimal instruction. Range-of-motion exercises can be active or passive. It is theorized that improved muscle support of the joint may retard the progression of OA.

Improved strength of the paraarticular structures resulting from exercise adds stability and support to the joint and appears to reduce symptoms. A supervised program of fitness walking and education improves functional status without worsening OA of the knee (54). Patients with OA should be encouraged to exercise. (Dispel the myth that any exercise worsens arthritis.) The onset of the exercise program should be carefully graded. If the regimen is advanced too quickly, symptoms may worsen and threaten compli-

ance. The patient should be advised that worsening pain is a warning sign that exercise tolerance has been reached.

There is no advantage to bed rest for patients with acute or chronic low back pain (55). The value of exercise for chronic low back pain should not be confused with the advantages of normal physical activities for acute low back pain (56).

Other muscle groups should be exercised. Strengthening of the quadriceps muscles in a patient with knee OA can improve function and decrease pain for up to 8 months (57). Indeed, there is some question as to whether the muscle weakness actually precedes the development of symptomatic OA. Care should be taken to choose exercises that maximize muscle strengthening while minimizing stress on the affected joints. Involvement in a particular sport or activity may need to be curtailed or replaced. Swimming is particularly effective in that it exercises multiple muscle groups and is useful in nearly all forms of OA. There are exceptions where specific exercises may actually worsen symptoms (e.g., chondromalacia patella may be worsened by bicycle riding; lumbar facet OA may be worsened by hyperextension of the spine, as in swimming).

Supportive devices are often of value as a supplement to the exercise program. They partially unload the joint and may improve symptoms. Some of these devices include canes, crutches, walkers, corsets, collars, and orthotics for shoes. Canes, when properly used, can increase the base of support, decrease loading, and reduce demands on the lower limb and its joints (58). As a consequence, such devices as canes, forearm crutches, crutches, and walkers can improve balance and decrease pain. The total length of a properly measured cane should be equal to the distance between the upper border of the greater trochanter of the femur and the bottom of the heel of the shoe. This should result in elbow flexion of about 20 degrees. The cane should be held in the hand contralateral to and moved together with the affected limb. The healthier limb should precede the affected limb when climbing up stairs; when climbing down stairs, the cane and the affected limb should be advanced first. The cane can unload the affected hip by 60% (59).

Proper footwear and orthotic shoes can be of great value. A short leg that accentuates lumbar scoliosis may be helped through a unilateral heel or a sole lift. An orthotic device, or shoe insert, may help the patient with subluxed metatarsophalangeal joints (60). Walking ability and pain in early medial compartment OA of the knee can be improved by using a lateral-heel-wedged insole (61,62). Athletic shoes with good mediolateral support, good medial arch, and calcaneal cushion can be of benefit.

Knee braces may be of use in some patients with tibiofemoral disease (63), especially those with lateral instability and with a tendency for the knee to "give out."

All these supports and orthotics allow the patient more activities, improve compliance, and allow the patient to

TABLE 22.5. PHYSICAL MEASURES IN THE MANAGEMENT OF OSTEOARTHRITIS

Exercise
  Passive range of motion
  Rest periods
  Active: range of motion, isometric, isotonic, isokinetic
Support devices and orthotics
  Canes
  Crutches
  Collars
  Shoe insoles
  Medial taping of the patella
  Knee braces
Modified activities of daily living
  Proper positioning and support when sitting, sleeping, or
    driving a car
  Adjusting ways of performing such activities as getting
    dressed, etc.
  Adjusting furnishings around the house or at work (e.g.,
    raising the level of a chair or toilet seat)
Thermal modalities
  Superficial heat (e.g., hot packs, paraffin baths)
  Deep heat (e.g., ultrasound)
  Cold applications (e.g., cold packs, vapocoolant sprays)
Miscellaneous
  Pulsed electromagnetic fields
  TENS
  Acupuncture
  Chiropractic
  Spa, massage, and yoga therapy

From Lozada CJ, Altman RD. In: Koopman WJ, ed. *Arthritis and allied conditions: a textbook of rheumatology*, 14th ed. Philadelphia: Lippincott Williams & Wilkins, 2001:2246–2263, with permission.

retain functional independence. The devices should be frequently monitored to ensure proper use. Examples of this include use of cervical collars intermittently at the start, proper sizing of the collar, and proper orientation of the collar. Cane/crutch tips should be changed when worn, in order to avoid slipping on smooth or wet surfaces.

There may be a need to alter some *activities of daily living.* Simple instructions on adjusting daily activities may be very helpful in decreasing symptomatology. For example, patients with back pain should be instructed not to sit on soft couches or recliners. They should also not lie in bed with a pillow under the knees or read in bed. Patients with back pain should be advised to sit in straight-back chairs with good structural support (cushions allowed). Raising the level of a chair or toilet seat can be helpful, since the hip and knee are subjected to the highest pressures during the initial phase of rising from the seated position (64). However, lift chairs are very rarely helpful or necessary. The patient should also be advised to use a firm bed, perhaps with a bed board, and not to slouch, even when driving. The car seat should be placed forward so that the knees are flexed during driving. Stress on low back structures from slouching or sitting in soft chairs/recliners often becomes manifest the next morning when the patient has pain upon rising from bed.

Thermal modalities can be particularly effective. Superficial heat modalities have no advantage over cold applications (65). The use of heat, cold, or alternating heat and cold is based on patient preference. Traditionally, the more acute the process, the more likely cold applications will be of benefit (66). Heat can be subdivided into superficial and deep, with no proven advantage of one over the other (67–69). Hot packs, paraffin baths, hydrotherapy, and radiant heat are vehicles for providing superficial heat. Deep heat can be provided by using ultrasound, usually for larger joints, such as hips. The therapeutic value of applying heat includes decreasing joint stiffness, alleviating pain, relieving muscle spasm, and preventing contractures. Heat modalities should be used with caution in anesthetized, somnolent, or obtunded patients. The use of heat is contraindicated over tissues with inadequate vascular supply, bleeding, or cancer. Heat should also be avoided in areas close to the testicles or near developing fetuses (70). The range of temperatures used is from 40° to 45°C (104° to 113°F) (71) for 3 to 30 minutes. Cold is mostly used in the form of cold packs or vapocoolant sprays to relieve muscle spasm, decrease swelling in acute trauma, and relieve pain from inflammation.

There are several *miscellaneous* physical modalities, such as massage, yoga therapy (72), acupressure, acupuncture (73), magnets, pulsed electromagnetic fields (74), transcutaneous neural stimulation (TENS) (75), and spa therapy (balneotherapy). Many of these programs are of unproven value and work through unclear mechanisms. Chiropractic or other forms of manipulation often relieve the pain of muscle spasm transiently; repeated manipulations are often needed because of the short-lived benefit.

Psychosocial Measures

Pain and disability are not solely related to physical and mechanical impairment. Psychosocial factors are very much intertwined with the perception of pain and associated disability. Several factors have been linked to disability in patients with musculoskeletal complaints. These include older age, lower educational level, lower income, and unmarried status (76).

Reassurance, counseling, and education by the physician are important in trying to minimize the negative effects of psychosocial factors. Patients should be encouraged to participate in their care and understand their disease. This should lead the patient to better acceptance, adaptation, and compliance. Periodic telephone support has been found to be beneficial and to promote self-care among patients with OA (77).

Another potential need for psychosocial intervention is with obese patients. Weight loss groups and a stable social support system may be helpful in a concerted effort at weight reduction.

Patients can often have sexual problems secondary to the symptomatology from their OA but may be reluctant to discuss these unless specifically queried (78). Psychosocial intervention and counseling can be effective in this area as well.

Depression must be recognized and treated.

Medication-Based Symptomatic Therapy

Medications used to treat symptoms in OA can be divided into categories of topical agents, systemic oral agents, adjuvant therapies (e.g., antispasmodics and psychoactive drugs), intraarticular agents, and structure-/disease-modifying drugs (no agents yet proven to belong in this latter category) (Table 22.6). These categories of agents are individualized for each patient and are often used in combinations.

Patients frequently inquire about the benefits of diets, vitamins, and minerals. At this time there is no adequate evidence that any of these improve the symptoms or underlying disease. That is, they do not seem to affect the metabolism of cartilage or the natural history of OA. Therefore ingestion of special diets, vitamins, zinc, or copper beyond the recommended daily requirements is not encouraged.

Topical Agents

Topical agents can be useful adjuncts in the treatment of OA. The use of capsaicin has been supported in double-blind trials (79,80). Capsaicin is derived from capsicum, the common pepper plant (81). It is available as a nonprescription agent over the counter in two strengths. It is applied from two to four times daily. It has also been used

TABLE 22.6. MEDICINAL MEASURES IN THE MANAGEMENT OF OSTEOARTHRITIS

Symptomatic therapy
 Nonsteroidal antiinflammatory agents
 COX-2 inhibitors
 Nonantiinflammatory analgesics (opioids, non-opioids)
 Glucosamine sulfate[a]
 Chondroitin sulfate[a]
 S-adenosylmethionine (SAMe)[a]
 Diacerein[a]
 Avocado/soy nonsaponifiables[a]
 Ginger extracts[a]
 Adjuvant Agents
  Antispasmodics
  Tricyclic antidepressants
 Intraarticular Agents
  Intraarticular depocorticosteroids
  Intraarticular hyaluronic acid
Potential structure/disease-modifying agents
 Tetracyclines[a]
 Collagenase inhibitors[a]
 Glycosaminoglycan polysulfuric acid (GAGPS)[a]
 Glycosaminoglycan-peptide complexes[a]
 Pentosan polysulfate[a]
 Growth factors and cytokines (e.g., TGF β)[a]
 Genetic therapy[a]
 Osteochondral grafts and stem cell transplantation[a]

[a]Investigational therapy.
COX, cyclooxygenase.
Modified from Lozada CJ, Altman RD. In: Koopman WJ, ed. *Arthritis and allied conditions: a textbook of rheumatology,* 14th ed. Philadelphia: Lippincott Williams & Wilkins, 2001:2246–2263.

in postherpetic neuralgia and diabetic neuropathy (82). Capsaicin traverses the skin and interferes with substance P–mediated pain transmission by reversibly depleting stores of substance P in unmyelinated C fiber afferent neurons (83). Over the first several days of administration, until the nerve endings are depleted of substance P, capsaicin applications are accompanied by a sensation of heat or burning in the area of the skin where it is applied. If not used continuously, the nerve endings will renew their supply of and sensitivity to substance P. Care should be taken to avoid inadvertently getting capsaicin in the eyes.

There are a variety of other topical analgesic agents. Menthol- and salicylate-based over-the-counter topical preparations are available in the United States, but despite their popularity, no published trials support their use in OA. Topical NSAIDs are in common use in many parts of the world (84,85).

Systemic Oral Agents

Nonantiinflammatory *analgesics* include drugs such as acetaminophen. Despite many years of research, the mechanisms of action of acetaminophen are still not understood. In animals, the actions appear to act at the cord and cerebral levels. Acetaminophen has minimal cyclooxygenase inhibitory effect. It was as effective as ibuprofen for the

treatment of pain in osteoarthritis of the knee (86). In contrast, ibuprofen 1,200 mg was more effective and as well tolerated as acetaminophen 4,000 mg in a 6 day study for those with more severe pain (87). Acetaminophen appears free of gastric adverse effects, but hepatotoxicity can occur when ingested at high doses. Epidemiologic evidence suggests possible renal toxicity even when ingested at the recommended dose (88).

Tramadol has mild suppressive effects on the μ opioid receptor and inhibits the uptake of norepinephrine and serotonin (89). Tramadol does not have significant addictive tendencies (90) and is not a controlled schedule prescription in the United States. There have been isolated reports of abuse by opioid-dependent patients. Seizures and allergic reactions have also been reported, mostly at higher than recommended doses (91). Nevertheless, tramadol appears to have a place in the therapy of OA (92) and may have NSAID-sparing properties (93). Tramadol can produce nausea and central nervous system side effects that can be reduced by starting with 50 mg twice daily for 3 days and slowly escalating the dose to the maximum or until the desired pain relief is achieved.

The pain of OA is generally responsive to narcotic analgesics. Mildly potent and minimally addictive narcotic analgesics, such as codeine and propoxyphene, have been used effectively in patients with OA, especially in combination with nonnarcotic analgesics (e.g., acetaminophen). However, propoxyphene is not recommended in the elderly and should be avoided if at all possible.

The chronic nature of the pain in OA and the addictive potential of the stronger opiates and opioids test the skill of the physician in the use of these agents. With great care and judgment, narcotic analgesics have a place in the care of many chronic pain states, even OA. There is still uncertainty on how to block nonnarcotic central nervous system pain receptors. Guidelines for the use of narcotics in patients with nonmalignant pain have been published (94).

Antiinflammatory drugs, of which NSAIDs are the most commonly prescribed (95), are used for treating both pain and inflammation in OA. In-depth discussions of the pharmacology and potential differences between these agents have been published elsewhere (96).

Traditionally, NSAIDs have had nonselective COX inhibition, although specific and selective COX-2 inhibitors are now in clinical use. With most traditional NSAIDs, analgesia can be achieved at smaller doses than are needed for antiinflammatory effects (97). Indeed, for most NSAIDs, the greater the dose, the greater the antiinflammatory effect (also the greater risk of an adverse reaction). Since inflammation is usually not severe in OA, only smaller doses of NSAIDs may be required. In OA, the NSAID can be titrated to the lowest effective dose. Also, since the pain of OA is often intermittent, the use of NSAIDs in OA can be intermittent. There is some indication that analgesics lacking significant antiinflammatory effects may be of benefit in many patients with OA (86).

The major potential adverse effects of nonselective NSAIDs are gastrointestinal (peptic ulcer disease, gastritis) (98) and renal (interstitial nephritis, prostaglandin-inhibition-related renal insufficiency). These adverse effects are more prevalent in the elderly (99), the population with the highest prevalence of OA.

Effective strategies have been developed to mitigate the gastrointestinal (GI) toxicity of the NSAIDs: use of low-dose NSAID, use of a nonacetylated salicylate, concomitant use of misoprostol or a proton pump inhibitor, use of a specific cyclooxygenase (COX)-2 inhibitor, topical analgesics, intraarticular therapy with a depocorticosteroid or hyaluronate.

The timing of the dose of the NSAID may be important; indomethacin administered at 8 P.M. caused fewer adverse reactions than when administered at 8 A.M. (100). The effects of NSAIDs on articular cartilage and the outcome of OA are controversial (101,102).

Misoprostol, a prostaglandin E1 analog, can be taken orally and reduces the incidence of major gastric adverse events in patients receiving NSAIDs (103). In several clinical trials, the incidence of gastroduodenal ulceration in patients taking NSAIDs has been reduced by misoprostol in doses ranging from 200 μg b.i.d. to q.i.d. (104). However, the incidence of diarrhea and abdominal pain are increased (105). Misoprostol is also available as a combination product with diclofenac (106).

Proton pump inhibitors such as omeprazole (20 mg p.o. q.d.) have also been shown to reduce the incidence of gastric and duodenal endoscopic ulceration when taken by patients on NSAIDs (107). Their endoscopic effect has been equivalent to that of full doses of misoprostol (200 μg q.i.d.) in some studies (108). Although effective for symptoms, other purported gastroprotective agents such as H_2 blockers have not been as effective (109).

Patients vary in their benefit and adverse reactions to the various NSAIDs. Difference in half-lives of the NSAIDs may influence patient compliance and dosing.

In selected patients, the nonacetylated salicylates may be of value, since they do not inhibit prostaglandins at the usual doses and have reduced effects on the gastric mucosa, renal function, and platelet adhesiveness.

The discovery of two isoforms of COX has quickly led to the development of novel therapeutic modalities. The original NSAIDs work through nonspecific inhibition of cyclooxygenase isoforms 1 and 2 (COX-1 and COX-2), although alternative modes of action have been proposed (110). COX-1 is constitutively expressed in platelets, kidneys, and GI tissues, among others. COX-2 is constitutive in the brain, ovaries, kidneys, and small and large bowels but is inducible at sites of inflammatory responses. Indeed, both pain and inflammation are in the domains of COX-2. In contrast, the GI (gastritis, peptic ulcer disease) adverse effects of NSAIDs are in the domain of COX-1 inhibition. Outcome studies have demonstrated a significant reduction in GI adverse events and serious GI adverse events with spe-

cific COX-2 inhibitors when compared with nonselective NSAIDs.

In addition, platelet aggregation and bleeding time are not affected by specific COX-2 inhibition. If an antiplatelet effect is desired, an agent such as aspirin can be added. Unfortunately, mammals, including humans, express COX-2 in the macula densa and medulla of the kidney (111,112). Therefore these drugs can have renal adverse event profiles similar to those of NSAIDs.

Several excellent reviews address the COX isoenzymes and their roles (113,114). The initially available specific COX-2 inhibitors are celecoxib and rofecoxib. A double-blind, placebo-controlled trial of rofecoxib in 672 patients with hip and knee OA showed superiority to placebo at 6 weeks as assessed by WOMAC (Western Ontario and MacMaster Universities Osteoarthritis Index) pain subscale, patient global assessment of response to therapy, and physician assessment of disease status (115). Subsequent studies have shown clinical efficacy comparable to diclofenac and ibuprofen using the WOMAC pain subscale as the primary endpoint (116,117).

A 12-week double-blind, placebo-controlled study in 1,004 patients with OA of the knee showed superiority of celecoxib to placebo and no statistical difference with naproxen in arthritis assessments (118). GI adverse events and withdrawal rates were similar to placebo.

Further studies have clinical efficacy of celecoxib comparable to diclofenac in rheumatoid arthritis (119) and lack of pharmacologic interaction with methotrexate and warfarin (120). However, both celecoxib and rofecoxib may prolong prothrombin time (PT) and International Normalized Ratio (INR) values in patients on warfarin by competing for protein binding sites.

Large, double-blind, placebo-controlled trials have shown each COX-2 specific inhibitor to be numerically and statistically superior to comparator NSAIDs in terms of composite GI adverse event endpoints that have included perforations, obstructions, GI bleeds, and symptomatic ulcers (121,122).

Meloxicam, a new NSAID, is said to be COX-2 selective (in contrast to COX-2 specific). Meloxicam was tested versus diclofenac in a 6-month, multicenter, double-blind study of 336 patients. Severe adverse events, treatment withdrawal, and clinically significant laboratory abnormalities were numerically but not statistically more common with diclofenac than with meloxicam (123,124). No endoscopic trials reporting on ulceration rates are available.

COX-2 inhibitors may have effects through modulation of nitric oxide pathways (125). This may point to an antiinflammatory role for NO and its derivatives in OA.

Diacerein is the acetylated form of the naturally occurring dihydroxyanthraquinone rhein, related to the senna compounds. Diacerein inhibits the synthesis of IL-1β on human OA synovium in vitro as well as the expression of IL-1 receptors on chondrocytes (126). IL-1-dependent stromelysin-1 production was also diminished. No effects were observed on TNF or its receptors. Other observed effects of diacerein have included inhibition of superoxide anion production, chemotaxis, and phagocytosis of neutrophils and macrophages. Collagenase production has also been reduced, and articular damage has been reduced by diacerein in animal models (127–129). In human clinical trials, oral diacerein at 50 mg twice daily improved pain scores as compared with placebo. Both diacerein and tenoxicam were superior to placebo in osteoarthritis of the hip (130). Diarrhea is the main potential side effect and can be observed in up to 30% of patients (131).

Nutraceuticals, or compounds that are considered nutritional supplements in the United States, have often been employed by patients in the absence of scientific evidence to support their therapeutic use. When evidence for their effects does exist, it is usually in the form of small, nonblinded studies. Recently, although little information is available, more attention has been paid to some of these compounds in an attempt to bridge the existing information gap relative to conventional therapies.

Glucosamine sulfate, an intermediate in mucopolysaccharide synthesis, has been tested orally and intramuscularly. Glucosamine sulfate 500 mg three times daily was compared with ibuprofen 400 mg three times daily in OA of the knee in a randomized, double-blind parallel-group, 4-week study. The response to ibuprofen was quicker, but at 4 weeks there was no statistically significant difference in the two agents (reduction of at least two points in the Lequesne Index) (132). A double-blind study in China tested 178 patients with OA of the knee on oral glucosamine sulfate 1,500 mg daily versus ibuprofen 1,200 mg daily for 4 weeks. Improvement in knee pain at 4 weeks was numerically but not statistically superior with glucosamine sulfate. Adverse drug reactions were reported in 6% of the glucosamine group and 16% of the ibuprofen group with no discontinuations in the glucosamine group and 10% discontinuations in the ibuprofen group (133).

The mechanism of action of glucosamine sulfate is unknown. Some in vitro experiments have shown stimulation of the synthesis of cartilage glycosaminoglycans and proteoglycans (134,135). Enhanced synovial production of hyaluronic acid (HA) has been proposed as a mechanism in one study (136). There is evidence of structure/disease modification in animal studies showing decreased cartilage erosion (137). Statistically significant structure modification as measured by anteroposterior films of the knee was demonstrated in a 3-year European multicenter study (138). This last study has been somewhat controversial because semiflexed films of the knees, the present standard for structure-modification studies, were not used. Confirmation of the findings in other studies will be necessary. If the findings are confirmed, glucosamine could be the first structure-/disease-modifying drug for OA.

There is less information on other nutraceuticals. Oral *chondroitin sulfate,* a glycosaminoglycan with a molecular mass of around 14,000, is composed of repeating units of *N*-acetyl galactosamine and glucuronic acid. One study compared chondroitin sulfate 1,200 mg daily for 3 months to diclofenac sodium 150 mg daily for 1 month, both followed by placebo to 6 months in a double dummy protocol. The diclofenac group had quicker response to therapy, whereas the chondroitin group had a more prolonged improvement as measured by the Lequesne Index, visual analog scale for pain, four-point scale for pain, and paracetamol use (rescue medication) (139).

A metaanalysis and quality assessment of the studies of glucosamine and chondroitin in OA of hip or knee concluded that insufficient information about study design and conduct has generally been provided with these trials to allow for a definitive evaluation of either agent (140). Larger studies with longer follow-up periods are needed.

One double-blind, placebo-controlled crossover trial evaluated men with pain and radiographic knee or low back pain OA on the combination of glucosamine HCl 1,500 mg/day, chondroitin sulfate 1,200 mg/day, and manganese ascorbate 228 mg/day. Thirty-four patients were enrolled on this 16-week trial. Patients with knee OA reported improvement in visual analog scale for pain, patient assessment of treatment effect, and a summary disease score (pain questionnaire, functional questionnaire, physical examination score, and running time). No benefit was reported on patients with spinal OA (141).

S-adenosylmethionine (SAM-e), a methyl group donor (142) and oxygen radical scavenger, has been used by intravenous loading and oral maintenance. In one study the two centers reported differing results. One center reported reductions in overall pain and rest pain over placebo; the other showed no significant difference between the test group and placebo but treated patients with more severe OA (143).

Methylsulfonylmethane (MSM) has been touted, especially through the Internet, as a "sulfate donor." This "natural" product is actually chemically manufactured. It is related to DMSO, a solvent that has also been proposed as a remedy for several different conditions. Very little, if any, information on the efficacy of MSM and/or toxicity is available in the peer-reviewed scientific literature.

Avocado/soybean unsaponifiables (that part of the oil that does not hydrolize and form soap and glycerin) may have potential as slow-acting symptom-relieving drugs for OA. Prior testing was in scleroderma (144). Avocado/soy nonsaponifiables may modulate chondrocyte synthetic and repair activity (145–147). In a 3-month prospective, multicenter, randomized, double-blind, placebo-controlled trial of 162 patients with OA of hip or knee, one daily tablet of avocado/soybean unsaponifiables was compared with placebo. NSAID use was 43% in the avocado/soybean group versus 70% in the placebo group (148). Pain scores were similar in both groups, but the Lequesne functional index was significantly improved in the avocado/soy unsaponifiable group, which was compared with placebo in a 6-month study of patients with OA of the hip or knee (149). The efficacy avocado/soy unsaponifiable group was measured by the Lequesne functional index and VAS pain scale. Those in this group had significant symptomatic improvement over those taking placebos, with the effect appearing after the second month of therapy. There was also less NSAID use in the active treatment group.

Ginger-based products have been used for OA in some areas and are currently in clinical trials (150). Still other nutraceuticals (e.g., "cat's claw" and shark cartilage) are entrenched in popular culture and are being used with increasing frequency and being sold over the counter in pharmacies and health food stores. There are no carefully performed trials to support their use.

Adjuvant Agents

Any analgesic program can be supplemented with *tricyclic antidepressants*. These agents make possible the analgesic effects of the other analgesics. In addition, they may exert part of their benefit in those patients having sleep disturbances due to nocturnal myoclonus and fibromyalgia-like complaints.

Antispasmodics are useful in reducing muscle pain and spasm in OA. Although the main treatment for muscle spasm is through the physical modalities noted earlier, pain associated with muscle spasm may be reduced with an injection of lidocaine with or without a depocorticosteroid. The value of oral medications in relieving the pain of muscle spasm is controversial. Clinical trials have not convincingly demonstrated any medication to be superior to placebo. However, centrally acting agents may be helpful for their sedating qualities and potential for disrupting neurologic transmission of the pain sensation. Sedation is of value to improve sleep patterns but is no longer proposed for most patients with muscle spasm (particularly related to low back pain).

Intraarticular Therapy

Oral corticosteroids are not indicated for the treatment of OA. In contrast, *intraarticular depocorticosteroids* are felt to be of value when there is evidence of synovial inflammation. Synovial effusions should be removed before injection. Infiltration of depocorticosteroids may also be helpful in case of periarticular soft-issue complications, such as anserine bursitis. They have not been consistently helpful in facet joints for treatment of chronic low back pain (151) but have been useful in many patients as epidural injections for symptomatic spinal stenosis. In spite of the impression of many clinicians that intraarticular depocorticosteroids are of benefit in OA, few published double-blind trials support

their benefit over aspiration alone (152). Some trials have shown short-term benefit (153,154). Despite the clinical impression that they are of value in the presence of inflammation, no consistent clinical predictors of response to intraarticular depocorticosteroids have been found to aid in patient selection for this therapy (155).

There is some evidence that depocorticosteroids may slow cartilage catabolism in vitro and in animal models (156). There is contradictory evidence that they may advance osteoarthritis (157). In general, depocorticosteroid injections should be limited to four injections to any single joint per year (158).

Complications of intraarticular depocorticosteroids, such as septic arthritis, are rare if proper aseptic technique is employed. Depocorticosteroids are crystalline and can induce a transient synovitis or "flare." A "flare" occurs within several hours of the injection. This is in contrast to infection, which most often happens 24 to 72 hours after the procedure. The application of cold compresses often reduces the pain until the "flare" resolves within several hours (159). The suspicion of infection should prompt immediate reaspiration with subsequent Gram stain and cultures.

Synthetic and naturally occurring *HA derivatives* are administered intraarticularly. They are prepared in a variety of molecular weights (range <100,000 to >1,000,000 Svedberg units). In general, they are reported to reduce pain for prolonged periods of time and may improve mobility (160,161). The mechanism(s) of action is unknown. However, there is some evidence for an antiinflammatory effect (particularly at high molecular weight), a short-term lubricant effect, an analgesic effect by directly buffering synovial nerve endings, and a stimulating effect on synovial lining cells into producing normal HA, perhaps through binding to the synovial cell CD44H receptors.

Three weekly HA (Synvisc; Genzyne, Cambridge, MA, U.S.A. and Wyeth, Madison, NJ, U.S.A.) intraarticular injections provided comparable pain relief to a single depocorticosteroid intraarticular injection at 1-week follow-up; at 45-day follow-up, HA was superior to the depocorticosteroid (162). An intraarticular HA (Hyalgan; Sanofi-Synthelabo Inc., New York, NY, U.S.A.) derivative was compared with oral naproxen or placebo in a 14-week double-blind study (163). Pain relief was prolonged with the HA, and at 6 months more than 60% of the completers had at least a 20% reduction of pain, with no pain in half of that group. Even though 40% of the placebo group improved, there was significant improvement in the HA-injected group when compared with placebo. The benefit compared favorably to naproxen with significantly fewer adverse effects (fewer GI complaints). In another study, three weekly intraarticular injections of HA (Synvisc) were compared with their combination with an NSAID, and with the NSAID alone. At 12- and a telephone 26-week follow-up, the groups receiving the HA were better in terms of rest pain and lateral joint tenderness (164). Other HA derivatives are under investigation (Artz, DHA, Orthovisc).

Surgical Intervention

The primary reason for elective orthopedic surgery is intractable pain. A secondary reason for surgery is restoration of compromised function. Interventions include removal of loose bodies, stabilization of joints, redistribution of joint forces (e.g., osteotomy), relief of neural impingement (e.g., spinal stenosis, herniated disc), and joint replacement (e.g., total knee replacement).

Total hip and knee arthroplasties have improved the morbidity and probably the indirect mortality of OA. Most series report good to excellent long-term results in more than 90% of patients undergoing either hip or knee replacement (132), with 85% success rates at 20-year follow-up of the Charnley total hip prosthesis. These procedures appear cost-effective when the improved quality of life and the alternatives are considered. Osteotomies may serve as alternatives to arthroplasty, in younger, overweight patients, and in unicompartmental disease of the knee. This may delay progression of disease (hence the need for total joint replacement). However, only 50% of patients with knee osteotomies have satisfactory results at 10 years (165). Hip osteotomies have less certain long-term results.

Arthroscopic intervention should be limited to patients in whom an additional diagnosis is suspected. Surgical arthroscopy is useful for repair and for partial removal of damaged menisci as discussed earlier. The value of synovectomy and debridement has not been established in OA (166).

Arthroscopic lavage has also been tried with some success. Large-bore needle lavage with saline may be of value in selected patients (167). It has been shown to be effective in the relief of pain in OA of the knees for up to 6 months (168).

Structure/Disease-Modifying Agents

Structure/disease-modifying agents for OA are intended to retard the progression of OA and/or enhance a normal reparative process (Table 22.6). Since OA is a disease of the entire joint, the prior term *chondroprotection* is inappropriate. It appears most difficult to establish the value of a structure-/disease-modifying drug in a disease process that progresses at variable rates and has no definable clinical or laboratory marker of activity/progression. Measures used to identify structure/disease modification include radiographic assessment of joint space, such as fluoroscopically positioned anteroposterior radiographs of the knee or MRI (169). Although several agents are being evaluated for these properties, none have been established as effective. Several of the agents discussed earlier have structure-/disease-modifying potential. Agents with structure-/disease-modifying

potential can be listed as follows: (a) growth factors and cytokines, (b) sulfated and nonsulfated sugars, (c) hormones and other steroids, (d) enzyme inhibitors. Particularly intriguing areas of investigation include glucosamine sulfate (already discussed), metalloproteinase inhibitors, such as the tetracyclines, growth factors/cytokines, and chondrocyte/stem cell transplantation.

Tetracyclines, apart from any antimicrobial effect, are inhibitors of tissue metalloproteinases. This could be due to their ability to chelate calcium and zinc ions. There has also been investigation into the potential role of nitric oxide in the mechanism of action of the tetracyclines (170). Doxycycline and, to a lesser extent, minocycline have blocked and reversed spontaneous and IL-1β-induced OA cartilage nitric oxide synthase (NOS) activity in *in vitro* experiments. More recently, however, tetracyclines have been shown to be capable of up-regulation of COX-2 and PGE2 production independently of any effects on nitric oxide (171). The clinical significance of this as human trials with tetracyclines in OA go forth is unclear. Minocycline has been used in the management of rheumatoid arthritis (172). Doxycycline, another tetracycline derivative, has been shown to inhibit articular cartilage collagenase and activity (173,174).

Doxycycline has also reduced the severity of OA in canine models (175).

A study of cartilage extracts from 21 human femoral heads from patients undergoing arthroplasty for end-stage hip OA showed that doxycycline at 100 mg b.i.d. inhibited both collagenase and gelatinase activity (176).

A multicenter, double-blind, placebo-controlled trial using doxycycline for "structure modification" in obese women with OA of the knee is ongoing. Other compounds with collagenase-inhibiting properties are being developed and investigated as structure-/disease-modifying agents not only in OA, but also in rheumatoid arthritis (177).

Growth factor and cytokine manipulation are areas of potential intervention (178). In an animal model, induction of repair in partial-thickness articular cartilage lesions by timed release of transforming growth factor (TGF)-β using liposomes has been attempted. The defects exhibited an increase in cellularity, being populated by cells of mesenchymal origin from the synovial membrane. The appearance of the repaired cartilage resembled hyaline cartilage and its integrity persisted for up to 1 year after surgery (179). Genetic therapy may also be in the future of OA. The control of genes such as the tissue inhibitor of metalloproteinases (TIMP) and the metalloproteinase (MMP) genes would, in theory, provide the opportunity to modulate the patients' disease. Expression of TGFβ has been achieved in chondrocytes and synoviocytes of guinea pigs using adenovirus as the vector (180). Using this same vector, temporary expression of the β galactosidase gene has been seen in human chondrocytes (181). Reduction in the macroscopic and histologic severity of cartilage lesions was achieved in an anterior cruciate ligament model of dog OA by transfecting the IL-1 receptor antagonist gene into synovial fibroblast-like cells (182).

In the future, better results and techniques may be achieved through the use of osteochondral grafts. Implantation of chondrocytes into cartilage defects has become possible in humans (183), and even implantation of stem cells into defects with eventual differentiation into bone and cartilage has been accomplished in a rabbit model (184). If these procedures become practical, they may radically alter the management of OA. They may lead not only to "chondroprotection" but also to the preservation of the entire joint organ.

Structure/disease modification has yet to be achieved in OA, and any claims are premature until well-designed, double-blind, placebo-controlled trials are demonstrated. Trials currently under way could provide an answer as to whether this is a realistic goal.

It is also possible that some of the drugs being tested now for structure/disease modification could provide symptom relief and could add to our armamentarium in that capacity, even if not successful as structure-/disease-modifying agents.

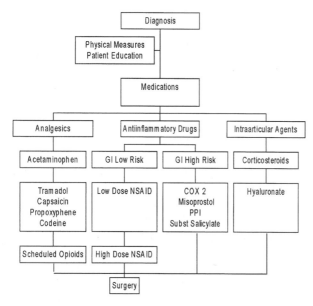

FIGURE 22.1. Flow chart for the therapy of osteoarthritis. Physical measures and patient education are the baseline of therapy and need to be continued throughout the program. Medications can be used singly or in combination. Surgery is an option when the physical and medicinal programs fail to provide adequate symptomatic relief. *COX-2,* cyclooxygenase 2 specific inhibitor; *GI,* risk of GI adverse event; *NSAID,* nonsteroidal antiinflammatory drug; *PPI,* protein pump inhibitor; *Subst Salicylate,* substituted (nonacetylated) salicylate. (From Lozada CJ, Altman RD. In: Koopman WJ, ed. *Arthritis and allied conditions: a textbook of rheumatology,* 14th ed. Philadelphia: Lippincott Williams & Wilkins, 2001:2246–2263, with permission.)

SUMMARY

OA is the most common articular disease. Age is its most notable risk factor. With the aging of the population of the developed world, there will be a growing need for better understanding of OA and for superior therapies. There is increasing appreciation for the role of inflammation in OA. There is also the realization that OA is a disease not only of cartilage but of the entire joint. This has led to increasing interest in structure/disease modification as the goal in OA therapy.

Presently, there are no proven structure-/disease-modifying interventions, Therefore current therapy is aimed at symptom relief. One must clinically attempt to define the cause of the symptoms, most often pain. This allows goal-directed therapy. Effective therapy combines many of the tools available, utilizing physical measures, medications, psychologic approaches, and surgery. An algorithm for the therapy of OA is reflected in Fig. 22.1.

REFERENCES

1. Lawrence RC, Hochberg MC, Kelsey JL, et al. Estimates of the prevalence of selected arthritic and musculoskeletal diseases in the United States. *J Rheumatol* 1989;16:427–441.
2. Kramer JS, Yelin EH, Epstein WV. Social and economic impacts of four musculoskeletal conditions: a study using national community-based data. *J Rheumatol* 1983;26:901–907.
3. Lozada CJ, Altman RD. Osteoarthritis: a comprehensive approach to management. *J Musculoskelet Med* 1997;14:26–38.
4. Hochberg MC, Altman RD, Brandt KD, et al. Guidelines for the medical management of osteoarthritis. Part II: osteoarthritis of the knee. *Arthritis Rheum* 1995;38:1541–1546.
5. Hochberg MC, Altman RD, Brandt RD, et al. Guidelines for the medical management of osteoarthritis. Part I: osteoarthritis of the hip. *Arthritis Rheum* 1995;38:1535–1540.
6. Altman R, Brandt K, Hochberg M, et al. Design and conduct of clinical trials in patients with osteoarthritis: recommendations from a task force of the Osteoarthritis Research Society. *Osteoarthritis Cart* 1996;4:217–243.
7. Hutton CW. Osteoarthritis: the cause, not result of joint failure? *Ann Rheum Dis* 1989;48:958–961.
8. Liang MH, Fortin P. Management of osteoarthritis of the hip and knee. Editorial *N Engl J Med* 1991;325:125–127.
9. Trock DH, Bollet AJ, Dyer RH Jr, et al. A double-blind trial of the clinical effects of pulsed electromagnetic fields in osteoarthritis. *J Rheumatol* 1993;20:456–460.
10. Lewis D, Lewis B, Sturrock RD. Transcutaneous electrical nerve stimulation in osteoarthrosis: a therapeutic alternative? *Ann Rheum Dis* 1984;43:47–49.
11. Altman R, Asch E, Bloch D, et al. Development of criteria for the classification and reporting of osteoarthritis: classification of osteoarthritis of the knee. *Arthritis Rheum* 1986;29:1039–1049.
12. Altman R, Alarcon G, Applerough D, et al. The American College of Rheumatology Criteria for the classification and reporting of osteoarthritis of the hand. *Arthritis Rheum* 1990;33:1601–1610.
13. Altman R, Alarcon G, Applerough D, et al. The American College of Rheumatology criteria for the classification and reporting of osteoarthritis of the hip. *Arthritis Rheum* 1991;34:505–514.

14. Roberts J, Burch TA. *Prevalence of osteoarthritis in adults by age, sex, race, and geographic area, United States—1960–1962.* National Center for Health Statistics: vital and health statistics: data from the national health survey. United States Public Health Service Publication No. 1000, Series 11, No. 15, 1966. Washington DC: U.S. Government Printing Office, 1966.

15. Felson DT. Epidemiology of hip and knee osteoarthritis. *Epidemiol Rev* 1988;10:1–18.

16. Peyron JG, Altman RD. The epidemiology of osteoarthritis. In: Moskowitz RW, Howell DS, Goldberg VM, et al., eds. *Osteoarthritis: diagnosis and management.* Philadelphia: WB Saunders, 1992:15–17.

17. Siegel DB, Gelberman RH, Smith R. Osteoarthritis of the hand and wrist. In: Moskowitz RW, Howell DS, Goldberg VM, et al., eds. *Osteoarthritis: diagnosis and management.* Philadelphia: WB Saunders, 1992:547–560.

18. Lawrence JS. Generalized osteoarthrosis in a population sample. *Am J Epidemiol* 1969;90:381–389.

19. Pattrick M, Manhire A, Ward AM, et al. HLA-A, B antigens and alpha$_1$-antitrypsin phenotypes in nodal generalized osteoarthritis and erosive osteoarthritis. *Ann Rheum Dis* 1989;48:470–475.

20. Knowlton RG, Katzenstein PL, Moskowitz RW, et al. Genetic linkage of a polymorphism in the type II pro-collagen gene (COL 2A) to primary osteoarthritis associated with mild chondrodysplasia. *N Engl J Med* 1990;322:526–530.

21. Vikkula M, Palotie A, Ritvaniemi P. Early-onset osteoarthritis linked to the type II procollagen gene. *Arthritis Rheum* 1993;36: 401–409.

22. Felson DT. The epidemiology of knee osteoarthritis: results from the Framingham osteoarthritis study. *Semin Arthritis Rheum* 1990;20:42–50.

23. Hubert HB, Bloch DA, Fries JF. Risk factors for physical disability in an aging cohort: the NHANES 1 epidemiologic followup study. *J Rheumatol* 1993;20:480–488.

24. Silberberg M, Silberberg R. Osteoarthritis in mice fed diets enriched with animal or vegetable fat. *Arch Pathol* 1960;70: 385–390.

25. Kellgren JH, Lawrence JS. Osteo-arthrosis and disk degeneration in an urban population. *Ann Rheum Dis* 1958;17:388–397.

26. Knight SM, Ring EFJ, Bhalla AK. Bone mineral density and osteoarthritis. *Ann Rheum Dis* 1992;51:1025–1026.

27. Reference deleted.

28. Pelletier JP, Martel-Pelletier J, Howell DS. Etiopathogenesis of osteoarthritis. In: Koopman WJ, ed. *Arthritis and allied conditions: a textbook of rheumatology,* 13th ed. Baltimore: Williams & Wilkins, 1997:1969–1984.

29. Brandt KD. Pain, synovitis, and articular cartilage changes in osteoarthritis. *Semin Arthritis Rheum* 1989;18(Suppl 2):77–80.

30. Kellgren JH, Lawrence RC. Radiological assessment of osteoarthrosis. *Ann Rheum Dis* 1957;16:494–501.

31. Hochberg MC, Lawrence RC, Everett DF, et al. Epidemiologic associations of pain in osteoarthritis of the knee: data from the National Health and Nutrition Examination-I Epidemiologic follow-up Survey. *Semin Arthritis Rheum* 1989;18(Suppl 2):4–9.

32. Altman R, Dean D. Pain in osteoarthritis: introduction and overview. *Semin Arthritis Rheum* 1989;18(Suppl 2):1–3.

33. Harkness IAL, Higgs ER, Dieppe PA. Osteoarthritis. In: Wall PD, Melzadk R, eds. *Textbook of pain.* London: Churchill Livingstone, 1984:215–224.

34. Wyke B. The neurology of joints: a review of general principles. *Clin Rheum Dis* 1981;7:223–239.

35. Altman RD, Dean D. Introduction and overview: pain in osteoarthritis. *Semin Arthritis Rheum* 1989;18(Suppl 2):1–3.

36. Kolasinski SL, Haines KA, Siegel EL, et al. Neuropeptides and inflammation: a somatostatin analog as a selective antagonist of neutrophil activation by substance P. *Arthritis Rheum* 1992;35: 369–375.

37. Badalamente MA, Cherney SB. Periosteal and vascular innervation of the human patella in degenerative joint disease. *Semin Arthritis Rheum* 1989;18(Suppl 2):61–66.

38. Kiaer T, Gronlund J, Sorensen KH. Intraosseous pressure and partial pressures of oxygen and carbon dioxide in osteoarthritis. *Semin Arthritis Rheum* 1989;18(Suppl 2):57–60.

39. Schumacher HR. The role of inflammation and crystals in the pain of osteoarthritis. *Semin Arthritis Rheum* 1989;18(Suppl 2):81–85.

40. Bellamy N, Sothern RB, Campbell J, et al. Circadian and circaseptan variation in pain perception in osteoarthritis of the knee. *J Rheumatol* 1990;17:364–372.

41. Felson DT. The epidemiology of knee osteoarthritis: results from the Framingham Osteoarthritis Study. *Semin Arthritis Rheum* 1990;20:42–50.

42. Hubert HB, Bloch DA, Fries JF. Risk factors for physical disability in an aging cohort: the NHANES 1 epidemiologic followup study. *J Rheumatol* 1993;20:480–488.

43. Hochberg MC, Lethbridge-Cejku M, Scott WW Jr, et al. The association of body weight, body fatness and body fat distribution with osteoarthritis of the knee: data from the Baltimore Longitudinal Study of Aging. *J Rheumatol* 1995;22:488–493.

44. Oliveira SA, Felson DT, Cirillo PA, et al. Body weight, body mass index, and incident symptomatic osteoarthritis of the hand, hip, and knee. *Epidemiology* 1999;10:161–166.

45. Carman WJ, Sowers M, Hawthorne VM, et al. Obesity as a risk factor for osteoarthritis of the hand and wrist: a prospective study. *Am J Epidemiol* 1994;139:119–129.

46. Leach RE, Baumgard S, Broom J. Obesity: its relationship to osteoarthritis of the knee. *Clin Orthop* 1973;93:271–273.

47. Hart DJ, Doyle DV, Spector TD. Association between metabolic factors and knee osteoarthritis in women: the Chingford Study. *J Rheumatol* 1995;22:1118–1123.

48. Martin K, Lethbridge-Cejku M, Muller DC, et al. Metabolic correlates of obesity and radiographic features of knee osteoarthritis: data from the Baltimore Longitudinal Study of Aging. *J Rhuematol* 1997;24:702–707.

49. Felson DT, Zhang Y, Anthony JM, et al. Weight loss reduces the risk for symptomatic knee osteoarthritis in women. *Ann Intern Med* 1992;116:535–539.

50. Toda Y, Toda T, Takemura S, et al. Change in body fat, but not body weight or metabolic correlates of obesity, is related to symptomatic relief of obese patients with knee osteoarthritis after a weight control program. *J Rheumatol* 1998;25:2181–2186.

51. Slemenda C, Heilman DK, Brandt KD, et al. Reduced quadriceps strength relative to body weight: a risk factor for knee osteoarthritis in women? *Arthritis Rheum* 1998;41:1951–1959.

52. Fisher NM, Pendergast DR, Gresham GE, et al. Muscle rehabilitation: its effect on muscular and functional performance of patients with knee osteoarthritis. *Arch Phys Med Rehabil* 1991;72:367–374.

53. Van Baar ME, Dekker J, Oostendorp RA, et al. The effectiveness of exercise therapy in patients with osteoarthritis of the hip or knee: a randomized clinical trial. *J Rheumatol* 1998;25:2432–2439.

54. Kovar PA, Allegrante JP, MacKenzie, R, et al. Supervised fitness walking in patients with osteoarthritis of the knee. *Ann Intern Med* 1992;116:529–534.

55. Waddell, G. A new clinical model for the treatment of low-back pain. *Spine* 1987;12:632–641.

56. Malmivaara A, Hakkinen V, Aro T, et al. The treatment of acute low back pain—bed rest, exercises, or ordinary activity? *N Engl J Med* 1995;332:351–355.

57. Fisher NM, Pendergast DR, Gresham GE, et al. Muscle rehabilitation: its effects on muscular and functional performance of

patients with knee osteoarthritis. *Arch Phys Med* 1991;72: 367–374.

58. Blount WP. Don't throw away the cane. *J Bone Joint Surg* 1956; 38A:695–708.

59. Brand SA, Crowninshield RD. The effect of cane use on hip contact force. *Clin Orthop* 1980;147:181–184.

60. Thompson JA, Jennings MB, Hodge W. Orthotic therapy in the management of osteoarthritis. *J Am Podiatr Med Assoc* 1992; 82:136–139.

61. Keating EM, Faris PM, Ritter MA, et al. Use of lateral heel and sole wedges in the treatment of medial osteoarthritis of the knee. *Orthop Rev* 1993;22:921–924.

62. Liang MH, Fortin P. Management of osteoarthritis of the hip and knee. *New Engl J Med* 1991;325:125–127.

63. Rubin G, Dixon M, Danisi M. Prescription procedures for knee orthosis and knee-ankle-foot orthosis. *Orthotics Prosthetics* 1977;31:15–25.

64. Kirk JA, Kersley GD. Heat and cold in the physical treatment of rheumatoid arthritis of the knee: a controlled clinical trial. *Ann Phys Med* 1967;9:270–274.

65. Felson DT, Zhang Y, Anthony JM, et al. Weight loss reduces the risk for symptomatic knee osteoarthritis in women. *Ann Intern Med* 1992;116:535–539.

66. Swezey RL. Essentials of physical management and rehabilitation in arthritis. *Semin Arthritis Rheum* 1974;3:349–368.

67. Fontain P, Gersten J, Sengir O. Decrease in muscle spasm produced by ultrasound, hot packs and infrared radiation. *Arch Phys Med Rehabil* 1960;41:293–298.

68. Cordray YM, Krusen EM. Use of hydrocollator packs in the treatment of neck and shoulder pains. *Arch Phys Med Rehabil* 1959;40:105.

69. Lehman JF, Brunner GD, Stow RW. Pain threshold measurements after therapeutic application of ultrasound, microwaves, and infrared. *Arch Phys Med Rehabil* 1958;39:560–565.

70. Lehman JF, DeLateur BJ. Diathermy and superficial heat, laser, and cold therapy. In: Kottke FJ, Lehman, JF eds. *Krusen's handbook of physical medicine and rehabilitation,* 4th ed. Philadelphia: WB Saunders, 1990:283–367.

71. Basford JR. Physical agents and biofeedback. In: DeLisa JA, et al., eds. *Rehabilitation medicine: principles and practice.* Philadelphia: JB Lippincott, 1988:257–275.

72. Garfinkel MS, Shumacher HR Jr, Husain A, et al. Evaluation of a Yoga-based regimen for treatment of osteoarthritis of the hands. *J Rheumatol* 1994;21:2341–2343.

73. Christensen BV, Iuhl IU, Bulow H-H, et al. Acupuncture treatment of severe knee osteoarthrosis: a long-term study. *Acta Anaesthesiol Scand* 1992;36:519–525.

74. Trock DH, Bollet AJ, Dyer RH Jr, et al. A double-blind trial of the clinical effects of pulsed electromagnetic fields in osteoarthritis. *J Rheumatol* 1993;20:456–460.

75. Lewis D, Lewis B, Sturrock RD. Transcutaneous electrical stimulation in osteoarthrosis: a therapeutic alternative? *Ann Rheum Dis* 1984;43:47–49.

76. Cunningham LS, Kelsy JL. Epidemiology of musculoskeletal impairments and associated disability. *Am J Pub Health* 1984; 74:574–579.

77. Rene J, Weinberger M, Mazzuca SA, et al. Reduction of joint pain in patients with knee osteoarthritis who have received monthly telephone calls from lay personnel and whose medical treatment regimens have remained stable. *Arthritis Rheum* 1992;35:511–515.

78. Currey LF. Osteoarthrosis of the hip joint and sexual activity. *Ann Rheum Dis* 1970;29:488–491.

79. McCarthy GM, McCarthy DJ. Effect of Topical Capsaicin in the Therapy of Painful osteoarthritis of the hands. *J Rheumatol* 1992;19:604–607.

80. Deal CL, Schnitzer TJ, Lipstein E, et al. Treatment of arthritis with topical capsaicin: a double-blind trial. *Clin Ther* 1991; 13:383–389.

81. Virus RM, Gebhart GF. Pharmacologic actions of capsaicin: apparent involvement of substance P and serotonin. *Life Sci* 1979;25:1273–1284.

82. Zhang WY, Li Wan Po A. The effectiveness of topically applied capsaicin: a meta-analysis. *Eur J Clin Pharmacol* 1994;46: 517–522.

83. Rains C, Bryson HM. Topical capsaicin. A review of its pharmacological properties and therapeutic potential in post-herpetic neuralgia, diabetic neuropathy and osteoarthritis. *Drugs Aging* 1995;7:317–328.

84. Dreiser RL, Tisne-Camus M. DHEP plasters as a topical treatment of knee osteoarthritis: a double-blind placebo-controlled study. *Drugs Exp Clin Res* 1993;19:117–123.

85. Rolf C, Engstrom B, Beauchard C, et al. Intra-articular absorption and distribution of ketoprofen after topical plaster application and oral intake in 100 patients undergoing knee arthroscopy. *Rheumatology* 1999;38:564–567.

86. Bradley JD, Brandt KD, Katz BP, et al. Comparison of an antiinflammatory dose of ibuprofen, an analgesic dose of ibuprofen, and acetaminophen in the treatment of patients with osteoarthritis of the knee. *N Engl J Med* 1991;325:87–91.

87. Altman RD, the IAP Study Group. Ibuprofen, acetaminophen and placebo in osteoarthritis of the knee: a six-day double-blind study (abstract). *Arthritis Rheum* 1999;42:(Suppl):S403.

88. Perneger TV, Whelton PK, Klag MJ. Risk of kidney failure associated with the use of acetaminophen, aspirin, and nonsteroidal antiinflammatory drugs. *N Engl J Med* 1994;331: 1675–1679.

89. Raffa, RB, Friederichs E, Reimann W, et al. Opioid and nonopioid components independently contribute to the mechanism of action of tramadol: an "atypical" opioid analgesic. *J Pharmacol Exp Ther* 1992;260:275–285.

90. Katz WA. Pharmacology and clinical experience with tramadol in osteoarthritis. *Drugs* 1996;52(Suppl 3):39–47.

91. Goeringer KE, Logan BK, Christian GD. Identification of tramadol and its metabolites in blood from drug-related deaths and drug-impaired drivers. *J Anal Toxicol* 1997;21:529–537.

92. Roth SH. Efficacy and safety of tramadol HCl in breakthrough musculoskeletal pain attributed to osteoarthritis. *J Rheumatol* 1998;25:1358–1363.

93. Schnitzer TJ, Kamin M, Olson WH. Tramadol allows reduction of naproxen dose among patients with naproxen-responsive osteoarthritis pain: a randomized, double-blind, placebo-controlled study. *Arthritis Rheum* 1999;42:1370–1377.

94. AGS Panel on Chronic Pain in Older Persons. The management of chronic pain in older persons. *J Am Geriatr Soc* 1998;46: 635–651.

95. McAlindon T, Dieppe P. The medical management of osteoarthritis of the knee: an inflammatory issue? *Br J Rheumatol* 1990;29:471–473.

96. Brooks PM, Day PO. Nonsteroidal antiinflammatory drugs: differences and similarities. *N Engl J Med* 1991;324:1716–1725.

97. Mazzuca SA, Brandt KD, Anderson SE, et al. The therapeutic approaches of community based primary care practitioners to osteoarthritis of the hip in an elderly patient. *J. Rheumatol* 1991;18:1593–1600.

98. Roth SH. Non-steroidal anti-inflammatory drugs: gastropathy, deaths, and medical practice. *Ann Intern Med* 1988;109: 353–354.

99. Griffin MR, Ray WA, Schaffner W. Nonsteroidal anti-inflammatory drug use and death from peptic ulcer in elderly persons. *Ann Intern Med* 1988;109:359–363.

100. Levi F, Le Louran C, Reinberg A. Timing optimizes sustained-

release indomethacin treatment of osteoarthritis. *Clin Pharmacol Ther* 1985;37:77–84.

101. Palmoski MJ, Brandt KD. Effects of some nonsteroidal antiinflammatory drugs on proteoglycan metabolism and organization in canine articular cartilage. *Arthritis Rheum* 1980;23:1010–1020.

102. Herman JH, Appel AM, Hess EV. Modulation of cartilage destruction by select non-steroidal anti-inflammatory drugs. *Arthritis Rheum* 1987;30:257–265.

103. Graham DY, Agrawal NM, Roth SH. Prevention of NSAID-induced gastric ulcer with misoprostol: multicenter, double-blind, placebo-controlled trial. *Lancet* 1988;2:1277–1280.

104. Agrawal NM, Van Kerckhove HE, Erhardt LJ, et al. Misoprostol coadministered with diclofenac for prevention of gastroduodenal ulcers. A one-year study. *Dig Dis Sci* 1995;40:1125–1131.

105. Melo Gomes JA, Roth SH, Zeeh J, et al. Double-blind comparison of efficacy and gastroduodenal safety of diclofenac/misoprostol, piroxicam, and naproxen in the treatment of osteoarthritis. *Ann Rheum Dis* 1993;52:881–885.

106. Bocanegra TS, Weaver AL, Tindall EA, et al. Diclofenac/misoprostol compared with diclofenac in the treatment of osteoarthritis of the knee or hip: a randomized, placebo controlled trial. *J Rheumatol* 1998;25:1602–1611.

107. Cullen D, Bardhan KD, Eisner M, et al. Primary gastroduodenal prophylaxis with omeprazole for non-steroidal anti-inflammatory drug users. *Aliment Pharmacol Ther* 1998;12:135–140.

108. Hawkey CJ, Karrasch JA, Szczepanski L, et al. Omeprazole compared with misoprostol for ulcers associated with non-steroidal antiinflammatory drugs. Omeprazole versus misoprostol for NSAID-induced ulcer management (OMINUM) Study Group. *N Engl J Med* 1998;338:727–734.

109. Yeomans ND, Tulassay Z, Juhasz L, et al. A comparison of omeprazole with ranitidine for ulcers associated with non-steroidal antiinflammatory drugs. Acid Suppression Trial: Ranitidine versus Omeprazole for NSAID-associated Ulcer Treatment (ASTRONAUT) Study Group. *N Engl J Med* 1998;338:719–726.

110. Abramson SB, Weissmann G. The mechanism of action of nonsteroidal antiinflammatory drugs. *Arthritis Rheum* 1989;32:1–9.

111. Harris RC, McKanna JA, Akai Y, et al. Cyclooxygenase-2 is associated with the macula densa in rat kidney and increases with salt restriction. *J Clin Invest* 1994;94:2504–2510.

112. Guan Y, Chang M, Cho W, et al. Cloning, expression, and regulation of rabbit cyclooxygenase-2 in renal medullary interstitial cells. *Am J Physiol* 1997;273:F18–F26.

113. Dubois RN, Abramson SB, Crofford L, et al. Cyclooxygenase in biology and disease. *FASEB J* 1998;12: 1063–1073.

114. Vane JR, Botting RM. Mechanism of action of aspirin-like drugs. *Semin Arthritis Rheum* 1997;26:2–10.

115. Ehrich E, Schnitzer T, Kivitz A, et al. MK-966, a highly selective COX-2 inhibitor, was effective in the treatment of osteoarthritis (OA) of the knee and hip in a 6-week placebo controlled study. *Arthritis Rheum* 1997;40:S85 (abs. 330).

116. Cannon G, Caldwell J, Holt P, et al. MK-0966, a specific COX-2 inhibitor, has clinical efficacy comparable to diclofenac in the treatment of knee and hip osteoarthritis (OA) in a 26-week controlled clinical trial. *Arthritis Rheum* 1998;41(Suppl):S196.

117. Saag K, Fisher C McKay J, et al. MK-0966, a specific COX-2 inhibitor, has clinical efficacy comparable to ibuprofen in the treatment of knee and hip osteoarthritis (OA) in a 6-week controlled clinical trial. *Arthritis Rheum* 1998;41(Suppl):S196.

118. Hubbard R, Geis GS, Woods E, et al. Efficacy, tolerability and safety of celecoxib, a specific COX-2 inhibitor in osteoarthritis. *Arthritis Rheum* 1998;41(Suppl):S196.

119. Geis GS, Stead H, Morant S, et al. Efficacy and safety of celecoxib, a specific COX-2 inhibitor, in patients with rheumatoid arthritis. *Arthritis Rheum* 1998;41(Suppl):S316.

120. Karin A, Tolbert D, Piergies A, et al. Celecoxib, a specific COX-2 inhibitor, lacks significant drug-drug interactions with methotrexate or warfarin. *Arthritis Rheum* 1998;41 (Suppl):S315.

121. Bombardier C, Laine L, Reicin A, et al. Comparison of upper gastrointestinal toxicity of rofecoxib and naproxen in patients with rheumatoid arthritis. VIGOR Study Group. *N Engl J Med* 2000;343:1520–1528.

122. Silverstein FE, Faich G, Goldstein JL, et al. Gastrointestinal toxicity with celecoxib vs. nonsteroidal anti-inflammatory drugs for osteoarthritis and rheumatoid arthritis: the CLASS Study. A randomized controlled trial. Celecoxib Long-term Arthritis Safety Study. *JAMA* 2000;284:1247–1255.

123. Hosie J, Distel M, Bluhmki E. Meloxicam in osteoarthritis: a 6-month, double-blind comparison with diclofenac sodium. *Br J Rheumatol* 1996;35(Suppl 1):39–43.

124. Linden B, Distel M, Bluhmki E. A double-blind study to compare the efficacy and safety of meloxicam 15 mg with piroxicam 20 mg in patients with osteoarthritis of the hip. *Br J Rheumatol* 1996;35(Suppl 1):35–38.

125. Amin AR, Attur M, Patel RN, et al. Superinduction of cyclooxygenase-2 activity in human osteoarthritis-affected cartilage: influence of nitric oxide. *J Clin Invest* 1997;99:1231–1237.

126. Martel-Pelletier J, Mineau F, Jolicoeur FC, et al. In vitro effects of diacerein and rhein on interleukin 1 and tumor necrosis factor-alpha systems in human osteoarthritic synovium and chondrocytes. *J Rheumatol* 1998;25:753–762.

127. Carney SL, Hicks CA, Tree B, et al. An in vivo investigation of the effect of anthraquinones on the turnover of aggrecans in spontaneous osteoarthritis in the guinea pig. *Inflamm Res* 1995;44:182–186.

128. Brun PH. Effect of diacetylrhein on the development of experimental osteoarthritis: a biochemical investigation [letter]. *Osteoarthritis Cartilage* 1997;5:289–291.

129. Brandt K, Smith G, Kang SY, Myers S, et al. Effects of diacerein in an accelerated canine model of osteoarthritis. *Osteoarthritis Cartilage* 1997;5:438–449.

130. Nguyen M, Dougados M, Berdah L, et al. Diacerein in the treatment of osteoarthritis of the hip. *Arthritis Rheum* 1994;37:529–537.

131. Spencer CM, Wilde MI. Diacerein. *Drugs* 1997;53:98–108.

132. Muller-Fabender H, Bach GL, Haase W, et al. Glucosamine sulfate compared to ibuprofen in osteoarthritis of the knee. *Osteoarthritis Cartilage* 1994;2:61–69.

133. Qiu GX, Gao SN, Giacovelli G, et al. Efficacy and safety of glucosamine sulfate versus ibuprofen in patients with knee osteoarthritis. *Arzneimittelforschung* 1998;48:469–474.

134. Karzel K, Domenjoz R. Effects of hexosamine derivatives and uronic acid derivatives on glycosaminoglycan metabolism of fibroblast cultures. *Pharmacology* 1971;5:337–345.

135. Bassleer C, Reginster JY, Franchimont P. Effects of glucosamine on differentiated human chondrocytes cultivated in clusters (abstract). *Rev Esp Reumatol* 1993;20(Suppl 1):96.

136. McCarty MF. Enhanced synovial production of hyaluronic acid may explain rapid clinical response to high–dose glucosamine in osteoarthritis. *Med Hypotheses* 1998;50:507–510.

137. Mathieu M, Piperno S, Annefeld M, et al. Glucosamine sulfate significantly reduced cartilage destruction in a rabbit model of osteoarthritis. *Arthritis Rheum* 1998;41(Suppl):S147.

138. Reginster JY, Deroisy R, Rovati LC, et al. Long-term effects of glucosamine sulphate on osteoarthritis progression: a randomized placebo-controlled clinical trial. *Lancet* 2001;357:251–256.

139. Morreale P, Manopulo R, Galati M, et al. Comparison of the antiinflammatory efficacy of chondroitin sulfate and diclofenac

sodium in patients with knee osteoarthritis. *J Rheumatol* 1996;23:1385–1391.

140. McAlindon TE, Gulin J, Felson DT. Glucosamine (GL) and chondroitin (CH) treatment for osteoarthritis (OA) of the knee or hip: meta-analysis and quality assessment of Clinical Trials. *Arthritis Rheum* 1998;41(Suppl):S198.

141. Leffler CT, Philippi AF, Leffler SG, et al. Glucosamine, chondroitin and manganese ascorbate for degenerative joint disease of the knee or low back: a randomized, double-blind, placebo-controlled pilot study. *Mil Med* 1999;164:85–91.

142. McCarty MF. The neglect of glucosamine as a treatment for osteoarthritis: a personal perspective. *Med Hypotheses* 1994;42: 323–327.

143. Bradley JD, Flusser D, Katz BP, et al. A randomized, double blind, placebo controlled trial of intravenous loading with S-adenosylmethionine (SAM) followed by oral SAM therapy in patients with knee osteoarthritis. *J Rheumatol* 1994;21:905–911.

144. Szczepanski A, Dabrowska H, Moskalewska K. An appraisal of the effect of Piascledine in the treatment of scleroderma. *Przegl Derm* 1975;LXII,4.

145. Harmand MF. Etude de l'action des insaponifiables d'avocat et de soja sur les cultures de chondrocytes articulaires. *Gazette Med France* 1985;92:No. 29.

146. Loyau G, Pujol JP, Mauviel A. Effet des insaponifiables d'avocat/soja aur l'activité collagénolytique de cultures de synoviocytes rhumatoïdes humains et de chondrocytes articulaires de lapin traités par l'interleukine-1. *Rev Rhumat* 1991;58:241–245.

147. Chevalier X, Feng XZ, Groult N, et al. Modulation of fibronectin biosynthesis, elastase activity, cell proliferation and cell phenotype of rabbit chondrocytes by soja and avocado extracts. Communication at the 12th European Congress on Rheumatology-Budapest 7/1991.

148. Blotman F, Maheu E, Wulwik A, et al. Efficacy and safety of avocado/soybean unsaponifiables in the treatment of symptomatic osteoarthritis of the knee and hip: a prospective, multicenter, three-month, randomized, double-blind, placebo-controlled trial. *Rev Rhum Engl Ed* 1997;64:825–834.

149. Maheu E, Mazieres B, Valat JP, et al. Symptomatic efficacy of avocado/soybean unsaponifiables in the treatment of the knee and hip: a prospective, randomized, double-blind, placebo-controlled, multicenter clinical trial with a six month treatment period and a two-month followup demonstrating a persistent effect. *Arthritis Rheum* 1998;41:81–91.

150. Srivasta KC, Mustafa T. Ginger (Zingiber officinale) in rheumatism and musculoskeletal disorders. *Med Hypotheses* 1992;39: 342–348.

151. Carette S, Marcoux S, Truchon R, et al. A controlled trial of corticosteroid injections into facet joints for chronic low back pain. *N Engl J Med* 1991;325:1002–1007.

152. Miller JH, White J, Norton TH. The value of intra-articular injections in osteoarthritis of the knee. *J Bone Joint Surg* 1958; 40A:636–643.

153. Dieppe PA, Sathapatayavongs B, Jones HE, et al. Intra-articular corticosteroids in osteoarthritis. *Rheumatol Rehabil* 1980;19: 212–217.

154. Ravaud P, Moulinier L, Giraudeau B, et al. Effects of joint lavage and steroid injection in patients with osteoarthritis of the knee: results of a multicenter, randomized, controlled trial. *Arthritis Rheum* 1999;42:475–482.

155. Jones A, Doherty M. Intra-articular corticosteroids are effective in osteoarthritis but there are no clinical predictors of response. *Ann Rheum Dis* 1996;55:829–832.

156. Pelletier JP, Martell-Pelletier J. Protective effects of corticosteroids on cartilage lesions and osteophyte formation in the Pond-Nuki dog model of osteoarthritis. *Arthritis Rheum* 1989; 32:181–193.

157. Wada J, Koshino T, Morii T, et al. Natural course of osteoarthritis of the knee treated with or without intraarticular corticosteroid injections. *Bull Hosp Jt Dis* 1993;53:45–48.

158. Schnitzer TJ. Osteoarthritis treatment update. *Postgrad Med* 1993;93:89–93.

159. Altman RD. Osteoarthritis: Aggravating factors and therapeutic measures. *Postgrad Med* 1986;80:150-163.

160. Peyron JG. Intraarticular hyaluronan injections in the treatment of osteoarthritis: state-of-the art review. *J Rheumatol* 1993;20(Suppl)39:10–15.

161. Dougados M, Nguyen M, Listrat V, et al. High molecular weight sodium hyaluronate (hyalectin) in osteoarthritis of the knee: a 1 year placebo-controlled trial. *Osteoarthritis Cartilage* 1993;1:97–103.

162. Leardini G, Mattara L, Franceschini M, et al. Intra-articular treatment of knee osteoarthritis: a comparative study between hyaluronic acid and 6-methyl prednisolone acetate. *Clin Exp Rheumatol* 1991;9:375–381.

163. Altman RD, Moskowitz R. Intraarticular sodium hyaluronate (Hyalgan) in the treatment of osteoarthritis of the knee: a randomized clinical trial. Hyalgan Study Group. *J Rheumatol* 1998;25:2203–2212.

164. Adams MF, Atkinson M, Lussler AJ, et al. Comparison of intra-articular Hyalgan G-F (Synvisc), a viscoelastic derivative of hyaluronan and continuous NSAID therapy in patients with osteoarthritis of the knee. *Arthritis Rheum* 1993;37:S165.

165. Oldenbring S, Egund N, Knutson K, et al. Revision after osteotomy for gonarthrosis: a 10–19-year follow-up of 314 cases. *Acta Orthop Scand* 1990;61:128–130.

166. Gibson JNA, White MD, Chapman VM, et al. Arthroscopic lavage and debridement for osteoarthritis of the knee. *J Bone Joint Surg (Br)* 1992;74-b:534–537.

167. Liveseley PJ, Doherty M, Needoff M, et al. Arthroscopic lavage of osteoarthritic knees. *J Bone Joint Surg (Br)* 1991;73-B: 922–926.

168. Ravaud P, Moulinier L, Giraudeau B, et al. Effects of joint lavage and steroid injection in patients with osteoarthritis of the knee. *Arthritis Rheum* 1999;42:475–482.

169. Lozada CJ, Altman RD. Chondroprotection in osteoarthritis. *Bull Rheum Dis* 1997;46:5–7.

170. Amin AR, Attur MG, Thakker GD, et al. A novel mechanism of action of tetracyclines: effects on nitric oxide synthases. *Proc Natl Acad Sci USA* 1996;93:14014–14019.

171. Amin AR, Patel RN, Attur MG, et al. Tetracyclines upregulate COX-2 expression and PGE2 production independently from the inhibition of nitric oxide. *Arthritis Rheum* 1998;41(Suppl):S342.

172. Tilley BC, Alarcon GS, Heyse SP, et al. Minocycline in rheumatoid arthritis: a 48-week, double-blind, placebo-controlled trial. *Ann Intern Med* 1995;122:81–89.

173. Cole AD, Chubinskaya S, Luchene LJ, et al. Doxycycline disrupts chondrocyte differentiation and inhibits cartilage matrix degradation. *Arthritis Rheum* 1994;32:1727–1734.

174. Yu LP Jr, Smith GN Jr, Hasty KA, et al. Doxycycline inhibits type XI collagenolytic activity of extracts from human osteoarthritic cartilage and of gelatinase. *J Rheumatol* 1991;18: 1450–1452.

175. Brandt KD, Yu LP, Amith G, et al. Therapeutic effect of doxycycline (doxy) in canine osteoarthritis (OA). *Osteoarthritis Cartilage* 1993;1:14.

176. Smith GN Jr, Yu LP Jr, Brandt KD, et al. Oral administration of doxycycline reduces collagenase and gelatinase activities in extracts of human osteoarthritic cartilage. *J Rheumatol* 1998; 25:532–535.

177. Lewis EJ, Bishop J, Bottomley D, et al. Ro32-3555, an orally active collagenase inhibitor, prevents cartilage breakdown in vitro and in vivo. *Br J Pharmacol* 1997;121:540–546.

178. Pelletier JP, Roughley PJ, DiBattista JA, et al. Are cytokines involved in osteoarthritic pathophysiology? *Semin Arthritis Rheum* 1991;20(Suppl 2):12–25.

179. Hunziker EB, Rosenberg L. Induction of repair in partial thickness articular cartilage lesions by timed release of TGF-beta. *Transactions of the 40th Annual Meeting of the Orthopaedic Research Society* 1994;19(Sec. 1):236.

180. Ikeda T, Kubo T, Arai Y, et al. Adenovirus mediated gene delivery to the joints of guinea pigs. *J Rheumatol* 1998;25:1666–1673.

181. Doherty PJ, Zhang H, Tramblay L, et al. Resurfacing of articular cartilage explants with genetically modified human chondrocytes in vitro. *Osteoarthritis Cartilage* 1998;6:153–159.

182. Pelletier JP, Caron JP, Evans C, et al. In vivo suppression of early experimental osteoarthritis by interleukin-1 receptor antagonist using gene therapy. *Arthritis Rheum* 1997;40:1012–1019.

183. Brittberg M, Lindahl A, Nilsson A, et al. Treatment of deep cartilage defect in the knee with autologous chondrocyte transplantation. *N Engl J Med* 1994;331:889–895.

184. Wakitani S, Goto T, Pineda SJ, et al. Mesenchymal cell-based repair of large, full-thickness defects of articular cartilage. *J Bone Joint Surg Am* 1994;76:579–592.

GOUT AND CRYSTAL-INDUCED SYNOVITIS

DENNIS W. BOULWARE
MICHAEL A. BECKER
N. LAWRENCE EDWARDS

Gout is a heterogeneous group of diseases resulting from tissue deposition of monosodium urate or uric acid crystals from supersaturated extracellular fluids. The range of clinical manifestations of urate deposition includes recurrent attacks of a unique type of acute inflammatory arthritis (acute gout); accumulation of potentially destructive crystalline aggregates (tophi), especially in connective-tissue structures; uric acid urolithiasis; and, infrequently, renal impairment (gouty nephropathy). Hyperuricemia (supersaturation for urate in serum) is the pathogenic common denominator through which people are predisposed to crystal deposition and the potential for clinical events. Although hyperuricemia is a necessary underlying feature of gout, it is in most instances insufficient for expression of the disorder. Thus the distinction between hyperuricemia, a biochemical aberration, and gout, a disease state, is essential. Recognition of this distinction, in conjunction with increasing evidence that hyperuricemia and gout are, at worst, only weak risk factors for the development of chronic renal insufficiency, has promoted conservatism in the use of drug therapy to treat asymptomatic hyperuricemia and even the early stages of gout.

PATHOGENESIS OF HYPERURICEMIA AND GOUT

Among mammalian species, only man and the great apes excrete uric acid as the end product of purine metabolism, reflecting the lack of the enzyme uricase, which catalyzes the degradation of uric acid to the readily excretable compound allantoin (1). Uric acid is a weak organic acid (pK_{a1} = 5.75) that is sparingly soluble both in the un-ionized acid form prevalent in normal urine and in the ionized urate form at the pH and sodium concentration of other extracellular fluids (2) (Fig. 23.1). The combination of lack of uricase and the solubility properties of uric acid conditions humans to the deposition of urate from super-

saturated (hyperuricemic) body fluids, with the consequent risk of clinical sequelae (gout). The magnitude of this problem is dramatized by the fact that, at least among normal adult white men, mean serum urate concentrations are within 1 mg/dL of the theoretic limit of urate solubility in serum. The factors determining who will develop hyperuricemia and, among this group, who will develop gout are diverse and are best understood in the context of how purine compounds are normally metabolized (Fig. 23.2) and the physiologic mechanisms maintaining uric acid homeostasis. Dietary purine ingestion and the endogenous pathway of de novo purine

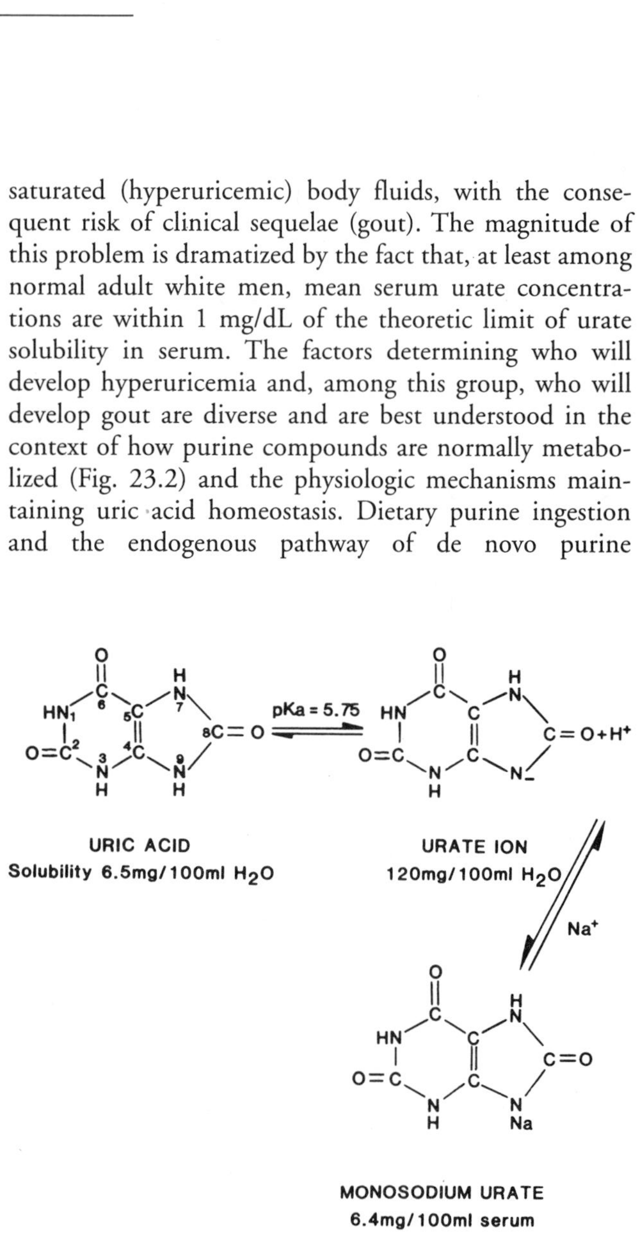

FIGURE 23.1. Solubility of uric acid species. (From Becker MA. Clinical gout and the pathogenesis of hyperuricemia. In: Koopman WJ, ed. *Arthritis and allied conditions: a textbook of rheumatology,* 14th ed. Philadelphia: Lippincott Williams & Wilkins, 2001:2281–2313, with permission.)

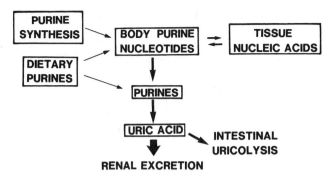

FIGURE 23.2. Human purine metabolism. (Courtesy of Dr. J. Edwin Seegmiller.) (From Becker MA. Clinical gout and the pathogenesis of hyperuricemia. In: Koopman WJ, ed. *Arthritis and allied conditions: a textbook of rheumatology,* 14th ed. Philadelphia: Lippincott Williams & Wilkins, 2001:2281–2313, with permission.)

nucleotide synthesis provide net contributions to body pools of purine compounds.

Overproduction

The overproduction of uric acid characterized by the excessive daily urinary uric acid excretion is demonstrable in 10% to 15% of patients with gout and primary hyperuricemia and in most patients whose hyperuricemia reflects increased cell turnover (e.g., a myelo- or lympho-proliferative disease) or a toxic state or pharmacologic intervention resulting in increased uric acid production (3) (Table 23.1). Two inborn errors of metabolism, HGPRT deficiency and PRPP synthetase superactivity, are both X-linked conditions, and together they account for only a small proportion (10% to 15%) of patients with primary uric acid overproduction (3). In another enzymatic disorder, glucose-6-phosphatase deficiency (glycogen storage disease, type I; von Gierke disease), hyperuricemia appears as early as infancy, and gout has been reported by the end of the first decade. Patients surviving into adulthood with this autosomal recessive disorder may then suffer tophaceous gout and gouty renal disease as major clinical problems unless effective management is instituted (4,5).

Underexcretion

In normal persons, approximately two-thirds of the uric acid produced daily is excreted by the kidney, one-third is eliminated by the gastrointestinal tract, and less than 1% is excreted in sweat (3,6). In gouty patients, decreased renal clearance commonly leads to hyperuricemia despite increased gastrointestinal urate excretion. A reduction of uric acid clearance may contribute to hyperuricemia in as many as 90% of patients with primary gout. Decreased urate clearance in primary gout could be due to reduced

TABLE 23.1. CAUSES OF HYPERURICEMIA IN MAN

Increased purine biosynthesis or urate production	Lead nephropathy
Inherited enzyme defects	Polycystic kidney disease
Hypoxanthine–guanine phosphoribosyltransferase deficiency	Hypertension
Phosphoribosylpyrophosphate synthetase overactivity	Dehydration
Glucose-6-phosphatase deficiency (glycogenosis I)	Salt restriction
Clinical disorders leading to purine overproduction	Starvation
Myeloproliferative disorders	Diabetic ketoacidosis
Lymphoproliferative disorders	Lactic acidosis
Polycythemia vera	Obesity
Malignant diseases	Hyperparathyroidism
Hemolytic disorders	Hypothyroidism
Psoriasis	Diabetes insipidus
Obesity	Sarcoidosis
Tissue hypoxia	Toxemia of pregnancy
Glycogenosis III, V, VII	Bartter syndrome
Drugs or dietary habits	Chronic beryllium disease
Ethanol	Down syndrome
Diet rich in purines	Drugs or dietary habits
Pancreatic extract	Ethanol
Fructose	Diuretics
Nicotinic acid	Low doses of salicylates
Ethylamino-1,3,4-thiadiazole	Ethambutol
4-Amino-5-imidazole carboxamide riboside	Pyrazinamide
Vitamin B_{12} (patients with pernicious anemia)	Laxative abuse (alkalosis)
Cytotoxic drugs	Levodopa
Warfarin	Methoxyflurane
Decreased Renal Clearance of Urate	Cyclosporine
Clinical disorders	
Chronic renal failure	

urate filtration, enhanced uric acid reabsorption, or decreased urate secretion.

CLINICAL FEATURES

Asymptomatic Hyperuricemia

The term *asymptomatic hyperuricemia* is applied to the state in which the serum urate concentration is abnormally high but symptoms have not occurred. In men, primary hyperuricemia frequently begins at puberty, whereas in women, it is usually delayed until menopause. Once developed, asymptomatic hyperuricemia frequently lasts a lifetime, but gout may develop in hyperuricemic individuals at any point. The prevalence of asymptomatic hyperuricemia among adult American males has been estimated at 5% to 8%, but even higher prevalence rates have been reported in Asian-Pacific populations (7,8). Management of hypertension and congestive heart failure with diuretics has expanded an already large population of individuals with asymptomatic hyperuricemia, particularly among elderly women.

Few studies have assessed the risks of asymptomatic hyperuricemia. In a cohort of 2,046 initially healthy men followed for 15 years with serial measurements of serum urate concentrations, the annual incidence of gout was 4.9% for a serum urate of 9 mg/dL or more (9). In contrast, the incidence rate was only 0.5% for values between 7.0 and 8.9 mg/dL, and 0.1% for values below 7.0 mg/dL. Throughout this prospective study, no evidence existed of renal deterioration attributable to hyperuricemia. This finding was confirmed by a study of 3,693 subjects enrolled in a hypertension detection and follow-up program (10). Therapy with thiazide-type diuretics increased both serum urate and creatinine concentrations. However, lowering urate values with drug therapy did not influence creatinine values. In addition, the incidence of gouty attacks in subjects at risk was only 2.7% over a 5-year period. Fessel concluded that hyperuricemia is of no clinical importance with respect to renal outcomes until serum urate levels reach at least 13 mg/dL in men and 10 mg/dL in women, limits beyond which little information is available (11). Urolithiasis was rare among previously asymptomatic hyperuricemic individuals, with an annualized incidence rate of 0.4% compared with 0.9% in gouty patients. In the Framingham study, gout developed in only 12% of patients with urate levels between 7 and 7.9 mg/dL over a period of 14 years (12). Values greater than 9 mg/dL had a sixfold greater predictive value but represented only 20% of the gouty population.

The available data thus do not justify therapy for most patients with asymptomatic hyperuricemia. Once a hyperuricemic individual experiences one of these complications, the asymptomatic phase is ended, and medical management of hyperuricemia may be indicated.

Clinical Gout

Acute gouty arthritis, intercritical gout, and chronic tophaceous gout represent the three classic stages in the natural history of progressive urate crystal deposition disease. Contemporary management modalities are highly efficient in interrupting the progression of the disorder and in reducing the frequency of acute gouty arthritis, urolithiasis, and tophus formation. Thus gout only infrequently unfolds in the classic manner at present, and this is largely among noncompliant individuals and patients in whom the management scheme has not been appropriately communicated or the diagnosis of gout has not been made.

Acute Gouty Arthritis

> The patient goes to bed and sleeps quietly till about two in the morning when he is awakened by a pain which usually seizes the great toe, but sometimes the heel, ankle, or instep. The pain resembles that of a dislocated bone . . . and is immediately preceded by a chillness and slight fever in proportion to the pain which is mild at first but grows gradually more violent every hour; sometimes resembling a laceration of ligaments, sometimes the gnawing of a dog, and sometimes a weight and constriction of the parts affected, which becomes so exquisitely painful as not to endure the weight of the clothes nor the shaking of the room from a person walking briskly there-in (from Sydenham, quoted in ref. 13).

The acute gouty attack so vividly described by Sydenham lasts from a few days to several weeks in untreated patients. With multiple recurrences, shorter intervals, separate attacks, and polyarticular involvement are more frequent. Chronic inflammation with superimposed acute exacerbations may progress to a crippling arthritis. Various studies, heavily weighted to male patients, cite the peak age of onset of gouty arthritis to be between the fourth and sixth decades (3,14), but in women initial episodes often arise in the sixth to eighth decades (15,16). Onset before age 30 or in a premenopausal woman should raise suspicion of an inherited enzyme defect, an inherited or toxic renal disease, or induction by a drug or toxic agent [such as ethanol or lead or even a chronically ingested diuretic (17)].

In older series describing the natural history of gout in men, fully 90% of patients experienced acute attacks at the base of the great toe (podagra) at some time during the course of their disease, and the first metatarsophalangeal joint was involved in about 50% of first attacks (3,14). Although it is generally accepted that about 80% of initial attacks are monoarticular, polyarticular first attacks are more common in elderly women and in patients with gout accompanying myeloproliferative disorders or the use of cyclosporine (18–22). Common initial sites of involvement include the instep, ankle, heel, knee, wrist, fingers, and elbows (olecranon bursa). Rarely involved sites include the shoulders, sternoclavicular joints, hips, spine, and sacroiliac joints. Conceptually, acute gout remains predominantly a disease of the lower extremity, and the more distal the site of involvement, the more typical the attack.

Trivial episodes of pain ("petite attacks") lasting only hours and sometimes recurrent over several years may precede the first dramatic gouty attack. The initial attack of gout often occurs with explosive suddenness, typically awakening the patient or becoming apparent as a foot is placed on the floor upon arising. The skin over the affected joint soon becomes reddened and warm; extreme tenderness of the affected joint and periarticular tissues is noted (Fig. 23.3). The slightest pressure produces exquisite pain. Fever, leukocytosis, and elevation of the erythrocyte sedimentation rate often occur. The skin over the joint may desquamate as the episode subsides.

The course of untreated acute gout is variable. Mild attacks may subside in several hours or may persist for only a few days and not reach the intensity described by Sydenham. Severe attacks may last many days to several weeks. A number of physiologic responses that contribute to the spontaneous and complete resolution of gouty arthritis have recently been reviewed (23,24).

On recovery, the patient reenters an asymptomatic phase termed the *intercritical period.* Even though the attack may have been incapacitating, with excruciating pain and swelling, resolution is usually complete, and the patient is once again well. This freedom from symptoms during the intercritical period is an important feature in the diagnosis of acute arthritis as gout.

Factors capable of provoking episodes of acute gouty arthritis include trauma, surgery, alcohol ingestion, starvation, overindulgence in foods with high purine content, and ingestion of drugs that cause changes in urate concentrations. The precise relationship of these factors to the attacks remains speculative.

Intercritical Gout and Recurrent Episodes

A clear and detailed history of an acute arthritic attack followed by a completely asymptomatic intercritical period before a recurrence is valuable in pointing toward the diagnosis of gout. During this period, aspiration of a previously inflamed joint can frequently corroborate the diagnosis of gout. For example, in an untreated gouty population, 36 of 37 synovial fluid aspirates obtained during intercritical periods yielded urate crystals if the knee aspirated had been subject to past gouty attacks (25). By comparison, the yield was only 22% if there was no history of prior acute involvement in the aspirated knee and was 50% in previously inflamed knees in patients on urate-lowering medication. Without therapy, most gouty patients will experience a second episode within 2 years. In one large series (3), 62% of patients had recurrences within the first year, and 78% within 2 years, with only 7% free of recurrences for 10 years or more (9).

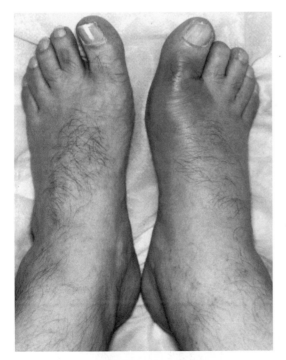
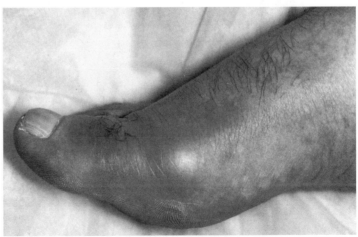

FIGURE 23.3. Acute gouty arthritis of the right first metatarsophalangeal joint. Note the swelling and hyperemia about the affected joint. (From Becker MA. Clinical gout and the pathogenesis of hyperuricemia. In: Koopman WJ, ed. *Arthritis and allied conditions: a textbook of rheumatology,* 14th ed. Philadelphia: Lippincott Williams & Wilkins, 2001:2281–2313, with permission.)

As the disease progresses in the untreated patient, acute attacks occur with increasing frequency and are often polyarticular, more severe, longer-lasting, and occasionally associated with a febrile course. Although affected joints may continue to recover completely, bony erosions may develop. As many as one-third of patients with late polyarticular attacks reported that their initial attack was also polyarticular (26). Joints may flare in sequence, in a migratory pattern, or, as in pseudogout, several neighboring joints may be involved simultaneously in a cluster attack. Frequently, periarticular sites such as bursae and tendons are also involved.

Eventually, the patient may suffer chronic polyarticular gout without pain-free intercritical periods. Gout at this stage may be confused with rheumatoid arthritis, especially if nodules (tophi) are mistaken for rheumatoid nodules. On occasion, the disease may progress from initial podagra to a rheumatoid arthritis–like chronic deforming arthritis without remissions but with synovial thickening and the early development of tophi. Unlike rheumatoid arthritis, in which polyarticular inflammation is most often synchronous, inflamed gouty joints are frequently out of phase—a flare in one joint may coincide with subsidence of inflammation in another joint. Conversely, subcutaneous nodules in patients with "rheumatoid nodulosis" are easily confused with tophi (27). Coexistence of gout and rheumatoid arthritis is rare, however, and the appropriate diagnosis is best established by demonstrating the presence or absence of urate crystals by aspiration of affected joints or tophaceous deposits.

Chronic Tophaceous Gout

Chronic tophaceous gout (Fig. 23.4) is characterized by the identifiable deposition of solid urate (tophi) in connective tissues, including articular structures, with ultimate development of a destructive arthropathy, often with secondary degenerative changes. The identification of tophi with or before the initial gouty attack, once considered rare in primary gout (28), has been documented more frequently in recent years (29,30). In patients without tophi, the mean serum urate concentration was 9.2 mg/dL. Values of 10 to 11 mg/dL were found in subjects with minimal-to-moderate deposits, and patients with extensive tophaceous deposits had urate concentrations in excess of 11 mg/dL. In untreated patients, the interval from the first gouty attack to the beginning of chronic arthritis or visible tophi is highly variable, ranging from 3 to 42 years, with an average of 11.6 years (3).

Tophaceous gout is often associated with an early age of onset, a long duration of active but untreated disease, frequent attacks, high serum urate values, and a predilection for upper-extremity and polyarticular episodes (31). Characteristics of the arthritis included asymmetric, ascending joint involvement in which chronic inflammation was typ-

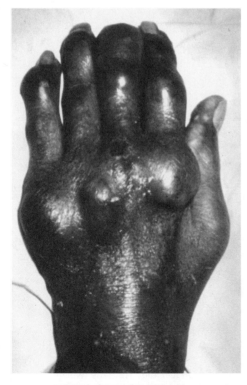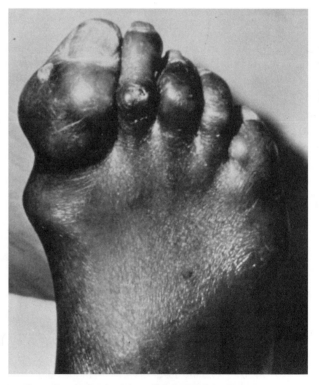

FIGURE 23.4. Chronic tophaceous gout manifested as multiple skin and joint deformities in a hand and a foot. (From Becker MA. Clinical gout and the pathogenesis of hyperuricemia. In: Koopman WJ, ed. *Arthritis and allied conditions: a textbook of rheumatology,* 14th ed. Philadelphia: Lippincott Williams & Wilkins, 2001:2281–2313, with permission.)

ical. Although ethanol consumption and diuretic use were frequently associated with gout in this population, suboptimal management and patient compliance were considered to be major factors in the progression from monoarticular gout to polyarticular status.

Organ transplant recipients treated with cyclosporine (and often diuretics as well) comprise another group at increased risk for the accelerated development of chronic tophaceous gout (18–22). Both renal and cardiac transplant patients, particularly those with compromised renal function, have developed severe and often difficult-to-manage complications of the effects of cyclosporine on renal urate clearance.

The helix of ear is a classic extraarticular location for tophaceous deposits, which take the form of small white excrescences (Fig. 23.5A). Other sites of predilection include the olecranon (Fig. 23.5B) and prepatellar bursae,

ulnar surfaces of the forearm, Achilles tendons, and finger pads, where urate crystal deposits may be intradermal as well as subcutaneous (32,33). Deposits may produce irregular and often grotesque tumescences on the hands or feet with accompanying joint destruction and crippling (Figs. 23.4, 23.6). The tense, shiny skin overlying the tophus may ulcerate and extrude white, chalky material composed of needle-shaped (acicular) urate crystals (Fig. 23.7). Ulcerated tophi rarely become secondarily infected. Bony ankylosis is also unusual (34).

As tophi and renal disease that is often associated advance, acute attacks may recur less frequently and may be milder. Late in the illness, they may disappear entirely or may be superimposed on indolently inflamed joints. Virtually all parenchymal organs except the brain have been sites of tophus formation in one or another report (35,36).

The availability of uricosuric agents and allopurinol has resulted in a significant decline in visible tophi and chronic gouty arthritis. Before the introduction of these drugs, tophaceous deposits were found in as many as 70% of gouty patients (3); more recent surveys report frequencies of less

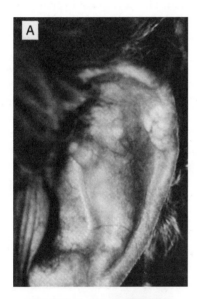
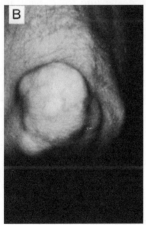

FIGURE 23.5. Tophi in helix of ear **(A)** and olecranon bursa **(B)**. (From Becker MA. Clinical gout and the pathogenesis of hyperuricemia. In: Koopman WJ, ed. *Arthritis and allied conditions: a textbook of rheumatology,* 14th ed. Philadelphia: Lippincott Williams & Wilkins, 2001:2281–2313, with permission.)

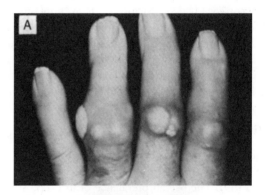
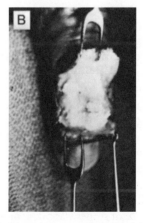

FIGURE 23.6. A: Impostumous gout involving osteoarthritic joints of an elderly woman on diuretic therapy for hypertension. **B:** Extensive urate deposits in periarticular tissue from a similar patient. (Courtesy of Dr. Michael Jablon. From Becker MA. Clinical gout and the pathogenesis of hyperuricemia. In: Koopman WJ, ed. *Arthritis and allied conditions: a textbook of rheumatology,* 14th ed. Philadelphia: Lippincott Williams & Wilkins, 2001: 2281–2313, with permission.)

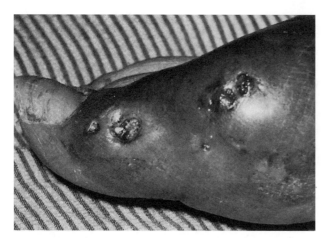

FIGURE 23.7. Ulcerated tophi. (Courtesy of Dr. Ira Melnicoff. From Becker MA. Clinical gout and the pathogenesis of hyperuricemia. In: Koopman WJ, ed. *Arthritis and allied conditions: a textbook of rheumatology,* 14th ed. Philadelphia: Lippincott Williams & Wilkins, 2001:2281–2313, with permission.

than 5% (37). In some population groups, however, residual frequencies of tophaceous gout approaching 50% have been reported (31,38). Factors such as noncompliance, poor physician–patient communication, misdiagnosis, aggressive management of hypertension with diuretics (especially in the elderly), and use of cyclosporine in transplant recipients make further reduction in the current low frequency of tophaceous gout unlikely in the future.

Urolithiasis and Gout

Uric acid stones account for 5% to 10% of all renal stones in the United States and Europe, and 40% of renal stones in Israel (39). The overall prevalence of uric acid stones in the adult U.S. population is estimated to be 0.01%, but in a series of 1,258 patients with primary gout and 59 patients with secondary gout the prevalence of renal lithiasis was 22% and 42%, respectively (40). More than 80% of calculi in these gouty patients consisted entirely of uric acid, with the remainder containing calcium oxalate or calcium phosphate, often with a central nidus of uric acid. The several-hundred-fold higher incidence of uric acid stones in gout patients is accompanied by a 10- to 30-fold increased incidence of calcium oxalate stones (41). In studies of gouty individuals, higher prevalence rates of uric acid urolithiasis are associated with increased uric acid excretion. In gouty patients with daily excretion of more than 1,100 mg of uric acid, the prevalence of stones was 50%, or 4.5 times greater than in patients excreting less than 300 mg/d (40). Many clinical circumstances result in hyperuricosuria, including inherited enzymatic defects and hematologic disorders that lead to accelerated purine biosynthesis, diets high in purine (42), and administration of uricosuric drugs (which cause only a transient increase in uric acid excretion).

Kidney Disease in Gout

Apart from arthritis and tophus formation, renal disease is the most frequently reported clinical association of hyperuricemia (3). Hyperuricemia may affect the kidney through (a) deposition of urate crystals in the renal interstitium, referred to as urate nephropathy; (b) deposition of uric acid crystals in the collecting tubules, an entity referred to as uric acid nephropathy; and (c) uric acid urolithiasis. Acute uric acid nephropathy with accompanying acute renal tubular damage and an obstructive uropathic clinical picture is very uncommon except in patients with malignancy and hyperuricemia treated by radiation or chemotherapy, or with inherited enzyme defects resulting in markedly increased uric acid excretion. In addition to these direct effects of hyperuricemia, other causes of renal dysfunction, such as hypertension, diabetes mellitus, alcohol abuse, nephrotoxic drug therapy, and lead nephropathy are also prevalent in the gouty population. The isolation of hyperuricemia or gout as primary risk factors for progressive renal disease is thus exceedingly difficult (9,11,43–45).

Significant impairment of renal function in up to 40% of patients with gout was reported in two older series of patients (3,46), and renal failure was the eventual cause of death in 18% to 25% of patients in one of these series (46). Recent evaluations, however, have deemphasized a primary causal relationship between hyperuricemia/gout and renal disease (11,43). The incidence of renal disease among gouty individuals is probably no greater than that in subjects of comparable age with similar degrees of hypertension, obesity, and primary renal disease.

DIAGNOSIS OF GOUTY ARTHRITIS

The diagnosis of gout should be established on firm criteria to ensure that expensive and toxic medications are not prescribed unnecessarily. Available data do not support therapeutic intervention for the great majority of patients with asymptomatic hyperuricemia. A definitive diagnosis of gout is established by demonstration of intracellular monosodium urate crystals in synovial fluid neutrophils by polarized compensated light microscopy (Fig. 23.8). It is, however, important to recall the occasional patient in whom acute gouty arthritis coexists with another type of joint disease such as septic arthritis, calcium pyrophosphate dihydrate (CPPD) crystal, deposition disease (pseudogout), or even basic calcium phosphate crystal deposition disease (47,48).

Extracellular urate crystals are also identifiable in synovial fluid from previously affected joints in 70% to 97% of gouty patients during asymptomatic intervals (25,49).

Demonstration of urate crystals in tophi is nearly as specific for gout as synovial fluid crystal identification. Because, however, tophi are found in only a minority of patients with gout, this diagnostic test is of limited sensitiv-

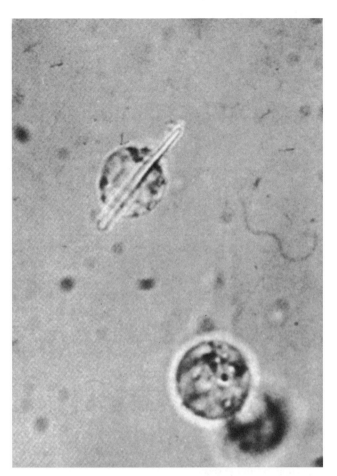

FIGURE 23.8. Polymorphonuclear leukocyte containing a phagocytized monosodium urate crystal. (From Becker MA. Clinical gout and the pathogenesis of hyperuricemia. In: Koopman WJ, ed. *Arthritis and allied conditions: a textbook of rheumatology,* 14th ed. Philadelphia: Lippincott Williams & Wilkins, 2001: 2281–2313, with permission.)

ity. In the absence of the means to identify urate crystals or a negative polarized light-microscopic study, the following combination of findings may be useful in suggesting a diagnosis of gout: (a) a classic history of monoarticular arthritis followed by an intercritical period completely free of symptoms; (b) rapid resolution of synovitis after colchicine therapy; and (c) hyperuricemia (50). Normouricemia does not preclude the diagnosis of gout, given that up to 40% of patients have normal serum urate levels at the time of acute attacks (51). Criteria for improvement resulting from colchicine therapy include major subsidence of objective joint inflammation within 48 hours and no recurrence of inflammation in any joint for at least 7 days (52). Arthritis alone in a hyperuricemic patient is insufficient to establish a diagnosis of gout.

Pseudogout (CPPD) and basic calcium phosphate crystal–induced inflammation are diseases difficult to differentiate clinically from acute gout. Self-limited attacks of acute inflammation in the first metatarsophalangeal joint

(pseudopodagra), resulting from transient amorphous calcific deposits, have been described in premenopausal women (47). Septic arthritis, cellulitis, and fractures are additional processes that often need careful exclusion in the clinical setting, suggesting acute gouty arthritis. The resemblance of gouty inflammation to cellulitis points up the diffuse, periarticular nature of gouty arthritis, which differentiates this process from primary synovitis disorders such as rheumatoid arthritis.

RADIOGRAPHIC FINDINGS IN GOUT

The major value of radiographic examination during the initial attack of gout is to exclude other types of arthritis. At this stage, the findings related to gout are nonspecific, usually in the form of soft-tissue swelling. The radiographic hallmarks of long-standing gout are those of an asymmetric, inflammatory, erosive arthritis often accompanied by soft-tissue nodules, but generally with retention of normal bone and periarticular density and joint spaces.

Sharply "punched-out," round, or oval defects situated in the marginal areas of the joint and surrounded by a sclerotic border suggest gout (Fig. 23.9). Bony (intraosseous)

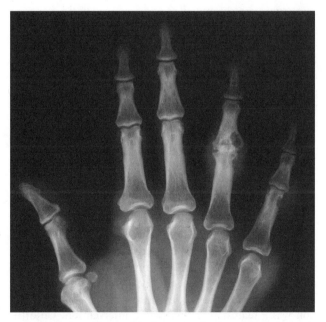

FIGURE 23.9. Radiographic features of gout are prominently displayed in the fourth and fifth proximal interphalangeal joints of the right hand of this individual. Soft-tissue swellings (tophi) surround both joints, and there are marginal erosions with sclerotic borders and overhanging edges as well as osseous cysts. Bony mineralization is generally well maintained, and the joint space of the fifth proximal interphalangeal joint remains intact. (Courtesy of Dr. Larry B. Dixon. From Becker MA. Clinical gout and the pathogenesis of hyperuricemia. In: Koopman WJ, ed. *Arthritis and allied conditions: a textbook of rheumatology,* 14th ed. Philadelphia: Lippincott Williams & Wilkins, 2001:2281–2313, with permission.)

tophaceous lesions almost always antedate subcutaneous tophi and may be seen in joints that have never been clinically inflamed (31). In about 40% of patients with gouty erosions in bone, an elevated margin extends outward into the soft-tissue covering the tophaceous nodule (53). This "overhanging margin" of bone, which may result from bony resorption beneath the enlarging tophus and periosteal apposition of the involved cortex, helps to distinguish gouty erosions from the "pocketed" erosions seen in rheumatoid arthritis. Bony erosions occur relatively late in gout, and many patients with repeated acute attacks show neither bone nor soft-tissue lesions. Another feature useful in distinguishing gout from rheumatoid arthritis is the infrequency of periarticular osteopenia in the former.

Bony erosions caused by deposits of urate crystals are related to both the duration and severity of gout. In patients with advanced chronic tophaceous gout, joint destruction may be extensive. Bony ankylosis with obliteration of the joint space has been observed but is rare except in the interphalangeal joints of the hands and feet and in the intercarpal region (34). In fact, the presence of a relatively normal joint space in a joint with extensive erosions is an important radiologic characteristic of gout.

Uric acid stones are radiolucent and appear radiologically as "filling defects." Cysteine, xanthine, and 2,8-dihydroxyadenine stones are also radiolucent, but most radiolucent stones are composed of uric acid. Uric acid stones or gravel may be white or pink ("brick dust") as a result of absorption of a pigment that has not been identified. Patients with brick dust urine may present with what they believe to be hematuria. Radiopaque stones also occur with greatly increased frequency in gouty subjects and are composed largely of calcium oxalate. These stones often contain a small amount of uric acid, which probably serves as a nidus for the deposition of calcium oxalate by epitaxial overgrowth.

TREATMENT

The stereotype of the gouty patient as a corpulent, hypertensive, overimbibing, middle-aged man is sufficiently accurate that usually there is an opportunity to modify the management of hyperuricemia and gout. Before the advent of effective uric acid–lowering agents, dietary purine restriction was a mainstay of therapeutic intervention. Unfortunately, even a severe reduction in purine intake rarely lowers serum urate levels by more than 1 mg/dL unless the patient has an unusually high consumption of purine-rich foods on a consistent basis. Other lifestyle modifications can also be helpful in treating hyperuricemia. Dietary counseling for weight loss in obese and hypertensive patients will help lower urate levels. Regular alcohol consumption should be discouraged, since it can stimulate increased purine production. Episodic acute intoxication can also

cause hyperuricemia on the basis of transient increased serum lactic acid levels and interference with renal uric acid excretion (54). Beer drinking can be especially problematic, since it not only exerts an ethanol effect on purine production and elimination but also is a purine-rich food.

Before initiating uric acid–lowering therapy, the physician should review the patient's current medications to determine if any might be contributing to the hyperuricemia (Table 23.2). Potential offending drugs (especially thiazide diuretics) should be replaced with alternatives. Several medications have a paradoxical effect on uric acid excretion (Table 23.3); this is to say, a low dose of these medications results in elevated serum urate levels, whereas a higher dose results in hypouricemia. The mechanism for this paradoxical effect has not been elucidated for all of these medications. For salicylate, a mechanism has been proposed that may, in general, be applicable to the other agents listed in Table 23.3. When aspirin is administered in low doses (<1.5 g/d), it is a competitive inhibitor of the urate secretory system, resulting in hyperuricemia. When

TABLE 23.2. CAUSES OF HYPERURICEMIA: DECREASED URIC ACID EXCRETION

Primary hyperuricemia
   Decreased filtered load
   Increased tubular reabsorption
   Decreased tubular secretion
Secondary hyperuricemia
   Reduced renal functional mass
      Chronic renal disease
   Increased tubular reabsorption: contraction of extracellular volume
      Dehydration
      Diabetes mellitus
      Diuretics
   Decreased tubular secretion: associated with increased organic acidemia
      Starvation
      Diabetic ketoacidosis
      Acute ethanol ingestion
      Toxemia of pregnancy
   Decreased tubular secretion: associated with drug administration
      Salicylates (<2 g/d)
      Phenylbutazone (<200 mg/d)
      Thiazide diuretics
      Cyclosporine
      Levodopa
      Ethambutol
      Nicotinic acid
   Mechanism not established
      Chronic lead exposure
      Berylliosis
      Sarcoidosis

From Becker MA. Clinical gout and the pathogenesis of hyperuricemia. In: Koopman WJ, ed. *Arthritis and allied conditions: a textbook of rheumatology,* 14th ed. Philadelphia: Lippincott Williams & Wilkins, 2001:2281–2313, with permission.

TABLE 23.3. DRUGS WITH PARADOXIC EFFECTS ON URATE EXCRETION

Salicylate	Ethacrinic acid
Probenecid	Acetazolamide
Phenylbutazone	Pyrazinamide

From Becker MA. Clinical gout and the pathogenesis of hyperuricemia. In: Koopman WJ, ed. *Arthritis and allied conditions: a textbook of rheumatology,* 14th edition. Philadelphia: Lippincott Williams & Wilkins, 2001:2281–2313, with permission.

aspirin intake is increased to 4.8 g/d (approximately 14 tablets), salicylate inhibits tubular reabsorption of urate at the early and, possibly, late sites, resulting in uricosuria and hypouricemia (55).

Urate-Lowering Drugs

Reduction of the serum urate concentration is achieved pharmacologically by (a) increasing the renal excretion of uric acid or (b) decreasing uric acid synthesis. The urate-lowering drugs (ULDs) most widely used in the United States are the uricosuric agents probenecid and sulfinpyrazone, and the uric acid synthesis inhibitor allopurinol. The antiinflammatory agent diflunisal and the angiotensin II receptor antagonist losartan both have uricosuric effects that may, in selected patients, have clinical utility.

Uricosuric Agents

Uricosuric agents are successful 70% to 80% of the time in achieving optimal serum urate levels. These drugs lose effectiveness as renal function deteriorates and are completely ineffective when the glomerular filtration rate reaches ≤30 mL/min. Probenecid and sulfinpyrazone require multiple doses per day and may interfere with other medications being used by the patient. For these reasons compliance becomes a problem in the chronic use of these agents. A reasonable candidate for treatment with uricosuric agents might be a gouty subject with the features described in Table 23.4.

TABLE 23.4. INDICATIONS FOR USE OF URICOSURIC AGENTS

Hyperuricemia with uric acid urinary excretion of less than 800 mg/d on a regular diet
Satisfactory renal function (creatinine clearance greater than 50 mL/min)
No history of renal calculi
Younger than 60 years
Lack of polypharmacy

From Becker MA. Clinical gout and the pathogenesis of hyperuricemia. In: Koopman WJ, ed. *Arthritis and allied conditions: a textbook of rheumatology,* 14th ed. Philadelphia: Lippincott Williams & Wilkins, 2001:2281–2313, with permission.

Probenecid

Probenecid is rapidly and completely absorbed by the gastrointestinal tract and is more than 70% eliminated from the circulation in 24 hours (56). The biologic half-life is between 6 and 12 hours and is dose dependent. The uricosuric activity of probenecid is due largely to inhibition of renal tubular reabsorption of uric acid at the postsecretory reabsorptive site (Fig. 23.10).

Therapy is begun at 250 mg twice each day and is increased as necessary up to 3 g/d. Optimal serum urate control can be achieved with 1 g/d or less in 50% of gouty patients and in 85% with 2 g/d or less (57). Because of the serum half-life of 6 to 12 hours, probenecid should be taken in 2 or 3 evenly spaced doses.

Probenecid is generally well tolerated with approximately 5% of patients developing complications such as rash, fever, gastric irritation, or precipitation of acute gout or nephrolithiasis. Acute gouty arthritis can usually be avoided by the concomitant use of colchicine or a nonsteroidal antiinflammatory drug. Renal stones can be avoided by maintaining adequate urine volume and an alkaline urine pH, as well as a slow escalation of the probenecid dose. Taking the medication with meals usually abates gastric irritation. Probenecid influences the metabolism and elimination of multiple other medications (Table 23.5).

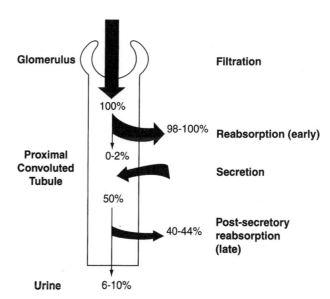

FIGURE 23.10. The four-component model of urate handling by the kidney. Uric acid is filtered at the glomerulus and then undergoes bidirectional transport within the proximal convoluted tubule. The percentages represent the fraction of urate filtered at the glomerulus that is subsequently transported. (From Edwards NL. Management of hyperuricemia. In: Koopman WJ, ed. *Arthritis and allied conditions: a textbook of rheumatology,* 14th ed. Philadelphia: Lippincott Williams & Wilkins, 2001: 2314–2328, with permission.)

TABLE 23.5. DRUG–DRUG INTERACTIONS WITH PROBENECID

Ampicillin	Salicylates
Penicillin	Indomethacin
Nafcillin	Heparin
Cephradine	Dapsone
Cephaloridine	Rifampicin

From Becker MA. Clinical gout and the pathogenesis of hyperuricemia. In: Koopman WJ, ed. *Arthritis and allied conditions: a textbook of rheumatology,* 14th ed. Philadelphia: Lippincott Williams & Wilkins, 2001:2281–2313, with permission.

Sulfinpyrazone

Sulfinpyrazone is an analog of the antiinflammatory drug phenylbutazone. Sulfinpyrazone has no antiinflammatory activity but is a potent uricosuric and exerts an antiplatelet effect. Like probenecid, it is rapidly absorbed in the gastrointestinal tract, although its plasma half-life is much shorter at 1 to 3 hours (58). Renal insufficiency lessens the effectiveness of sulfinpyrazone, but not to the same extent as with probenecid. Its mechanism of action is the same as that of probenecid.

In the treatment of gout, sulfinpyrazone is initiated at a dose of 50 mg, twice a day with incremental increases to 100 mg and then 200 mg twice daily as needed to achieve optimal urate control. This medication is generally well tolerated with many of the same complications as probenecid. Gastrointestinal side effects are found in 10% to 15% of treated subjects. Bone marrow toxicity has been reported (59) and drug–drug interactions with oral hypoglycemic agents and sulfa drugs have also been described (60).

Diflunisal

Diflunisal (Dolobid) is a fluorinated salicylate that is commonly used as a nonsteroidal antiinflammatory drug. From the time of its release, diflunisal was known to have moderate uricosuric effects at all dose levels studied (61,62). Dosing at 500 to 1,000 mg/d in divided doses is effective for both analgesic and uricosuric effects.

Losartan

Losartan is a member of a new class of antihypertensive agents—the angiotensin II receptor antagonists. It is as effective as angiotensin-converting enzyme (ACE) inhibitors, calcium channel blockers, or β-blockers in lowering blood pressure, but losartan also possesses uricosuric activity (63). Investigators have found this drug useful in treating cyclosporine-induced hyperuricemia in renal and heart transplant recipients (64). In patients with recalcitrant hyperuricemia because of dependency on diuretics, the addition of ACE inhibitors is also helpful in lowering serum urate levels (65).

Inhibitors of Urate Synthesis

Allopurinol

Allopurinol is the most commonly prescribed ULD because of its easy dosing regimen, its broad range of efficacy, and its generally good safety profile. Allopurinol is a structural analog of hypoxanthine, originally designed to be an antitumor agent, but its primary biologic activity is to inhibit the uric acid generating enzyme xanthine oxidase (66). The plasma half-life of allopurinol is only 1 to 3 hours, as it is extensively catabolized to oxypurinol. Oxypurinol has a half-life of 17 to 40 hours, depending on renal function, and is a potent inhibitor of xanthine oxidase. The formation of oxypurinol provides a more stable level of xanthine oxidase inhibition, as well as a once-a-day dosing schedule for the parent drug, allopurinol.

Within 1 to 2 days of allopurinol administration, the serum urate concentration begins to fall, reaching a nadir within 7 to 14 days. A marked drop in urinary uric acid excretion accompanies this decline in serum urate level. This is an important difference from the urate-lowering activities of the uricosuric agents. Hypoxanthine and xanthine levels rise in both serum and urine as a result of allopurinol therapy. Both of these compounds are more soluble and readily excretable than uric acid.

Allopurinol is a potent ULD for virtually all causes of hyperuricemia, but it is particularly indicated for patients with the following conditions: (a) gout and either renal insufficiency and/or a 24-hour urinary uric acid excretion of greater than 1,000 mg/d, (b) noncompliance with uricosuric agents, (c) allergy or failure to respond to uricosuric agents, (d) a history of renal calculi of any type and a urinary uric acid of greater than 600 mg/d, and (e) prophylaxis or treatment of tumor lysis syndrome.

Caution should be exercised in the initiation of allopurinol in patients with renal failure or in patients taking azathioprine (Imuran), 6-mercaptopurinol (Purinethol), or other purine-based antimetabolites. In fact, there has been a widely accepted trend over the last decade to initiate allopurinol at a low dose in all patients and gradually increase the dose until the optimal serum urate level is achieved. The traditional approach had been to start all gouty subjects on 300 mg/d as a "standard" dose. Starting all patients at 100 mg/d and gradually increasing the dose every 4 weeks until a target serum urate level is reached greatly decreases the chances of precipitating an acute gouty attack or of triggering a severe hypersensitivity reaction. The exception to this scheme is the patient with a creatinine clearance of less than 20 mL/min. In this case, a starting dose of 100 mg every other day or even every third day is recommended. But even in these more extreme cases of renal failure, the dose of allopurinol frequently needs to be escalated to achieve normouricemia. Even after allopurinol has been started, it is important to continue to look for and correct any secondary causes of hyperuricemia. This may include lifestyle modifications or changes in other medications.

Allopurinol may interfere with the metabolism of drugs other than the purine derivatives mentioned above. Increased levels of theophylline and warfarin may occur in patients taking allopurinol due to altered hepatic metabolism. Cyclophosphamide toxicity and bone marrow suppression are enhanced with allopurinol, although the mechanism for this is unclear (67). A 20% incidence of skin rash has been reported in patients on allopurinol taking either ampicillin or amoxicillin (68). Table 23.6 lists other drugs potentially affected by allopurinol therapy.

Side effects of allopurinol are infrequent and generally mild. The most frequently encountered problems include rashes, gastrointestinal distress, diarrhea, and headache. Mild rashes may occur in 2% of patients taking allopurinol. In most cases, a reduction in dose will allow the rash to clear. In subjects with more persistent rashes or other mild allergic responses to allopurinol, desensitization by either oral or intravenous routes can be attempted (67,69).

A severe hypersensitivity reaction to allopurinol is rare but potentially life-threatening. The true incidence of this immunologically mediated syndrome is unknown but estimates of 0.1% to 0.4% are reported (70,71). There is a characteristic setting for this hypersensitivity reaction and special precautions may help avoid it. Fever, rash, hepatitis, leukocytosis with eosinophilia, and worsening renal function (72,73) characterize the allopurinol hypersensitivity syndrome (AHS). Death is reported in 25% to 30% of these cases, even when allopurinol is quickly discontinued. Fever and rash are present acutely in 95% of AHS cases. The fever is usually in the range of 39.0° to 39.5°C (102° to 103°F). The skin involvement may include generalized

exfoliative erythroderma, marked palmar/plantar hyperkeratosis, Stevens-Johnson syndrome, or toxic epidermal necrolysis ("scalded skin" syndrome). Eighty percent to 90% of patients with AHS will have elevated serum transaminase levels that may occasionally progress into hepatic failure. A leukocytosis is observed in 40% and is frequently associated with eosinophilia and lymphopenia (74). A peripheral eosinophilia is found in 75% of AHS cases. The causes of death in AHS include acute renal and hepatic failure, gastrointestinal bleeding, and sepsis associated with skin exfoliation.

The clinical setting for AHS is consistent in most published series. Eighty percent have mild renal dysfunction and 50% are taking thiazide diuretics at the time allopurinol is initiated. Most AHS patients develop their symptoms soon after starting a "standard" dose (300 mg/d) of allopurinol. The mean duration from start of therapy to onset of symptoms is 3 weeks (70). Tragically, over half of the patients who develop this life-threatening reaction have no clear indication for being started on allopurinol.

By recognizing the risk factors of mild renal dysfunction combined with the use of thiazide diuretics and by adopting the "go low, go slow" approach to initial allopurinol dosing, AHS can be prevented in many cases. Treatment of AHS consists of early recognition, withdrawal of allopurinol, and supportive measures. The benefit of using corticosteroids in treating AHS is controversial (72,75).

Oxypurinol

Oxypurinol is the active product of allopurinol oxidation and has pharmacologic effects similar to those of allopurinol. In direct comparative studies, allopurinol is more effective due to better gastrointestinal absorption (60). Although neither the oral nor intravenous forms of oxypurinol are commercially available in the United States, it has been used on a compassionate basis for many years in individuals with severe allopurinol hypersensitivity who experience acute urate overload from tumor lysis syndrome. However, cross-reactivity between allopurinol and oxypurinol is reported at 30%.

When to Start Urate-Lowering Drugs

Asymptomatic Hyperuricemia

Most subjects with chronic hyperuricemia will never develop symptoms of urate deposition. It is therefore generally not advisable to begin ULDs on the basis of elevated serum urate alone. It is universally advised to evaluate patients thoroughly with the markedly elevated urate levels for the underlying diseases or medications listed in Tables 23.2 and 23.7.

TABLE 23.6. DRUG–DRUG INTERACTIONS WITH ALLOPURINOL

Ampicillin/Amoxicillin	6-Mercaptopurine
Azathioprine	Probenecid
Chlorpropamide	Vidarabine
Cyclophosphamide	Warfarin
Dilantin	ACE inhibitors[a]

[a]Suspected.
ACE, angiotensin-converting enzyme.
From Becker MA. Clinical gout and the pathogenesis of hyperuricemia. In: Koopman WJ, ed. *Arthritis and allied conditions: a textbook of rheumatology,* 14th ed. Philadelphia: Lippincott Williams & Wilkins, 2001:2281–2313, with permission.

TABLE 23.7. CAUSES OF HYPERURICEMIA: INCREASED URIC ACID PRODUCTION

Primary hyperuricemia
  HPRT deficiency
    Complete: Lesch–Nyhan syndrome
    Partial: Kelley–Seegmiller syndrome
  PP-ribose-P synthetase overactivity
Secondary hyperuricemia
  Increased ATP degradation
    Glucose-6-phosphatase deficiency
    Tissue hypoxia
    Ethanol consumption
  Increased nucleic acid turnover
    Blood dyscrasias
    Malignancy
    Infectious mononucleosis
    Psoriasis
    Tumor lysis syndrome

ATP, adenosine triphosphate; HPRT, hypoxanthine-guanine phosphoribosyl transferase; PP-ribose-P synthetase, 5-phosphoribosyl-1 pyrophosphate synthetase.
From Becker MA. Clinical gout and the pathogenesis of hyperuricemia. In: Koopman WJ, ed. *Arthritis and allied conditions: a textbook of rheumatology,* 14th ed. Philadelphia: Lippincott Williams & Wilkins, 2001:2281–2313, with permission.

Gout

Urate-lowering drugs are indicated in all patients with chronic gouty arthritis, with or without tophi. From the first episode of acute gout, however, it may take years or decades to reach this stage of chronic nonremitting arthritis. There has been considerable controversy as to when to initiate UDLs during this long period of "intermittent gout." There is no evidence of bony destruction early in the course of intermittent gout. As episodes of acute gout recur in the same joint, bony destruction takes place. As many as 42% of subjects with intermittent gout will demonstrate radiographic evidence of joint deterioration prior to the development of subcutaneous tophi or chronic arthritis (76,77). If the goal of therapy in gout is to prevent destructive changes in bones and joints, then clearly ULDs need to be started sometime between the stages of asymptomatic hyperuricemia and chronic tophaceous gout. Serial monitoring for radiographic changes has been proposed as a useful mechanism for determining when to begin ULDs (78). The cost-effectiveness of urate-lowering therapy has been analyzed by comparing treated and nontreated groups (79). Treatment of patients who had two or more gouty attacks per year resulted in an overall cost savings when compared with the costs avoided by not having to treat acute episodes or the complications of NSAID use.

The optimal target range for serum urate reduction is another area dominated by opinions rather than controlled studies. Preventing recurrent gouty attacks can usually be achieved by reducing the serum urate to between 5 and 6 mg/dL (300 μmol/L and 360 μmol/L), respectively (80,81). Resorption of subcutaneous tophi may require a serum urate reduction of less than 5 mg/dL (77,80).

The decision regarding which type of ULD to choose as the initial urate-lowering therapy is dictated by the indications and contraindications for uricosurics and allopurinol discussed earlier. In gouty subjects who excrete less than 800 mg of uric acid per day, reduction in serum urate can be achieved with either allopurinol or the uricosuric agents. They may rarely require both types of ULDs. Early studies found no clear advantage for allopurinol compared with uricosurics (82), while subsequent reports demonstrated better long-term treatment outcomes with allopurinol (83,84). Despite a lack of compelling, well-controlled data on the long-term treatment of hyperuricemia in gout, a strong bias toward the initial use of allopurinol has emerged.

Nephrolithiasis

Uric acid calculi occur frequently in patients with gout but can occur in subjects with no previous evidence of uric acid–related symptoms. The development of gout and tophi correlates closely with serum urate levels. Uric acid stone disease, on the other hand, is correlated with urinary uric acid concentration and urine pH. In urine, uric acid becomes insoluble at acid pH but has more than ten times greater solubility with pH of more than 7.0. Regardless of serum urate concentration, patients who present with renal calculi should have a 24-hour urine examined for pH, volume, and uric acid excretion. Volume deficits and acidic pH should be corrected. Patients with renal calculi who have daily urinary uric acid excretion of more than 800 mg should be placed on allopurinol regardless of the composition of the stone. Potassium citrate (30 to 80 mEq/d orally in divided doses) is a good approach for correcting a consistently acid urine. It can be used alone or in combination with allopurinol (85).

When to Stop Urate-Lowering Drugs

For patients with chronic tophaceous gout who have experienced resolution of tophi and complete abatement of arthritis through the use of ULDs, the traditional approach is to continue the ULD indefinitely (80). Given the cost of medications and their monitoring, the possibilities of side effects, and the burden of taking drugs on a daily basis, alternatives to lifelong use of ULDs have been investigated.

The effect of discontinuing ULDs in gouty subjects in remission has been studied on several occasions (86–88). Recurrent arthritis was observed in approximately 50% of patients within 2 to 3 years of ULD stoppage. In one study that selectively enrolled patients who formerly had chronic tophaceous gouty arthritis, 81% had recurrent arthritis and 43% redeveloped tophi within 3 years (88).

Clinical factors that might predict early recurrence of arthritis and tophi after ULDs are stopped include severity of basal hyperuricemia, duration of gouty symptoms, duration of ULD therapy, and obesity. These, however, have not been studied in a systematic fashion.

Special Considerations

Transplantation Gout

Hyperuricemia and gout are common occurrences in subjects who have undergone solid organ transplantation and are receiving cyclosporine to prevent rejection (89). Allopurinol is the most frequently used ULD following renal or cardiac transplantation (90). Of concern, however, is the drug–drug interaction between allopurinol and azathioprine, a common co-therapy with cyclosporine. A general guideline for initiating allopurinol therapy in the presence of azathioprine has been published (90). Allopurinol is begun at 50 mg/d and the dose of azathioprine is reduced by 50%. Serum urate, cyclosporine levels, and white blood cell count are monitored weekly. The dose of allopurinol is escalated in 50-mg increments every 2 to 3 weeks. As the serum urate level drops toward the target range of 5 to 6 mg/dL, the azathioprine is reduced to about 25% of the initial dose. Markers of rejection need to be monitored closely.

The uricosuric properties of the angiotensin II receptor antagonist losartan provide a possible alternative to allopurinol, as long as the urinary uric acid excretion does not exceed 800 mg/d and the patient can maintain good hydration (64).

Tumor Lysis Syndrome

Tumor lysis syndrome describes a constellation of metabolic abnormalities associated with lymphoproliferative malignancies following spontaneous or chemotherapy-induced cytolysis (91). The biochemical aberrations include hyperphosphatemia, hyperkalemia, hypocalcemia, and azotemia, but the most clinically important is hyperuricemia. Early prophylactic measures can greatly reduce the frequency and severity of complications associated with tumor lysis syndrome. Allopurinol in full doses is given to prevent uric acid formation. Vigorous hydration to ensure good renal blood flow and urine volume are important in preventing acute renal failure. Alkalization of the urine with sodium bicarbonate is important to improve uric acid solubility. The alkalization should, however, not be overly zealous, since massive phosphate crystalluria might occur (92). A target urine pH of 6.5 to 7.0 is adequate in this setting. In severe cases of tumor lysis syndrome, hemodialysis may be an important salvage technique, since uric acid is readily dialyzable.

REFERENCES

1. Hitchings GH. Uric acid: chemistry and synthesis. In: Weiner IM, Kelley WN, eds. *Uric acid: handbook of experimental pharmacology,* Vol 51. New York: Springer-Verlag, 1978:1–20.
2. Loeb J. The influence of temperature on the solubility of monosodium urate. *Arthritis Rheum* 1972;15:189–192.
3. Wyngaarden JB, Kelley WN. *Gout and hyperuricemia.* New York: Grune and Stratton, 1976.
4. Chen Y-T, Burchell A. Glycogen storage diseases. In: Scriver CR, Beaudet AL, Sly WS, et al., eds. *The metabolic and molecular bases of inherited disease,* 7th ed. New York: McGraw-Hill, 1995:935–965.
5. Reitsma-Bierens WCC. Renal complications in glycogen storage disease type I. *Eur J Pediat* 1993;152:S60–S62.
6. Sorensen LB. The elimination of uric acid in man studied by means of ^{14}C-labelled uric acid. *Scand J Clin Lab Invest* 1960;12(Suppl):1–214.
7. Gibson T, Waterworth R, Hatfield P, et al. Hyperuricemia, gout and kidney function in New Zealand Maori men. *Br J Rheumatol* 1984;23:276–282.
8. Darmavan J, Valkenburg HA, Muirden KD, et al. The epidemiology of gout and hyperuricemia in a rural population of Java. *J Rheumatol* 1992;19:1595–1599.
9. Campion EW, Glynn RJ, DeLabry LO. Asymptomatic hyperuricemia: risks and consequences in the normative aging study. *Am J Med* 1987;82:421–426.
10. Langford HG, Blaufox MD, Borhani NO, et al. Is thiazide-produced uric acid elevation harmful? Analysis of data from the hypertension detection and follow-up program. *Arch Intern Med* 1987;147:645–649.
11. Fessel JW. Renal outcomes of gout and hyperuricemia. *Am J Med* 1979;67:74–82.
12. Hall AP, Barry PE, Dawber TR, et al. Epidemiology of gout and hyperuricemia: a long-term population study. *Am J Med* 1967;42:27–37.
13. Copeman WSC. *A short history of the gout and the rheumatic diseases.* Berkeley: University of California Press, 1964;66–79.
14. Grahame R, Scott JT. Clinical survey of 354 patients with gout. *Ann Rheum Dis* 1970;29:461–468.
15. Macfarlane DG, Dieppe PA. Diuretic-induced gout in elderly women. *Br J Rheumatol* 1985;24:155–157.
16. Meyers OL, Monteagudo FSE. Gout in females: an analysis of 92 patients. *Clin Exp Rheumatol* 1985;3:105–109.
17. Hayem G, Delahousse M, Meyer O, et al. Female premenopausal tophaceous gout induced by long term diuretic abuse. *J Rheumatol* 1996;23:2166–2167.
18. Scott JT. Drug-induced gout. *Bailliere's Clin Rheumatol* 1991;5:39–60.
19. Kahl LE, Thompson ME, Griffith BP. Gout in the heart transplant recipient: physiologic puzzle and therapeutic challenge. *Am J Med* 1989;87:289–294.
20. Lin HY, Rocher LL, McQuillan MA, et al. Cyclosporine-induced hyperuricemia and gout. *N Engl J Med* 1989;321:287–292.
21. Burack DA, Griffith BP, Thompson ME, et al. Hyperuricemia and gout among heart transplant recipients receiving cyclosporine. *Am J Med* 1992;92:141–146.
22. Baethge BA, Work J, Landreneau MD, et al. Tophaceous gout in patients with renal transplants treated with cyclosporine A. *J Rheumatol* 1993;20:718–720.
23. Terkeltaub RA, Dyer CA, Martin J, et al. Apolipoprotein (apo) E inhibits the capacity of monosodium urate crystals to stimulate neutrophils: characterization of intraarticular apo E and demonstration of apo E binding to urate crystals in vivo. *J Clin Invest* 1991;87:20–26.

24. Terkeltaub RA. What stops a gouty attack? *J Rheumatol* 1992; 19:8–10.

25. Pascual E. Persistence of monosodium urate crystals and low-grade inflammation in the synovial fluid of patients with untreated gout. *Arthritis Rheum* 1991;34:141–145.

26. Raddatz DA, Mahowald ML, Bilka PJ. Acute polyarticular gout. *Ann Rheum Dis* 1983;42:117–122.

27. Ginsberg MH, Genant HK, Yü T-F, et al. Rheumatoid nodulosis: an unusual variant of rheumatoid disease. *Arthritis Rheum* 1975;18:49–58.

28. Wernick R, Winkler C, Campbell S. Tophi as the initial manifestation of gout: report of six cases and review of the literature. *Arch Intern Med* 1992;152:873–876.

29. Iglesias A, Londono JC, Saaibi DL, et al. Gouty nodulosis: widespread subcutaneous deposits without gout. *Arthritis Care Res* 1996;9:74–77.

30. Liu K, Moffatt EJ, Hudson ER, et al. Gouty tophus presenting as a soft-tissue mass diagnosed by fine needle aspiration: a case report. *Diagn Cytopathol* 1996;15:246–249.

31. Nakayama DA, Barthelemy C, Carrera G, et al. Tophaceous gout: a clinical and radiographic assessment. *Arthritis Rheum* 1984;27:468–471.

32. Holland NW, Jost D, Beutler A, et al. Finger pad tophi in gout. *J Rheumatol* 1996;23:690–692.

33. Fam AG, Assad D. Intradermal urate tophi. *J Rheumatol* 1997; 24:1126–1131.

34. Good AE, Rapp R. Bony ankylosis: a rare manifestation of gout. *J Rheumatol* 1978;5:335–337.

35. Lichtenstein L, Scott HW, Levin MH. Pathologic changes in gout: survey of 11 necropsied cases. *Am J Pathol* 1956;32: 871–895.

36. Stark TW, Hirokawa RH. Gout and its manifestations in the head and neck. *Otolaryngol Clin North Am* 1982;15:659–664.

37. O'Duffy JD, Hunder GG, Kelly PJ. Decreasing prevalence of tophaceous gout. *Mayo Clin Proc* 1975;50:227–228.

38. Lawry GV II, Fan PT, Bluestone R. Polyarticular versus monoarticular gout: a prospective comparative analysis of clinical features. *Medicine* 1988;67:335–343.

39. Yü T-F. Uric acid nephrolithiasis. In: Weiner IM, Kelley WN, eds. *Uric acid: handbook of experimental pharmacology,* Vol 51. New York: Springer-Verlag, 1978:397–422.

40. Yü T-F, Gutman AB. Uric acid nephrolithiasis in gout: predisposing factors. *Ann Intern Med* 1967;67:1133–1148.

41. Coe FL, Kavalach AG. Hypercalciuria and hyperuricosuria in patients with calcium nephrolithiasis. *N Engl J Med* 1974;291: 1344–1350.

42. Zollner N, Griebsch A. Diet and gout. *Adv Exp Med Biol* 1974; 41B:435–442.

43. Berger L, Yü T-F. Renal function in gout: 4. An analysis of 524 gouty subjects including long-term follow-up studies. *Am J Med* 1975;59:605–613.

44. Reif MC, Constantiner A, Levitt MF. Chronic gouty nephropathy: a vanishing syndrome? *N Engl J Med* 1981;304:535–536.

45. Liang MH, Fries JF. Asymptomatic hyperuricemia: the case for conservative management. *Ann Intern Med* 1978;88:666–670.

46. Talbott JH, Terplan KL. The kidney in gout. *Medicine* 1960;39: 405–468.

47. Fam AG, Rubenstein J. Hydroxyapatite pseudopodagra: a syndrome of young women. *Arthritis Rheum* 1989;32:741–747.

48. Mines D, Abduhl SB. Hydroxyapatite pseudopodagra: acute calcific periarthritis of the first metatarsophalangeal joint. *Am J Emerg Med* 1996;14:180–182.

49. Rouault T, Caldwell DS, Holmes EW. Aspiration of the asymptomatic metatarsophalangeal joint in gout patients and hyperuricemic controls. *Arthritis Rheum* 1982;25:209–212.

50. Wallace SL, Robinson H, Masi AT, et al. Preliminary criteria for the classification of the acute arthritis of primary gout. *Arthritis Rheum* 1977;20:895–900.

51. Logan JA, Morrison E, McGill P. Serum uric acid in acute gout. *Ann Rheum Dis* 1997;56:696–697.

52. Wallace SL, Bernstein D, Diamond H. Diagnostic value of colchicine therapeutic trial. *JAMA* 1967;199:525–528.

53. Martel W. The overhanging margin of bone: a roentgenologic manifestation of gout. *Radiology* 1968;91:755–756.

54. MacLachlan MJ, Rodnan GP. Effect of food, fast, and alcohol on serum uric acid and acute attacks of gout. *Am J Med* 1967; 42:38–57.

55. Diamond HS, Sterba G, Jayadeven K, et al. On the mechanism of the paradoxical effect of salicylate on urate excretion. *Adv Exp Med Biol* 1980;122A:221–231.

56. Dayton PG, Yu T-F, Chen W, et al. The physiological disposition of probenecid, including renal clearance in man, studied by an improved method for its estimation in biological material. *J Pharm Exp Ther* 1963;140:278–291.

57. Gutman AB, Yu T-F. Protracted uricosuric therapy in tophaceous gout. *Lancet* 1957;111b:1258–1260.

58. Emmerson BT. A comparison of uricosuric agents in gout with special reference to sulfinpyrazone. *Med J Aust* 1963;1:839–844.

59. Gutman AB. Uricosuric drugs with special reference to probenecid and sulfinpyrazone. *Adv Pharmacol* 1966;4:91–142.

60. Khawaja AT, Diamond HS. Hypouricemic drugs. In: Smyth CV, Holers VM, eds. *Gout, hyperuricemia, and other crystal-associated arthropathies.* New York: Marcel Dekker, 1999:219–240.

61. Dresse A, Fischer P, Gerard MA, et al. Uricosuric properties of diflunisal in man. *Br J Clin Pharmacol* 1979;7:267–272.

62. Van Loenhout JWA, van de Putte LBA, Gribnau FWJ, et al. Persistent hypouricemic effect of long-term diflunisal administration. *J Rheumatol* 1981;8:639–642.

63. Burnier M, Rutschmann B, Nussberger J, et al. Salt dependent renal effects of an angiotensin II antagonist in healthy subjects. *Hypertension* 1993;22:339–347.

64. Minghelli G, Seydoux C, Goy J-J, Burnier M. Uricosuric effect of the angiotensin II receptor antagonist Losartan in heart transplant recipients. *Transplantation* 1998;66:268–271.

65. Leary WP, Reyes AJ. Angiotensin I converting enzyme inhibitors and the renal excretion of urate. *Cardiovasc Drugs Ther* 1987; 1:29–38.

66. Elion GB, Callahan S, Nathan H, et al. Potentiation by inhibition of drug degradation: 6-substituted purines and xanthine oxidase. *Biochem Pharmacol* 1963;12:85–98.

67. Fam AG, Lewtas J, Stein J, et al. Desensitization to allopurinol in patients with gout and cutaneous reactions. *Am J Med* 1992; 93:299–302.

68. Boston Collaborative Drug Surveillance Program. Excess of ampicillin rashes associated with allopurinol therapy or hyperuricemia. *N Engl J Med* 1972;286:505–507.

69. Walz-LeBlanc BAE, Reynolds WJ, MacFadden DK. Allopurinol sensitivity in a patient with chronic tophaceous gout: success of intravenous desensitization after failure of oral desensitization. *Arthritis Rheum* 1991;34:1329–1331.

70. Hande KR, Noone RM, Stone WJ. Severe allopurinol toxicity: description and guidelines for prevention in patients with renal insufficiency. *Am J Med* 1984;76:47–56.

71. McInnes GT, Lawson DH, Jick H. Acute adverse reactions attributed to allopurinol in hospitalized patients. *Ann Rheum Dis* 1981;40:245–249.

72. Arellano F, Sacristan JA. Allopurinol hypersensitivity syndrome: a review. *Ann Pharmacother* 1993;27:337–343.

73. Edwards NL. Allopurinol hypersensitivity. In: Klippel JH, Dieppe PA, eds. *Rheumatology,* 2nd ed. St Louis: CV Mosby, 1998:8:19.11–19.12.

74. Lockard O, Harmon C, Nolph K, et al. Allergic reactions to

allopurinol with cross-reactivity to oxypurinol. *Ann Intern Med* 1976;85:333–335.

75. Lang PG. Severe hypersensitivity reactions to allopurinol. *South Med J* 1979;72:1361–1368.

76. Nakayama DA, Barthelemy C, Carrera GF, et al. Tophaceous gout: a clinical and radiographic assessment. *Arthritis Rheum* 1984;27:468–471.

77. McCarthy GM, Barthelenay CR, Veum JA, et al. Influence of antihyperuricemic therapy on the clinical and radiographic progression of gout. *Arthritis Rheum* 1991;34:1489–1494.

78. Barthelemy CR, Nakayama DA, Carrera GF, et al. Gouty arthritis: a prospective radiographic evaluation of sixty patients. *Skeletal Radiol* 1984;11:1–8.

79. Ferraz MB, O'Brien B. A cost effectiveness analysis of urate lowering drugs in nontophaceous recurrent gouty arthritis. *J Rheumatol* 1995;22:908–914.

80. Emmerson BT. The management of gout. *N Engl J Med* 1996;334:445–451.

81. Howe S, Edwards NL. Hyperuricemia and gout. In: Rakel RE, ed. *Conn's current therapy.* Philadelphia: WB Saunders, 1995: 503–505.

82. Scott JT. Comparison of allopurinol to probenecid. *Ann Rheum Dis* 1966;25:623–626.

83. Weinberger A, Schreiber M, Sperling O, et al. Comparative eval-uation of uricosuric and allopurinol treatment in a series of 183 patients. *Intern Rev Rheum* 1975;5:681–692.

84. Rundles RW, Metz EN, Silberman HR . Allopurinol in the treatment of gout. *Ann Intern Med* 1966;64:229–258.

85. Pak CYC, Sakhaee K, Fuller C. Successful management of uric acid nephrolithiasis with potassium citrate. *Kidney Int* 1986; 30:422–428.

86. Loebl WY, Scott JT. Withdrawal of allopurinol in patients with gout. *Ann Rheum Dis* 1974;33:304–307.

87. Gast LF. Withdrawal of long term antihyperuricemic therapy in tophaceous gout. *Clin Rheumatol* 1987;6:70–73.

88. Van Lieshout-Zuidema MF, Breedveld FC. Withdrawal of long term antihyperuricemic therapy in tophaceous gout. *J Rheumatol* 1993;20:1383–1385.

89. Lin H, Rocher LL, McQuillan MA, et al. Cycolsporine induced hyperuricemia and gout. *N Engl J Med* 1989;321:287–292.

90. Howe S, Edwards NL. Controlling hyperuricemia and gout in cardiac transplant recipients. *J Musculoskel Med* 1995;12:15–24.

91. Jones DP, Mahmoud H, Chesney RW. Tumor lysis syndrome: pathogenesis and management. *Pediatr Nephrol* 1995;9: 206–212.

92. Stapleton FB, Strother DR, Roy S, et al. Acute renal failure at onset of therapy for advanced stage Burkitt lymphoma and B cell acute lymphoblastic leukemia. *Pediatrics* 1988;82:863–869.

OSTEOPENIC BONE DISEASES

KENNETH G. SAAG
SARAH L. MORGAN
BRUCE A. JULIAN

OSTEOPOROSIS

Epidemiology

Definition of Osteoporosis

According to the World Health Organization (WHO), "Osteoporosis is a systemic skeletal disease characterized by low bone mass and microarchitectural deterioration of bone tissue with a consequent increase in bone fragility and susceptibility to fracture." The WHO's definitions of *osteoporosis* are based on epidemiologic data that relate incidence of fracture to bone mineral density (BMD) in white women (Table 24.1).

By the age of 60 to 70 years, one in three non-Hispanic white women will have osteoporosis; the remainder, osteopenia. By 80 years of age, 70% will have osteoporosis. Figure 24.1 shows the prevalence of osteoporosis and osteopenia at the femoral neck in non-Hispanic white, non-Hispanic black, and Mexican-American men and women.

Incidence, Prevalence, Burden, and Ethnicity Distribution of Fracture

The estimated number of fractures among North American women was more than 200,000 in 1990 and is expected to increase to 469,000 in 2025 and to be more than 500,000 in 2050. The percentage of fractures attributable to osteoporosis is less for nonwhites than for whites, and less for men than for women. The incidence rate for hip fractures is approximately two per 1,000 patient-years at the age of 65 to 69 years in white and nonwhite women, and increases to about 26 per 1,000 patient-years at the age of 80 to 84 years. The incidence and prevalence of vertebral fractures is low before 50 years of age and rises almost exponentially thereafter. Among American women, the incidence of wrist fractures increases rapidly at the time of menopause and plateaus at about 700 per 100,000 person-years after age 60.

The lifetime risk of any fracture in the hip, spine, or distal forearm is about 40% in white women more than 50 years of age and 13% in white men of similar age. Table 24.2 gives the estimated lifetime risk for fracture at various sites in 50-year-old white men and women.

The Impact of Osteoporosis on Society

Osteoporosis and consequent fractures are major public health concerns in the United States. The economic costs of osteoporotic fractures are large and somewhat difficult to assess because the total includes expenses for surgery and hospitalization, rehabilitation, long-term care, loss of productivity, and medications. Other burdens associated with fracture include poor resultant functional status, pain, diminished quality of life, loss of independence, fear, and depression.

Hip fractures result in more than 7 million days of restricted activity and 6,000 admissions to nursing homes annually in the United States; 74% of all nursing home admissions are related to osteoporosis. For hip fractures, about half of the health care costs reflect nursing home expenses. There is an approximately 20% mortality within 1 year of hip fracture, and 50% of survivors never fully recover. The mortality associated with vertebral fractures was also greater than expected in the general population, and the mortality of patients with wrist fractures was similar.

TABLE 24.1. WHO CRITERIA FOR THE DIAGNOSIS OF OSTEOPENIC BONE DISEASE BASED UPON *T*-SCORE

Category	Definition
Normal	BMD better than 1 SD below the mean value of peak bone mass in young white women
Osteopenia	BMD between 1 and 2.5 SDs below the mean peak value
Osteoporosis	BMD more than 2.5 SDs below the peak value
Severe osteoporosis	BMD criteria for osteoporosis and fracture

BMD, bone mineral density; SD, standard deviation; WHO, World Health Organization.

A. OSTEOPENIA

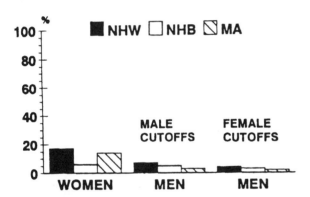

B. OSTEOPOROSIS

FIGURE 24.1. Age-adjusted prevalence of low femur neck bone mineral density by race or ethnicity, ages 50+ years. *MA,* Mexican American; *NHB,* non-Hispanic black; *NHW,* non-Hispanic white. (From Looker AC, Orwoll ES, Johnston CC, et al. Prevalence of low femoral bone density in older US adults from NHANES III.*J Bone Miner Res* 1997;12:1761–1768, with permission. Reprinted in Morgan SL, Saag KC, Julian BA, et al. Osteopenic bone diseases. In: Koopman WJ, ed. *Arthritis and allied conditions: a textbook of rheumatology,* 14th ed. Philadelphia: Lippincott Williams & Wilkins, 2001:2449–2513.)

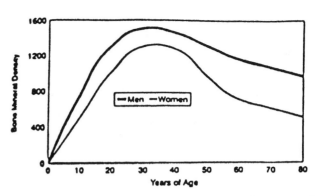

FIGURE 24.2. Age-related bone mineral density for men and women. (From Christenson RH. Biochemical markers of bone metabolism: an overview. *Clin Biochem* 1997;30:573–593, with permission. Reprinted in Morgan SL, Saag KC, Julian BA, et al. Osteopenic bone diseases. In: Koopman WJ, ed. *Arthritis and allied conditions: a textbook of rheumatology,* 14th ed. Philadelphia: Lippincott Williams & Wilkins, 2001:2449–2513.)

Pathophysiology/Pathogenesis

Patterns of Acquisition and Loss of Bone Mineral Density

Figure 24.2 shows the lifetime accrual and loss of bone mineral density (BMD) in men and women. Peak BMD is the maximum possible with normal growth and represents a genetically and environmentally determined apex from which future losses occur. Most skeletal density (both trabecular and cortical) is accumulated by age 18. Some skeletal sites, such as the skull, increase in density until menopause. In cortical bone, a slow phase of loss begins at age 40, ranging from 0.3% to 0.5% per year in men and women. At menopause in women not taking hormone replacement therapy, losses average about 1% per year but may approach 3% to 5% per year. After this accelerated loss for about 8 to 10 years, the rate decreases in another slow phase. A longitudinal population-based study in Australia of men and women approximately 60 years of age reported a loss in the femoral

TABLE 24.2. ESTIMATED LIFETIME FRACTURE RISK IN 50-YEAR-OLD WHITE WOMEN AND MEN[a,b]

Site	Women (%; 95% Confidence Interval)	Men (%; 95% Confidence Interval)
Proximal femur	17.5 (16.8, 18.2)	6.0 (5.6, 6.5)
Vertebral fracture	15.6 (14.8, 16.3)	5.0 (4.6, 5.4)
Distal forearm fracture	16.0 (15.2, 16.7)	2.5 (2.2, 3.1)
Any fracture	39.7 (38.7, 40.6)	13.1 (12.4, 13.7)

[a]Age 50 years was chosen because this is about the average age of menopause in women.
[b]Using incidence of clinically diagnosed fractures only.
From Melton LJ, Chrischilles EA, Cooper C, et al. Perspective: How many women have osteoporosis? *J Bone Miner Res* 1992;7:1005–1010, with permission.

neck of 0.9% per year in women and 0.82% per year in men. The rate increased with age in both genders. never reaching a plateau. The cumulative lifetime losses of bone may be as much as 30% to 40% of peak BMD in women and 20% to 30% in men.

Genetics of Osteoporosis

BMD at any particular age is an interplay of endogenous factors such as genetics and exogenous environmental fac-

tors. About 46% to 62% of BMD is attributable to inherited factors, as shown in twin and family studies.

Allelic variations of many genes alter bone mass and likely contribute to the pathogenesis of osteoporosis. Candidate genes include those for the vitamin D receptor, estrogen receptor, transforming growth factor β, interleukin 6, collagen type I, and collagenase. Polymorphisms in the vitamin D receptor have been associated with variations in BMD, but the significance is controversial. Lifestyle risk factors modify the genetic influence on

TABLE 24.3. DISEASES AND DRUG THERAPIES ASSOCIATED WITH OSTEOPENIA AND FRACTURE

Unique to Women
  Natural menopause
  Pregnancy
  Hypogonadism
    Agonist for gonadotropin-releasing hormone or Depo-Provera
    Gonadal dysgenesis (e.g., Turner syndrome)
    Endometriosis
Unique to Men
  Hypogonadism
    Constitutional delay of puberty
    Hemochromatosis [due either to infiltration of testes (hypergonadotropic) or pituitary (hypogonadotropic)]
    Kallman syndrome (isolated gonadotropin deficiency)
    Klinefelter syndrome (genotype XXY)
    Orchitis, viral
Men and Women
  Age-related bone loss
  Connective-tissue diseases
    Ankylosing spondylitis
    Osteogenesis imperfecta
    Rheumatoid arthritis
    Spinal cord injury
  Endocrine causes
    Acromegaly
    Adrenal trophy and Addison's disease
    Cushing syndrome
    Diabetes mellitus type 1
    Glucocorticoid excess (endogenous and exogenous)
    Gonadotroph cell adenoma
    Hyperparathyroidism (primary and secondary)
    Hyperprolactinemia (as a cause of hypogonadism)
    Hyperthyroidism
    Hypocalcitoninemia?
    Hypogonadism (primary, secondary, or surgical)
    Panhypopituitarism
    Thyrotoxicosis
  Gastrointestinal diseases
    Cholestatic liver disease (especially primary biliary cirrhosis)
    Gastrectomy
    Inflammatory bowel disease (especially regional enteritis)
    Postgastrectomy
  Lifestyle/genetic factors
    Excessive alcohol
    Excessive caffeine?
    Excessive exercise (impairment of hypothalamic-pituitary axis)

    Excessive protein intake
    Immobilization or microgravity
    Low calcium or vitamin D intake
    Sedentary lifestyle
    Smoking
  Malignancy
    Lymphoproliferative and myeloproliferative diseases (lymphoma and leukemia)
    Multiple myeloma
    Systemic mastocytosis
    Tumor secretion of parathyroid hormone-related peptide
  Nutritional disorders
    Eating disorders such as anorexia nervosa
    Osteomalacia
    Malabsorption syndromes
    Parenteral nutrition
    Pernicious anemia
  Other diseases
    Chronic obstructive pulmonary disease (often secondary to glucocorticoid usage)
    Chronic renal failure
    Congenital porphyria
    Epidermolysis bullosa
    Hemochromatosis
    Hemophilia
    Homocystinuria
    Hypophosphatasia
    Idiopathic scoliosis
    Multiple sclerosis
    Sarcoidosis
    Thalassemia
Medications
  Aluminum
  Antiepileptics (some)
  Chemotherapeutic agents that cause chemical castration
  Cyclosporine A and tacrolimus
  Cytotoxic drugs
  Glucocorticoids and adrenocorticotropin
  Heparin (perhaps less severe with low-molecular-weight compounds)
  Lithium
  Methotrexate?
  Tamoxifen (premenopausal use)
  Thyroid hormone (in excess)
  Warfarin?

From Morgan SC, Saag KG, Julian BA, et al. Osteopenic bone disease. In: Koopman WJ, ed. *Arthritis and allied conditions: a textbook of rheumatology,* 14th edition. Philadelphia: Lippincott Williams & Wilkins, 2001:2449–2513.

BMD. For example, among individuals with a vitamin D receptor genotype associated with low spinal BMD (a restriction site within the vitamin D receptor designated bb), greater calcium intake and weight-bearing physical activity appeared to improve BMD. In addition, specific genes that regulate bone mass, bone turnover, and bone loss likely play roles in determining BMD. Recent studies have shown the importance of genetic influences on type 1 collagen synthesis. Certain COL1A1 gene polymorphisms have been associated with a lower BMD and an increased fracture rate.

Clinical Features

The clinical evaluation of osteoporosis should identify lifestyle risk factors and pertinent physical findings, and assess secondary causes of osteopenia. Table 24.3 lists conditions associated with osteopenia/osteoporosis.

History/Symptoms

A careful evaluation of osteoporosis includes *identification* of a family history of metabolic bone disease, lifestyle risk factors, history of change in height and weight, history of previous fractures, reproductive history (evidence of hypogonadism), endocrine history, dietary factors (including lifetime and current consumption of calcium, vitamin D, sodium, and caffeine), a smoking history, alcohol intake, exercise, history of renal or hepatic failure, and past and current medications and supplements. In addition, factors that increase the risk of falls, such as neuromuscular disease and unsafe living conditions, should be sought. A history of bone pain is useful; however, osteoporosis is not painful unless fractures develop. Further, a large proportion of vertebral fractures may occur without overt symptoms.

Physical Examination/Signs

Height measured with a stadiometer is a vital part of the physical examination at each visit. Comparison of current height with that on the driver's license is helpful in uncovering height loss. Loss of 2 inches is a fairly sensitive indicator of vertebral compression. The spine should be examined for conformation, and spinal and paraspinous tenderness. If kyphosis is present, the possibility of pulmonary compromise should be considered. A "buffalo hump," easy bruisability, and striae suggest Cushing syndrome. Blue sclerae indicate osteogenesis imperfecta. The number of missing teeth has been correlated to the severity of loss in BMD. A joint assessment may suggest rheumatologic causes of low BMD. The neurologic examination is important because muscular weakness predisposes for falls and an underlying neurologic problem may be discovered. A gynecologic examination or prostatic examination should be included if hormone replacement therapy is considered.

Clinical Evaluation

Laboratory Evaluation

The laboratory assessment seeks possible secondary causes of loss of BMD. Table 24.4 lists tests that may be appropriate. Many are not cost-effective if obtained for every patient. Intact parathyroid hormone (PTH) concentration, for example, should be measured if the calcium concentration is elevated and the phosphorus concentration is low, or if clinical suspicion is high for hyperparathyroidism.

Bone Turnover Markers
Biochemical markers of bone turnover are sometimes used in the management of osteoporosis. While bone formation and resorption are usually "coupled," net imbalances can be

TABLE 24.4. LABORATORY EVALUATION OF DECREASED BONE MASS

Test	Diagnosis Ruled In or Ruled Out
Serum protein electrophoresis/complete blood count	Multiple myeloma
Serum calcium and phosphorus	Hyperparathyroidism
Serum intact parathyroid hormone	Hyperparathyroidism
Serum creatinine	Renal failure
Liver enzymes	Liver failure
24-hour urine free cortisol or dexamethasone suppression test	Cushing syndrome
Thyroid-stimulating hormone	Hyperthyroidism
Follicle-stimulating hormone	Menopause
Free testosterone	Male hypogonadism
Urine calcium/creatinine ratio	Hypercalciuria
25-monohydroxy vitamin D_3 and alkaline phosphatase	Vitamin D deficiency or osteomalacia

From Morgan SL, Saag KC, Julian BA, et al. Osteopenic bone diseases. In: Koopman WJ, ed. *Arthritis and allied conditions: a textbook of rheumatology*, 14th ed. Philadelphia: Lippincott Williams & Wilkins, 2001:2449–2513.

TABLE 24.5. BIOCHEMICAL MARKERS OF BONE TURNOVER

Formation	Resorption
From osteoblasts, in serum Bone alkaline phosphatase Osteocalcin	From osteoclasts Tartrate-resistant acid phosphatase
From Bone Matrix, in Serum	
Procollagen I carboxyterminal propeptide Procollagen I aminoterminal propeptide	Aminoterminal telopeptide of type I collagen Carboxyterminal telopeptide of type I collagen
From Bone Matrix, in Urine	
	Pyridinoline and deoxypyridinoline cross-links Aminoterminal telopeptide of type I collagen Hydroxyproline from collagen degradation

From Rosalki SB. Biochemical markers of bone turnover. *Int J Clin Pract* 1998;52:255–256, with permission.

evaluated with these assays. Table 24.5 lists bone turnover markers that can be classified as indices of bone formation or resorption. *Bone balance* is the net difference between formation and resorption.

Imaging

Dual-energy x-ray absorptiometry (DXA) is currently the "gold standard" for patient care and clinical investigation for osteoporosis. On DXA, bone mass is reported as an absolute value in g/cm², a comparison to age- and sex-matched reference range (the Z-score), and a comparison to mean bone mass of young adult normal individuals (the T-score or young adult Z-score) (Fig. 24.3). T-scores are used to predict fracture risk and classify disease status. A change of one standard deviation in the T-score correlates with a change of approximately 0.06 g/cm², or about 10% of BMD. Although the Z-score is of less clinical value than the T-score, Z-scores significantly deviating from normal may indicate alternative causes of metabolic bone disease. Modern DXAs also produce a density-based image useful in interpreting scan quality (Fig. 24.3 and later).

DXA readings are compared with the National Health and Nutrition Examination Survey (NHANES) III database. In a large clinical referral population, this change from manufacturers to NHANES III databases resulted in a 21% reduction in prevalence of osteoporosis diagnoses at the femoral neck and 20% reduction at the total hip.

DXA measures bone mass at central and peripheral sites. The choice of site(s) scanned should depend on the anticipated rates of change in bone mass within these skeletal locations and precision of the testing device at these sites. The central DXA sites of the hip and spine, followed by peripheral sites of the wrist and heel, are the most desired imaging locations. Central DXA of the spine and hip has excellent precision and good accuracy. Central DXA is generally preferred because the quantity of cancellous bone of central sites is highly indicative of the osteoporosis burden and fracture risk. In osteoporosis, the earliest bone loss begins in cancellous bone. A higher proportion of early postmenopausal women have lower cancellous BMD than cortical BMD. Approximately a third of the spongy trabecular bone of the hip and spine remodels each year, as opposed to only 3% turnover of compact cortical bone comprising a greater pro-

FIGURE 24.3. Dual x-ray absorptiometry (DXA) printout for a 70-year-old white woman. **A:** DXA of this patient's lumbar spine showing imaging windows for vertebrae L1 to L4. Estimated vertebral areas, bone mineral content (*BMC*), and bone mineral density (*BMD*) are shown (*middle*). BMD is plotted against a lumbar spine reference database showing the patient's current value as well as previous readings indicated by crosses (*right, top*). The dark (*top*) bar of the graph indicates two standard deviations above normal and the *lighter* (*bottom*) *bar* two standard deviations below normal for age. The *dashed line* corresponds to two standard deviations below peak bone mass. T-scores (peak bone mass matched) show that the patient is well below the World Health Organization definition of osteoporosis (T-score less than –2.5) at each vertebral level and for the lumbar spine overall. The Z-score is an age-matched measurement. **B:** Similar parameters are shown for the left hip and, based on T-scores, there is osteoporosis at both the femoral neck and total hip. **C:** At both the hip and lumbar spine, there has been significant 3-year improvement in BMD. The serial plot (*left*) and table show a nearly 12% increase at the left hip. The *asterisk* signifies a significant increase or decline between two values. An 18.4% increase in BMD was also seen at the lumbar spine (data not shown). (From Morgan SL, Saag KC, Julian BA, et al. Osteopenic bone diseases. In: Koopman WJ, ed. *Arthritis and allied conditions: a textbook of rheumatology,* 14th ed. Philadelphia: Lippincott Williams & Wilkins, 2001:2449–2513, with permission.)

The Kirklin Clinic

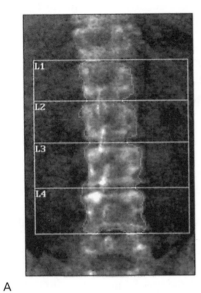

011109917   Wed Nov 10 15:28 1999
Name: PRINT OUT
Comment: osteoporosis
I.D.:   Sex: F
S.S.#:   00   Ethnic: W
ZIP Code: 35209   Height:5' 1"
Operator: BA   Weight: 111
BirthDate: 12/06/28   Age: 70

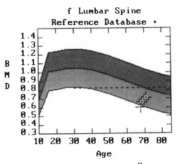

f Lumbar Spine
Reference Database •

BMD(L1-L4) = 0.705 g/cm²

Region	Est.Area (cm²)	Est.BMC (grams)	BMD (gms/cm²)
L1	10.32	6.20	0.601
L2	11.46	8.00	0.698
L3	12.91	9.73	0.753
L4	14.39	10.67	0.741
TOTAL	49.08	34.59	0.705

Region	BMD	T(30.0)		Z	
L1	0.601	-2.94	65%	-1.03	84%
L2	0.698	-3.00	68%	-0.87	88%
L3	0.753	-3.01	69%	-0.77	90%
L4	0.741	-3.41	66%	-1.10	86%
L1-L4	0.705	-3.11	67%	-0.95	87%

A

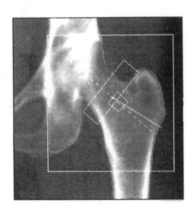

Region	Est.Area (cm²)	Est.BMC (grams)	BMD (gms/cm²)
Neck	4.88	2.66	0.546
Troch	9.71	4.73	0.487
Inter	14.55	9.55	0.657
TOTAL	29.14	16.95	0.582
Ward's	1.24	0.50	0.403

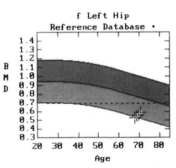

f Left Hip
Reference Database •

BMD(Total[L]) = 0.582 g/cm²

Region	BMD	T		Z	
Neck	0.546	-2.73 (25.0)	64%	-0.88	85%
Troch	0.487	-2.13 (25.0)	69%	-0.77	86%
Inter	0.657	-2.86 (35.0)	60%	-1.55	73%
TOTAL	0.582	-2.95 (25.0)	62%	-1.40	77%
Ward's	0.403	-2.83 (25.0)	55%	-0.23	94%

B

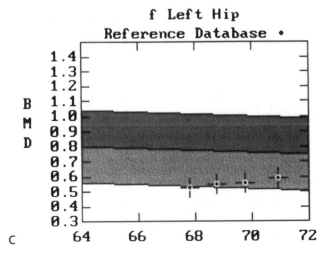

f Left Hip
Reference Database •

C

Total[L]

	09/25/96	09/17/97
09/17/97	4.1%	
09/23/98	5.3%*	1.2%
11/10/99	11.7%*	7.3%*

portion of peripheral skeleton. At the spine, DXA measures an individual vertebra as well as average BMD of the LI to L4 (Fig. 24.3). At the hip, femoral neck, trochanter, and total hip are the three measurement sites of greatest clinical interest. Ward's triangle, the site of lowest BMD in the hip that is nearly exclusively trabecular bone, is an area with less predictive value and reproducibility than the other locations. Total body BMD also can be measured with some instruments and can be used to calculate total body bone mineral content. Central measurements are used to diagnose osteoporosis, assess fracture risk, and follow up the response to antiosteoporotic therapies.

The ability to detect significant serial changes in DXA depends on the rate of change in BMD at a particular site (Fig. 24.3). A 2.8% change is required between two successive DXA studies to achieve a statistically significant difference with 95% confidence. To determine the amount of BMD change that is needed to indicate a significant improvement or worsening in BMD at the 95% confidence level, this change value is then multiplied by the precision error (coefficient of variation) of the measuring device. For example, if the instrument has a 2% precision error, a change in BMD greater than 5.6% is needed to be confident that this is not due to chance or precision error.

Peripheral DXA of the forearm is moderately correlated with central DXA results and thus can be used as an alternative to predict fracture risk. Heel DXA correlates well with other heel-imaging technologies and adequately discriminates osteoporotic from normal young subjects. However, the much slower rate of bone remodeling at sites such as the heel limits this technology for monitoring the response to therapy. The enhanced portability of dedicated peripheral bone mass measurement instruments and their lower cost render them increasingly attractive for community osteoporosis screening.

Fracture Risk Prediction

BMD measured by DXA is the best predictive factor of the risk of hip and spinal fractures. Spinal fracture is inversely proportional to bone mineral content. For each decline of about one standard deviation of bone mass there is a 1.3- to 2.5-fold increase in fracture risk of any site. Although fracture risk at any site can be accurately assessed using a variety of noninvasive bone mass measurements done at any site, BMD at the femoral neck is better than BMD at the spine, radius, and calcaneus to predict hip fracture. Decreases of two standard deviations in radial and calcaneal bone mass are associated with four- to sixfold increases in risk for vertebral fracture. Increasing age and decreasing BMD of the radius predict subsequent nonspinal fractures. It is estimated that a 50-year-old woman has a 19% lifetime risk of fracture if radial bone mass is in the tenth percentile, compared with an 11% lifetime risk if the measurement is in the ninetieth percentile.

Population-based studies show that hip fractures are uncommon among women with femoral neck BMD greater than 1.0 g/cm^2. A 30% loss of BMD from peak BMD at the hip is necessary before hip fractures occur after moderate trauma.

Potential Pitfalls in Dual-Energy X-Ray Absorptiometry Measurement

Osteoporosis occurs inhomogeneously throughout the body, dependent on age and underlying cause of bone loss. A 15% or greater discordance between sites, more common in the elderly, means that imaging only one site, particularly using a peripheral device, may be misleading. Measurement at multiple sites increases the chances of successfully detecting osteoporosis. Because of the high prevalence of facet and posterior element spinal osteoarthritis among adults more than 65 years of age, measurement of spinal DXA in the posterior–anterior projection may be falsely elevated. In older adults, measurement of the hip or lateral DXA imaging of the spine may circumvent this problem. Regression to the mean, a common phenomenon of nearly all numerical tests, can lead to misleading conclusions from a single follow-up measurement.

The visual image of the regions of interest allows the DXA reader to screen for artifacts (e.g., calcium pills in the gut, metal objects on clothing, objects in pockets, etc.), positioning errors (e.g., wrong vertebra imaged, hip malrotated), and anatomic deformities or changes (e.g., severe scoliosis, calcified aorta, vertebral crush fractures) that may limit precision and accuracy of the scan.

Prevention and Treatment

Although decrements in BMD may accurately predict fracture risk, when evaluating prevention and treatment studies, the effect of an intervention on fracture incidence is the most critical outcome.

Numerous general medical and specialty societies have promulgated guidelines for osteoporosis prevention and treatment. In 1998 the National Osteoporosis Foundation (NOF) issued guidelines in collaboration with ten medical organizations. These recommendations are based on age, BMD *T*-score, and whether there are accompanying risk factors. The NOF guidelines advocate pharmacologic intervention to reduce the risk of fractures in

- Women with BMD *T*-scores below −2 in the absence of risk factors (see earlier)
- Women with BMD *T*-scores below −1.5 if other risk factors are present
- Women more than 70 years of age with multiple risk factors (especially those with previous nonhip, nonspine fractures) are at high enough risk to initiate treatment without BMD testing

Nonpharmacologic

Exercise

Moderate to intensive weight-bearing exercise can lead to modest increases of about 1% to 3% in BMD. For an exercise to be effective in altering BMD, it must strain the skeletal site being evaluated. For example, bone mass gains are particularly notable in the tibia in runners and in the spine among weight lifters. Older women may demonstrate lumbar BMD gains with regular vigorous weight bearing performed multiple times per week. Continued physical activity is required to maintain observed BMD gains. Spinal extension exercises are preferred over flexion maneuvers, which may lead to spinal compression deformities.

Hip Protectors

Protective hip pads worn in specialized undergarments have effectively reduced fracture rates in nursing home patients.

Pharmacologic

Calcium and Vitamin D

Calcium alone may somewhat reduce, but not fully prevent, bone loss early after menopause. In postmenopausal women, sufficient calcium provided through dietary and exogenous sources decrease appendicular skeletal bone loss by 1% to 3%, compared with women who do not consume adequate calcium. Calcium may be most beneficial for women after menopause. However, even among younger women and men, calcium supplementation prevents bone loss at various skeletal sites.

Varying amounts of elemental calcium are found in different food groups and nutritional supplements (Table 24.6). Calcium is equally well absorbed (25% to 30%) from either milk products or calcium carbonate. However, cal-

cium is not equally bioavailable in all foods; certain leafy vegetables (e.g., spinach) have poor calcium bioavailability because of high oxalate content. Although some studies suggest that calcium citrate has slightly higher absorption than other preparations, other investigations indicate that they are equally well absorbed.

One area of controversy concerns the use of calcium supplements in patients with a history of nephrolithiasis. High intake of dietary calcium appears to decrease the risk of stones, whereas intake of high doses of supplemental calcium may modestly increase risk. Dietary calcium may beneficially bind oxalate, the primary component in most renal stones.

Although many patients tolerate calcium supplements well, constipation (in about 10% of users) and dyspepsia limit long-term adherence. Individual trials of different preparations and times of administration may maximize patient satisfaction. Consensus recommendations for daily doses of elemental calcium are 1,200 to 1,500 mg/d in postmenopausal women not on hormone replacement therapy (HRT) and 1,000 to 1,200 mg in premenopausal women, men, and postmenopausal women on HRT. The increasing variety of food and beverage products available in the United States that are calcium-fortified have reduced the reliance on exogenous calcium salt supplements to achieve daily requirements.

Vitamin D is a group of fat-soluble sterols that includes ergocalciferol (vitamin D_2) and cholecalciferol (vitamin D_3). Most potent among vitamin D analogs is the active metabolite calcitriol. Calcitriol is 1,25-dihydroxyvitamin D_3, a synthetic active metabolite of vitamin D. Calcitriol increases calcium absorption and may prevent spinal bone loss, particularly among older women. Despite BMD gains, several studies have not shown a beneficial effect of active vitamin D metabolites on fracture rate. The potential for

TABLE 24.6. FOOD SOURCES OF BIOAVAILABLE CALCIUM

Food	Serving Size (g)	Calcium Content[a] (mg)	Fractional Absorption[b] (%)	Estimated Absorbable Ca/Serving (mg)	Servings Needed to Equal 1 Glass of Milk
Milk (or 1 glass yogurt or 1½ oz. cheddar cheese)	240	300	32.1	96.3	1.0
Beans, dried	177	50	15.6	7.8	12.3
Broccoli	71	35	61.3	21.5	4.5
Cabbage	85	79	52.7	41.6	2.3
Kale	65	47	58.8	27.6	3.5
Spinach	90	122	5.1	6.2	15.5
Tofu, calcium set	126	258	31.0	80.0	1.2

[a]Adjusted for load; for milk, this is fractional absorption (Fx abs) = 0.889 − 0.0964 in load; for low-oxalate vegetables, after adjusting by the ratio of fractional absorption determined for kale relative to milk at the same load, the equation becomes Fx abs = 0.959 − 0.0964 in load.
[b]Calcium content (mg) × Fx abs.
From Weaver CM, Heaney RP, Shils ME, et al., eds. *Modern nutrition in health and disease,* 9th ed. Baltimore: Williams & Wilkins, 1999:147, with permission.

hypercalciuria and hypercalcemia with active vitamin D preparations limits their routine use and requires careful serum and urine monitoring. If calcitriol is used, it is important to moderate calcium supplementation.

Inactivated vitamin D analogs also have beneficial effects on bone. Cholecalciferol 800 IU/d increased femoral BMD by 2.7% and lowered the risk of hip and other nonvertebral fractures among elderly women in a large study. Older men and women receiving calcium plus vitamin D_3 showed reduced bone loss and decreased incidence of nonvertebral fractures in some, but not all, studies. It is recommended that older adults be supplemented with 400 to 1,000 IU of vitamin D_3, the amount found in many multivitamins. In individuals with documented vitamin D deficiency or calcium malabsorption, more vitamin D supplementation is needed.

Estrogen

Because of the accelerated rate of bone loss at menopause, estrogen replacement therapy (ERT) has been used in postmenopausal women for prevention of osteoporosis. ERT is most effective in decreasing bone loss when initiated soon after menopause and used continuously. Lumbar spine BMD increases by 1% to 4 % in women receiving conjugated estrogen at 0.3 to 0.625 mg/d in combination with calcium for 1 year. The Postmenopausal Estrogen/Progestin Intervention (PEPI) trial showed about a 2% increase in hip BMD after 1 year in patients randomized to treatment with conjugated estrogen, 0.625 mg/d.

Use of a transdermal patch resulted in a 5.3% increase in lumbar BMD and a trend toward a reduction in vertebral fractures among older women with documented osteoporosis. No clinical trial confirmed a significant effect on vertebral fractures or showed a lower risk of nonvertebral fractures.

ERT raises high-density lipoproteins and lowers low-density lipids in postmenopausal women. Observational studies have reported a 35% to 80% reduction in cardiovascular events and prolonged survival among women with coronary heart disease (CHD) compared with nonusers. However, results from the Heart and Estrogen/Progestin Replacement Study (HERS), a randomized blinded, placebo-controlled study of secondary cardiovascular prevention among women with prior vascular disease, identified an increase in coronary heart disease (CHD) events in the first year of therapy. A reduction in CHD events was seen in years 4 and 5 of the trial. Venous thromboembolic events are three to four times more common among estrogen users than among nonusers (absolute risk of about 0.4%). Estrogen causes endometrial thickening, an effect offset by concomitant administration of progestin. Daily administration of estrogen with continuous low-dose progestin (e.g., medroxyprogesterone 2.5 mg/d) is generally well tolerated, with rare breakthrough bleeding and no documented increase in the endometrial thickness. Although many studies have failed to find an increased risk for breast cancer with ERT, a combined analysis of 51 studies indicated that a relative risk of 1.35 for

breast cancer is attributable to 5 years of estrogen compared with never-use. Results from the Women's Health Institute (WHI) confirm an increased risk of breast cancer and cardiovascular disease and hip fracture risk reduction. Although ERT in women with a family history of breast cancer was not associated with increased incidence in one large population-based cohort study, a strong family history of breast cancer continues to be a relative contraindication for estrogen use.

Ultimately, the decision to initiate ERT needs to be individualized and based on a balanced assessment of risk and benefits. The absence of definitive fracture reduction data, a probable small increased risk for breast cancer, potential for hypercoagulability, an increasing concern about an absence of cardiovascular benefit, and the use of alternative, more potent bone-protective agents have attenuated enthusiasm for estrogens as antiosteoporotic agents.

Selective Estrogen Receptor Modulators

Selective estrogen receptor modulators (SERMs) are nonsteroidal synthetic compounds that have estrogen-like properties in the bone and cardiovascular systems yet are estrogen antagonists to the breast and, in some cases, the endometrium. Raloxifene is the first SERM licensed in the United States for osteoporosis. It significantly lowers biochemical markers of bone remodeling to levels equivalent to conjugated estrogens. In postmenopausal women, after 6 months of raloxifene 60 mg/d, bone mass in the lumbar spine and total hip increased significantly by 2.4%. Low-density lipoproteins, total cholesterol, and triglycerides all declined, and high-density lipoproteins increased. After 3 years of follow-up in the Multiple Outcomes of Raloxifene Evaluation (MORE), a multicenter study of more than 7,700 postmenopausal women with at least one vertebral fracture or osteoporosis on the basis of a T-score of less than or equal to −2.5, 60 mg/d raloxifene increased BMD of the spine by 2.6% and femoral neck BMD by 2.1%, and reduced vertebral fracture risk by 30%. To date, raloxifene has not been proved to prevent fractures at nonvertebral sites. The risk of invasive breast cancer was decreased by 76% during the MORE study. In contrast to estrogen, hot flashes and other menopausal symptoms may recur with raloxifene. Similar to estrogen, with raloxifene there is an increase in lower-extremity edema and a threefold increased risk of deep venous thrombosis.

Calcitonin

When used for prevention or treatment of osteoporosis, synthetic calcitonin (derived from salmon) is administered either subcutaneously (up 100 IU daily for osteoporosis) or, more commonly, intranasally (200 IU daily). Calcitonin should be given with adequate calcium (at least 1 g) and vitamin D (400 IU day). Randomized controlled trials of injectable and intranasal calcitonin for treatment of established postmenopausal osteoporosis have consistently shown either stabilization of BMD or small but significant increases in vertebral bone mineral density of approximately 1% to 3%. Beneficial BMD effects at the hip have not yet been reported.

A 5-year multicenter study designed to assess whether calcitonin nasal spray reduced vertebral fractures among postmenopausal women with established osteoporosis and at least one prevalent fracture (Prevention of Recurrent Osteoporotic Fractures, or PROOF) showed a 36% reduction in vertebral fractures in the 200-IU but not in the 100- or 400-IU groups. Interpretation of the study was limited by an approximately 50% dropout rate.

Calcitonin may also have analgesic efficacy for acute compression fracture pain. The exact mechanism of this putative effect is not well understood.

Nasal calcitonin is generally well tolerated, aside from occasional rhinitis minimized by alternating nostrils each day. Headache, flushing, nausea, and diarrhea have been reported more commonly with subcutaneous than with intranasal calcitonin.

Bisphosphonates

Bisphosphonates comprise a class of antiresorptive agents characterized by a phosphorus–carbon–phosphorus bond. They are recognized as potent inhibitors of bone resorption and reduce risks for fractures when administered orally or by intravenous infusion. Variations in the structure of their amino side chains alter the pharmacologic activity. (See the comparative structures in Fig. 24.4.) Oral bisphosphonates are poorly absorbed, with bioavailability of less than 1%, and are bound by divalent cations. Thus they should be taken on an empty stomach to maximize absorption. In bone, these agents bind tightly to hydroxyapatite crystals in the resorption lacunae of bone, where they have a long skeletal retention (about 10 years for alendronate).

Bisphosphonates may cause gastrointestinal intolerance, particularly at low gastric pH. There have been rare reports of severe esophagitis. Some studies suggest that GI safety may be better for particular agents. Recommendations to reduce gastrointestinal symptoms and maximize absorption include ingesting pills with 8 oz of water, remaining upright for at least 30 minutes after swallowing the tablet, and having nothing to eat or drink for 30 to 60 minutes before and after ingesting each pill. Achalasia and esophageal strictures are contraindications to bisphosphonate therapy. Two bisphosphonates, alendronate and risedronate, are licensed in the United States for treatment of osteoporosis and both are now approved for once-weekly dosing.

Alendronate

Alendronate inhibits bone resorption without detrimental effects on mineralization. Studies of postmenopausal women receiving 10 mg daily showed that lumbar spine BMD increased by 7% to 9% over a 2-year period. In early postmenopausal women, 5 mg/d prevented loss of BMD at

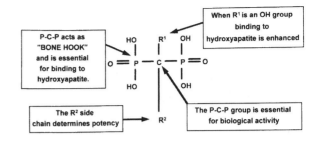

BISPHOSPHONATE	R1	R2
Etidronate*	OH	CH$_3$
Clodronate*	Cl	Cl
Pamidronate*	OH	CH$_2$CH$_2$ NH$_2$
Alendronate*	OH	(CH$_2$)$_3$ NH$_2$
Risedronate*	OH	CH$_2$-3-pyridine
Tiludronate*	H	CH$_2$-S-phenyl-Cl
Ibandronate*	OH	CH$_2$CH$_2$ N(CH$_3$) (pentyl)
Zoledronate	OH	CH$_2$-imidazole
YH529	OH	CH$_2$-2-imidazo-pyridinyl
Incadronate (YM175)	H	N-(cyclo-heptyl)
Olpadronate	OH	CH$_2$CH$_2$ N(CH$_3$)$_2$
Neridronate	OH	(CH$_2$)$_5$ NH$_2$
EB-1053	OH	CH$_2$-1-pyrrolidinyl

FIGURE 24.4. Structures of bisphosphonates used in clinical studies and under development. *Asterisks* indicate bisphosphonates already approved for one or more indications in one or more countries. Pamidronate is the most extensively used for Paget disease. (From Graham R, Russell G, Rogers JJ, et al. The pharmacology of bisphosphonates and new insights into their mechanisms of action. *J Bone Miner Res* 1999;14:53–65, with permission. Reprinted in Morgan SL, Saag KC, Julian BA, et al. Osteopenic bone diseases. In: Koopman WJ, ed. *Arthritis and allied conditions: a textbook of rheumatology*, 14th ed. Philadelphia: Lippincott Williams & Wilkins, 2001:2449–2513.)

the spine, hip, and total body. Among more than 2,000 older women with at least one prior vertebral fracture and low femoral neck BMD in the Fracture Intervention Trial (FIT), alendronate significantly reduced vertebral and hip fractures by 47% and 51%, respectively. In FIT subjects without prevalent vertebral fractures, alendronate 10 mg/d decreased radiographic vertebral fractures by 44%. A multinational study of alendronate similarly identified a 47% risk reduction for nonvertebral fractures. In postmenopausal women with low BMD despite ongoing ERT, addition of alendronate significantly increased BMD in the lumbar spine and hip trochanter. Safety has been acceptable in clinical trials, with no significant increases in serious adverse effects or significant gastrointestinal adverse effects between treatment and placebo groups.

Risedronate

Treatment with 5 mg daily of risedronate significantly lowered the risk of new vertebral (41% reduction) and nonvertebral (39% reduction) fractures over a 3-year period in women with at least one prior vertebral fracture. A beneficial effect of each treatment on hip fractures among women with very low bone mass has also been demonstrated. Risedronate is generally well tolerated, with no significant differences in upper gastrointestinal adverse events compared with those receiving placebo.

Based on the documented efficacy of alendronate and risedronate, bisphosphonates are considered by many to be the most effective antiresorptive agents currently available.

Sodium Fluoride

Fluoride has not gained widespread acceptance in the United States due in part to a narrow therapeutic window and studies reporting no protective effect or even a heightened risk of both vertebral and nonvertebral fractures.

Parathyroid Hormone

In contrast to its perceived catabolic action on bone, exogenously administered PTH can increase bone turnover and increase BMD in rodents and, more recently, in humans. Estrogen-deficient perimenopausal women receiving PTH (amino acids 1–34) had less bone loss from the proximal femur and increased their BMD in the spine. Osteoporotic men treated with PTH and 1,25 dihydroxyvitamin D also showed improved spinal bone mass. In postmenopausal women on estrogen, PTH (amino acids 1–34) given as subcutaneous injections significantly increased BMD by 13% at the lumbar spine and decreased the incidence of vertebral fractures of the spine. The effects of PTH appear to be preserved, even when potent antiresorptive agents (such as alendronate) are given concomitantly. Although not yet FDA approved, PTH has considerable promise as a bone anabolic agent.

Surgical

Percutaneous vertebroplasty and kyphoplasty, procedures that inject polymethylmethacrylate into the vertebral body, have been explored for treatment of painful vertebral compression deformities. Rigorous studies demonstrating sustained efficacy are lacking. However, case reports and an open-label study of 26 patients described acute pain relief in most recipients. The mechanism of pain relief of this proposed technique and its long-term efficacy and safety merit further investigation.

GLUCOCORTICOID-INDUCED OSTEOPOROSIS

Epidemiology

Osteoporosis is a well-recognized complication of supraphysiologic levels of glucocorticoids. Glucocorticoid-induced osteoporosis (GIOP) is second in frequency only to the osteoporosis after menopause and is the most common form of drug-induced osteoporosis.

During the first 6 to 12 months of glucocorticoid therapy, there is an initial rapid loss of 3% to 27% of BMD. Trabecular bone is preferentially affected, followed ultimately by losses in cortical bone. Cumulative steroid dose is the primary predictor of bone loss. Alternate-day dosing does not spare bone. Following approximately 2 years of glucocorticoid therapy, rate of bone loss slows in many patients. However, BMD continues to be lost at a rate higher than that with normal aging.

Individuals who already have very low bone mass (such as postmenopausal women who have not taken hormone replacement therapy) reach a fracture threshold sooner on glucocorticoids. In addition to older women, significant bone loss may occur in men and in premenopausal women on long-term glucocorticoids.

Studies of steroid-dose effects are confounded by the variable timing of glucocorticoid administration, differing disease processes, variable alternative osteoporosis risk factors (independent of glucocorticoid use), and the fact that fracture risk is ultimately determined by factors other than only BMD. Glucocorticoids increase risk of fractures roughly twofold, independent of age, gender, and rheumatoid arthritis. Women with RA taking low-dose prednisone have a nearly 33% chance of a self-reporting a clinical fracture after 5 years. Although safer for bone than oral or enteral glucocorticoids, even nonsystemically administered glucocorticoids may have biologic effects on bone.

Pathogenesis

The etiology of GIOP is multifactorial and occurs, in many cases, concomitantly with normal age- and menopause-associated bone loss. There are two major pathways by which patients on glucocorticoids develop abnormalities in bone metabolism: reduced bone formation and increased bone resorption. Controversy exists surrounding the relative importance of these mechanisms on bone loss among glucocorticoid users.

Clinical Evaluation

There should be a high suspicion for potential bone loss among all patients initiating or chronically using glucocorticoids. The most effective way to determine a glucocorticoid-user's osteoporosis status and risk for future bone loss is to assess BMD by DXA or an alternate bone mass measurement technique. Current recommendations for bone-mass measurement of patients on glucocorticoids have been proposed by the U.S. Bone Mass Measurement Act and by different medical societies and federal agencies. Most guidelines suggest assessing BMD if the patient will receive more than 7.5 mg prednisone or its equivalent for at least 1 to 6 months.

It is also important to consider gonadal status in chronic glucocorticoid users. In perimenopausal women, measurement of follicle-stimulating hormone (FSH) and estradiol levels may provide further clarification. Premenopausal women with severe RA also may be estrogen deficient, often manifested by oligo- or amenorrhea. Because of the well-defined association between RA and male hypogonadism, measurement of free testosterone in men on chronic glucocorticoids, or those with symptoms of gonadal insufficiency, is warranted.

Prevention and Treatment

The most effective intervention to prevent bone loss and fractures among glucocorticoid users is discontinuation of treatment or, at a minimum, reducing the dose. Practically, this is not always possible because of the severity of many chronic inflammatory diseases.

Calcium and Vitamin D

Supplements of elemental calcium 1,200 to 1,500 mg/d are necessary, although generally not sufficient as a sole therapy, for most patients on glucocorticoids. Vitamin D can be administered in a variety of formulations that have been investigated for GIOP prevention and treatment. Subjects who received a combination containing calcitriol, calcium, and calcitonin experienced significantly less bone loss in the spine than those receiving calcium alone. Inactivated vitamin D preparations also have merit. One thousand milligrams of calcium carbonate coupled with 500 IU of vitamin D partially prevents bone loss in the lumbar spine and trochanter in some studies. Data are more equivocal with respect to ergocalciferol, typically administered as 50,000 IU orally once weekly. Because of impairment in calcium absorption mediated by glucocorticoids and the common occurrence of vitamin D deficiency among housebound patients suffering with chronic inflammatory conditions, vitamin D should be prescribed for all glucocorticoid users. This can be easily accomplished with 800 IU/d vitamin D_3, available in many multivitamins and in many vitamin D–supplemented calcium preparations. With careful use of exogenous calcium and monitoring of urine and serum calcium, vitamin D can be administered alternatively as calcitriol.

Calcitonin

Calcitonin is weakly effective at both preventing and treating GIOP. Spinal BMD declines less in newly treated patients who also received calcitonin. In one of three treatment studies, placebo patients lost 8% BMD over 2 years, whereas those on nasal calcitonin showed an increase of 2.8%. For GIOP, calcitonin is a relatively weak antiresorptive agent. It may maintain bone mass, but in most studies calcitonin did not significantly increase BMD. Calcitonin treatment did not reduce fracture rates in GIOP.

Estrogen and Testosterone

In postmenopausal women with RA receiving ERT (transdermal estradiol approximately 50 mg/d) or calcium supplementation (400 mg/d) women on ERT had higher BMD in the spine than those receiving calcium alone after 2 years. Two small observational studies of ERT demonstrated reduced bone loss in the spine among chronic glucocorticoid users. Testosterone also increases BMD of the lumbar spine significantly in hypogonadal use.

Hormonally deficient women and men should be offered appropriate hormonal replacement therapy, because of its benefit on bone as well as other potential health benefits. Hormonal replacement therapy is indicated not only in older women but also in premenopausal women who are oligomenorrheic or amenorrheic (associated with their chronic inflammatory diseases) and in hypogonadal men (because of their underlying disorders and/or glucocorticoid effects). Selective estrogen receptor modulators (SERMs) may offer an as yet unproven therapeutic option in glucocorticoid-induced osteoporosis.

Bisphosphonates

When administered over 1 or 2 years to patients on glucocorticoids for a variety of chronic inflammatory disorders, alendronate and risedronate prevent and/or reverse bone loss at the spine and of the hip.

Alendronate has proven efficacy in preventing and treating bone loss associated with glucocorticoid therapy and in preventing vertebral fractures. Glucocorticoid users have about a 3% increase in BMD on 10 mg alendronate. Similar effects are seen at the trochanter, and smaller but significant gains in BMD are noted at the femoral neck. A second-year extension to this study showed a 90% reduction in an overall small number of incident vertebral fractures.

Similar to alendronate, risedronate at 2.5 or 5.0 mg/d maintains or increases bone mass at the lumbar spine, trochanter, and femoral neck in patients beginning glucocorticoids. In patients on long-term glucocorticoids, 2.5 and 5.0 mg risedronate maintained or increased bone mass at the lumbar spine, trochanter, and femoral neck. Risedronate and alendronate decrease vertebral fractures by 70% to 90% when used for a year or more.

Treatment Algorithm

A treatment algorithm is proposed in Fig. 24.5. Given the accumulating data on the efficacy of bisphosphonates for preventing and treating GIOP, initial administration of a bisphosphonate should be strongly considered in all high-risk patients. While this algorithm represents a rational

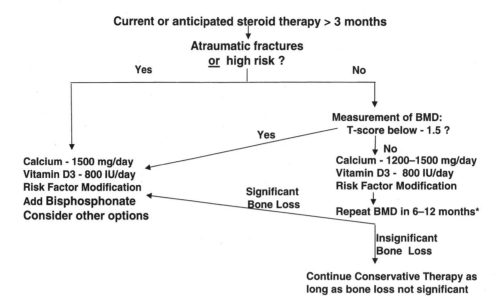

FIGURE 24.5. Treatment algorithm for the management of glucocorticoid-associated bone disease. *Asterisks* indicate during the first 2 years of therapy and then less regularly. (Adapted from Rosen HN, Rosenblatt M. Prevention and treatment of glucocorticoid-induced osteoporosis. In: Rose B, ed. *UpToDate,* Vol 6, No. 3. Wellesley, MA: UpToDate, 1998. Reprinted in Morgan SL, Saag KC, Julian BA, et al. Osteopenic bone diseases. In: Koopman WJ, ed. *Arthritis and allied conditions: a textbook of rheumatology,* 14th ed. Philadelphia: Lippincott Williams & Wilkins, 2001:2449–2513.)

approach, GIOP management is rapidly changing and will be further refined, based on emerging literature as well as societal cost-effectiveness considerations.

MALE OSTEOPOROSIS

Osteoporosis in men is common. About 20% of all osteoporotic fractures occur in men. As the population ages, osteoporosis in men is becoming an even greater public health problem.

Epidemiology

In North America, men 50 years of age have a 13% lifetime risk for fracture of the hip, spine, or forearm. In the United States, the incidence of hip fracture in men older than 65 years is four or five in 1,000, about half that in women of similar age. Incidence of hip fracture in men differs between different ethnic groups. African-American men have a rate about half that of whites, and Japanese men living in Japan or Hawaii may have a lower frequency than white American men.

Osteoporotic vertebral fractures in men are more common in the low thoracic region but may occur at any level. Elderly men less often fracture more than one vertebral body. Most fractures are the anterior compression type; crush fractures occur less commonly than in women, thereby accounting for less kyphosis in men.

Pathogenesis

The greater bone mass in men than in women is mostly related to body size, with the exception of a few sites such as the radius. After attaining peak bone mass, men maintain a stable BMD during middle age, and then lose bone at an accelerating rate into old age. This rate may reach 5% to 10% per decade, and is greater in trabecular than in cortical bone.

As many as 20% to 40% of men with an osteoporotic fracture have no identifiable medical condition or risk factor associated with osteoporosis; they are designated as having primary osteoporosis to distinguish them from men who have lost substantial bone mass secondary to any of various conditions.

Clinical Evaluation

In men with clinical features or findings suggestive of metabolic bone disease (such as radiographic osteopenia, low-trauma fractures, or disorders associated with bone loss), measurement of BMD should be considered. These measurements may be used to confirm low bone mass, gauge its severity, and serve as a baseline to assess the progression of disease or therapeutic response. Criteria to define osteoporosis in men are not as clear as they are for women. The average young adult man has greater total bone mineral content than the young adult woman. Estimates of fracture risk derived from measurements of women may not apply to men. Lower bone density is associated with an increased risk for fracture, and measurements can be used to monitor serial changes in bone mass.

The initial history and physical examination should be undertaken with knowledge of conditions associated with osteoporosis. Special attention should be given to signs of genetic, nutritional, and lifestyle factors (alcohol or tobacco), systemic illness, and medication usage. If the cause of osteoporosis remains undefined, measurement of serum thyroid-stimulating hormone, and 24-hour urinary calcium and cortisol, and perhaps serum estradiol, should be considered. Measurement of luteinizing hormone, FSH, and prolactin levels will assess whether a pituitary tumor is present. A transiliac bone biopsy is generally performed only in special circumstances because of its cost and invasiveness, but may be undertaken to identify unusual causes of osteoporosis diagnosed only by histologic studies (such as mastocytosis) or to ensure that osteomalacia is not present.

Treatment

To achieve maximal adult bone mass, adolescent boys should be encouraged to ingest 1,200 to 1,500 mg calcium daily in their diets, participate in regular weight-bearing exercise, maintain ideal body weight, and avoid use of tobacco and excessive alcohol. Extending this approach into adulthood, it is recommended that men 25 to 65 years of age consume 1,000 mg of calcium daily and that men over the age of 65 years consume 1,500 mg daily.

Testosterone increases BMD in hypogonadal men or those on glucocorticoid therapy, and has been used empirically in eugonadal men, albeit in short-term trials. The most effective, safe, practical, and inexpensive supplements are intramuscular testosterone enanthate or cyprionate. The usual dose is 200 mg every 14 days, but this may be tailored for individual patients to range from 100 mg weekly to 300 mg every 3 weeks. Some patients dislike the variations in the sense of well-being, sexual activity, and emotional stability that parallel swings in testosterone levels. Transdermal patches gel can be applied to nongenital or shaved scrotal skin. Oral testosterone undecanoate entails the inconvenience of three daily doses. The goal of therapy is a physiologic testosterone profile. Side effects generally are not serious. Excessive libido is uncommon. Weight may increase due to anabolic effects on lean mass or salt and water retention, particularly in men with cardiac disease, cirrhosis, or nephrotic syndrome. Urinary retention is uncommon in the absence of prostatic cancer, and there is generally no significant effect on serum prostatic-specific antigen or prostate volume. Whether the likelihood for prostatic cancer increases must await large clinical trials. Some men develop erythrocytosis due to augmented erythropoiesis. Levels of total and HDL cholesterol frequently decrease. Gynecomastia may develop due to aromatization of testosterone to estradiol. 17 α-

Alkylated androgens should be avoided because of greater risks for increased liver enzymes, cholestasis, and liver tumors. Contraindications to androgen therapy include prostatic cancer, prostatic hypertrophy, sleep apnea, inappropriate sexual behavior, and breast cancer.

Among other therapies, bisphosphonates currently offer substantial promise, although experience is limited. Calcitonin reduced loss of bone mass after orchiectomy and attenuates bone loss when combined with calcium supplements. Correction of hypercalciuria with hydrochlorothiazide can significantly increase bone mass. Supplementation with vitamin D and calcium should be encouraged, since they are relatively inexpensive and safe, may have modest independent benefits to bone, and may allow other therapeutic interventions.

ORGAN TRANSPLANTATION

Epidemiology

Solid-organ transplantation has become established as the best therapy for patients with end-stage renal, hepatic, cardiac, and pulmonary disease. Bone marrow transplantation has been increasingly used for patients with hematopoietic and breast malignancies. Unfortunately, transplant recipients frequently are afflicted with symptomatic osteoporosis and other musculoskeletal complications that reduce their quality of life and potential for rehabilitation.

Pathogenesis and Clinical Presentation

Osteoporosis after organ transplantation develops from a complex interplay of skeletal toxicities of immunosuppressants, complications unique to failure of the particular organ, and other factors that contribute to bone loss in the general population. Glucocorticoids continue to be an integral component of most long-term immunosuppressive regimens and are the cornerstone for treatment of acute rejection. Cyclosporine and tacrolimus greatly accelerate bone turnover in experimental animals, and the amount of trabecular bone lost within a month is substantial. In animals given cyclosporine, bone loss can be prevented by antiresorptive agents, including bisphosphonates, estrogen, and calcitonin. Other immunosuppressants have no clinically important skeletal toxicity (azathioprine) or have not been sufficiently evaluated (mycophenolate mofetil, and sirolimus).

The relative risks and clinical manifestations of loss of BMD after transplant vary greatly by the organ engrafted. Patients with severe renal insufficiency are at increased risk for decreased bone mass, and may have any of several histologic derangements, secondary to hyperparathyroidism, osteomalacia, a dynamic (aplastic) bone disease, or more than one disorder. These patients are frequently hypogonadal. White patients with end-stage renal disease have a higher prevalence of osteoporosis than blacks, independent of the type of renal osteodystrophy. The loss of bone mass after renal transplantation is greatest in the first 6 months, during which time it may average 7%. This loss occurs even in the setting of mild pretransplant hyperparathyroidism, relatively modest doses of glucocorticoids, and excellent allograft function. Fractures may occur in atypical locations (e.g., in metatarsals and, less commonly, in long bones); vertebral fractures are relatively uncommon. The highest fracture rate is in patients with diabetic renal disease, who comprise about a third of newly transplanted patients in many centers. Bone loss after renal engraftment may contribute to osteonecrosis of the hips, knees, or humeral heads, a complication detectable by magnetic resonance imaging in 5% to 10% of recipients within 3 to 6 months of engraftment.

Recipients of hepatic, cardiac, lung, and bone marrow transplants have a higher prevalence of osteoporosis before engraftment than renal allograft recipients. Some cholestatic hepatic disorders (e.g., primary biliary cirrhosis) are especially associated with severe osteoporosis. Bone marrow recipients frequently have undergone treatment with radiation or alkylating agents that render them hypogonadal.

Prevention and Treatment

Bone loss is a common complication for many potential recipients awaiting organ transplantation. Measurement of bone mass by DXA identifies patients who will benefit from therapy designed to maintain or improve bone mass and, it is hoped, reduce risk for osteoporotic fracture after engraftment. All patients should ingest 1,000 to 1,500 mg calcium daily (depending upon age, use of glucocorticoids, and menopausal status) and vitamin D analogs. A regular walking exercise program and abstinence from smoking and excessive ethanol should be encouraged.

Few studies have directly examined treatment of solid-organ transplant recipients, and the current approaches have been extrapolated from experiences with glucocorticoid-induced bone losses (see earlier). Continuing hormonal replacement therapy in hypogonadal patients and the general approach outlined previously for transplantation candidates seem reasonable. Preliminary data from the treatment of liver, heart, and renal allograft recipients with bisphosphonates have been encouraging. The results with calcitonin have been less conclusive.

OSTEOMALACIA

Epidemiology and Pathogenesis

Normal bone growth and mineralization require adequate vitamin D, calcium, and phosphorus. A prolonged deficiency of any of these leads to accumulation of unmineralized bone matrix, or osteoid, and slow bone formation.

Decreased mineralization in young patients causes rickets due to damage of growth plates (epiphyses) and newly formed trabecular and cortical bone. Strength of the bone matrix is decreased, leading to structural deformities in weight-bearing bones such as bowing. In older individuals in whom epiphyses have closed and only bone is affected, this defective mineralization is called osteomalacia.

Insufficient mineralization of bone may develop because of hypovitaminosis D as a result of chronic dietary intake of less than 70 IU (rare in the United States because of supplementation of food products such as milk); decreased synthesis because of minimal exposure to sunlight (bed-bound institutionalized patients); reduced vitamin D absorption because of biliary, pancreatic, proximal small bowel mucosal disease, or bile acid-binding resins; increased urinary excretion of vitamin D metabolites in patients with nephrotic syndrome and normal renal clearance function; and increased vitamin D catabolism by medications that activate hepatic drug-metabolizing enzymes (e.g., phenytoin, barbiturates, and rifampin). Clinically significant chronic hypophosphatemia may result from renal wasting due to Fanconi syndrome, renal tubular acidosis, monoclonal gammopathy, phosphotonin (a humeral substance secreted by some tumors, most commonly mesenchymal in origin), decreased intestinal absorption due to antacid abuse, or chronic total parenteral nutrition if inadequate phosphorus is provided.

Clinical Evaluation

Clinical manifestations of osteomalacia may mimic rheumatic disorders with generalized aching bone pain, easy fatigue, proximal weakness, and periarticular tenderness. These symptoms promptly resolve with treatment to correct the mineralization defect. Radiographs of patients with rickets may show general demineralization with thinning of cortical surfaces of long bones, widening, fraying, and cupping of distal ends of the shaft, and loss of the zone of provisional cartilaginous calcification. Some patients with osteomalacia exhibit thin cortical radiolucent lines (stress fractures) perpendicular to the bone shaft that are often symmetric and bilateral (called Looser zones); other patients may have multiple old rib fractures with poor callus formation.

Laboratory features of vitamin D deficiency osteomalacia are low or normal serum calcium level, hypophosphatemia, increased serum alkaline phosphatase level, normal serum osteocalcin level, increased serum parathyroid hormone level (if hypocalcemia is present), and a low serum 25-hydroxyvitamin D level. Secondary hyperparathyroidism and hypophosphatemia stimulate renal synthesis of 1,25-dihydroxyvitamin D to maintain normal serum levels. Urinary calcium excretion is decreased. In calcium deficiency osteomalacia, parathyroid hormone levels are increased, 1,25-dihydroxyvitamin D levels are normal, and serum phosphorus levels may be low or normal. In osteomalacia resulting from hyperphosphaturia, levels of serum calcium, osteocalcin, parathyroid hormone, and 1,25-hydroxyvitamin D are normal; serum alkaline phosphatase levels are usually increased; serum phosphorus and 1,25-dihydroxyvitamin D levels are low; and urinary phosphorus excretion is very high. Patients with type II renal tubular acidosis have defective reabsorption of bicarbonate and manifest hyperchloremic, hypokalemic acidosis with hypophosphatemia caused by augmented phosphaturia. Low serum 1,25-dihydroxyvitamin D levels in some patients may be the consequence of abnormal proximal tubular metabolism. Patients with renal tubular acidosis and Fanconi syndrome may also excrete excessive amounts of calcium, magnesium, potassium, as well as uric acid, glucose, amino acids, and citrate. Nephrocalcinosis may reduce the glomerular filtration rate. Hypophosphatasia is a rare autosomal dominant disorder with decreased serum bone alkaline phosphatase level. Serum calcium, phosphorus, 25-hydroxyvitamin D, and 1,25-dihydroxyvitamin D levels are not reduced. No treatment is available.

Treatment

Adults consuming diets low in vitamin D–fortified foods may take 1,500 to 5,000 IU vitamin D_2 per day orally until serum chemistries and urinary calcium excretion return to normal, after which 400 IU daily will suffice. In patients with intestinal fat malabsorption, treatment should include control of the primary disease and use of a more polar vitamin D compound such as 25-hydroxyvitamin D, 20 to 30 pg/d, or 1,25-dihydroxyvitamin D, 0.15 to 0.50 pg/d, given orally, or ergocalciferol 10,000 to 50,000 IU given intramuscularly and titrated to the response in serum chemistries. Supplemental calcium, 1,000 to 2,000 mg/d, should also be provided. Treatment for several months may be necessary for the serum chemistries to return to normal. Patients should be carefully monitored for hypercalcemia or hypercalciuria. To prevent vitamin D deficiency in settings other than malabsorption, daily 30-minute exposure to sunlight, ultraviolet B irradiation of the back with a suberythemal dosage for 3 to 7 minutes three times a week, consumption of 400 IU/d in fortified foods, or a dietary supplement is recommended.

In patients with renal tubular acidosis, restoration of the serum bicarbonate level to normal using sodium bicarbonate supplements reverses bone resorption and hypercalciuria. Patients with osteomalacia due to hyperphosphaturia in Fanconi syndrome need oral phosphate supplements, generally 14 g/d given in four to six doses, and may benefit from treatment with 1,25-dihydroxyvitamin D, 0.15 to 0.50 μg/d. Calcium supplements may be necessary to avoid symptomatic hypocalcemia but should not be taken concomitantly with a phosphorus supplement. Once the bone disease has healed, the vitamin D can be discontinued.

PRIMARY HYPERPARATHYROIDISM

Primary hyperparathyroidism and malignancy are the two most common causes of hypercalcemia, accounting for more than 90% of patients with hypercalcemia. The prevalence of primary hyperparathyroidism ranges from 1 in 400 to 1 in 1,000, and has increased severalfold in the last 25 years because of the more common use of multichannel autoanalyzers for blood tests. Most individuals are between 40 and 60 years of age, and the female-to-male ratio is about 3:1. A parathyroid adenoma is the cause in about 80% of patients, whereas hyperplasia of all glands is found in about 15% to 20% of patients, and parathyroid carcinoma, in less than 0.5%. If the disorder appears in childhood, a familial hyperparathyroid syndrome such as a multiple endocrine neoplasia should be considered.

Oversecretion of parathyroid hormone primarily affects the skeleton and kidneys. Pronounced osseous manifestations, such as subperiosteal resorption of the middle phalanges and distal clavicle, "salt-and-pepper" skull, and bone cysts are now relatively uncommon. More frequent is loss of bone mass, preferentially in sites rich in cortical bone such as the distal third of the forearm or femoral neck. Nephrolithiasis develops in about 5% of patients. Diffuse deposition of calcium phosphate complexes may cause nephrocalcinosis that can lead to interstitial fibrosis and reduce renal clearance. About 25% to 30% of patients have hypercalciuria. Complications due to severe hypercalcemia, such as proximal weakness in the legs, weight loss, nausea, constipation, pancreatitis, and band keratopathy, are now rare. Most patients are asymptomatic and are discovered after routine laboratory screening shows a serum calcium concentration of not more than 1 mg/dL above normal.

The diagnosis is generally established by an increased serum intact parathyroid hormone concentration in a patient with hypercalcemia. Occasionally, a patient with familial hypocalciuric hypercalcemia has an increased serum parathyroid hormone level, but the very low urinary calcium/creatinine ratio, less than 0.01, distinguishes this condition from primary hyperparathyroidism. The serum phosphorus concentration is low normal or low, and some patients exhibit a mild nongap hyperchloremic metabolic acidosis. Patients with significant bone disease may have increased levels of markers of bone formation. Patients with humoral hypercalcemia of malignancy have low serum parathyroid hormone concentrations; the increased parathyroid-hormone-related peptide does not cross-react in assays for intact parathyroid hormone.

The cure for hyperparathyroidism is surgical removal of the parathyroid adenoma or carcinoma, or most of the hyperplastic tissue, after which bone mass often increases for several years. The general guidelines for recommending surgery in patients without carcinoma are a serum calcium concentration more than 1 mg/dL above the upper limit of normal, a significant complication (overt bone disease, nephrolithiasis), marked hypercalciuria (more than 400 mg daily), BMD Z-score of the distal radius worse than −2.0, and age less than 50 years. Postoperatively, hypocalcemia may develop due to increased skeletal uptake, the "hungry bone" syndrome. For preoperative management or for patients deemed unable to undergo parathyroid surgery, medical management includes adequate hydration and moderate intake of calcium, avoidance of thiazide diuretics that may increase serum calcium concentrations, and regular ambulatory exercise. Calcitonin offers substantial benefit for management of acute hypercalcemia, but resistance to the drug limits long-term therapy. Estrogen supplements for postmenopausal women and bisphosphonates also can be considered. Bisphosphonates may be more effective when given cyclically rather than continuously; with the latter therapy, a compensatory increase in parathyroid hormone raises the serum calcium concentration back to pretreatment levels after about 3 months. Treatment in the future may include calcimimetic agents acting on the calcium-sensing receptor to suppress synthesis of parathyroid hormone.

SECONDARY HYPERPARATHYROIDISM

Secondary hyperparathyroidism is relatively common in the elderly and may cause enough bone loss to contribute to the genesis of osteoporosis. Glucocorticoid therapy, fat malabsorption, loop diuretic therapy, and renal insufficiency may cause secondary hyperparathyroidism. Treatment generally includes calcium supplements and doses of calcitriol or vitamin D to increase intestinal absorption of calcium, and is monitored by serial measurements of serum PTH.

OSTEOGENESIS IMPERFECTA

Occasionally, an adult with multiple fractures, especially in the long bones of the legs, and radiographic osteopenia has osteogenesis imperfecta. A genetically determined inability to form quantitatively or qualitatively normal collagen characterizes this group of disorders. Several mutations in the gene for type 1 procollagen have been identified. All result in formation of unstable collagen helices. Most patients develop fractures in childhood. Some are deaf or have blue sclera, but others have only osseous manifestations.

If no phenotypic characteristic of osteogenesis imperfecta is present except for fragile bones, diagnosis can be difficult. A positive family history and a history of multiple fractures in childhood are suggestive. Radiographs show thinning of cortical and trabecular areas of bones, especially metacarpals and metatarsals. Platybasia of the skull and bone islands in the cranium suggest osteogenesis imperfecta. Bone biopsy shows diminished quantities of osteoid and excessive osteocyte numbers. Therapy with bisphosphonates, sodium fluoride, calcitonin, or gonadal hormones has been advocated. The most compelling rate is with bisphosphonates.

HYPERTHYROIDISM

Bone disease of hyperthyroidism is a type of high-turnover osteoporosis. Serum triiodothyronine levels inversely correlate with bone mass. Patients may have bone pain and fracture, in addition to other features of hyperthyroidism. Radiographs may show diffuse osteopenia; abnormal striations of cortical bone are observed occasionally. Biochemical parameters usually include normal or mildly increased serum calcium levels and increased serum alkaline phosphatase levels. Urinary excretion of calcium and collagen breakdown fragments are often increased.

Correction of the hyperthyroid state often restores bone mass. Estrogen for women or bisphosphonates may be considered if an accelerated rate of bone loss or decreased bone mass is present.

METABOLIC BONE MANIFESTATIONS OF GASTROINTESTINAL DISEASES

Patients afflicted with gastrointestinal disorders may develop a spectrum of bone disease, ranging from osteoporosis to osteomalacia. Several pathogenic mechanisms contribute: (a) calcium malabsorption, alone or combined with malabsorption of vitamin D, leading to secondary hyperparathyroidism; (b) impaired absorption of vitamin D, altered metabolism of vitamin D, or reduced enterohepatic circulation of vitamin D metabolites; and (c) glucocorticoid treatment of inflammatory bowel disease. Although early reports suggested that the bone disorder in patients with primary biliary cirrhosis was predominantly osteomalacia, subsequent histomorphometric studies showed that osteoporosis was more common. Bone disease after gastrectomy is also more commonly osteoporosis than osteomalacia. Calcium malabsorption is more likely due to loss of duodenal absorptive surface than to achlorhydria. Celiac sprue has long been known to cause rickets in children and osteomalacia in adults. Some patients with gluten-sensitive enteropathy develop secondary hyperparathyroidism, presumably because of calcium malabsorption. These skeletal complications develop even without steatorrhea or frequent bowel movements. Patients with inflammatory bowel disease may have decreased BMD due to osteomalacia or osteoporosis, and the risk is greater for Crohn disease than for ulcerative colitis.

BONE COMPLICATIONS OF MALIGNANCY

In malignancy, osteoporosis can develop as a result of skeletal effects of various cytokines, rather than localized bone destruction caused by metastatic disease. In multiple myeloma, abnormal plasma cells secrete several osteoclast-stimulating factors, including interleukin-1, interleukin-6, lymphotoxin, and parathyroid hormone-related protein. Biochemical markers for bone resorption are often increased, whereas serum alkaline phosphatase may not be. Other neoplasms also may produce hormones that alter bone metabolism and cause hypercalcemia, most commonly parathyroid-hormone-related peptide in solid malignancies, 1,25-dihydroxyvitamin D in lymphomas and benign granulomas, and, rarely, parathyroid hormone. However, the prevalence of osteoporosis in these settings is uncertain.

BIBLIOGRAPHY

Bauer DC, Gluer CC, Cauley JA, et al. Broadband ultrasound attenuation predicts fractures strongly and independently of densitometry in older women. A prospective study. *Arch Intern Med* 1997; 157:629–634.

Bonnick SL. *Bone densitometry in clinical practice.* Totowa, NJ: Humana, 1998.

Chapuy MC, Arlot ME, Duboeuf F, et al. Vitamin D3 and calcium to prevent hip fractures in the elderly woman. *N Engl J Med* 1992;327:1637–1643.

Chesnut CH, Silverman S, Andriano K, et al. Prospective, randomized trial of nasal spray calcitonin in postmenopausal women with established osteoporosis: the PROOF study. *Am J Med* 2000;109: 267–276.

Conference Report. Consensus Development Conference: diagnosis, prophylaxis and treatment of osteoporosis. *Am J Med* 1993;94: 646–650.

Cummings SR. Black DM, Thompson DE, et al. Effect of alendronate on risk of fracture in women with low bone density but without vertebral fractures: results from the Fracture Intervention Trial. *JAMA* 1998;280:2077–2082.

Cummings SR. Browner WS, Bauer D, et al. Endogenous hormones and the risk of hip and vertebral fractures among older women. *N Engl J Med* 1998;339:733–738.

Dawson-Hughes B, Harris SS, Krall EA, et al. Effect of calcium and vitamin D supplementation on bone density in men and women 65 years of age or older. *N Engl J Med* 1997;337: 670–676.

Ettinger B, Black DM, Mitlak BH, et al. Reduction of vertebral fracture risk in post-menopausal women with osteoporosis treated with raloxifene. *JAMA* 1999;282:637–645.

Favus MJ, eds. *Primer on the metabolic bone diseases and disorders of mineral metabolism,* 4th ed. Philadelphia: Lippincott Williams & Wilkins, 1999.

Harris ST, Watts NB, Genant HK, et al. Effects of risedronate treatment on vertebral and nonvertebral fractures in women with post-menopausal osteoporosis. *JAMA* 1999;282:1344–1352.

Kleerekoper M, Sins E, McClung M. *The bone and mineral manual: a practical guide.* San Diego: Academic Press, 1999.

Morgan SL, Saag KG, Julian BA, et al. Osteopenic bone diseases in arthritis and allied conditions. In: Koopman WJ, ed. *Arthritis and allied conditions,* 14th ed. Philadelphia: Lippincott Williams & Wilkins, 2001:2449–2513.

NIH Consensus Development Panel on Osteoporosis Prevention, Diagnosis, and Therapy. Osteoporosis prevention, diagnosis, and therapy. *JAMA* 2001;285:785–795.

Orwoll ES. Osteoporosis in men. *Endocrinol Metab Clin North Am* 1998;27:349–367.

Parfitt AM, Rao DS, Kleerekoper M. Asymptomatic hyperparathyroidism discovered by multichannel biochemical screening: clinical course and considerations bearing on the need for surgical intervention. *J Bone Miner Res* 1991;6(Suppl 2):S97–S101.

Riggs BL, Khosla S, Melton LJ III. A unitary model for involutional osteoporosis. *J Bone Miner Res* 1998;13:763–773.

Rodino MA, Shane E. Osteoporosis after organ transplantation. *Am J Med* 1998;104:459–469.

OSTEONECROSIS

KENNETH A. JAFFE

·Osteonecrosis (ON) is a disease caused by ischemic death of the bony and marrow tissues. Other synonyms for *osteonecrosis* are *ischemic bone necrosis, avascular necrosis,* and *aseptic necrosis* (1). ON usually is not a specific diagnostic entity, but rather the final common pathway of a series of derangements that produce a decrease in blood flow leading to cellular death. It has been identified in multiple locations in the axial and appendicular skeleton and has been associated with a large number of medical conditions and with injury.

The condition may occur in up to 30% of patients with certain medical conditions and is the underlying diagnosis in 5% to 18% of the more than 500,000 total hip arthroplasties performed yearly in the United States and Western Europe (2). Despite the recognition of between 10,000 and 20,000 new cases of ON each year (3), the true prevalence of the condition remains difficult to define.

ETIOLOGY

Many causes and risk factors can lead to ON. The resulting pathologic findings are similar in all patients. Bone death as the result of diminished arterial blood supply can be reproduced in experimental animals. If blood flow is completely interrupted and not restored, bone death inevitably ensues (1).

In a canine model, Nakamura et al. (4) have shown that the process of ON may begin early after vascular change. At 3 days, edema with decreased cell population and bleeding within the bone marrow were observed. At 1 week, histologic changes consistent with necrosis of the femoral head but no evidence of creeping substitution were observed. ON was observed in all dogs studied at 4 weeks. These changes included empty lacunae and appositional bone in trabecular bone and mature fibrous tissue in the bone marrow (4).

Ischemia may also occur as a result of intra- and extravascular pathology within the bone itself. Small-vessel vasculitis, intravascular arteriolar thrombosis venous occlusion, and microembolism are well-recognized causes of ischemia. Increased intraosseous pressure has been postulated as another mechanism of inducing ON. The increased pressure either initiated as a primary (infiltrative) process or as a secondary (altered blood flow) results in ischemia and cell damage. The presence of increased intraosseous pressure has been used in the past as a diagnostic tool for ON.

Other factors, such as cytotoxicity, may play an important role in the pathogenesis of ON. The high-dose corticosteroid therapy used for immunosuppression after transplantation, as well as for treating rheumatologic and autoimmune diseases, has been implicated as a risk factor for development of atraumatic ON (3,5,6). The cause-and-effect relationship between steroid use and ON has been difficult to establish because of the multiplicity of confounding factors (7). Most patients who take steroids also have other risk factors. It is still unclear whether the resulting osteonecrosis is due to the underlying disease or to the use of steroids (8). The results of initial studies indicated that high doses (>30 mg/d) and longer duration of treatment were the most important predictors of development of osteonecrosis (8,9). Nonrheumatologic conditions treated with long-term low-dose corticosteroid therapy (e.g., ulcerative colitis, asthma, skin disorders) do not present with a high incidence of atraumatic ON (8).

The mechanism postulated for steroid-induced ON is unclear. A disorder in fat metabolism has been implicated as a possible mechanism (10). Fat cells within the bone marrow increase in size, leading to the disorder (10). Cell hypertrophy increases pressure inside the bone, resulting in sinusoidal vascular collapse and finally necrosis. The exact mechanism of the cell hypertrophy remains elusive. Patients undergoing steroid treatment may be in a hyperlipidemic state, which can increase the fat content in the bone and increase intracortical pressure, producing sinusoidal collapse and necrosis (11). Other investigators have proposed that this hyperlipidemic state may lead to fat embolism that occludes the microvasculature and initiates the pathophysiologic process (12).

High alcohol consumption has been implicated as a risk factor for developing ON (3,5,13,14). The exact amount of alcohol intake that can induce ON is unknown. The pathophysiologic process of alcohol-induced osteonecrosis is not completely understood. Both a direct toxic effect and alteration of lipid metabolism have been proposed. Excess alcohol can change fat metabolism, which then allows small fat emboli from the liver to occlude the vasculature, decreasing blood flow and leading to osteonecrosis. Alcohol consumption may produce an accumulation of lipids inside the osteocytes (14). These cells hypertrophy and compress the nuclei of the osteocytes, resulting in cell death (15,16).

OTHER FACTORS

Other etiologic factors and clinical conditions that have been proposed as causes of osteonecrosis include sickle cell anemia, Gaucher disease, thrombophilia, and hypofibrinolysis. Caisson disease, or dysbaric osteonecrosis, is a form of ON that occurs in deep-sea divers and miners. Environmental conditions with exposure to hyperbaric conditions can cause an occlusion of blood vessels by circulating nitrogen bubbles that are induced in response to a reduction in ambient pressure during decompression (17).

Sickle cell anemia has been reported to be an important risk factor for the development of ON. The prevalence of ON in patients with sickle cell anemia has been estimated to range from 3% to 41% (18,19). Patients with sickle cell trait can also be affected. Intravascular sickling within sinusoids associated with a hyperviscosity syndrome produced by high hemoglobin concentrations produces short, temporary occlusions of blood flow, which leads to ON and eventually to collapse (19). The distinctive histologic pattern is characterized by rows of necrotic bone separated by fibroadipose tissue.

Disorders in fat metabolism may also lead to fat emboli and immune complex deposition. The resulting microvascular obstruction can result in hemorrhage and death of bone (14,15,20). Type I Gaucher disease is an autosomal recessive genetic disease that affects primarily Ashkenazi Jews and is caused by an enzymatic deficiency of glucocerebroside hydrolase (21). It results in accumulation of sphingolipids within macrophages and other reticuloendothelial cells and can affect bone as well as other solid organs. Compression of the cellular and vascular elements and increased pressure within the rigid cortical bone decrease blood flow, leading to osteonecrosis (22).

Arterial disorders have also been associated with osteocytes and bone marrow necrosis. The specific mechanism that results in damage to the tunica intima and tunica media is unknown. However, investigators have noted pathologic changes in arteries in hemorrhage zones surrounding areas of necrosis (23,24).

For this reason this entity should not be considered a simple lesion, but rather a multifactorial disease process that can be produced by a diverse group of disorders leading to a common finding—necrosis and inevitable collapse. The pathologic alterations are similar in all patients with ON.

PATHOPHYSIOLOGY

When the affected site is small, reparative processes are initiated rapidly, replacing dead bone with normal new bone. Pluripotential cells within the bone are recruited in the repair process. Osteoclasts are stimulated to resorb dead bone, and osteoblasts lay down new bone over necrotic areas, creating the characteristic appearance termed *creeping substitution* (7).

However, as the necrotic area enlarges, the histologic appearance changes. At the periphery of the lesion, a zone of vascular in-growth is produced, with replacement of bone and bone marrow, leading to marked thickening and increased density of its borders (4). Because vascular structures cannot penetrate deep inside the avascular lesion, repair is interrupted. In periarticular regions such as the femoral head, the dead bone then fractures, although the superior articular surface does not collapse, owing to the strength of the subchondral bone. The radiolucent space produced under the subchondral bone is called the "crescent sign." In time, this fragile structure collapses and the femoral head flattens. After deformation, abnormal stresses on the articular cartilage and subchondral bone lead to sclerosis, cyst formation, and marginal osteophyte formation. Advancing degeneration leads to obliteration of the joint space.

CLASSIFICATION

The prognoses for and success of different treatments for ON of the femoral head or any other bone are related to the stage of the disease (25–27). Comparison of different therapeutic strategies is possible only through the use of an accurate standard classification system.

The Association Research Circulation Osseous (ARCO) has proposed a classification system that incorporates the Pennsylvania system based on lesion size and the Japanese system based on lesion location (28). Imaging modalities utilized include radiographs, computed tomography (CT), bone scans, and MRI (29,30). Quantitation (percentage of area involvement of femoral head, length of crescent sign, percentage of surface collapse, and dome depression) and location of the lesion (medial, central, or lateral) (28) represent important prognostic factors.

CORRELATION OF PATHOMORPHOLOGY AND IMAGING FINDINGS

To understand the patterns of ON seen on the different imaging modalities, the pathomorphologic changes can be described in five phases (31) (Fig. 25.1 and Table 25.1).

STAGE	0	1	2	3	4
FINDINGS	All present techniques normal or non-diagnostic	X-ray and CT are normal. At least ONE of the below is positive	NO CRESCENT SIGN: X-RAY ABNORMAL: sclerosis, lysis, focal porosis	CRESCENT SIGN on the X-ray and/or flattening of articular surface of femoral head	OSTEOARTHRITIS joint space narrowing, acetabular changes, joint destruction
TECHNIQUES	X-ray CT Scintigraph MRI	Scintigraph MRI *QUANTITATE on MRI	X-ray, CT Scintigraph MRI *QUANTITATE MRI & X-ray	X-ray, CT ONLY *QUANTITATE on X-ray	X-ray ONLY
LOCATION	NO	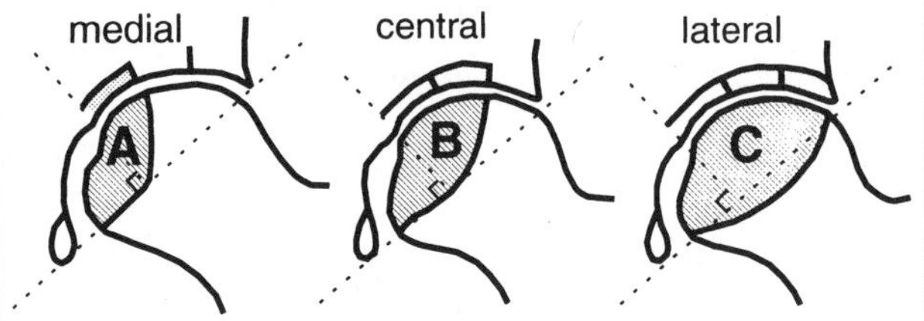	medial / central / lateral		NO
SIZE	NO	QUANTITATION		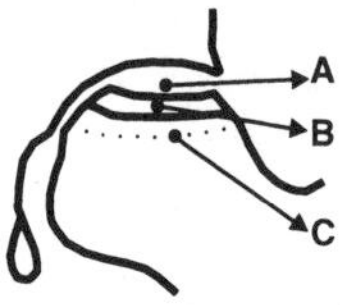	NO

QUANTITATION

% AREA INVOLVEMENT
minimal   A < 15%
moderate B 15-30%
extensive C > 30%

LENGTH of CRESCENT
A < 15%
B 15-30%
C > 30%

% SURFACE COLLAPSE & DOME DEPRESSION
A < 2 mm
B 2-4 mm
C > 4 mm

FIGURE 25.1. Schematic modified outline of the five-stage Association Research Circulation Osseous (ARCO) international classification for osteonecrosis of the femoral head. *CT,* computerized tomography; *MRI,* magnetic resonance imaging. (From Jones JP Jr. Osteonecrosis. In: Koopman WJ, ed. *Arthritis and allied conditions: a textbook of rheumatology,* 14th ed. Philadelphia: Lippincott Williams & Wilkins, 2001:2143–2163, with permission.)

TABLE 25.1. ARCO OSTEONECROSIS CLASSIFICATION: CLINICAL, RADIOGRAPHIC, AND MORPHOLOGIC CORRELATION

Finding	ARCO Stage (Histologic Phase)				
	0 (I)	1 (II)	2 (III)	3 (IV)	4 (V)
Clinical	Normally no pain	Normally no pain	May have pain	Pain	Pain
Radiograph	Normal	Normal	Mottled and sclerotic rim	CrescentCollapse sign and/or flattening	
CT	Normal	Normal	Mottled and sclerotic rim	Subchondral fracture	Collapse
Bone scan	Normal	Cold spot	Cold in hot spot	Cold in hot spot	Hot in hot spot
MRI	Normal	Necrotic area and reactive interface	Necrotic area and reactive interface	CrescentCollapse sign	
Histology	Plasmostasis and marrow	Bone necrosis and inflammanecrosistory response	Reactive interface repair	Resorption and subchondral fracture	Flattening and cartilage destruction

ARCO, *Association* Research Circulation Osseous; CT, computed tomography; MRI, magnetic resonance imaging.
From Hofmann S, Kramer J, Plenk H, et al. Osteonecrosis: imaging of osteonecrosis. In: Urbaniak JR, Jones JP Jr, eds. *Osteonecrosis: etiology, diagnosis, and treatment.* Chicago: American Academy of Orthopaedic Surgeons, 1997:213–223, with permission.

Stage 0

In the initial phase of ON, the patient is asymptomatic and all imaging techniques are normal or nondiagnostic. Only medullary changes occur during the first 7 days. Radiographs and CT cannot detect these early bone marrow changes. Conventional MRI does not show any signal alterations in this very early stage of dead bone without repair, because as long as the fat cells have their cellular integrity, they give a normal signal on MRI. This initial phase of ON may be detected as a photopenic ischemic "cold spot" with focal decreased tracer uptake in the bone scan (32) and reduced contrast enhancement in dynamic contrast-enhanced MRI studies (33). If ischemia does not persist, the morphologic changes in stage 0 may be sufficiently repaired, and the ischemic damage may be reversible.

Stage 1

Normally, the patient is asymptomatic, but bone scans and/or MRI may show nonspecific patterns of ON, and radiographs and CT are still normal. On histology, bone marrow becomes necrotic. At this point, termination of the ischemic event in combination with a sufficient repair capacity makes the necrotic lesion still reversible. Several factors (e.g., the size of the lesion, risk factors, and repair capacity) determine whether this process ends with a focal subchondral necrosis or repair of the lesion (31,34,35). Radiographs and CT cannot detect these early stage 1 changes. Bone scans show a "hot spot," indicating the high vascularity of the repair process. On MRI the focal subchondral necrotic defect may show the pattern of bone marrow edema with low signal on T1-weighted images and high signal intensity on T2-weighted images (31,35). There is still controversy as to whether bone marrow edema syndrome (BMES), or so-called transient osteoporosis or algodystrophy, represents an early reversible ON (36,37). Some authorities argue that BMES represents a subgroup of patients in ARCO stage 1 with joint pain and a diffuse lesion instead of the focal lesion of true ON (38).

Stage 2

In stage 2 the patient usually is still asymptomatic. However, a pathognomonic ON pattern can be observed in CT, bone scans, and MRI; radiographs show only unspecific changes (39).

On histology, an insufficient repair mechanism produces a band of increased vascularity, granulation tissue, and new bone formation, which borders the defect at the periphery of the necrotic lesion. The repair mechanism may revascularize some parts of the necrotic lesion, but only focal creeping substitution occurs (31,34,35,40).

On plain radiographs, the sclerotic rim surrounding the lesion may be clearly visible, but in stage 2 it usually can be detected by CT only (31,41). The combination of mottled osteolytic and sclerotic subchondral lesion, surrounded by a distinct sclerotic rim, represents the characteristic radiographic and CT pattern of ON. On bone scan, an area of decreased tracer uptake can be surrounded by increased tracer accumulation. The "cold in hot" spot is nearly pathognomonic of ON. However, in most cases, the increased tracer uptake of the repair mechanism covers the small cold spot of the necrotic lesion, and only a nonspecific hot spot is observed, which is the most common but unspecific bone scan finding in ON. The cold-in-hot scintigraphic lesions are best detected by single photon emission tomography (SPECT) (42). On MRI, the subchondral necrotic defect shows different signal alternations (43). These signal changes are surrounded by a band of low signal intensity on T1-weighted images, which represents new bone formation in the reactive interface. In most of the cases, a high signal line central to the low signal line can be observed in the reactive interface on T2-weighted images, indicating the well-vascularized granulation tissue. This "double-line sign" represents the sclerotic rim (outer dark line) and the hypervascularity of the repair zone (inner high signal line) (31). The reactive interface and the double-line sign have been considered to be pathognomonic of ON (43).

Stage 3

Acute onset of joint pain, usually aggravated by weight-bearing and relieved by rest, is the clinical sign of stage 3. In the ARCO classification system, stage 3 lesions reveal a crescent sign and/or flattening of the articular surface. On histology, these pathognomonic changes for ON can be identified on plain radiographs and CTs, whereas only indirect patterns can be found on bone scans and MRI. The combination of osteoclastic resorption induced by the repair process and microfractures induced by shear forces at the chondroosseous junction is the pathomorphologic cause of this subchondral fracture (31). On radiographs, this pathognomonic subchondral fracture line can be best identified on lateral views as a crescent sign. Earlier in the course of ON, the subchondral fracture at the chondroosseous junction can be detected more accurately by CT. It cannot be detected by bone scan. In some cases, the penetration of joint fluid into the subchondral fracture gap may produce a high-intensity line, the so-called MRI crescent sign, on T2-weighted MRI images (43).

Stage 4

Continuous progressive joint pain, even at rest, in combination with stiffness and weakness, are the clinical signs of stage 4 disease. Nonspecific secondary osteoarthritic changes can be identified in all imaging modalities. Collapse and secondary osteoarthritic joint destruction with subchondral cysts on the femoral and acetabular side of the joint are seen histologically. The histomorphologic changes cannot be differentiated from osteoarthritis at this stage. On bone scans, the mechanical effect of the collapse and the hypervascularization at the chondroosseous junction of the collapse may produce a "hot-in-hot" spot (44). MRI can identify the joint effusion and the original ON lesion.

TREATMENT

Femoral Head

No single method or combination of methods has been demonstrated to universally prevent disease progression. The natural history of ON is one of subchondral fractures leading to collapse and painful disabling arthrosis. Studies have shown that when management is limited to observation alone or restricted weight-bearing, collapse of the femoral head will eventually occur in at least 80% of cases (7,45–47). Several treatment modalities are currently available. Their use is based on the stage of the disease: In the early stages, prophylactic measures are instituted to prevent further progression of disease; in later stages, when collapse and significant distortion of the head are present, reconstruction is the procedure of choice.

Early Stages

Conservative treatment involving non-weight-bearing status with the use of crutches or a cane has proved ineffective except for the treatment of small, asymptomatic lesions located outside the major weight-bearing areas. An appropriate pharmacologic treatment for osteonecrosis is still being sought.

Core decompression, as described by Arlet and Ficat in 1964, was first used as part of a diagnostic protocol in which a portion of the femoral head (8 to 10 mm) was removed to obtain tissue for histologic studies (3). Because patients who underwent this procedure reported lessening of pain, it was instituted as a treatment modality, with the rationale that elevated intraosseous pressure was reduced when holes were drilled into the diseased femoral head. In addition, removal of one or more cores may stimulate repair of the sclerotic areas by promoting vascular in-growth. Success rates of 96% for stage I disease, 74% for stage II disease, and 35% for stage III disease have been reported (9). However, these encouraging results have not always been obtained by other investigators.

Although the effectiveness of core decompression continues to be controversial, the larger, better-controlled series report a low incidence of complications and superior results when compared with conservative management. Patients who undergo core decompression benefit from pain relief, preservation of the femoral head, and delay of arthroplasty (7).

Bone-grafting procedures are used as treatment for osteonecrosis, alone or in combination with other procedures, such as core decompression. Both cortical bone and cancellous bone are used for structural support and to promote vascular in-growth in the healing bone. A vascularized fibular bone grafting requires a microvascular anastomosis between the vessels of the graft and the branches of the femoral artery that supply the hip joint. The procedure is technically difficult. There is some morbidity at the graft donor site. Complications included contractures of the flexor hallucis longus and deep venous thrombosis (48).

Osteotomies of the proximal femur are aimed at shifting the affected areas of the femoral head away from the major weight-bearing regions of the joint. Their effectiveness is still under evaluation (6,49).

Late Stages

When collapse and deformation of the femoral head occur and painful arthrosis is refractory to medical treatment, reconstruction arthroplasty is the procedure of choice. The choices in reconstructive arthroplasty are hemiarthroplasty (reconstruction of the femoral head) or total hip arthroplasty [(THA) reconstruction of the acetabular and femoral head]. The results of conventional unipolar and bipolar prostheses have been unsatisfactory. It appears that these prostheses are of historic interest only (50,51).

The two types of procedures in arthroplasty surgery are surface replacement or total hip replacement for ON.

Surface replacement has some advantages over total hip arthroplasty because the former procedure leads to preservation of the femoral head and neck, and allows for a future total hip replacement if necessary. Several investigators have suggested that this procedure is effective in cases in which the femoral head is not extensively involved, permitting the prostheses to be fit on structurally viable bone.

Amstutz et al. (52) reported on the results of surface hemiarthroplasties using cemented titanium-6 aluminum components in young adult patients with ON of the femoral head. The authors concluded that hemiarthroplasty provided a conservative solution to the problem of the young patient with a stage III ON of the femoral head. It appears that even in the worst of instances it allowed patients to buy some time before more radical procedures, such as conventional arthroplasty, became necessary.

The hemiresurfacing can provide a satisfactory interim solution and should be something to consider, particularly in the very young patient with stage III disease. The available literature on total hip arthroplasty for ON indicates that the results appear to be somewhat worse than those reported for other diagnoses, such as degenerative joint disease.

Early reports on the use of total hip replacement (THA) for treatment of ON showed a high incidence of unsatisfactory results. Stauffer (53) reported a 50% failure with a follow-up of 10 years, whereas Salvati and Cornell (54) reported a 37% failure with 8 years of follow-up. These prostheses were all inserted using cement. The use of cementless prostheses has produced varying results (55,56).

Several authors have compared long-term outcomes between OA and ON undergoing THA. Ritter and Meding (57) reported on a comparison of 64 THAs for ON and 615 for degenerative disease. After a minimum follow-up of 3 years, there was no difference in the incidence of lucencies, loosening, pain, or revision, but there appeared to be a higher death rate in patients with ON, perhaps related to the original diagnosis, and a higher incidence of heterotopic ossification in patients with osteoarthritis. Saito et al. (58) reported on 20 THAs for ON and 63 for osteoarthritis and followed up for 7 years. The clinical results were inferior in ON, and the incidence of loosening and revision was higher in these diagnoses. Ortiguera et al. (59) analyzed 188 THAs with 10 to 25 years of follow-up to try to answer the question of difference between ON and degenerative disease. There was a significantly high dislocation rate in patients with ON, and in patients younger than 50 years of age, the incidence of revision or loosening was statistically higher in patients with ON. Thus it appears that the results of cemented THA for ON in the young patient are less favorable than those for degenerative joint disease.

The results of THA in patients with ON depend on the etiology of the ON. THAs in patients who have had kidney transplants and in patients with SLE provide adequate results. However, THA should be considered only with caution in patients with sickle cell disease. The outcome of THA in patients with ON are inferior to those in patients with degenerative joint disease. Finally, the choice of fixation in THA for ON should be the same as that for other diagnoses (50).

Other Bones

ON most commonly affects the hip (proximal femur) (60), but it also can affect other epiphyseal areas, including the knee (distal femur, proximal tibia) (61–63), shoulder (proximal humerus) (64,65), and ankle (talus, distal tibia) as well as other locations on rare occasions. Treatment options for the knee have included nonsurgical therapy, such as restricted weight-bearing, analgesics, and observation (63). Unfortunately, these treatment methods have led to a greater than 80% clinical failure rate.

There have been few reports specifically focusing on the surgical treatment of this problem. Some authors have advocated joint-preserving surgical treatment modalities, including arthroscopic debridement (66), core decompression (61,63), vascularized bone grafting (67,68), and resurfacing with osteoarticular allografts (69,70). These procedures have been most successful for patients with early stages of the disease (before condylar collapse). Patients who have second arthrosis from severe disease have few options

other than unicompartmental (71) or total knee arthroplasty (62,72) despite their young age.

The pathophysiology of ON of the proximal humerus is similar to that of the disease in other locations. Objectives of nonsurgical treatment are the relief of pain and preservation of passive motion. Surgical treatment has traditionally been reserved for patients with severe disabling pain.

Arthroscopic debridement may be appropriate in certain patient populations, just as arthroplasty may be inappropriate in younger patients. Many of these patients still have significant mechanical symptoms relating to the shoulder in the form of painful locking, popping, and catching related to radiographic evidence of osteochondral fracture or loose body. Hemiarthroplasty or, in the presence of glenoid involvement, total shoulder arthroplasty has been the mainstay of therapy.

One of the well-recognized complications of severe ankle trauma is ON of the talus (73,74). This disease entity has also been reported with other nontraumatic entities and progresses through sequential stages similar to those of femoral head lesions.

The options for symptomatic ON of the talus are analgesics, bracing, and restricted weight-bearing. Core decompression provides a satisfactory solution for symptomatic precollapse lesions. Unfortunately, a few surgical options that include various arthrodesis procedures are utilized if all else fails, although they are technically challenging and involved longer time to fusion than with osteoarthritis.

ON is a complex entity that requires a specific treatment regimen after accurate diagnosis. Early diagnosis is crucial. MR imaging is the gold standard tool. Preservation of bone is the primary goal of any intervention modality. Improved diagnostic techniques have made it possible to intervene before segmental collapse occurs, but no one technique has been completely satisfactory.

REFERENCES

1. Alarcón GS. Osteonecrosis. In: Klippel JH, Weyand CM, Wortmann RL, eds. *Primer on the rheumatic diseases*, 11th edition. Atlanta: Arthritis Foundation, 1997:378–381.
2. Vail TP, Covington DB. The incidence of osteonecrosis. In: Urbaniak JR, Jones JP Jr, eds. *Osteonecrosis: etiology, diagnosis and treatment.* Chicago: American Academy of Orthopaedic Surgeons, 1997:43.
3. Mont MA, Hungerford DS. Non-traumatic avascular necrosis of the femoral head. *J Bone Joint Surg Am* 1995;77:459–474.
4. Nakamura T, Matsumoto T, Nishino M, et al. Early magnetic resonance imaging and histologic findings in a model of femoral head necrosis. *Clin Orthop* 1997;334:68–72.
5. Hungerford DS, Zizic TM. Alcoholism associated ischemic necrosis of the femoral head: early diagnosis and treatment. *Clin Orthop* 1978;130:144–153.
6. Kerboul M, Thomine J, Postel M, et al. The conservative surgical treatment of idiopathic aseptic necrosis of the femoral head. *J Bone Joint Surg Br* 1974;56:291–296.
7. Lavernia CJ, Sierra RJ, Grieco FR. Osteonecrosis of the femoral head. *J Am Acad Orthop Surg* 1999;7:250–261.

8. Colwell CW Jr, Robinson CA, Stevenson DD, et al. Osteonecrosis of the femoral head in patients with inflammatory arthritis or asthma receiving corticosteroid therapy. *Orthopedics* 1996;19: 941–946.

9. Hungerford DS. Treatment of avascular necrosis in the young patient. *Orthopedics* 1995;18:822–823.

10. Johnson LC. Histiogenesis of avascular necrosis. Presented at the Conference on Aseptic Necrosis of the Femoral Head, St. Louis, 1964.

11. Jaffe WL, Epstein M, Heyman N, et al. The effect of cortisone on femoral and humeral heads in rabbits. *Clin Orthop* 1972; 82:221–228.

12. Jones JP Jr. Fat embolism, intravascular coagulation, and osteonecrosis. *Clin Orthop* 1993;292:294–308.

13. Matsuo K, Hirohata T, Sugioka Y, et al. Influence of alcohol intake, cigarette smoking, and occupational status on idiopathic osteonecrosis of the femoral head. *Clin Orthop* 1988;234: 115–123.

14. Schroeder WC. Current concepts on the pathogenesis of osteonecrosis of the femoral head. *Orthop Rev* 1994;23:487–497.

15. Nishimura T, Matsumoto T, Nishino M, et al. Histopathologic study of veins in steroid treated rabbits. *Clin Orthop* 1997;334: 37–42.

16. Kenzora JE, Glimcher MJ. Accumulative cell stress. The multi-factorial etiology of idiopathic osteonecrosis. *Orthop Clin North Am* 1985;16:669–679.

17. Lehner CE, Adams WM, Dubielzig RR, et al. Dysbaric osteonecrosis in divers and caisson workers: an animal model. *Clin Orthop* 1997;344:320–332.

18. Moran MC. Osteonecrosis of the hip is sickle cell hemoglobinopathy. *Am J Orthop* 1995;24:18–24.

19. Styles LA, Vichinsky EP. Core decompression in avascular necrosis of the hip in sickle-cell disease. *Am J Hematol* 1996;52: 103–107.

20. Moskal JT, Topping RE, Franklin LL. Hypercholesterolemia: an association with osteonecrosis of the femoral head. *Am J Orthop* 1997;26:609–612.

21. Katz K, Horev G, Grunebaum M, et al. The natural history of osteonecrosis of the femoral head in children and adolescents who have Gaucher disease. *J Bone Joint Surg Am* 1996;781: 14–19.

22. Tauber C, Tauber T. Gaucher disease. The orthopaedic aspect: report of seven cases. *Arch Orthop Trauma Surg* 1995;114: 179–182.

23. Saito S, Ohzono K, Ono K. Early arteriopathy and postulated pathogenesis of osteonecrosis of the femoral head: the intracapital arterioles. *Clin Orthop* 1992;277:98–110.

24. Saito S, Inoue A, Ono K. Intramedullary haemorrhage as a possible cause of avascular necrosis of the femoral head: the histology of 16 femoral heads at the silent stage. *J Bone Joint Surg Br* 1987;69:346–351.

25. Steinberg ME, Hayken GD, Steinberg DR. A quantitative system for staging avascular necrosis. *J Bone Joint Surg Am* 1995; 77B:34–41.

26. Stulberg BN, Levine M, Bauer TW, et al. Multi-modality approach to osteonecrosis of the femoral head. *Clin Orthop* 1989; 240:181–193.

27. Hungerford DS, Jones LC. Diagnosis of osteonecrosis of the femoral head. In: Schoutens A, Arlet J, Gardeniers JWM, et al., eds. *Bone circulation and vascularization in normal and pathological conditions*. New York: Plenum Press, 1993:265–275.

28. Ohzono K, Saito M, Sugano N, et al. The fate of nontraumatic avascular necrosis of the femoral head: a radiologic classification to formulate prognosis. *Clin Orthop* 1992;277:73–78.

29. Mont MA, Glueck CJ, Pacheco IH, et al. Risk factors for osteonecrosis in systemic lupus erythematosus. *J Rhematol* 1997; 24:654–662.

30. Gardeniers JWM. ARCO international classification of osteonecrosis. *ARCO Newsletter* 1993;5:79–82.

31. Hofmann S, Kramer J, Leder K, et al. The non-traumatic femur head necrosis in the adult. I. Pathophysiology, clinical picture and therapeutic options. *Radiologe* 1994;34:1–10.

32. Jones JP Jr. Concepts of etiology and early pathogenesis of osteonecrosis. In: Schafer M, Instructional Course Lectures 43. Chicago: American Academy of Orthopaedic Surgeons, 1994; 499–512.

33. Nadel SN, Debatin JF, Richardson WJ, et al. Detection of acute avascular necrosis of the femoral head in dogs: dynamic contrast-enhanced MR imaging vs spin-echo and STIR sequences. *Am J Roentgenol* 1992;159:1255–1261.

34. Arlet J. Nontraumatic avascular necrosis of the femoral head: past, present, and future. *Clin Orthop* 1992;277:12–21.

35. Hauzeur JP, Pasteels JL, Schoutens A, et al. The diagnostic value of magnetic resonance imaging in non-traumatic osteonecrosis of the femoral head. *J Bone Joint Surg Am* 1989;71A:641–A649.

36. Guerra JJ, Steinberg ME. Distinguishing transient osteoporosis from avascular necrosis of the hip. *J Bone Joint Surg Am* 1995; 77A:616–624.

37. Conway WF, Hayes CW, Daniel WW. Bone marrow edema pattern on MR images: transient osteoporosis or early osteonecrosis of bone? In: Weissman BN, ed. *Syllabus, A categorical course in musculoskeletal radiology*. Oakbrook, IL: Radiological Society of North America, 1993:141–154.

38. Hofmann S, Fialka V, Kramer J, et al. The bone marrow oedema syndrome of the hip and its relationship with avascular necrosis and reflex sympathetic dystrophy. *Bailliere's Clin Orthop* 1996;2: 291–314.

39. Hofmann S, Kramer J, Plenk H, et al. Osteonecrosis: imaging of osteonecrosis. In: Urbaniak JR, Jones JP Jr, eds. *Osteonecrosis: Etiology, diagnosis, and treatment*. Chicago: American Academy of Orthopaedic Surgeons, 1997:213–223.

40. Ficat RP. Idiopathic bone necrosis of the femoral head. Early diagnosis and treatment. *J Bone Joint Surg* 1989;67B:3–9.

41. Dihlmann W. CT analysis of the upper end of the femur: the asterisk sign and ischemic bone necrosis of the femoral head. *Skelet Radiol* 1982;8:251–258.

42. Freeman LM, Blaufox MD. Single photon emission computed tomography (SPECT). *Semin Nucl Med* 1987;17:247–266.

43. Mitchell DG, Steinberg MR, Dalinka MK, et al. Magnetic resonance imaging of the ischemic hip: alterations within the osteonecrotic, viable, and reactive zones. *Clin Orthop* 1989;244: 60–77.

44. Kramer J, Hofmann S, Imhof H. The non-traumatic femur head necrosis in the adult. II. Radiologic diagnosis and staging. *Radiologe* 1994;34:11–20.

45. Mont MA, Carbone JJ, Fairbank AC. Core decompression versus nonoperative management for osteonecrosis of the hip. *Clin Orthop* 1996;324:169–178.

46. Steinberg ME, Brighton CT, Corces A, et al. Osteonecrosis of the femoral head. Results of core decompression and grafting with and without electrical stimulation. *Clin Orthop* 1989;249: 199–208.

47. Ohzono K, Saito M, Takaoka K, et al. Natural history of non-traumatic avascular necrosis of the femoral head. *J Bone Joint Surg Br* 1991;73B:68–72.

48. Sotereanos DG, Plakseychuk AY, Rubash HE. Free vascularized fibula grafting for the treatment of osteonecrosis of the femoral head. *Clin Orthop* 1997;344:243–256.

49. Sugioka Y, Hotokebuchi T, Tsutsui H. Transtrochanteric anterior rotational osteotomy for idiopathic and steroid-induced necrosis

of the femoral head. Indications and long-term results. *Clin Orthop* 1992;227:111–120.

50. Cabanela M. Hip arthroplasty in osteonecrosis of the femoral head. In: Urbaniak JR, Jones JP Jr, eds. *Osteonecrosis.* Chicago: American Academy of Orthopaedic Surgeons, 1997.

51. Lachiewicz PF, Desman SM. The bipolar endoprosthesis in avascular necrosis of the femoral head. *J Arthroplasty* 1988;3:131–138.

52. Amstutz HC, Grigoris P, Safran MR, et al. Precision-fit surface hemiarthroplasty for femoral head osteonecrosis: long-term results. *J Bone Joint Surg Am Br* 1994;76B:423–427.

53. Stauffer RN. Ten-year follow-up study of total hip replacement. *J Bone Joint Surg Am* 1982;64A:983–990.

54. Salvati EA, Cornell CN. Long-term follow-up of total hip replacement in patients with avascular necrosis. In: Bassett FH III, ed. *Instructional Course Lectures XXXVII.* Park Ridge, IL: American Academy of Orthopaedic Surgeons, 1988:67–73.

55. Brinker MR, Rosenberg AG, Kull L, et al. Primary total hip arthroplasty using noncemented porous-coated femoral components in patients with osteonecrosis of the femoral head. *J Arthroplasty* 1994;9:457–468.

56. Piston RW, Engh CA, DeCarvalho PI, et al. Osteonecrosis of the femoral head treated with total hip arthroplasty without cement. *J Bone Joint Surg Am* 1994;76A:202–214.

57. Ritter MA, Meding JB. A comparison of osteonecrosis and osteoarthritis patients following total hip arthroplasty: a long-term follow-up study. *Clin Orthop* 1986;206:139–146.

58. Saito S, Saito M, Nishina T, et al. Long-term results of total hip arthroplasty for osteonecrosis of the femoral head: a comparison with osteoarthritis. *Clin Orthop* 1989;244:198–207.

59. Ortiguera CJ, Pulliam I, Cabanela ME. Abstract. Total hip arthroplasty for osteonecrosis: a matched pair analysis of 188 hips with 10- to 25-year follow-up. *Proceedings of the American Academy of Orthopaedic Surgeons 64th Annual Meeting,* San Francisco. Chicago: American Academy of Orthopaedic Surgeons, 1997:113.

60. Mont MA, Maar DC, Urquhart MW, et al. Avascular necrosis of the humeral head treated by core decompression: a retrospective review. *J Bone Joint Surg Am* 1993;75B:785–788.

61. Jacobs MA, Loeb PE, Hungerford DS. Core decompression of the distal femur for avascular necrosis of the knee. *J Bone Joint Surg Am* 1989;71B:583–587.

62. Mont MA, Myers TH, Krackow KA, et al. Total knee arthroplasty for osteonecrosis. *Clin Orthop* 1997;334:91–97.

63. Mont MA, Tomek IM, Hungerford DS. Core decompression for avascular necrosis of the distal femur: long-term follow-up. *Clin Orthop* 1997;334:124–130.

64. Mont MA, Hungerford DS. Non-traumatic avascular necrosis of the femoral head. *J Bone Joint Surg Am* 1995;77A:459–474.

65. Mont MA, Hungerford DS, Mohan V, et al. Abstract. Demographic characterization of avascular necrosis of the proximal humerus. *ARCO Trans* 1996;8:103.

66. Miller GK, Maylahn DJ, Drennan DB. The treatment of idiopathic osteonecrosis of the medial femoral condyle with arthroscopic debridement. *Arthroscopy* 1986;2:21–29.

67. Ochi M, Kimori K, Sumen Y, et al. A case of steroid-induced osteonecrosis of femoral condyle treated surgically. *Clin Orthop* 1995;312:226–231.

68. Rindell K. Muscle pedicled bone graft in revascularization of aseptic necrosis of the humeral head. *Ann Chir Gynaecol* 1987;76:283–285.

69. Flynn JN, Springfield DS, Mankin HJ. Osteoarticular allografts to treat distal femoral osteonecrosis. *Clin Orthop* 1994;303: 38–43.

70. Meyers MH, Akeson W, Convery FR. Resurfacing of the knee with fresh osteochondral allograft. *J Bone Joint Surg Am* 1989; 71A:704–713.

71. Marmor L. Unicompartmental arthroplasty for osteonecrosis of the knee joint. *Clin Orthop* 1993;294:247–253.

72. Bergman NR, Rand JA. Total knee arthroplasty in osteonecrosis. *Clin Orthop* 1991;273:77–82.

73. Blair HC. Comminuted fractures and fracture dislocations of the body of the astragalus: operative treatment. *Am J Surg* 1943;59: 37–43.

74. Dennis MD, Tullos HS. Blair tibiotalar arthrodesis for injuries to the talus. *J Bone Joint Surg Am* 1980;62A:103–107.

ARTHROPATHIES ASSOCIATED WITH SYSTEMIC DISEASES

JANET M. KIM

Rheumatology is a multidisciplinary specialty that requires knowledge of almost every organ system. In addition to musculoskeletal features, the diffuse connective-tissue diseases and many of the inflammatory arthritides have significant systemic manifestations. Conversely, a wide range of systemic diseases has musculoskeletal manifestations that occasionally may be the most prominent and presenting symptom. Several of these disorders can closely resemble various rheumatic diseases and confound diagnosis. This chapter discusses some of these systemic disorders but is not intended to be a comprehensive review. Other systemic diseases are discussed elsewhere in this book.

AMYLOIDOSIS

The amyloidoses are a group of protein deposition diseases that are distinguished by the fibrillar nature and specific staining properties of the tissue deposits, called amyloid. Deposition of amyloid interferes with normal tissue structure and function, and can result in localized or systemic disease. There are four major types of systemic amyloidosis (Table 26.1) associated with different diseases. Inflammatory arthritides are one class of disorders associated with the development of amyloidosis, which is likely the reason that this disease is often assigned to the rheumatologist. Pathologic features of amyloid deposits include composition of fibrils with a diameter of 8 to 10 nm that form a beta-pleated sheet structure (Fig. 26.1). Amyloid typically binds Congo Red and demonstrates yellow/green birefringence when viewed under polarized light. It is uncertain what causes a protein to become amyloidogenic. At least 15 different types of amyloidosis have been identified, each characterized by a specific fibril subunit protein causing distinctly separate diseases. A second protein, amyloid P component, is found among all types. Common to all the amyloidoses is the accumulation of the insoluble protein deposits in the extracellular matrix.

Expression of disease is determined by the extent of the tissues and organs involved (1).

Clinical Manifestations

Immunoglobulin (Primary) Amyloidosis

Immunoglobulin, or primary (AL), amyloidosis is the most common form of systemic amyloidosis in the United States. The amyloid fibrils are composed of kappa or lambda immunoglobulin light chain. It is associated with a monoclonal plasma cell dyscrasia, such as multiple myeloma, Waldenström macroglobulinemia, or benign monoclonal gammopathy. Serum protein electrophoresis may differentiate this type of amyloidosis from others. However, 10% to 20% of patients with AL amyloidosis show absence of detectable light chains in the serum or urine at the time of initial presentation. AL amyloidosis is associated with multisystem involvement, rapid progression, and poorer prognosis. Five-year survival is approximately 20%.

The usual presentation is proteinuria or renal failure. Urinary protein losses can be mild to massive and may exceed 25 g/d. The nephrotic syndrome may precede renal insufficiency by 1 or 2 years. Azotemia may then progress rapidly to renal failure.

Cardiac involvement is the second most common presentation and is usually detected after significant impairment has occurred. Restrictive cardiomyopathy is the hallmark of myocardial amyloidosis. Echocardiographic findings include thickening of the intraventricular septum, left atrial enlargement, and a sparkling appearance of the ventricular myocardium. Tachyarrhythmias and heart failure may result.

Musculoskeletal and articular manifestations arise from infiltration of skeletal muscle or periarticular structures. Macroglossia occurs in up to 10% of patients and is pathognomonic for AL amyloidosis (Fig. 26.2). In addition to organomegaly, the tongue exhibits firmness to palpation and indentations from the teeth. The "shoulder

TABLE 26.1. SYSTEMIC AMYLOIDOSES

Type	Clinical Names	Subunit Protein	Distinguishing Feature
Immunoglobulin (AL)	Primary Myeloma-associated	Ig light chains (kappa or lambda)	Monoclonal immunoglobulin
Reactive (AA)	Secondary	Amyloid A	Inflammatory disease
Hereditary	Familial	Transthyretin	Autosomal dominant
	Heredofamilial	Apolipoprotein AI	
	FAP	Gelsolin	
		Fibrinogen Aα chain	
		Lysozyme	
		Cystatin C	
β_2-microglobulin (β_2M)	Dialysis	β_2-microglobulin	Renal dialysis

FAP, familial amyloid polyneuropathy.
From Benson MD. Amyloidosis. In: Koopman WJ, ed. *Arthritis and allied conditions: a textbook of rheumatology,* 14th ed., Philadelphia: Lippincott Williams & Wilkins, 2001:1866–1895, with permission.

FIGURE 26.1. High magnification showing typical fibrillar nature of amyloid deposit (×68, 125). (From Benson MD. Amyloidosis. In: Koopman WJ, ed. *Arthritis and allied conditions: a textbook of rheumatology,* 14th ed. Philadelphia: Lippincott Williams & Wilkins, 2001:1866–1895, with permission.)

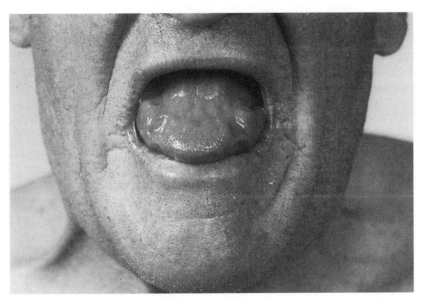

FIGURE 26.2. Macroglossia in primary (AL) amyloidosis. The tongue is firm to palpation. Note deep nonreducible impressions in the tongue caused by the teeth. (From Benson MD. Amyloidosis. In: Koopman WJ, ed. *Arthritis and allied conditions: a textbook of rheumatology,* 14th ed. Philadelphia: Lippincott Williams & Wilkins, 2001:1866–1895, with permission.)

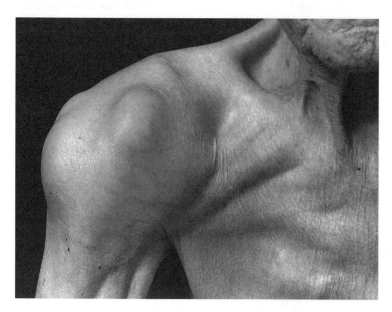

FIGURE 26.3. Articular amyloid infiltration in a 70-year-old man with primary (AL) amyloidosis. The subunit protein extracted from amyloid in the shoulder joint was a kappa III immunoglobulin light chain. (From Benson MD. Amyloidosis. In: Koopman WJ, ed. *Arthritis and allied conditions: a textbook of rheumatology,* 14th ed. Philadelphia: Lippincott Williams & Wilkins, 2001: 1866–1895, with permission.)

pad sign" (Fig. 26.3) is the most striking articular physical finding and may cause limited motion and significant pain. Carpal tunnel syndrome is frequent and may occur several years before systemic manifestations.

Nearly every organ system can be involved. Peripheral neuropathy occurs in approximately 20% of affected individuals and may precede visceral manifestations by months to years. Autonomic neuropathy is also common. Liver infiltration may lead to significant hepatomegaly. Gastrointestinal involvement is relatively common and usually manifests as motility disorders or bleeding. Other involved organs include spleen, thyroid, adrenals, lymph nodes, lungs, and skin. Purpura can occur from minor trauma such as rubbing the eyes. Additionally, acquired factor X deficiency may occur in AL amyloidosis.

Reactive (Secondary) Amyloidosis

Reactive, or secondary (AA), amyloidosis is usually associated with chronic inflammatory disease such as rheumatoid arthritis and familial Mediterranean fever. It can occur in association with other chronic inflammatory conditions such as ankylosing spondylitis, psoriatic arthritis, cystic fibrosis, and granulomatous bowel disease, as well as chronic infections such as osteomyelitis and leprosy. The precursor protein of the AA amyloid fibril is serum amyloid A (SAA), an acute-phase reactant. Fortunately, the incidence of reactive amyloidosis in patients with rheumatoid arthritis is low, probably no more than 1% or 2%. Improved ability to control and treat inflammatory diseases has significantly contributed to decreasing this association.

Patients most commonly present with the nephrotic syndrome. Usually, the patient has had long-standing inflammatory arthritis for at least 10 years. The proteinuria gradually progresses, leading to renal insufficiency, then failure, which is the usual cause of death. Gastrointestinal hemorrhage may also be a presenting symptom. Splenomegaly, hepatomegaly, and autonomic neuropathy are relatively common. Cardiomyopathy rarely occurs. Musculoskeletal manifestations due to amyloidosis are not seen. Reactive amyloidosis is slowly progressive, and patients often survive more than 10 years.

β2-Microglobulin Amyloidosis

β2-Microglobulin amyloidosis is associated with chronic renal failure and occurs predominantly in patients on long-term dialysis. The amyloid fibril is β2-microglobulin, an integral part of the major histocompatibility complex class I molecules. This protein is normally catabolized by the kidney but is too large to pass through older, less permeable dialysis membranes. Like AL amyloidosis, this type of amyloidosis can significantly involve articular structures, which is its principal manifestation of disease. Patients often present with carpal tunnel syndrome. Diffuse arthralgia and persistent effusions are common and usually involve the large joints. The amyloid deposition is destructive, frequently causing bone erosions and cystic bone lesions in the shoulders, hips, and wrists with increased risk of pathologic fracture.

Hereditary Amyloidosis

Hereditary amyloidosis includes a number of rare autosomal dominant disorders that are associated with mutations in specific plasma proteins, including transthyretin, apoliprotein A-1, gelsolin, fibrinogen, and lysozyme. The transthyretin amyloidoses are the most common form of systemic hereditary amyloidosis in the United States. Patients usually present in middle to late life with peripheral neuropathy. Clinical manifestations are similar to AL amyloidosis and can include cardiomyopathy, nephropathy, and peripheral and autonomic neuropathy. Vitreous opacities occur commonly (approximately 25%) and are pathognomonic for transthyretin amyloidosis (1,2).

Diagnosis of Systemic Amyloidosis

Systemic amyloidosis should be suspected whenever a patient presents with functional abnormalities of more than one organ system, especially those with nephrotic syndrome, cardiomyopathy, and peripheral neuropathy. The diagnosis of amyloidosis is made by tissue biopsy. Abdominal fat aspiration is the least invasive technique and is positive in 60% to 90% of patients. If the result is negative but clinical suspicion for disease remains, a more invasive biopsy of a tissue site suspected to be involved is recommended. Other sites for biopsy include rectal, gastric or duodenal, cardiac, renal, and hepatic tissues with relatively high yield. The biopsy material should demonstrate staining characteristics of amyloid by binding Congo Red and exhibit the typical apple-green birefringence when viewed under polarized light microscopy. Once a diagnosis is made, an extensive evaluation for the underlying type of amyloid and degree of organ involvement should be performed because of the varied course and prognosis among the systemic amyloidoses. Evaluation for a plasma cell dyscrasia, underlying inflammatory disorder, and obtaining extensive information regarding family history and ethnicity may greatly aid diagnosis. If hereditary amyloidosis is suspected, DNA testing confirms the diagnosis but is only available for a fraction of the mutations. Nuclear scanning using radiolabeled amyloid P component has been used to determine the presence and extent of deposits in patients, and may help assess extent of disease and response to therapy (3).

Treatment of Amyloidosis

A thorough evaluation of organ system involvement is critical in managing the patient and providing prognostic information. Chemotherapy is the only specific treatment for AL amyloidosis. The most common regimen is melphalan and prednisone, which has been used for multiple myeloma and may increase survival in some patients with amyloidosis. High-dose chemotherapy with stem cell rescue has been used in some patients with promising results. Therapy of reactive AA amyloidosis is directed toward optimal management of the underlying inflammatory condition. In patients with familial Mediterranean fever, daily colchicine administration is used successfully for the prevention of amyloidosis as well as its treatment. Specific treatment of dialysis-associated amyloidosis involves

removal of the β_2-microglobulin molecule that former dialysis membranes have precluded because of its large size. As dialysis technology has progressed over the last decade, use of highly permeable, biocompatible synthetic membranes, ultrapure dialysate, and high-flux dialyzers has allowed removal of significant β_2-microglobulin and likely lowered rates of amyloid development. Renal transplantation normalizes β_2-microglobulin levels and can improve symptoms. For the hereditary transthyretin amyloidoses, liver transplantation is the only specific treatment. Nonspecific therapies are an important aspect of managing all the systemic amyloidoses and include supportive measures such as dialysis for renal failure. Treatment of systemic manifestations can prolong survival and can significantly improve outcome (3,4).

SARCOIDOSIS

Sarcoidosis is a systemic inflammatory disease of unknown etiology characterized by noncaseating granulomata at sites of involvement. It most frequently affects the lungs, lymph nodes, skin, and eyes but may involve multiple other organs. Sarcoidosis is most commonly diagnosed in the third and fourth decades, although it can begin in infancy, and has a slightly female predominance. The incidence of sarcoidosis is increased in blacks. Although an infectious etiology has long been speculated, the cause of sarcoidosis is still unknown. The characteristic histopathologic features of the sarcoid granuloma are noncaseating central follicles of epithelioid cells and multinucleated giant cells surrounded by macrophages and activated CD4$^+$ helper T cells (Fig. 26.4). T cells are believed to play a significant role in the initial inflammatory response.

Clinical Manifestations

The presentation and severity of disease can be quite varied. Patients most commonly present with pulmonary complaints, including cough, dyspnea, and chest pain. Approximately 25% of patients present with constitutional symptoms such as fatigue, malaise, or weight loss. Extrathoracic involvement is also common throughout the course of the disease. Arthritis occurs in 10% to 15% of patients. The acute presentation of Lofgren syndrome, hilar adenopathy, fever, erythema nodosum, and acute arthritis is associated with an excellent prognosis, with remission occurring in 90% of patients. At presentation, more than 90% of patients have an abnormal chest roentgenogram. Sarcoidosis is staged according to characteristic abnormalities on the chest radiograph. Prognostically, patients with parenchymal involvement have much lower rates of remission and require more chronic treatment (5).

Musculoskeletal manifestations occur and can be an early sign of disease. The most frequent complaint is arthritis or

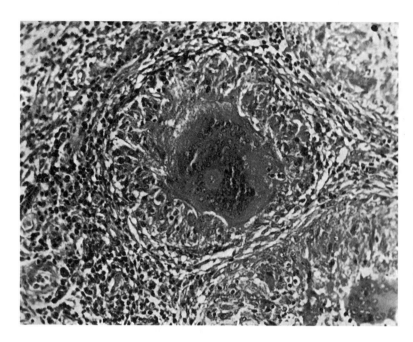

FIGURE 26.4. Multinucleated giant cell in the center of a tubercle of epithelioid cells. Surrounding the tubercle is a layer of fibroblasts and a cuff of lymphocytes, plasma cells, and mononuclear cells (×175). (From Sokoloff L, Bunim JJ. Clinical and pathological studies of joint involvement in sarcoidosis. *N Engl J Med* 1959;260:842–847. Used with permission.)

arthralgia. Two different patterns of sarcoid arthropathy are recognized, based upon whether the arthritis occurs within the first 6 months of disease or later. Acute arthropathy is the more common type and may be the presenting symptom of sarcoidosis, with arthritis heralding the other symptoms of Lofgren syndrome by several weeks. The ankles are the most frequent site of involvement, followed by the knees. Arthritis usually involves more than one joint and can be progressive in an additive fashion. In addition to synovitis, periarticular swelling and tenosynovitis can occur. Joint effusions are only mildly inflammatory. The joint manifestations of acute sarcoidosis are often self-limited, with most episodes resolving within a couple of weeks to months. Patients generally have an excellent prognosis and rarely develop bony erosions.

Late sarcoid arthritis is much less common and begins more than 6 months after onset of disease. Fewer joints are typically involved and include most commonly the knees, followed by the ankles and proximal interphalangeal joints. Arthritis can be evanescent or protracted. Even in cases of chronic synovitis, joint destruction is infrequent.

However, bony changes can occur in sarcoidosis and include cysts, sclerosis, and diffuse trabecular changes. Cystic lytic lesions and sclerosis typically occur in the middle portion of the phalanx (Fig. 26.5). These findings are sometimes associated with diffuse swelling of the finger, dactylitis, or overlying erythematous nodular masses, called lupus pernio. Some patients demonstrate these bony changes without any symptoms of arthritis.

Sarcoidosis can also affect the muscles, and often the granulomas are asymptomatic. However, involvement of skeletal muscles can present in a manner similar to polymyositis, with progressive proximal weakness and elevated creatine kinase levels (6).

Other manifestations of sarcoidosis may mimic rheumatic diseases. Sarcoid involvement of lacrimal and parotid glands can cause keratoconjunctivitis sicca and resemble Sjögren syndrome. Ocular involvement is fairly common and usually manifests as uveitis. Lymphadenopa-

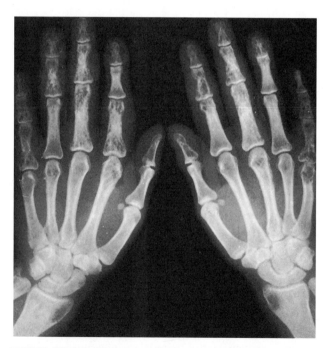

FIGURE 26.5. Radiographs of the hands showing unusually severe bone lesions of sarcoidosis. The bone cysts have not broken through the articular cortex. (From Schumacher HR Jr. Sarcoidosis. In: Koopman WJ, ed. *Arthritis and allied conditions: a textbook of rheumatology,* 14th ed. Philadelphia: Lippincott Williams & Wilkins, 2001:1896–1902, with permission.)

thy, which occurs in most patients; fever; and skin changes (e.g., erythema nodosum) are also seen in diffuse connective-tissue disorders (CTD). In addition, sarcoidosis can occur in association with CTDs and has been reported with systemic lupus erythematosus, rheumatoid arthritis, and scleroderma, among others (7).

Diagnosis

As there is no diagnostic test pathognomonic for sarcoidosis, the diagnosis is established by compatible clinical findings, exclusion of other causes, and demonstration of noncaseating granulomas. Serum angiotensin-converting enzyme levels may be elevated but are not specific. In patients with typical Lofgren syndrome or asymptomatic hilar adenopathy, biopsy may be deferred.

Treatment

Many patients with minimal symptoms require no treatment. Corticosteroids at moderately high doses (40 to 60 mg/d prednisone) are indicated for severe organ involvement, including lung, liver, eye, central nervous system, and hypercalcemia. Arthritis can usually be managed with nonsteroidal antiinflammatory drugs. Colchicine can shorten attacks of acute sarcoid arthritis. Low-dose methotrexate has been used in some patients with chronic persistent arthritis. Antimalarial drugs may improve cutaneous disease. Other immunosuppressives have been used in refractory sarcoidosis, but their efficacy has not yet been established.

HEMATOLOGIC DISORDERS

Malignancies

A wide range of hematologic disorders may be associated with rheumatic manifestations that may sometimes be the presenting symptom. Hematologic malignancies are associated with various musculoskeletal symptoms. Among patients with leukemia, they occur most frequently in children but are reported in 13.5% of adults. Symptoms include bone pain, arthralgia, and arthritis. Arthritis may present with symmetric involvement of the hands, shoulders, knees, and ankles, and may resemble rheumatoid arthritis. It can also be migratory and asymmetric. The underlying mechanisms of synovitis are not clearly understood but in some cases involve infiltration of leukemic cells into synovium or a paraneoplastic syndrome.

Skeletal manifestations are common to the malignant lymphomas. Bone pain usually manifests at regions of active bone destruction and may involve the skull, vertebrae, ribs, pelvis, and long bones. Pain is typically constant, worse at night, and unrelieved by rest. Radiographic abnormalities include osteolytic lesions, pathologic fractures, periostitis, and cortical destruction.

Therapy of the cancer-related rheumatologic symptoms involves treating the underlying malignancy and use of supportive measures (8).

Multiple Myeloma

Multiple myeloma is a relatively common plasma cell dyscrasia associated with various musculoskeletal complaints. Patients will frequently present with bone pain as a prominent symptom. It usually begins gradually but may be acute in onset if fracture occurs. Infiltration of malignant plasma cells into bone marrow and cytokine release cause bone resorption and osteoporosis. Radiographic findings classically show well-circumscribed lytic lesions in the proximal long bones, sternum, ribs, vertebrae, skull, or pelvis. A radiographic skeletal survey is the standard method for determining extent of bony involvement. Laboratory evaluation reveals a monoclonal gammaglobulin spike or excessive excretion of light chain in the urine. Multiple myeloma may be complicated by amyloidosis (see earlier). Treatment includes pain management for symptom relief and chemotherapy for myeloma (9).

Hemoglobinopathies

Musculoskeletal manifestations are a significant feature of the hemoglobinopathies. More than 80% of patients with sickle cell anemia report musculoskeletal symptoms. Pain may be bony, may be periarticular, or may involve the true joint; it is presumably due to ischemic injury or marrow hyperplasia. Arthritis is usually self-limited, resolving spontaneously within 1 to 2 weeks with hydration, analgesia, and rest. Joint effusions can occur and are usually noninflammatory. Infants 6 months to 2 years of age with sickle cell anemia may develop "hand–foot syndrome," or sickle cell dactylitis, with severe painful swelling, warmth, and erythema of the hands and feet. Long bone infarcts can be seen in all types of sickle cell disease, as can avascular necrosis. Osteonecrosis of the femur is the most disabling musculoskeletal complication of sickle cell disease. Approximately 50% of adults with sickle cell disease are hyperuricemic, but only a minority develops gout.

Patients with sickle cell disease have an increased susceptibility to bacterial infection. Osteomyelitis occurs approximately 100 times more frequently and may be initially difficult to distinguish from bone infarct. Salmonella is the most common pathogen in these patients. Myonecrosis has also been reported to occur.

Radiographic abnormalities associated with sickle cell disease include cupping of the vertebral bodies, thinning of cortices and trabeculae, and widening of medullary cavities. Treatment is directed toward management of the underlying cause of the manifestation. The β-thalassemia syndromes are also associated with skeletal abnormalities, such as osteoporosis, pathologic fractures, and growth disturbances with epiphyseal deformities. In contrast to sickle cell disease, osteonecrosis of the hip is rare. Ankle pain exacerbated by weight-bearing due to microfractures has been described. A chronic, pauciarticular, asymmetric arthropathy may occur. Because of the chronic need for blood transfusions and resulting iron overload, secondary hemochromatosis may develop (10).

Hemophilic Arthropathy

The functional deficiencies of clotting factors in the hemophilias result in disorders of blood coagulation and are associated with musculoskeletal manifestations. Severity and frequency of bleeding complications are determined by the quantity of clotting factor. Recurrent spontaneous and traumatic hemarthroses occur frequently in patients with severe disease, whereas those with moderate hemophilia usually have bleeding as a result of trauma but may have occasional spontaneous hemarthrosis. Hemarthrosis most commonly involves the large weight-bearing joints such as the knees,

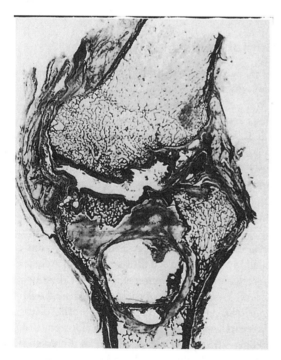

FIGURE 26.6. Sagittal section of the knee joint of a 49-year-old man with advanced hemophilic arthropathy. The femoral condyle appears flattened and the patella has virtually disappeared. The head of the tibia has undergone massive cystic resorption. The articular cartilage has disappeared from most of the joint surfaces, which have undergone partial fibrous ankylosis on the popliteal aspect on the right and have been replaced by fibrous tissue. The cyst in the tibia is lined by loose-textured fibrous tissue. The synovial and capsular tissues are thickened and infiltrated with many hemosiderin-laden mononuclear cells. (From Heck LW Jr. Arthritis associated with hematologic disorders, storage diseases, disorders of lipid metabolism, and dysproteinemias. In: Koopman WJ, ed. *Arthritis and allied conditions: a textbook of rheumatology,* 14th ed. Philadelphia: Lippincott Williams & Wilkins, 1997:1903–1924, with permission.)

followed by the ankles and elbows. Acute symptoms of hemarthrosis include erythema, stiffness, swelling, significant pain, and often low-grade fever. Weight-bearing is often intolerable, and the joint is held in flexion due to the increased volume and intraarticular pressure. Recurrent bleeding may result in chronic arthritis (Fig. 26.6) and eventually development of flexion contractures that significantly limit function. Hemorrhage into muscle and soft tissues may lead to complications, including myonecrosis, scarring, and flexion contractures. Compartment syndrome may also occur. Bleeding into bony structures may result in pseudotumors.

Treatment of acute hemarthrosis requires immediate transfusion of factor VIII. Arthrocentesis is generally not indicated unless infection is suspected, and the clotting factor should be replaced before procedure. Supportive measures—including rest, analgesics, and short-term use of NSAIDs—may help alleviate symptoms. Flexion contractures should be avoided; the joint should be put in as much extension as is comfortable, with physical therapy as an adjunctive measure once bleeding has subsided. Intraarticular corticosteroids are not advised. For patients with frequent recurrent hemorrhage, prophylactic administration of clotting factor is recommended. Arthroscopic synovectomy for chronic synovitis and total joint replacement for end-stage arthropathy have been used successfully (11).

LIPID STORAGE DISEASES

Gaucher disease is an autosomal recessive glycolipid storage disease in which enzyme deficiency of lysosomal glucocerebrosidase results in the accumulation of glucocerebroside in cells of the reticuloendothelial system. The disease is categorized into three types based on the presence and severity of central nervous system involvement. Infiltration of bone marrow by glucocerebroside-laden macrophages results in the musculoskeletal features. Severe bone pain may be a disabling manifestation of disease in young children and adults. Attacks are episodic and involve the hips, shoulders, and vertebrae. Other skeletal features include osteoporosis and vertebral collapse, osteonecrosis of the femoral head, and radiographic "Erlenmeyer flask" deformity with widening of the distal femur.

Fabry disease is an X-linked disorder caused by a deficiency of α-galactosidase activity and resulting in the accumulation of glycosphingolipids in lysosomes of various tissues. Vascular glycolipid deposition in the target organ leads to the clinical manifestations. The kidneys are the most common target organ. Skin involvement with red or dark blue angiokeratomas or telangiectasias, cardiovascular disease, and cerebrovascular disease can also occur. Pain of the palms and soles of the feet is seen and can be associated with paresthesias and hypohidrosis. Polyarthritis with swelling of the fingers and flexion contractures of the distal interphalangeal joints can develop. Osteonecrosis of the femoral head or talus may occur. Disease is usually slowly progressive.

Farber disease is a rare autosomal recessive disorder of infancy due to a deficiency of lysosomal acid ceramidase. Accumulation of ceramide in the lungs and in the cardiovascular and nervous systems usually results in death by 2 to 4 years of age. Painful polyarthritis and subcutaneous nodules may be prominent features of disease.

Diagnosis of a lipid storage disorder is confirmed by biochemical quantitation of the suspected deficient enzyme activity in leukocytes and cultured skin fibroblasts. The treatment of Gaucher disease is enzyme replacement therapy. Fabry disease is managed by supportive measures, including antiplatelet medications and renal transplantation or dialysis for renal failure (12).

MULTICENTRIC HISTIOCYTOSIS

Multicentric histiocytosis is a rare disorder of unknown etiology characterized by accumulation of lipid-laden histiocytes and multinucleated giant cells in skin, synovia, and other tissues. It typically presents as a symmetric inflamma-

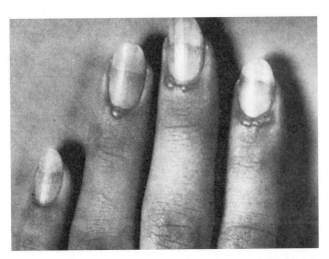

FIGURE 26.7. The fingers of a 16-year-old girl who had polyarthritis for 8 months and reddish brown "coral beads" around the nailfold for 5 months. Typical infiltrates of multicentric reticulohistiocytosis were found in biopsy specimens of both skin and synovium. (From Heck LW Jr. Arthritis associated with hematologic disorders, storage diseases, disorders of lipid metabolism, and dysproteinemias. In: Koopman WJ, ed. *Arthritis and allied conditions: a textbook of rheumatology,* 14th ed. Philadelphia: Lippincott Williams & Wilkins, 2001:1903–1924, with permission.)

tory polyarthritis mimicking rheumatoid arthritis, and most commonly involves the distal interphalangeal joints. The arthritis is painful, destructive, and potentially disabling. Skin nodules occur most frequently over the face, dorsum of the hands, ears, neck, forearm, and elbows. Clustering of small "coral bead"–like papules around the nailfolds is characteristic (Fig. 26.7). Mucosal lesions may also occur. Less frequently, involvement of cardiac, muscle, or neurologic tissues occurs. Rheumatoid factor is negative. Diagnosis is based upon histopathologic findings. There is no specific treatment for this disorder. Therapies ranging from nonsteroidal antiinflammatory drugs to alkylating agents have been used. Some patients may experience spontaneous remission (13).

REFERENCES

1. Benson MD. Amyloidosis. In: Koopman WJ, ed. *Arthritis and allied conditions: a textbook of rheumatology,* 13th ed. Baltimore: Williams & Wilkins, 1997:1661–1687.
2. Falk RH. Comenzo RL, Skinner M. The systemic amyloidoses. *N Engl J Med* 1997;337:898–909.
3. Husby G. Treatment of amyloidosis and the rheumatologist: state of the art and perspectives for the future. *Scand J Rheumatol* 1998;27:161–165.
4. Tan SY, Pepys MB, Hawkins PN. Treatment of amyloidosis. *Am J Kidney Dis* 1995;26:267–285.
5. Schumacher HR. Sarcoidosis. In: Koopman WJ, ed. *Arthritis and allied conditions: a textbook of rheumatology,* 13th ed. Baltimore: Williams & Wilkins, 1997:1689–1695.
6. Pettersson T. Rheumatic features of sarcoidosis. *Curr Opin Rheumatol* 1997;9:62–67.
7. Enzenauer RJ, West SG. Sarcoidosis in autoimmune disease. *Semin Arthritis Rheum* 1992;22:1–17.
8. Ehrenfeld M, Gur H, Shoenfeld Y. Rheumatologic features of hematologic disorders. *Curr Opin Rheumatol* 1999;11:62–67.
9. Heck LW. Arthritis associated with hematologic disorders, storage diseases, disorders of lipid metabolism, and dysproteinemias. In: Koopman WJ, ed. *Arthritis and allied conditions: a textbook of rheumatology,* 13th ed. Baltimore: Williams & Wilkins, 1997: 1697–1717.
10. Porter DR, Stubbock RD. Rheumatologic complications of sickle cell disease. *Bailliere's Clin Rheumatol* 1991;5:221–230.
11. Hilgartner MW. Hemophilic arthropathy. *Adv Pediatr* 1997;21: 139–165.
12. Rooney PJ. Hyperlipidemias, lipid storage disorders, metal storage disorders, and ochronosis. *Curr Opin Rheumatol* 1991;3: 166–171.
13. Gorman JD, Danning C, Schumacher HR, et al. Multicentric reticulohistiocytosis: case report with immunohistochemical analysis and literature review. *Arthritis Rheum* 2000;43: 930–938.

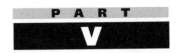

INFECTIOUS ARTHRITIS

BACTERIAL ARTHRITIS

ARTHUR KAVANAUGH

Bacterial arthritis is a significant condition that can be associated with substantial morbidity and accelerated mortality. Despite the advances in antimicrobial therapy, diagnostic testing, and general medical care in recent years, the prognosis for patients with bacterial arthritis continues to be guarded. Perhaps the most important factor regarding the outcome of patients with bacterial arthritis is the speed with which appropriate therapy is instituted. Therefore it remains as true at the start of the new millennium as it has for more than half a century: clinical suspicion of the diagnosis of bacterial arthritis is the most critical consideration for the clinician.

ETIOLOGY

Most cases of bacterial arthritis result from hematogenous dissemination of bacteria into the joint. Parenthetically, it is of note that in the vast majority of cases of bacteremia, septic arthritis does not develop. This highlights the critical roles of joint integrity and host defense in preventing this condition. Indeed, the most important factors associated with increased risk of bacterial arthritis are articular damage and immunosuppression. Joints that have been damaged by arthritis (e.g., rheumatoid arthritis, osteoarthritis, crystalline arthritis) or other conditions (e.g., trauma, sickle cell disease) are more susceptible to infection than normal joints. Likewise, joints with prosthetic components (e.g., after joint replacement) may be more likely to become infected during bacteremic episodes. Factors that interfere with host defense, such as primary immunodeficiencies (e.g., hypogammaglobulinemia) and the much more common secondary immunodeficiencies, may also predispose to bacterial arthritis. Important acquired immunodeficiencies include those associated with systemic illness (e.g., diabetes mellitus, AIDS, chronic liver disease, cancer, renal failure, rheumatoid arthritis), advancing age, and the use of immunosuppressive medications (e.g., corticosteroids, cytotoxic agents). Overall, the vast majority of cases of bacterial arthritis occur among patients with some degree of impaired structural integrity of the joint and suboptimal immune responsiveness.

In addition to hematogenous spread, bacterial arthritis may result from spread from contiguous structures (e.g., from adjacent foci of osteomyelitis, cellulitis, or septic bursitis). For that reason it is critical that penetration into a joint never be attempted through skin or surrounding structures suspected to be infected. Direct inoculation of bacteria (e.g., during arthroscopy or joint injection) is another potential avenue for causing bacterial arthritis.

DIAGNOSIS

The most important aspect of the diagnosis of bacterial arthritis is a high index of clinical suspicion in susceptible persons. The presentation of bacterial arthritis is usually that of acute, inflammatory, monoarticular arthritis. Although *acute* is typically defined as "having less than 6 weeks of involvement," some patients with bacterial arthritis may have symptoms presenting over a longer duration (e.g., if there was a delay in establishing the diagnosis). In any patient presenting with monoarticular arthritis, septic arthritis must be high on the differential diagnosis list. Likewise, patients known to have other forms of arthritis (e.g., someone with established RA) who present with new symptoms in one joint that are out of proportion to the arthritis elsewhere should be suspected of having bacterial arthritis. Because bacterial arthritis is an inflammatory type of arthritis, the diagnosis will be facilitated if the clinician is confident in his or her physical examination skills regarding differentiation of arthritis from involvement of structures surrounding the joint (e.g., skin, bursae, tendons). Although most cases of bacterial arthritis are monoarticular, a third or more may be polyarticular. Thus polyarticular involvement should never be considered to exclude the diagnosis of bacterial arthritis. In addition to complaints referred to involved joints, many patients with bacterial arthritis present with systemic symptoms indicative of an active ongoing infection, such as fever, malaise, and weight loss. However, patients may be afebrile and lack any other symptoms. The lack of associated symptoms and the potential for atypical presentations contribute to the delay in diagnosis that often leads to severe complications. Therefore a high degree of clinical suspicion, particularly when encountering patients with the predisposing factors described earlier, is key to the timely diagnosis of bacterial arthritis.

The cornerstone of the diagnosis of bacterial arthritis is aspiration and analysis of synovial fluid (Table 27.1). Although it is possible to obtain numerous types of tests on synovial fluid samples, the only tests of proven value are the white blood cell (WBC) count and differential, the Gram stain and culture, and crystal analysis (1). The WBC count will establish whether the synovial fluid is inflammatory (i.e., >2,000 WBC/mm³; or >75% neutrophils) or noninflammatory. In general, synovial fluids from patients with bacterial arthritis often appear more purulent and have higher WBC counts (e.g., >50,000 WBC/mm³) than those from patients with autoimmune inflammatory arthritis, such as rheumatoid arthritis. However, for an individual patient this generality may not be useful, and suspected bacterial arthritis should always be investigated with culture. Gram staining of synovial fluids from patients with bacterial arthritis is often positive and may be helpful in guiding initial antibiotic therapy. However, a negative Gram stain does not exclude infection. Culture is definitive and is positive in most cases of bacterial arthritis (with the important exception of gonococcal arthritis; see later). Nevertheless, false-negative cultures can occur (e.g., in patients who have received prior antibiotic therapy). Concomitant blood cultures may be helpful (e.g., if technical problems occurred during obtaining or processing the synovial fluid specimens). If there is suspicion for organisms with fastidious growth characteristics, the laboratory should be alerted so that cultures can be appropriately processed. Analysis of synovial fluid for crystals (e.g., monosodium urate, calcium pyrophosphate) is relevant, as crystalline arthritis (e.g., gout, pseudogout) figures prominently in the differential diagnosis of patients with acute monoarticular inflammatory arthritis. Moreover, among noninfectious causes of inflammatory arthritis, synovial fluid WBC counts are often markedly elevated in patients with crystalline arthritis. However, the presence of crystals in a synovial fluid specimen does not exclude the possibility of concomitant infection; if there is clinical suspicion, appropriate culture should be obtained.

Imaging studies are often of limited value in the diagnosis of bacterial arthritis early in the disease course. Bony changes on plain radiographs take 2 to 3 weeks or more to develop. X-rays obtained at earlier time points may show only soft-tissue swelling. In more chronic cases, plain radiographs demonstrate destructive changes that are characteristic of bacterial arthritis and highlight its rapid and pernicious course (Fig. 27.1). Erosions that have relatively indistinct margins may be indicative of septic arthritis, as opposed to other conditions that can be associated with bony erosions (e.g., gout, RA), which may have erosions with more clearly defined edges. For patients with prosthetic joints, bone respiration, lucency at the bone–implant interface, and periosteal reaction on radiographs suggest the possibility of septic arthritis. CT scanning provides greater detail but is subject to similar limitations as conventional radiography. Radionuclide scintigraphy (i.e., bone scanning) will typically demonstrate rapidly increased uptake in septic joints; however, it cannot definitely establish or exclude bacterial arthritis. Similarly, magnetic resonance imaging (MRI) is very sensitive for identifying inflammatory changes in articular tissues. Whether it can be useful in establishing the diagnosis of bacterial arthritis remains to be established.

MICROBIOLOGY

The microbiology of bacterial arthritis can be divided into infections caused by gonococci and those caused by other organisms. Overall, gonococcal arthritis accounts for about 20% of cases of bacterial arthritis. Affected patients are often younger and healthier than patients with other bacterial arthritis. A number of other characteristics of disease are disparate between gonococcal arthritis and bacterial arthritis from other causes (see the following section).

The largest series of cases of bacterial arthritis come from studies of elderly persons, patients with rheumatoid arthritis, and patients who have undergone arthroplasty (Tables 27.2 and 27.3) (2,3). Data from these studies show that the

---

TABLE 27.1. SUSPECTED BACTERIAL ARTHRITIS: KEY POINTS IN JOINT ASPIRATION

Never aspirate a joint through infected skin or soft tissues
Obtain white blood cell (WBC) count with differential, Gram stain and culture, and possibly crystal analysis from the aspirated synovial fluid
When there is clinical suspicion of infection, initiate antimicrobial therapy immediately after aspiration
Joint aspiration may be performed serially to remove infected fluid and assess WBC counts over time to help gauge clinical response to therapy
Consider orthopedic consultation for prosthetic joints, hip joints (particularly in children), or open drainage if clinical response is suboptimal
Use extreme care aspirating a prosthetic joint

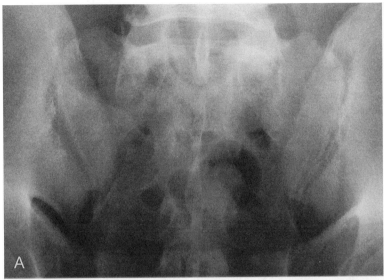

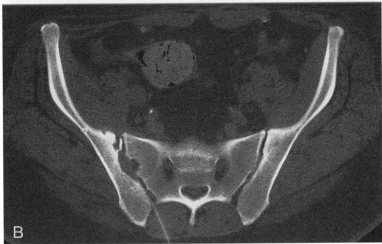

FIGURE 27.1. Sacroiliac joint infection with *Staphylococcus aureus* in a hemodialysis patient. Plain radiograph **(A)** shows joint widening and indistinct joint margins of the right sacroiliac joint. Computerized tomogram **(B)** shows bony erosion and fragmentation about the right sacroiliac joint. The patient had symptoms of pain in the region for 10 weeks before diagnostic aspiration. (From Ike RW. Bacterial arthritis. In: Koopman WJ, ed. *Arthritis and allied conditions: a textbook of rheumatology,* 14th ed. Philadelphia: Lippincott Williams & Wilkins, 2001:2570–2599, with permission.)

TABLE 27.2. CHARACTERISTICS OF BACTERIAL ARTHRITIS IN THE ELDERLY[a] IN PERCENT

Underlying joint disease	66
Knee involvement	50
Shoulder involvement	25
Associated mortality	30
Culture results	
Staphylococcus aureus infections	66
Gram negative infections	20

[a]Mean age 70 years.

TABLE 27.3. BACTERIAL ARTHRITIS IN RHEUMATOID ARTHRITIS PATIENTS[a] IN PERCENT

Systemic corticosteroids	53
Fever	42
Hypothermia	22
Prosthetic joint	8
Polyarticular	34
Fatal outcome	27
Culture results	
Staphylococci	58
Streptococci/pneumococci	18
Gram negative bacteria	16
Positive blood cultures	60

[a]Mean age: 60 years. Duration of rheumatoid arthritis: 14 years.

most important organisms causing nongonococcal arthritis are the Gram-positive cocci. *Staphylococcus* species, predominantly *S. aureus* but also coagulase-negative organisms (e.g., *S. epidermidis*), account for half to two-thirds of cases of bacterial arthritis in the elderly. These organisms also are responsible for approximately three-quarters of cases of bacterial arthritis in RA patients, and 75% to 90% of cases in patients with prosthetic joints. Because they are such a frequent cause of bacterial arthritis, the increasing prevalence of methicillin-resistant staphylococci is an important consideration when empirically treating bacterial arthritis (i.e., before culture and sensitivity results are known). Infections with staphylococci can lead to extensive, rapid destruction of the joint if the infections are not promptly diagnosed and aggressively treated (Fig. 27.1).

After staphylococci, the most common cause of bacterial arthritis comes from the streptococci, which account for 15% to 30% of cases of nongonococcal arthritis. Overall, the outcome following joint infection with streptococci tends to be more benign than that seen with staphylococcal infections. However, certain subtypes of streptococci may have a more aggressive course. Early diagnosis and prompt treatment are still essential.

Gram-negative bacilli account for as many as a quarter of cases of bacterial arthritis. In many cases, Gram-negative joint infections develop in patients with serious systemic illnesses, in patients with suppressed immune systems (e.g., chemotherapy-induced neutropenia), or in intravenous drug users. Commonly isolated organisms include *Pseudomonas aeruginosa, Escherichia coli,* and *Proteus mirabilis.* Related in part to the subset of patients affected, the response to therapy among patients with Gram-negative bacterial arthritis is often suboptimal, and the outcomes poor.

Anaerobic bacteria comprise less than 1% of cases of bacterial arthritis, although they may be involved in 5% or more of infections in prosthetic joints. This may be an underestimate, as such bacteria have historically been difficult to isolate in routine clinical practice. Organisms commonly implicated in anaerobic bacterial arthritis include fusobacterium, *Bacteroides fragilis,* and clostridium. Adequate drainage of the affected area is a key adjunct to antimicrobial therapy in such cases.

Brucellosis appears to be increasing in importance as a cause of infectious arthritis. Humans are exposed to brucella via consumption of unpasteurized milk or dairy products, or direct contact with infected animals. The major joint manifestation in brucellosis is sacroiliac involvement, typically unilateral and nondestructive. Peripheral arthritis occurs in about a third of cases, most often monoarthritis of the hip or knee. Concomitant systemic symptoms such as fever, arthralgias, and headache are often prominent. Culture of organisms from affected synovial fluid is slow (taking 3 to 4 weeks) and of low yield (positive in fewer than 50% of cases). Therefore serologic testing for brucella specific antibodies can be useful in supporting the diagnosis.

A variety of other bacteria can be associated with infectious arthritis (4). Uncommon causes should be considered in the appropriate clinical setting, or if appropriate testing fails to demonstrate one of the more common etiologic agents.

GONOCOCCAL ARTHRITIS

As opposed to other causes of bacterial arthritis, disseminated gonococcal infection tends to occur in younger, healthier patients. Diagnosis can be difficult, as only 25% of patients recall a history suggestive of urethritis or cervicitis. Women tend to have asymptomatic genital infection more commonly than men. Common clinical characteristics of disseminated gonococcal infection are shown in Table 27.4 (5). Migratory arthralgias are common, but because they are nonspecific they are often unhelpful diagnostically. Tenosynovitis can be an important diagnostic clue. It is uncommon in other forms of infectious or noninfectious inflammatory arthritis, with the exception of gout; however, the populations at risk for gout and gonococcal arthritis are often distinct. The dorsum of the wrist is a frequently involved area, as is the ankle. Skin lesions, which are typically painless, usually present as multiple small macules on the extremities.

Diagnosis of gonococcal arthritis is made much more difficult by the infrequent positive culture results. Even with attention to proper culture technique (chocolate agar, rapid plating, etc.) most synovial and blood samples will not demonstrate growth of gonococcus (Table 27.4). Culture from genitourinary sites has a higher yield, and this is therefore an important adjunct in establishing a presumptive diagnosis of gonococcal arthritis. More sensitive techniques for identification of gonococci, such as the polymerase chain reaction (PCR) with specific primers, may offer additional sensitivity for analysis of synovial samples in the near future.

Because of the potential difficulty in diagnosing gonococcal arthritis, a number of cases go untreated. Although

TABLE 27.4. CHARACTERISTICS OF DISSEMINATED GONOCOCCAL INFECTION (IN PERCENT)

Migratory polyarthralgia	70
Tenosynovitis	67
Skin lesions	67
Fever	63
Purulent arthritis	42
Monoarticular	32
Polyarticular	10
Positive culture results	
Genitourinary tract	80
Synovial fluid	27
Rectum	21
Pharynx	10
Blood	5
Skin	0

joint symptoms tend to wax and wane, joint destruction can occur if the infection is not appropriately treated.

SPECIAL CIRCUMSTANCES

Bacterial Arthritis in Children

Several characteristics of bacterial arthritis in children are distinct from that in adults (6). More children develop bacterial arthritis from contiguous osteomyelitis than do adults. The spectrum of common pathogens causing bacterial arthritis in young children include streptococci and *Haemophilus influenzae,* which derives in part from the relative inefficiency of antibody-mediated immune defenses in that age group. Bacterial joint infections in children prominently involve the large joints of the lower extremities. Of note, bacterial arthritis of the hip in children typically requires open surgical drainage. Finally, because children's bones are still in the process of growing and developing, destructive sequel from untreated septic arthritis can have even more profound implications with regard to body habitus and functional status.

Bacterial Arthritis in Immunocompromised Patients

Impairments in immune defense are important factors in the development of bacterial arthritis in most affected patients. In addition, patients with defects in specific components of the immune response tend to develop particular infections reflective of their immunodeficiency. For example, patients with defects in antibody mediated responses (e.g., common variable immunodeficiency, X-linked agammaglobulinemia) are more susceptible to infection by encapsulated organisms (e.g., pneumococci, *H. influenzae*). Patients with defects in cellular immunity (e.g., AIDS) are particularly susceptible to infection with intracellular organisms, including viruses, mycobacteria, and listeria, among others. Patients with impaired neutrophil function are more susceptible to infection with staphylococci and Gram-negative bacilli. Thus patients with known immunodeficiencies should be considered at particular risk for certain organisms.

Prosthetic Joint Infections

Infections in prosthetic joints pose a particularly vexing clinical problem. Patients can present with an acute arthritis, but not infrequently they have a prolonged, indolent course with no signs of systemic toxicity. Prosthetic joints have different risk for postoperative infections, with the elbow having the highest risk, followed by the knee and the hip.

Microbiology of prosthetic joint infections is associated with timing of surgery. Close to surgery (first 2 or 3 months) the most common pathogens include skin flora, most notably

S. aureus and *S. epidermidis.* Occasionally, hospital pathogens, such as Gram-negative organisms, can cause wound infections with subsequent joint involvement. Infections occurring after this initial time period are almost universally related to hematogenous seeding of the prosthetic valve. Although *S. aureus* remains the most common pathogen, urinary tract and gastrointestinal tract pathogens are occasionally implicated. Although conservative approaches have theoretical appeal, removal of the prosthesis followed by subsequent reimplantation may offer the best overall outcome (7). In cases of suspected infection of joint prostheses, consultation with an orthopedist should be strongly considered.

DIFFERENTIAL DIAGNOSIS OF BACTERIAL ARTHRITIS

Bacterial arthritis may be confused with other conditions that can present with an acute monoarticular or oligoarticular inflammatory arthritis (Table 27.5). In addition to these conditions, arthritis that typically manifests with polyarticular involvement, such as rheumatoid arthritis, can present initially in a more limited fashion.

PRINCIPLES OF TREATMENT

Appropriate antibiotic therapy is the mainstay of therapy for bacterial arthritis. The choice of agent as well as the duration of therapy will depend on the etiologic organism. Empiric antibiotic therapy should be based upon the most likely organisms, given the characteristics of the affected patient. Depending upon local conditions, the prevalence of resistance of some bacteria to standard therapy (e.g., methicillin-resistant staphylococci, penicillin-resistant streptococci, penicillin-resistant *Neisseria*) needs to be considered.

TABLE 27.5. DIFFERENTIAL DIAGNOSIS OF BACTERIAL ARTHRITIS

Other infectious arthritis
Viral arthritis
Mycobacterial arthritis
Fungal arthritis
Lyme disease
Crystalline arthritis
Gout
Pseudogout
Spondyloarthropathies
Reiter syndrome
Ankylosing spondylitis
Reactive arthritis (e.g., poststreptococcal)
Nonarthritic conditions
Cellulitis
Bursitis
Fracture
Foreign-body reaction

Drainage of joints affected by bacterial arthritis has been a time-honored approach to minimizing the damage associated with infection as well as aiding the response to antimicrobial therapy. For most joints, repeated needle arthrocentesis is sufficient, and open drainage is unnecessary. Serial evaluation of synovial fluid WBC counts has been shown to correlate with outcome. Progressive decrement in WBC numbers is typically seen as an infection resolves, whereas persistent elevation in counts tends to indicate poor response to therapy.

CONCLUSION

Bacterial arthritis continues to be an important health problem. Clinical suspicion, rapid diagnosis, and prompt therapy are key to improving outcomes.

REFERENCES

1. Schmerling RH, Delbanco ML, Tosteson AN, et al. Synovial fluid tests: What should be ordered? *JAMA* 1990;264:1009–1014.
2. Ho G, Su EY. Therapy of septic arthritis. *JAMA* 1982;247:797–800.
3. Dubost JJ, Fis I, Sorbier M, et al. Septic arthritis in patients with rheumatoid arthritis: a review of twenty-four cases and of the medical literature. *Rev Rhum (Engl Ed)* 1994;61:143–156.
4. Ike RW. Bacterial arthritis. In: Koopman WJ, ed. *Arthritis and allied conditions: a textbook of rheumatology,* 14th ed. Philadelphia: Lippincott Williams & Wilkins, 2001:2570–2599.
5. O'Brien JP, Goldenberg DL, Rice PA. Disseminated gonococcal infection: a prospective analysis of 49 patients and a review of pathophysiology and immune mechanisms. *Medicine (Baltimore).* 1983;62:395–406.
6. Fink CW, Nelson JD. Septic arthritis and osteomyelitis in children. *Clin Rheum Dis* 1986;12:423–435.
7. Ivey FM, Hicks CA, Calhoun JH, et al. Treatment options for infected knee arthroplasties. *Rev Infect Dis* 1990;12:468–478.

ARTHRITIS DUE TO MYCOBACTERIA, FUNGI, AND PARASITES

MAREN LAWSON MAHOWALD

The clinical presentations of tuberculous, fungal, and parasitic infections of the musculoskeletal system are very similar to noninfectious chronic inflammatory musculoskeletal disorders. These infections may not be considered initially; therefore the correct diagnosis is often delayed. The incidence of mycobacterial and fungal infections that are normally restricted to certain geographic regions is increasing in nonendemic areas because of immigration and travel from developing countries. The clinical importance of fungal infections is greater today because of the increasing numbers of susceptible individuals: immunocompromised patients as a result of human immunodeficiency virus (HIV) infection, malignancy, chemotherapy, immunosuppressive therapy for organ transplantation, and the expanding population of elderly patients with chronic debilitating diseases. Timely diagnosis requires a high index of suspicion based on the knowledge of the typical features as well as unusual clinical presentations. These infections should be sought in patients with chronic monoarticular or pauciarticular arthritis and should be considered in other situations, such as spondylitis, spondylodiscitis, tendonitis, and erythema nodosum. Definitive diagnosis depends on identification of the organism in synovial fluid, synovial tissue, abscesses, or osseous tissue.

MYCOBACTERIAL INFECTIONS

Mycobacterium Tuberculosis

Epidemiology

An estimated 8 million people worldwide are infected with *Mycobacterium tuberculosis* and 2 million deaths were attributed to tuberculosis (TB) in 1998 (1,2). In the United States there was a resurgence of TB until 1992 (26,673 cases) that was associated with the HIV epidemic; increased immigration from TB-endemic countries; increased TB transmission in nursing homes, hospitals, and prisons, and among the homeless; and emergence of multidrug-resistant

strains (3). From 1992 to 1998 the number of TB cases in the United States declined 31% to 18,361 (case rate 6.8/100,000) largely because of more effective TB control programs (4) (Fig. 28.1). Nevertheless, approximately 15 million persons in the United States have latent TB infection and are at risk for future disease. Since the mid-1980s the proportion of TB cases increased among foreign-born residents from Asia, Africa, and Latin America, where TB rates are five to 30 times higher than those in the United States (5). HIV-infected people are at much higher risk for active TB disease and have higher rates of infection with multidrug-resistant strains (6,7). During 1998, 8.1% of TB cases were infected with strains resistant to isoniazid and 1.1% were multidrug resistant (8).

Extrapulmonary TB can involve almost any organ system (Fig. 28.2) and remains a cause of fever of unknown origin (9,10). In 1997 there were 3,554 cases of extrapulmonary TB (17.9% of 19,851 total TB cases) (11). Approximately 11% of extrapulmonary TB involves bones and joints (about 2% of all TB cases). Extrapulmonary TB occurs more often in racial and ethnic minorities, those with HIV infection, immigrants from high-prevalence countries, the elderly, children less than 15 years of age, and others who are immunocompromised. In persons with HIV infection, the incidence of TB is 500 times that of the general population, and 25% to 50% of new TB patients are HIV positive (12,13). The proportion of extrapulmonary TB is increased in this group of patients, and the time from infection to disease is decreased. The control of TB is further complicated by the emergence of multidrug-resistant organisms. Most new infections with multidrug-resistant TB are seen in individuals from developing countries and those who are also infected with HIV (14).

Pathophysiology

Infection with *M. tuberculosis* occurs via inhalation of aerosolized bacteria from the index case with pulmonary

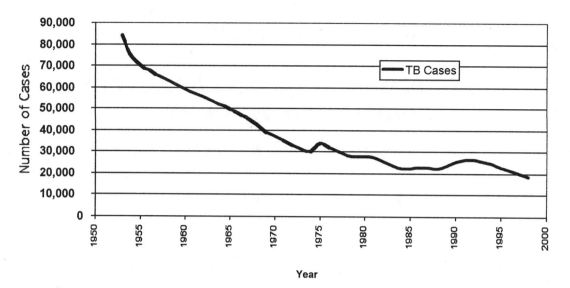

FIGURE 28.1. Cases of tuberculosis in the United States. (From Progress toward the elimination of tuberculosis: United States, 1998. *MMWR*1999;48:732–736, and Summary of notifiable diseases, United States, 1997. *MMWR* 1998;46:1–87, with permission. Reprinted in Mahowald ML. Arthritis due to mycobacteria, fungi, and parasites. In: Koopman WJ, ed. *Arthritis and allied conditions: a textbook of rheumatology,*14th ed., Philadelphia: Lippincott Williams & Wilkins, 2001:2607–2628.)

TB. *De novo* infection in the nonimmunized host depends on the number of organisms that survive phagocytosis by alveolar macrophages. Mycobacteria multiply intracellularly and rupture the alveolar macrophage. Hematogenous dissemination to distant organs may produce metastatic foci capable of recrudescence of active infection at later times. Other organisms reach the lymphatic

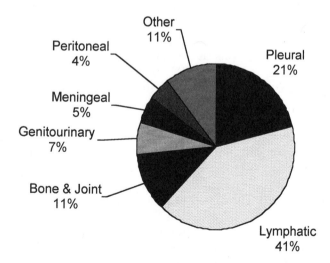

FIGURE 28.2. Extrapulmonary tuberculosis in the United States. (From Division of TB Elimination, CDC Surveillance Reports. *Reported tuberculosis in the US, 1996 and 1997, June 21, 1999 update.* Atlanta: Centers for Disease Control, 1999, with permission. Reprinted in Mahowald ML. Arthritis due to mycobacteria, fungi, and parasites. In: Koopman WJ, ed. *Arthritis and allied conditions: a textbook of rheumatology,*14th ed. Philadelphia: Lippincott Williams & Wilkins, 2001:2607–2628.)

system and regional lymph nodes, where cellular immunity is generated. CD4+ T cells provide protective immune responses in the lung, help B cells and CD8+ cytotoxic suppressor cells, and produce cytokines that recruit more monocytes and participate in granuloma formation (Ghon lesion). Humoral immunity plays a negligible role against TB, but genetic susceptibility to infection appears to be real. In nursing homes and prisons, the TB infection rate is twofold greater in blacks than in whites (15).

Clinical TB represents failure of the local immune defense. If the initial lesion is not sterilized by the inflammatory response, tuberculous pneumonia develops. In patients who are positive for purified protein derivative (PPD), clinical disease results from reactivation rather than from reinfection. Trauma or local factors appear to play a role in the reactivation of disease (16,17), and rates of reactivation are higher in immunocompromised individuals (18,19). Osteoarticular TB tends to be a disease of children in developing countries and a disease of the elderly and immunocompromised individuals in Western countries. Skeletal infection can develop by hematogenous or lymphatic spread from chronic pleural, renal, or lymph node foci, or by reactivation of latent infection at sites seeded in the primary illness (20,21).

In the United States osteoarticular TB usually results from recrudescence of latent infection. The rarity of bone and joint TB in Western countries has lowered the index of suspicion in the medical community, often resulting in unfortunate delays in diagnosis for many months or years (22), or misdiagnosis as osteoarthritis, rheumatoid arthritis, and bone metastases. Articular TB typically develops when a focus of osteomyelitis in adjacent subchondral epiphyseal bone erodes through the articular surface into the joint space. Rarely, the synovium may be seeded directly via the bloodstream. An initial inflammatory reaction is followed by formation of granulation tissue, effusion, and production of a pannus. Mycobacteria do not produce collagenase, so the articular surface is not rapidly destroyed as in pyogenic infections. The proliferative synovial pannus destroys the cartilage at the periphery of the joint, erodes into subchondral cancellous bone, and produces demineralization and necrosis, destroying the support structure of the articular cartilage. Ultimately, the process results in severe destruction of bone, formation of paraarticular cold abscesses, and spontaneous external fistulization. Healing takes place by the formation of fibrous tissue, which often produces fibrous ankylosis of the joint (23).

Pathogenic mechanisms leading to spinal TB include (a) hematogenous dissemination during the initial infection that produces granulomas in bone, causing bone destruction; (b) spread of infection to bone via lymphatic drainage from another focus of TB (e.g., from pleural or kidney via paraaortic lymph nodes to erode into the vertebral body), or (c) recrudescence of an old pulmonary infection with hematogenous spread to the spine, in which case the patient will also have signs of pulmonary TB infection (24). Patterns of tuberculous spinal involvement include paradiscal, anterior, and central (25). In the paradiscal or spondylodiscitis form, infection typically starts in the anterior portion of the vertebral bodies and invades the disc space early. As the disc and anterior vertebrae are destroyed, the characteristic anterior wedging of two adjacent vertebrae with disc space loss produces the kyphotic gibbus deformity. Anterior lesions develop under the anterior spinal ligament to involve several vertebrae. Central lesions (spondylitis without disc involvement) involve the entire vertebral body, resulting in significant deformity. Abscesses are common and may dissect for long distances along fascial planes to form abscesses remote from the spinal infection. There are several mechanisms of neurologic injury in spinal TB. Paraspinal abscesses may exert ischemic pressure on the subjacent spinal cord, whereas posterior extrusion of caseous or granulation tissue may cause anterior cord compression or inflammatory vasculitis with thrombosis of the spinal vessels. Sudden cord transection with severe spinal instability may occur rarely. Spinal root compression may occur with arachnoiditis or extension of paraosseous abscess through the dura.

Clinical Features

Tuberculous infection of diarthrodial joints produces chronic low-grade pain, swelling, and stiffness with slowly progressive loss of function and eventual abscess formation (26). In endemic regions, the weight-bearing joints are most commonly affected (60% to 90%), whereas in nonendemic areas, upper-extremity joints may be involved almost as frequently as lower-extremity joints. The arthritis presents as chronic monoarticular disease in approximately 85% of patients. Involvement of three or more joints is very rare (27,28). The peak incidence of peripheral arthritis is in the fourth and fifth decades in developed countries, where it is rare in patients in the first decade of life, and the incidence in males and nonwhites is much higher than that in females and whites. Tuberculous arthritis in children may be difficult to distinguish from juvenile inflammatory arthritis, resulting in delayed diagnosis unless a tuberculin skin test is performed during the evaluation of chronic monoarthritis (29,30). A poly- or oligoarticular pattern of TB may be seen in the elderly, immunocompromised individuals, those on corticosteroids, or those who have experienced trauma (31,32).

Multifocal TB of bone is rare and tends to be seen in individuals from endemic areas who are immunosuppressed, on chronic corticosteroid treatment, alcoholic, or elderly. Cases with multifocal osteoarticular TB may be misdiagnosed as malignant disease, especially in nonendemic areas (33). Half the patients may have no evidence for pulmonary TB and may have a negative tuberculin skin test (34). The most common presentation is chronic progressive joint pain and swelling without warmth or erythema, loss of motion, and often periarticular abscess formation and spontaneous drainage. Systemic symptoms that may occur include fever, night sweats, weight loss, anorexia, cough, and dyspnea. However, as many as 42% may be afebrile, and a third of patients may have no systemic symptoms (35). In one large series, Garrido et al. (20) reported radiographic changes in peripheral TB infection that included soft-tissue swelling (90%), osteopenia (72%), joint space narrowing (66%), erosions (64%), cysts (66%), bony sclerosis (20%), periostitis (15%), and calcifications (5%).

In the hip, tubercle bacilli may localize in the synovium, acetabulum, or proximal femur. Bony destruction is seen most commonly in the acetabulum. The femoral neck and capital and trochanteric epiphysis, or trochanteric bursa may also be involved (36,37). Symptoms include mild-to-moderate pain in the groin, knee, or thigh, and limitation of motion. A limp is the most common presenting complaint in children. Atrophy of the gluteal muscles and tenderness in the groin are often present. At rest, the hip is held in flexion and abduction. Later, severe destruction of the femoral neck and acetabulum occurs with formation of a cold abscess and sinus tract, which usually points to the outer thigh.

In the knee, pain is insidious in onset and may be present for years before the patient seeks medical attention.

About 20% of patients describe swelling, and 10% have stiffness as the initial complaint. Localized heat and muscular wasting are usually present on examination. A limp, synovial swelling, and limitation of motion are common. Although pure synovial infection does occur, most patients have involvement of both synovium and bone (38). In the ankle, elbow, and wrist, joint damage results in marked joint instability that usually requires arthrodesis or spontaneous fusion for functional restoration after antituberculous therapy (39).

TB infection of prosthetic joints is usually due to reactivation of previous osteoarticular infection and occurs years after implantation or may be identified at the time of arthroplasty (40). Clinically, joint pain is slowly progressive, and joint aspiration usually does not yield fluid. Multiple samples of tissue should be obtained for histologic and culture studies. Infection may be eradicated without removing the prosthesis but requires prolonged multidrug therapy (41,42). Soft-tissue sites of tuberculous infection (the synovial tissue in tendon sheaths; bursa; muscle; or deep fascia) are uncommon but may mimic common local inflammatory disorders and are therefore likely to be misdiagnosed (43). Soft-tissue infections cause focal swelling, which may or may not be painful and often coexist with involvement of adjacent bony structures. Reported cases often had a history of rheumatic diseases and had been treated with corticosteroids and immunosuppressive drugs, or were on dialysis (44). A history of antecedent local trauma may be obtained (45). Diagnosis may be delayed because a bursal injection of corticosteroid may produce a temporary decrease in the swelling or pain. TB involving tendons in the hand and wrist may cause a carpal tunnel syndrome (46). Infection of the trochanteric bursa and subdeltoid bursa have also been reported.

Tuberculous rheumatism, or Poncet disease, was reported in 1887. Poncet described inflammatory polyarthritis of the hands and feet in 12 patients with a past or current history of visceral TB. He called it tuberculous rheumatism; however, there was no evidence of bacteriologic involvement of the joints themselves. The concept of a reactive arthritis to TB has remained controversial because the rigor with which foci of TB infection were sought in these cases has been variable (47–50).

In the early twentieth century, TB of the spine was common and caused severe disability (51). Since the advent of antituberculous drugs characteristic spinal deformities and neurologic damage have declined. Spinal TB accounts for 50% of skeletal TB. Recently, in the United Kingdom and France, up to 70% of patients with spinal TB were foreign-born patients from developing countries (52). In endemic regions, spinal TB (Pott disease) is seen primarily in children and young adults. In the United States and Europe most patients are more than 20 years of age (mean, 49; range, 24 to 76). The clinical presentation is usually that of insidious pain with a history of weight loss, fever, malaise associated with neurologic deficits, abscesses, or sinus tracts. Approximately one-third of patients with spinal TB have no evidence of extraspinal TB, but two-thirds have pulmonary TB, and half of these have disseminated disease (53). Patients may also have symptoms from affected organ systems, such as the urinary, pulmonary, and lymphatic systems. The thoracic spine is most commonly involved, followed by the lumbar spine, and cervical spine. More than one vertebral body (average, two and one-half; range, one to five) and the disc space are usually involved. Skip areas with radiographically normal vertebrae in between occur in about 10% of patients. Paraspinous abscesses are common (50% to 96%) and may involve the neck, groin, chest wall, or sternum. The incidence of neurologic symptoms caused by cord compression in spinal TB (Pott paraplegia) varies from 12% to 50% in different series. Epidural compression of the cord or cauda equina may occur, and coexistent cord and root compression may cause both upper and lower motor neuron weakness. In the United States, patients with spinal TB are predominantly male (70%), 50% are immigrants, 45% are homeless, 25% are HIV-infected, and 25% are intravenous drug users.

Other notable sites of TB of the axial skeleton are the sacroiliac joints and the ribs. Rib lesions are often associated with a local soft-tissue mass and pain. They generally occur in patients with other skeletal involvement, particularly in the spine. Sacroiliac joint involvement, usually unilateral, occurs in about 7% of patients with skeletal TB. With sacroiliac joint infection the chief complaint is buttock and low back pain for 2 weeks to more than 1 year, described as continuous and severe enough to awaken from sleep at night. Most patients have constitutional symptoms and tenderness to direct palpation of the sacroiliac joint (54,55).

A mycotic aneurysm of the aorta, created when a paraspinous abscess penetrates the vessel wall, may occasionally complicate spinal TB. The resulting hematoma walls off to form a false aneurysm. Penetration of the abscess into the arterial blood may lead to secondary hematogenous spread and miliary disease (56).

Clinical Evaluation

Diagnosis of tuberculous arthritis requires a high index of suspicion and acquisition of material for histologic examination and culture. Microbiologic and histologic studies are complementary for maximum diagnostic yield. The quickest and most reliable method of diagnosis is biopsy. A positive diagnosis can be made by either histology or culture of synovial tissue in more than 90% of specimens.

Synovial fluid culture is positive in approximately 25% to 80%, and smear is positive in 20% to 40% of cases. Synovial fluid protein is always elevated, and 60% of patients have fluid with low glucose levels. The synovial white blood cell count varies widely but is usually between 10,000 and 20,000/mm³ with more than 75% polymorphonuclear leukocytes. In the case of spinal disease, material for culture is best obtained with a needle biopsy guided by fluoroscopy or CT.

Laboratory Testing

Peripheral white blood cell count is usually normal, and the sedimentation rate is usually elevated. The tuberculin skin test with PPD (5-TU) may be helpful. A positive reaction of greater than 10 mm induration at 48 hours occurs in 50% to 90% of individuals infected with *M. tuberculosis*. Reactions of 5 to 10 mm may be seen with other mycobacterial infections, prior *Bacillus Calmette–Guérin* (BCG) immunization, and HIV-infected patients who are infected with *M. tuberculosis*. False-negative tuberculin tests are seen in 15% to 20% of patients with active infection who are elderly, immunocompromised, or malnourished. Two-step testing can be carried out if the initial test is negative and a second test is administered 1 to 3 weeks later. A positive second test is likely due to a boosted reaction resulting from TB infection that occurred a long time ago (57).

Major advances have been made in TB diagnostics, including methods with reduced time to detect growth of *M. tuberculosis* in specimens and rapid-detection methods using nucleic acid amplification techniques that provide results in hours (58). The BACTEC radiometric culture system (Becton, Dickinson and Company, Franklin Lakes, NJ, U.S.A.) contains radioactive palmitate as the sole carbon source and can detect the organism's metabolism in 2 to 6 days, thus reducing the time to detection of mycobacterial growth. Two new tests can identify *M. tuberculosis* ribosomal RNA (MTD, Gen-Probe, San Diego, CA, U.S.A.) and DNA (Amplicor; Roche Molecular Systems; Branchburg, NJ, U.S.A.) in clinical specimens within 24 hours (59) and have high sensitivity and specificity (60,61). However, these rapid tests do not replace acid-fast staining and culture of the tissues. Culture of the organism is necessary for drug susceptibility testing. Restriction fragment length polymorphism analyses are used to identify specific strains in localized outbreaks of infection (62). Direct amplification tests based on the polymerase chain reaction (PCR) have not had extensive testing with osteoarticular tissues (63). False-positive results can occur with contamination and false-negative results can occur if PCR inhibitors are present in infected tissues. PCR-based DATs have also been used to detect other mycobacterial and fungal infections.

Imaging Studies in Osteoarticular Tuberculosis

There are no pathognomonic roentgenographic signs of skeletal TB (64,65). In general, TB causes destruction of bone without stimulating much reactive new bone formation. Destructive osseous lesions adjacent to joints are often oval with clear margins (Fig. 28.3). As they expand and erode the cortex, some periosteal reaction occurs. Sequestrum of necrotic cancellous bone may occur. When the joint itself is involved, local osteopenia and soft-tissue swelling are early signs. Later, small, subchondral erosions appear at the margins of the joint (Fig. 28.4). The cartilage space tends to be preserved until extensive destruction of adjacent cortical bone has occurred (Fig. 28.5). With advanced disease, total destruction of the joint can occur. Destruction is not accompanied by osteophyte formation, but the shadow of a cold abscess containing calcified debris may be seen.

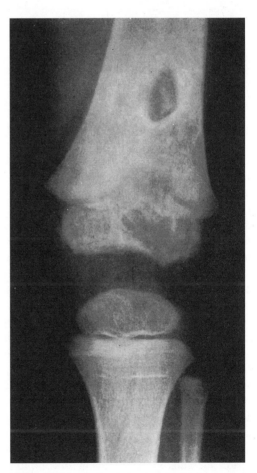

FIGURE 28.3. Tuberculosis of the knee and femur in a child. (From Mahowald ML. Arthritis due to mycobacteria, fungi, and parasites. In: Koopman WJ, ed. *Arthritis and allied conditions: a textbook of rheumatology,*14th ed. Philadelphia: Lippincott Williams & Wilkins, 2001:2607–2628, with permission.)

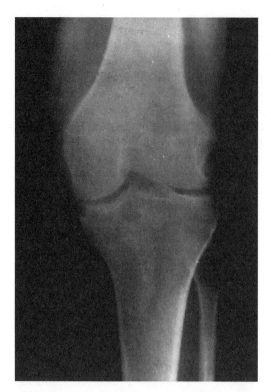

FIGURE 28.4. Tuberculosis of the knee in an adult. (Courtesy of Donald Resnick, MD. Reprinted in Mahowald ML. Arthritis due to mycobacteria, fungi, and parasites. In: Koopman WJ, ed. *Arthritis and allied conditions: a textbook of rheumatology,*14th ed., Philadelphia: Lippincott Williams & Wilkins, 2001:2607–2628.)

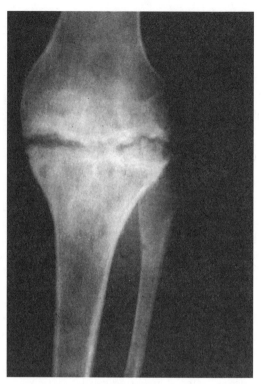

FIGURE 28.5. Advanced tuberculosis of the knee. (Courtesy of Donald Resnick, MD. Reprinted in Mahowald ML. Arthritis due to mycobacteria, fungi, and parasites. In: Koopman WJ, ed. *Arthritis and allied conditions: a textbook of rheumatology,*14th ed. Philadelphia: Lippincott Williams & Wilkins, 2001:2607–2628.)

Juxtaarticular osteopenia and cortical cyst formation may be complicated by spontaneous fractures.

In the spine, the classic picture is narrowing of the disc space with vertebral collapse and a paraspinous abscess. Scalloping of the anterior vertebral surface is common. Occasional infection of the central portion of the vertebrae may cause extensive bone destruction without disc space invasion. In about 10% of patients, productive or sclerotic changes, which are difficult to see radiographically, may occur in infected vertebrae. In the sacroiliac joint, TB infection produces joint space widening as a result of bony erosions in the sacral and iliac joint margins. Juxtaarticular sclerosis or osteopenia are equally prevalent. Bone scans may show increased uptake of ^{99m}Tc-pyrophosphate in early lesions; however, imaging may be insensitive with low-grade indolent or severely destructive lesions. Therefore a negative bone scan does not rule out the diagnosis of tuberculous bone infection. CT scanning is useful in delineating the extent of bone destruction and adjacent soft-tissue masses and in guiding percutaneous needle biopsy and drainage. MRI is useful in delineating the extent of disease, especially along the spinal cord.

Definitive diagnosis of spinal TB is made by biopsy guided by computed tomography (CT) to demonstrate a positive acid-fast smear, positive AFB culture, or granulomatous inflammation on histologic examination (66,67). The CT scan also defines the anatomy of the bony damage and paraspinal masses. Magnetic resonance imaging (MRI) is needed to evaluate compression of neural elements. If MRI is unavailable, a CT myelogram can be used. Plain radiographs are used to localize lesions and to measure alignment and deformity. Spinal deformity is present in most patients with thoracic and cervical lesions, and is less common in lumbar lesions (68,69). Bone scans may be negative in approximately one-third of cases.

In multifocal osteoarticular TB, lesions often have mild periosteal reaction, bone sclerosis, and severe bone destruction. Imaging with ^{99m}Tc is usually abnormal. The initial diagnosis is often malignancy, with correct diagnosis made on the biopsy.

Prevention and Therapy

Medical Treatment of Tuberculosis

For children with bone and joint TB, treatment should last at least 12 months. For adults treatment should be for 6 months. However, if the response is inadequate or slow, treatment should be prolonged to 12 months. The initial phase of treatment should be 8 weeks with four drugs: isoniazid (5 mg/kg, up to 300 mg orally daily), rifampin (10 mg/kg, up to 600 mg orally daily), pyrazinamide (15 to 30 mg/kg, up to 2 g daily), and ethambutol (15 to 25 mg/kg) or streptomycin (15 mg/kg up to 1 g daily) until susceptibility to INH and rifampin are shown. The continuation phase of treatment includes INH and rifampin daily for 16 to 44 weeks. If the incidence of multidrug-resistant TB is less than 4%, ethambutol or streptomycin may be unnecessary for patients with no individual risk factors for drug resistance (70,71). Updated recommendations for drug therapy can be readily obtained from the CDC World Wide Web site for the Morbidity and Mortality Weekly reports: http://www.cdc.gov/ (go to Publications and Scientific Data, then Morbidity and Mortality Weekly Report (MMWR). The major contraindication to the combined use of isoniazid and rifampin is the presence of active liver disease. Pyrazinamide and streptomycin should not be given to pregnant women. The optimum duration of treatment of osseous TB has not been defined. Response to treatment must be evaluated in each case (72). In articular TB with absent or minimal bone involvement, drug therapy alone may be effective (73).

Immobilization should be used early to relieve pain and prevent deformity or hip dislocation, especially in the young child. Joints should be repeatedly aspirated to remove purulent effusion, and joint lavage or arthroscopy should be used to ensure adequate drainage. If periarticular bone involvement is extensive, debridement of the foci of bone infection may hasten healing. Synovectomy with curettage may be important in children with hip disease (74). When articular destruction is extensive in weight-bearing joints, arthrodesis has been the procedure of choice to restore function in those too young for arthroplasty of joints such as ankles and wrists. In developing countries where sitting cross-legged and squatting are important, Girdlestone excision arthroplasty has been used effectively for hip disease. Total joint arthroplasty may be successful if the active infection is controlled (75).

Treatment options for spinal TB are selected based on the presence or absence of spinal instability, neurologic deficits, and level of surgical expertise available. In the preantibiotic era spinal TB was treated with prolonged immobilization and body casting. The mortality was 20%, and 20% to 30% had recurrence of infection. The initial success with chemotherapy in the 1960s prompted use of surgery to drain abscesses and markedly decreased the period of immobilization (76). In 1963 the Medical Research Council of Great Britain (MRC) began a multinational, clinical trial of five types of mechanical therapy combined with two chemotherapeutic regimens (PAS and INH for 18 months with or without streptomycin for the first 3 months). The five types of mechanical treatment included: (a) no restraints, (b) body cast in ambulant patients, (c) bed rest for 6 months, (d) minimal debridement, and (e) radical anterior excision with bone grafting (the "Hong Kong Operation"). A recent report summarizes the 20-year experience (77). Eighteen months of INH and PAS in ambulant outpatients was successful in most patients. The addition of streptomycin did not improve results, nor did casting or initial bed rest. The minimal debridement operation did not add any benefit to medical treatment alone. The radical resection of diseased bone and repair of the defect with bone grafts resulted in earlier bony fusion and less increase in the kyphosis. This favorable initial outcome was sustained up to the 20-year report. The MRC trial did not include patients with paraplegia or involvement of more than three vertebrae. The patients were younger and had a relatively acute disease course. In nonendemic areas, ambulant chemotherapy alone has had poorer results than in the MRC trial. In the United States, indications for surgery include a neurologic deficit, spinal instability, spinal deformity with more than 50% vertebral collapse or deformity of more than 5 degrees, nonresponse or noncompliance with medical therapy, or a nondiagnostic needle biopsy (78,79).

Today in the United States there is general agreement that Pott paraplegia should be treated with combined medical and surgical treatment. Spinal instability and angulation, once present, are likely to progress without surgery. In patients with neurologic deficits, debridement removes necrotic tissue, preventing progression and resulting in resolution of neurologic deficits (80). If surgical resources are limited, medical treatment alone may still be effective. A large study from Korea demonstrated that treatment with two drugs (INH, ethambutol, or PAS) and physical therapy resulted in resolution of paraplegia in 78% of cases within 6 months (81).

Mycobacteria Bovis and Bacillus Calmette–Guérin

Epidemiology

In the first half of the twentieth century, *Mycobacteria bovis* accounted for 11% of osteoarticular TB. During World War II as much as 25% of TB was caused by *M. bovis*. With elimination of bovine TB and widespread pasteurization of milk, infection with *M. bovis* has become rare, usually occurring in elderly individuals exposed to infected milk as children or those emigrating from regions still endemic for bovine TB, such as Mexico (82). BCG is an *M. bovis* attenuated by subculture, which is used for vaccination against TB and as an adjuvant immunostimulator for bladder cancer and other malignancies.

Pathophysiology

M. bovis in milk from infected cows enters humans via tonsils or the intestinal mucosa, produces lesions in cervical and abdominal lymph nodes, and has an affinity for bone. Although the strain has been attenuated, tuberculous osteomyelitis may occur in children who were immunized as infants (83). The use of BCG as adjuvant immunostimulatory treatment for bladder cancer can produce a local granulomatous reaction in the bladder and is associated with systemic symptoms and a reactive type of arthritis. This may be due to a transient infection or an adjuvant induced immune reaction. Rarely, BCG vaccination or immunotherapy can be complicated by progressive systemic BCG infection, including monarthritis with positive synovial cultures for *M. bovis,* infection of a joint prosthesis (84,85), or vertebral osteomyelitis (86). Additionally, a seronegative, asymmetric oligoarthritis with morning stiffness, local inflammation, and elevated sedimentation rate can occur (87,88). Some of these patients are human leukocyte antigen B27–positive, suggesting a reactive form of arthritis similar to adjuvant disease in rodents (89).

Clinical Features

The clinical features of osteoarticular infection with *M. bovis* are similar to those with *M. tuberculosis.* Several rheumatic syndromes have been reported in association with BCG immunotherapy (90,91). Intravesicular BCG for superficial bladder cancer is associated with granulomatous cystitis, dysuria, hematuria, malaise, fever, and transient arthritis or migratory arthralgias in up to 3% of patients. The symptoms occur after the first few treatments, increase in severity with additional treatments, and can be prevented with INH prophylaxis. (BCG is resistant to pyrazinamide.)

Nontuberculous Mycobacteria

Epidemiology

Nontuberculous mycobacteria (NTM) are ubiquitous worldwide and are cultured from human and nonhuman hosts, as well as from reservoirs in soil, water, vegetables, and dust (92). The nontuberculous mycobacteria are classified by pigment production. About one-quarter of patients with nontuberculous mycobacterial infections have an underlying illness, such as HIV infection (93) or another form of arthritis, such as degenerative joint disease, rheumatoid arthritis, or systemic lupus erythematosus. Approximately one-half of musculoskeletal infections in patients with HIV infection are due to nontuberculous mycobacteria.

Pathophysiology

Formerly regarded as harmless saprophytic organisms with low pathogenicity for man (94), nontuberculous mycobacteria have become opportunistic pathogens in immunocompromised individuals. A history of prior trauma or operation has been obtained in about half the patients, and 36% to 58% have had prior intraarticular injection of corticosteroids.

Clinical Features

Nontuberculous mycobacteria produce pulmonary disease resembling typical TB and can infect joints, tendons, bursae, and bones (Table 28.1). The infections are indolent, causing an insidious onset of joint pain and swelling often with periarticular cystic masses or chronically draining wounds. Constitutional symptoms are present only in 8%, and fewer than 15% of joints are red and warm. Patients with arthritis rarely have active pulmonary disease. Com-

TABLE 28.1. OSTEOARTICULAR TUBERCULOUS AND NONTUBERCULOUS MYCOBACTERIAL INFECTIONS

Organism	Bone	Joint	Tenosynovium or Soft Tissues	Comments
Mycobacterium tuberculosis	Usual	Uncommon	Rare	Can infect prostheses Can disseminate
M. kansasii	Uncommon	Usual	Usual	Can be multifocal in immunoincompetent
M. marinum (fish tuberculosis)	Very rare	Usual	Most common	Skin ulcer and local spread. Very rare dissemination
M. avium intracellulare	Rare	Uncommon	Uncommon	Dissemination in immunosuppressed and HIV infection
M. fortuitum; M. chelonei	Uncommon	Usual	Rare	Infection by direct injection and can infect prostheses
M. haemophilum	Usual	Usual	Rare	Dissemination in immunoincompetent, skin lesions mimic Kaposi
M. leprae	Uncommon	Usual	Rare	Erythema nodosum leprosum + swollen hand and forearm, can mimic rheumatic arthritis Charcot joints, wrists, or ankles with sensory loss

Adapted from Mahowald ML. Arthritis due to mycobacteria, fungi, and parasites. In: Koopman WJ, ed. *Arthritis and allied conditions: a textbook of rheumatology,* 14th ed. Philadelphia: Lippincott Williams & Wilkins, 2001:2607–2628.

mon sites of infection include the hand (53%), wrist (19%), and knee (18%). Infection of the hip, elbow, ankle, and prepatellar and olecranon bursae, as well as of periarticular tissue simulating arthritis, has also been described, and 17% of cases are polyarticular. Patients with flexor tendonitis at the wrist may develop carpal tunnel syndrome.

Clinical Evaluation

Pathologic changes in nontuberculous mycobacterial infections are indistinguishable from *M. tuberculosis* infections (95). Synovial and osseous tissue cultures for acid-fast bacilli may be positive when synovial fluid cultures are negative. Radiographic changes in nontuberculous mycobacterial infections demonstrate preservation of central joint spaces with sclerotic borders of marginal erosions. Patchy lytic lesions and periosteal new bone formation indicate osteomyelitis (96). Microscopic examination of synovial fluid or biopsy material may reveal granuloma and acid-fast bacilli, but definitive diagnosis requires culture.

Prevention and Therapy

These organisms are often resistant to the standard anti-TB drug regimen, and recurrence of infection is common. Selection of therapy for nontuberculous mycobacterial infections should be based on species identified, host immunocompetence, and extent of infection. Interpretation of in vitro sensitivity testing of nontuberculous mycobacteria isolates is controversial and may not accurately predict clinical efficacy (97). A combination of four or five drugs and synovectomy may be necessary (98). Generally, surgical debridement or excision is needed for extensive or deep infections, and amputation may be required to control infection. Empiric treatments recommended later must be modified based on both sensitivity tests and clinical response.

Clinical Features

There are more than 50 species of nontuberculous mycobacteria, but only a few are important human pathogens (99). The group I photochromogens (produce yellow pigment after exposure to light), *M. kansasii* and *M. marinum*, are the most frequent organisms causing osteoarticular nontuberculous mycobacterial infections (56%). These are followed by the group III nonphotochromogens (17%), including the *M. avium* and *M. intracellularis* complex (MAC) (100,101). The group II scotochromogens (produce yellow pigment when grown in the dark) (9%) (*M. gordonae, M. scrofulaceum, M. szulgae, M. xenopi*) are usually disregarded as contaminants, but sporadic cases of osteomyelitis and of bursal, tendon sheath, and prosthesis infections have been identified

(102,103). The group IV rapid growers (*M. chelonae* and *M. fortuitum*) cause 11% of nontuberculous mycobacterial osteoarticular infections and are found in water taps. These organisms are from human sources (*M. chelonae*) or animals, soil, and water (*M. fortuitum*), and have been recovered from postoperative slow-healing wounds, sinus tracts, and joints.

M. kansasii is found in milk, meat, and water supplies. It occasionally causes an indolent and often nondestructive arthritis or tenosynovitis in the hand, wrist, knee, ankle, or elbow in healthy individuals. In those with comorbid conditions (transplants, rheumatoid arthritis, systemic lupus erythematosus, or steroids) bone infection and joint destruction are more frequent (104). In the immunocompromised patients, pulmonary disease is often interstitial with endobronchitis, and dissemination with multifocal osteoarticular disease may occur (105). Treatment with INH, ethambutol, and rifampin for 18 to 24 months is recommended.

M. marinum causes TB in fish. Human infection presents as a superficial nodule, ulcerated skin plaque (swimming pool granuloma), synovitis, or tenosynovitis in fingers (61%) and hands (14%) or the knee (18%) (106). Predilection for the extremities is thought to be related to cooler body temperature. A history of penetrating trauma during occupational or recreational exposure to salt or fresh water or timber splinters is often present. Delay in diagnosis is common (mean, 5 months), and infections are often misdiagnosed as rheumatoid arthritis or gout. More than half the patients are initially treated with intraarticular steroid treatment before diagnosis. Local spread occurs in 20% to 25%, but the infection rarely disseminates (2%). There is a single case report of *M. marinum* as a cause of osteoarticular infection in an immunocompromised patient that was associated with severe bone and joint involvement (107). Treatment with rifampin and ethambutol or sulfonamide with trimethoprim is recommended for 3 to 6 months or longer, based on clinical response. Surgical debridement is recommended for joint infection.

Individuals with HIV infection, chronic pulmonary disease, or immunosuppression due to corticosteroids are at risk for disseminated *M. avium* complex (MAC) infection (108). Intermittent MAC bacteremias may infect every organ and tissue, including bone, tendon sheath, bursa, and joint, producing a clinical picture with insidious onset and progression (109). Patients develop night sweats, wasting, diarrhea and abdominal pain, hepatosplenomegaly, anemia, and elevated alkaline phosphatase. Bone lesions cause localized pain, focal abnormalities on x-ray, and abnormal bone scans (110). Surgical debridement and multidrug therapy are needed but are often limited by side effects and drug interactions. MAC strains are resistant to first-line anti-TB drugs. A multidrug treatment regimen that includes ethambutol plus rifampin (rifampin cannot be used with protease inhibitors) or rifabutin; ciprofloxacin, amikacin, or clofazimine; and clarithromycin or azithromycin is recommended for 1 year after cultures become negative in HIV-negative patients and for life in HIV-infected patients.

M. fortuitum, a group IV rapid grower, is found in soil, water, and fish, and can cause pulmonary disease, corneal ulcerations, and infection of bones, joints, and prosthetic joint. It causes joint infection by direct penetration and was identified in an iatrogenic outbreak due to contaminated needles used for joint injections as well as a joint infection following a dog bite (111). *M. fortuitum* is resistant to antituberculous drugs. Treatment requires both surgical debridement and chemotherapy with amikacin and cefoxitin or a combination of two drugs, including ofloxacin or ciprofloxacin, doxycycline, sulfamethoxazole, or clarithromycin (112).

M. haemophilum is a slow-growing, fastidious organism requiring low culture temperature and iron-supplemented medium. It is a rare but emerging human pathogen primarily in immunoincompetent hosts (113). It can cause painful ulcerating cutaneous lesions, bacteremia, and infection of lung, bone, and joints (ankles, knees, and wrists). Skin lesions may masquerade as Kaposi sarcoma. More than half the patients have osteoarticular sites of infection. The optimum drug regimen is currently uncertain, but resistance to INH and ethambutol has been reported (114).

Leprosy

Epidemiology

Over the past decade there have been dramatic changes in the prevalence of leprosy since the introduction of multidrug therapy and widespread BCG immunization of children in endemic areas (BCG immunization induces 50% protective efficacy). The number registered for treatment has decreased from 12 million to 1 million, with approximately 600,000 new cases per year. Eighty-one percent of the total disease burden occurs in five countries: India (57%), Brazil, Indonesia, Myanmar, and Nigeria (115,116). In the United States, there are about 7,000 patients, with 200 new cases diagnosed annually, mostly in immigrants and some armadillo handlers (117).

Pathophysiology

Leprosy presents as a spectrum between lepromatous leprosy, with a high bacillary load and defective cellular immunity, and tuberculoid leprosy with a small bacillary load and effective cellular immunity. Intermediate between lepromatous leprosy and tuberculoid leprosy are forms of borderline leprosy, borderline lepromatous leprosy, and borderline tuberculoid leprosy. The indolent

course of leprosy is punctuated by reactions wherein inflammation develops at sites of infection, often after therapy has started.

Clinical Features

Joint involvement can be subdivided into several distinct rheumatic syndromes (118,119). In lepromatous leprosy absence of specific cellular immunity results in a systemic disease with bacteremia and widespread organ infiltration causing fever, arthralgias, pitting edema of the hands from the metacarpal joints to mid-forearm, erythema nodosum leprosum (crops of inflamed subcutaneous nodules due to vasculitis or panniculitis), or a rheumatoid arthritis–like polyarthritis in proximal interphalangeal joints, metacarpophalangeal joints, wrists, metatarsophalangeal joints, ankles, and knees. In tuberculoid leprosy (TL) or borderline leprosy (BL) a vigorous cellular immunity localizes the bacilli and produces asymmetric macules or skin plaques and involvement of cutaneous nerves. TL may be accompanied by swelling of hands, knees, and ankles, and BL may be accompanied by a subacute symmetric polyarthritis of the small joints of the hands. Another type of chronic arthritis with recurrent swelling of large and small joints is independent of reactions or the type of leprosy (120). This arthritis begins insidiously months to years after the first symptoms of leprosy and involves the wrists, small joints of the hands and feet, and the knees. It is associated with morning stiffness and erosions on radiographs (121). It responds poorly to nonsteroidal antiinflammatory drugs but improves with treatment of the underlying disease (122). The most common joint deformities in leprosy occur secondary to disease in the peripheral nerves. Neurotrophic changes lead to absorption of bones, especially in the distal ends of the metatarsals. Sensory loss and repeated trauma are responsible for infection in soft tissues and bone, and are responsible for loss of terminal digits and severe deformities of the hands and feet. The claw hand that occurs secondary to nerve damage can further compound the disability. True neuropathic joints with complete disorganization of the weight-bearing surfaces and supporting bone may also occur. Charcot joints are most frequently seen at the wrist and ankle. Another form of arthritis occurs secondary to bone disease. In addition to arthritis, a necrotizing vasculitis, the Lucio phenomenon, may occur as large recurrent ulcerations in the lower legs.

Clinical Evaluation

In lepromatous leprosy, the erythrocyte sedimentation rate is elevated, anemia is common, and positive rheumatoid factors (RF) tests occur in 15% to 35 % of patients, and erosions may be seen in radiographs of the small joints (123). Synovial biopsy reveals an acute inflammatory reaction; however, lepra organisms are not detected in the synovium, and the synovial fluid is a transudate. It has been postulated that this form of arthritis is immune mediated rather than infectious. In tuberculoid leprosy, RF and antinuclear antibodies (ANA) are usually negative, and synovial fluid is purulent and contains lepra cells with ingested organisms, indicating a true septic arthritis. Additionally, infection of the nasal mucosa and cartilage may lead to septal collapse and a "saddle nose deformity" (124).

The diagnosis of leprosy rests on demonstration of acid-fast bacilli in skin smears and other tissues, including peripheral nerves. From a clinical standpoint, the cardinal sign is anesthesia of the skin. Typically, thermal and tactile sensation is lost before pain and pressure sensation. The ulnar and peroneal nerves frequently are involved early.

Prevention and Treatment

Treatment of leprosy requires a coordinated effort that includes attention to the social needs of the patient as well as specialized drug therapy and physical measures to protect the skin and joints and to reduce contractures. In response to the increasing incidence of primary and secondary dapsone resistance, the World Health Organization now recommends the use of three drugs for 2 to 5 years in patients with multibacillary disease (dapsone, rifampin, and clofazimine; minocycline or newer fluoroquinolones). Dapsone and rifampin for 6 months are recommended for those with paucibacillary disease. In the United States, patients with leprosy are entitled to treatment by the U.S. Public Health Service.

FUNGAL DISEASES

Fungi that cause primary infection in humans have a typical geographic distribution (blastomycosis, coccidioidomycosis, histoplasmosis); however, travelers may not manifest symptoms until they have returned to a nonendemic area. In immunoincompetent individuals systemic fungal infections become more chronic and often more widespread. In addition, fungi that are not normally pathogenic become opportunistic infections (such as those caused by candida, aspergillus, nocardia, cryptococcus). There are many fungal immunoserologic tests, but only a few are clinically helpful: antigen tests for cryptococcus and histoplasma, anticoccidioidal antibodies. Therefore diagnosis requires isolation of the organism from synovial fluid, synovial tissue, or other tissue site of infection. Treatments include amphotericin B, azole derivatives, and flucytosine plus surgical drainage and debridement of localized sites of infection. Typical features of the osteoarticular syndromes associated with fungal infections and treatment considerations are presented in

Table 28.2 for coccidioidomycosis (125) with desert rheumatism (126,127) and focal septic arthritis (128–131); blastomycosis (132–135); cryptococcosis (136–138); histoplasmosis (139–141); sporotrichosis (142–145); and candidiasis.

Candida species that are pathogenic for humans are also commensal organisms yet account for approximately 80% of systemic fungal infections. Since the introduction of antibiotics in the 1940s there has been a sharp increase in candidal infections. With the introduction of antifungal agents, nonalbicans candidal species resistant to these drugs are increasing. Nosocomial candidemia most often arises from an endogenous source because of colonization. Neutrophils rather than macrophages are the first line of defense against candidal organisms. Hence the increased risk for systemic candidiasis in neutropenic patients, whereas impaired cellular immunity is associated with a chronic mucocutaneous form of infection. Additional risk factors for candidemia include indwelling catheters, prolonged antibiotic use, parenteral hyperalimentation, extensive burns, major surgery, previous colonization of mucosal sites, intravenous drug abuse, corticosteroids, bone marrow transplantation, cancer chemotherapy, diabetes, and very low birth weight in neonates (146).

In recent case series, candidal species were found in approximately 5% of septic arthritis cases in children (147), and they account for less than 1% of septic arthritis cases in adults. In adults several distinct clinical syndromes have been described: chronic monoarthritis, prosthetic joint infection, and an acute or subacute monoarthritis or polyarthritis (148). An indolent chronic monoarticular arthritis occurs following direct inoculation of candidal organisms into the joint. This may occur after repeated joint aspiration or intraarticular injection of corticosteroids. These patients have a mean age of 62, are almost always afebrile, and usually have underlying osteoarthritis or rheumatoid arthritis. The knee is the most frequently involved joint, and the positive synovial fluid culture is often a surprise. Fungal infections of joint prostheses are extremely rare but usually due to nonalbicans candidal species (149–152). Most of these patients had no evidence of disseminated fungal infection and are in their 60s. About half have additional risk factors such as treatment with antibiotics or immunosuppressive drugs. The average interval between surgery and onset of symptoms is 14 months. Pain and limited range of motion are more frequent presenting symptoms in the patients with joint replacement and may be associated with loosening of the prosthesis. Candida arthritis may also occur secondary to hematogenous spread from the gastrointestinal or genital tracts. Common exogenous sources are hyperalimentation and intravenous drug abuse. Most have a serious illness, such as cancer, renal failure, sepsis, or a connective tissue disease. Antibiotics,

TABLE 28.2. SYSTEMIC FUNGAL INFECTIONS

Organism and Resulting Disease	Epidemiology	Pathogenesis	Clinical Features	Evaluation	Prevention and Treatment	Comment
Coccidioidomycosis *Coccidioides immitis* Valley fever San Joaquin fever	In soil Semiarid areas Southern California, Arizona, New Mexico, western Texas, northern Mexico, Argentina	Inhalation of spores to pulmonary infection Asymptomatic or mild respiratory illness, hypersensitivity rxn produces "desert rheumatism" (nondeforming) or disseminates	Self-limited fever, malaise, cough, or chest pain, "desert rheumatism"—polyarthritis, conjunctivitis, erythema nodosum or erythema multiforme 1% disseminate; may infect bone or joints: destructive, indolent monoarthritis of knee; may fistulate, with low-grade fever, anorexia, weight loss x-ray: erosions, bone destruction Bone scan may show asymptomatic sites	Synovial fluid/tissue culture Spherules in SF Granulomatous synovium with spherules packed with endospores (silver or PAS stain) Coccidioidin skin test + in 80% Serologic tests often positive: IgM abs early, high IgG abs with dissemination and bone and joint disease	Surgical drainage, debridement Itraconazole, fluconazole, ketoconazole, or amphotericin B for severe disease	Higher risk for dissemination with corticosteroids, HIV, late pregnancy, elderly age Coccidioidin skin test is positive in most who live in an endemic area but can use to monitor response to treatment
Blastomycosis *Blastomyces dermatidis*	A mold in soil with decaying material Ohio and Mississippi River valleys, Middle Atlantic states, southeastern states, upstate New York, southern Canada, Africa, Israel, Lebanon, Mexico, Venezuela	Inhalation of spores that convert to yeast and infect lung; may be asymptomatic, show mild symptoms, or cavitate and disseminate via blood and lymphatics to skin and bone and other tissues May infect dogs	Self-limited, cough, chest pain, high fever, infiltrates on x-ray; may cavitate; acute monoarthritis (knee, elbow, ankle, hand) in systemically ill person with pulmonary and extrapulmonary disease; osteomyelitis with red, tender overlying skin or asymptomatic until invades joint One or many enlarging skin papules with central atrophy Spinal blastomycosis destroys disc space, and anterior vertebral body; and extends as paraspinal abscess	SF KOH treated smears reveal large yeast with broad-based buds (silver or PAS +) Definite diagnosis by culture Immunodiffusion test with A antigen very sensitive but less specific and cross-reacts with *Histoplasma*	Amphotericin B for severe disease For milder cases: ketoconazole, itraconazole, fluconazole May need debridement and drainage Good prognosis	Increased incidence and severity in immuno-compromised individuals, especially those with HIV
Cryptococcosis *Cryptococcus neoformans* (torulosis)	Worldwide pigeon droppings	Inhalation of yeast, pulmonary infection (self-limited, subacute, or chronic course) Rare dissemination to skin, bone, brain, organs	Usually asymptomatic or mild respiratory illness Dissemination: skin papules, pustules that ulcerate, subcutaneous nodules Osteomyelitis, long bones, vertebrae (paraspinal abscesses), ribs, tarsal and carpal bones; progressive lytic lesions or eroding into joint infection (knee), usually in immunosuppressed person (severe disease in HIV)	SF/tissue: encapsulated yeast with narrow based buds (mucicarmine +) Latex fixation for capsular antigen x-ray: lytic bone lesion, scalloped margins, no periosteal reaction	No treatment if mild If immunosuppressed or extrapulmonary sites: amphotericin B with or without flucytosine	Predisposing conditions for opportunistic infection: HIV, transplantation, corticosteroids, lymphoma, sarcoidosis

Organism/Disease	Epidemiology	Transmission/Pathogenesis	Clinical features	Diagnosis	Treatment	Comments
Histoplasmosis *Histoplasma capsulatum* *H. duboisii* (Africa)	Most common pulmonary fungal infection worldwide; in the United States: Ohio, St. Lawrence, Mississippi, Rio Grande river valleys; northern Maryland; southern Pennsylvania; central New York, Texas; South America; southern Mexico; Indonesia; Philippines; Turkey; Africa	Mold in dirt contaminated with bird (chickens, starlings) or bat excreta; infects a yeast form when inhaled; disseminated if cell-mediated immunity defective; *H. duboisii* has predilection for bone	Three forms of disease: *Acute pneumonia:* asymptomatic or mild fever, cough, malaise. *Disseminated disease:* liver, spleen enlargement; lymphadenopathy; mucosal ulcers; fatigue; weakness; night sweats; malaise; weight loss. In 10% acute additive polyarthralgia/arthritis, e nodosum or e multiforme, clears without deformity. Rare indolent infection of knee or tenosynovitis causing carpal tunnel syndrome. *Cavitary disease:* apical cavities, progressive respiratory dysfunction	Culture SF/tissue, blood, sputum, bone marrow, liver, or lymph node. Histology: clusters of oval yeast cells in PMNs or macrophages (silver & PAS +). *Histoplasma* antigen in body fluids	Amphotericin B itraconazole Relapses common Surgical drainage and debridement of infected joints advised	Severe disease if exposure heavy or prolonged Progressive dissemination with HIV, elderly, and immunocompromised individuals Skin test often positive in those living in endemic areas
Candidal osteoarticular infections	Increased colonization of commensal organism in GI or GU tract after antibiotics Contaminant of injectable solutions or surgical instruments	Direct inoculation of organism into joint or prosthesis during surgery, or via hematogenous route in neutropenic patient 5% of joint infections in a child, <1% in adults	Acute mono-, polyarthritis in neutropenic patient Subacute or chronic monoarthritis after i.a. steroid injection, afebrile Late postop pain and limited ROM in prosthetic joint	Positive candida culture of synovial fluid, often a surprise Prosthetic infections, often noncandidal species		Common infection in seriously ill patients who have received broad-spectrum antibiotics, hyperalimentaion, i.v. drug abuse, i.a. steroids, and joint prostheses
Sporothrix schenckii (North, Central, and South America; Australasia; Southeast Asia)	Temperate and tropical areas in soil and plant debris; sphagnum moss; Dimorphic: mold in nature and yeast in tissue sites	Rose thorns or wood splinters penetrate skin; granulomatous suppuration and necrosis; lymphadenitis, usually in upper extremity Rare inhalation causes pulmonary infection	Skin nodule spreads proximally via lymphatics, forming multiple ulcerating subcutaneous lesions or penetrating adjacent tissues (chronic monoarthritis); can fistulate Rare dissemination from lung to cause chronic granulomatous mono- or oligoarthritis or tenosynovitis in the hand	ESR elevated Must culture SF or synovial tissue Antibodies detected with latex slide test or ELISA X-ray: osteoporosis and erosions	Potassium iodide Amptericin B, itraconazole External heat Surgical debridement	In immunoincompetent individuals dissemination may cause multifocal infection of skin, bones, joints

ELISA, enzyme-linked immunosorbent assay; ESR, erythrocyte sedimentation rate; GI, gastrointestinal; GU, gastrourinary; HIV, human immunodeficiency virus; i.a., intra-articular; i.v., intravenous; KOH, potassium hydroxide; PAS, periodic acid-Schiff; ROM, range of motion; rxn, reaction; SF, synovial fluid.

chemotherapy, immunosuppressive treatment, or indwelling intravenous catheters are frequently involved. The arthritis is monoarticular in 75% and polyarticular in 25% of the cases. The knee is the most common site, followed by other large joints, the spine, and bursa. Two-thirds of patients have an acute onset of their arthritis with a painful course. Contaminated heroin has also been noted as a predisposing cause. A distinctive syndrome of follicular and nodular lesions of the scalp, beard, and pubis with ocular infection or multiple osteoarticular lesions of the intervertebral discs, knee, or chondrocostal junctions has been noted in this group (153). Most children with candidal arthritis have been less than 1 year old. All have had a serious underlying illness, and most were critically ill at the time the arthritis was diagnosed. As in adults, antibiotics, immunosuppression, and catheters were frequently implicated as predisposing causes. Candidal arthritis may occur in as many as 2% of infants receiving hyperalimentation (154,155). Multiple joint infections occur about twice as often in infants as in adults (35% vs. 15%), and coexistent metaphyseal osteomyelitis is more common in infants. Joint infection may follow fungal septicemia by intervals of 2 to 12 weeks. Symptoms include pain, tenderness, synovial thickening, and effusion, but red-hot joints are infrequent.

The synovial fluid contains a mean of 38,000 leukocytes/mm^3, with 80% polymorphonuclear leukocytes, but lower counts may be found in patients with leukemia. Synovial fluid glucose levels have been low in 70% of reported cases. Culture of synovial fluid is a highly reliable method for identifying candidal species. A new method to detect fungi more rapidly in blood and body fluid cultures is provided by the BACTEC and BacT/Alert systems, which should be specifically requested when fungal infection is suspected. Gram stain is not reliable, being negative in 80% of culture-positive samples. Serologic tests for anticandidal antibodies do not clearly differentiate local infection or colonization from systemic disease. Recognition of dermal lesions that occur in about 10% of disseminated candidiasis patients may help in the diagnosis. Various lesions have been described, including multiple discrete erythematous papules and nodules of varying size, purpuric lesions with pale centers, necrotic eschars, and nodular subcutaneous abscesses. A triad of fever, erythematous papules, and severe, diffuse muscle tenderness has also been reported with disseminated disease. Biopsy of the dermal lesions may provide a definitive diagnosis (156).

The relatively small number of reported cases makes it difficult to draw firm conclusions regarding optimum treatment. Amphotericin B alone has resulted in eradication of the infection in about 60% of cases in which it has been used. The combined use of intraarticular and intravenous amphotericin B has succeeded when intravenous treatment alone has failed. 5-Fluorocytosine should not be used alone but may be useful as a supplement to amphotericin B (157).

Recent reports indicate fluconazole (400 to 800 mg/d) alone can be as effective as amphotericin B and is less toxic (158,159). Ketoconazole has had varying success (160), but more encouraging results have been obtained with fluconazole (161,162). If fluconazole has been used as prophylaxis in a neutropenic patient, the species causing candidiasis is likely to be a relatively resistant *Candida krusei* or *C. glabrata*. Unfortunately, the utility of fungal antibiotic sensitivity testing is not yet fully established. In both neutropenic and nonneutropenic patients, the cytokine granulocyte-(macrophage)-colony stimulating factor (GM-CSF) appears to be a useful adjunct for invasive candidiasis.

Subcutaneous Fungal Infections

Mycetoma, or Madura foot (Table 28.3), is a slowly progressive, chronic suppurative infection that is endemic in Africa, India, southern Asia, Central and South America, Mexico, the southern United States, and parts of California (163,164). It is caused by more than 20 species of the bacteria *Actinomycetes* (60% of mycetoma) and filamentous fungi (true fungi or eumycetoma) that are saprophytes in the soil or on vegetation. Mycetoma is not contagious and has a uniform appearance regardless of the causative organisms (165,166). Distinction between eumycetoma and actinomycetoma in a patient with Madura foot is critical because eumycetoma are unresponsive to antibiotics and need surgical excision or amputation early to eradicate the infection (167,168). Actinomycetomas may respond to dapsone plus streptomycin or trimethoprim/sulfamethoxazole plus streptomycin or rifampin. In addition to Madura foot, *Pseudallescheria boydii*, a soil and polluted water saprophyte, can rarely cause an indolent monoarticular or oligoarthritis in peripheral joints (169,170). Nocardia rarely infects healthy persons but is an opportunistic infection in those who are immunocompromised (171).

PARASITES

Parasitic infections may cause arthritis by direct invasion of the joints or through secondary immune mechanisms. They may also involve periarticular tissues and produce soft-tissue rheumatic syndromes (Table 28.4). These mechanisms are not mutually exclusive (172). Joint involvement is relatively rare in these diseases, but a large number of people in developing countries have parasitic infections. For example, 600 million people are estimated to have schistosomiasis or filariasis. Thus even a low incidence of arthritis may result in a significant number of cases in these populations. Parasitic intestinal infections may be accompanied by a reactive type of oligoarthritis and spondylitis that resolve if the underlying infection is eradicated. See Table 28.4 for features of the individual infections (173–175).

TABLE 28.3. OSTEOARTICULAR INFECTIONS WITH SUBCUTANEOUS FUNGAL INFECTIONS

Organism and Resulting Disease	Epidemiology	Pathogenesis	Clinical Features	Evaluation	Prevention and Treatment	Comment
Mycetoma ("tumor" caused by a fungal infection)	Tropical and subtropical. Organisms are saprophytes of soil and vegetation	Mean age 20–40 years. Organism enters via skin break or splinter—feet, hands, back (carrying contaminated loads). Suppurative granulomatous tissue response	No systemic symptoms. Small papule and subcutaneous abscess enlarges and fistulates. Progressive extension and destruction of bone, joint, tendons, muscle, and multiple draining tracts. Bacterial superinfection common	Microscopy and culture of "grains" (sclerotia). X-ray periosteal reaction, sclerosis, erosions, joint destruction	Prevention is impracticable. Treatment depends on distinction between eumycetoma or actinomycetoma. Surgical debridement or amputation	Mycetoma are not contagious. Better prognosis with actinomycotic than eumycotic infection. CT scan useful to define extent of the lesion
Actinomycetoma *Actinomadura madura* *Actinomadura pelletieri* *Streptomyces somaliensis*	Causes 60% of mycetoma		Indolent tumefaction and fistulation at site of penetration. More rapid course than eumycetoma	Gram positive filamentous organisms	Potentially curable with antibiotics	Treatment may take years
A. israelii	Normal oral commensal organism	Enters via decaying teeth or after jaw injury, forming abscesses, drain into mouth, aspiration and pulmonary infection, chest wall fistuae	Cervicofacial tumefaction (lumpy jaw) fistulates and direct extension into bone. Rare dissemination to skin, brain, abdominal organs, or vertebrae, causing back pain and fever	Gram positive filaments in pus. Often infection is polymicrobial	Repeated debridement, 2–12 months of antibiotics (penicillin, tetracycline, clindamycin, erythromycin)	
Nocardia *N. brasiliensis* (tropical climates, Mexico, South America) *N. asteroides* (United States, Europe, Japan) *N. caviae*	Worldwide distribution in composting vegetation. Gram-positive and partially acid fast bacterium with filamentous growth	In immunoincompetent individuals, infection via inhalation, then hematogenous dissemination. Skin contamination leads to mycetoma	Articular involvement via direct extension of the mycetoma. Very rare nocardia synovitis via hematogenous spread. Pulmonary and brain abscesses in immunosuppressed	SF or tissue. Gram positive, variably acid fast. No serologic tests available	Costrimoxazole	Very uncommon infection in healthy persons. Opportunistic infection in those on steroids, chemotherapy, or HIV infection
Eumycetoma (true fungi) *Madurella mycetomatis* *M. grisea* (India and Africa)	Saprophytes in soil, vegetation, and sewage	Penetrates skin of foot, multiplies in subcutaneous tissues	Slowly enlarging subcutaneous abscess or skin placque; skin ulcerates and drains; very slow, painless extension into tendons, muscle, bone, and joint	Fungal species identification based on granules. Methenamine stain for hyphae	Many resistant to all amphotericin B and 5-fluocytosine. Need long-term itraconazole, ketoconazole; need debridement	Amputation often required
Pseudallesheria boydii (North America)	Soil, polluted water, sewage		No fever or systemic symptoms. Pain and enlargement of foot, draining sinuses. Rare indolent monarthritis or oligoarthritis in knee, foot, wrists, and small joints of the hand	White yellow large (2 mm) grains	Resistant to antifungals. Extensive debridement or amputation	

CT, computerized tomography; SF, synovial fluid.

TABLE 28.4. TYPICAL RHEUMATOLOGIC SYNDROMES ASSOCIATED WITH PARASITES

Organism	Epidemiology	Pathogenesis	Clinical Features	Evaluation	Prevention and Treatment	Comment
Filariasis *Wucheria bancrofti*	Mosquito-borne in tropic and subtropic regions; 90 million are infected	Worms reside in lymph nodes, damage lymphatics Transient brawny edema with ulcers Chronic elephantiasis	Recurrent episodes of acute knee arthritis, fever, lymphadenopathy for 7 to 10 days Insidious chronic synovitis, hip, knee, ankles; periarticular skin ulcers	ESR normal, RF negative Blood smear and chylous synovial fluid show microfilariae	Avoid contact with mosquitoes Diethylcarbamazine only partially effective Surgical drainage with node-venous shunt and elastic dressings for edema	
Drancunculus medinensis (guinea worm)	Infects millions in India, Pakistan, Africa, parts of South America, West Indies	Water-borne, ingestion and migration to subcutaneous tissues, causing skin ulcers	Leg ulcer draining larvae; if periarticular, worm may invade joint, causing severe inflammation and pain or secondary bacterial infection	SF exudative; see larvae, worm Calcified worms on x-ray	Filter drinking water Remove larvae and worm by rolling on a stick or with lavage Thiabendazole or metronidazole	Can also be caused by loa loa and onchocerciasis
Dirofilaria (dog heartworm)	Rarely infects humans	Enters skin or inhaled; skin or pulmonary nodules contain the worm	Self-limited, intermittent, oligoarthritis		Duration of arthritis shortened by removing subcuatneous nodule with the worm	
Trichinosis *Trichinella spiralis*	Worldwide distribution Tissue dwelling roundworm, transmission by eating contaminated meat	Systemic invasion of larvae 2 weeks after ingestion of adult worm causes myositis	Myalgia, weakness, and muscle swelling with fever, periorbital edema, and headache May have chronic myalgia and low-grade fevers	Elevated muscle enzymes ESR normal Eosinophilia	Thorough cooking or freezing of meat Antihelminth drugs kill worms but not cysts	Eosinophilic myositis with larvae seen on muscle biopsy

	Epidemiology	Transmission/Pathogenesis	Clinical Features	Diagnosis	Treatment/Prevention	Comments
Schistosomiasis (Trematodes, blood flukes)	Africa, Asia, South America, Caribbean Infect fish and mollusks	Flukes penetrate skin and parasitize venous channels, produce eggs, and cause granuloma reaction Chronic GI and GU tract infection	Two forms of arthritis: Acute symmetrical polyarthritis with myalgias (? Immune complex mediated) Chronic oligoarthritis, enthesopathy, back pain (reactive arthropathy)	Eosinophilia RF negative SynBx may see ova, chronic synovitis ~40% abnormal sacroiliac x-ray	Avoid contaminated water; praziquantel Acute polyarthritis resolves with treatment for flukes	Schistosomal myeloradiculopathy: back pain with rapid weakness and autonomic dysfunction, intraspinal eggs
Cestodes *Taenia solium* (pork tapeworm)	Latin America, South Africa, India; rare in United States (usually immigrants)	Invasive phase with systemic symptoms Late cysticerci in subcutaneous tissue and muscle	Fever and myalgias Epilepsy Late skin and muscle nodules, rare joint involvement	Eosinophilia Calcified cysts on x-ray	Avoid undercooked pork Pain resolves with treating underlying infection with praziquantel	"Parasitic rheumatism" also reported with *Strongyloides stercoralis, Taenia saginata, Toxocara canis*
Intestinal Protozoa *Entamoeba histolytica* (lower GI tract infection) *Trichomonas* *Giardia lablia* (small bowel infect) *Cryptosporidium* (small bowel infect)	Worldwide distribution Common in United States in mental institutions, day-care centers, nosocomial outbreaks	Water-borne, fecal/oral transmission	Mild or severe diarrhea Diarrhea may be intractable in immunoincompetent Seronegative reactive type arthritis (knees, ankles, feet); may have fever, abdominal pains, headache, weight loss	Identify organism in stool Small bowel aspiration No organisms on synovial biopsy	Avoid contaminated water Musculoskeletal symptoms resolve with treatment of underlying bowel infection, metronidazole	Can be a STD
Extraintestinal Protozoa *Toxoplasma*	Birds and animals worldwide, can infect any nucleated cell	Transmit via cat feces, meat; transfusions; transplantation; transplacental transmission	Lymphadenopathy, fever, malaise, myalgias; self-limited in weeks to months Rare severe disseminated disease with polymyositis and rash Rare symmetric polyarthritis	Early IgM antibody, late IgG positive	Avoid undercooked meat Healthy patients usually don't need treatment	CNS toxoplasmosis common in HIV; need pyrimethamine plus sulfadiazine

CNS, central nervous system; ESR, erythrocyte sedimentation rate; GI, gastrointestinal; GU, genitourinary; HIV, human immunodeficiency virus; IgG, immunoglobulin G; IgM, immunoglobulin M; RF, rheumatoid factor; SF, synovial fluid; STD, sexually transmitted disease.

REFERENCES

1. World Health Organization. *The world health report 1999: making a difference.* Geneva: World Health Organization, 1999:116.
2. Snider GL. Tuberculosis then and now: a personal perspective on the last 50 years. *Ann Intern Med* 1997;126:237–243.
3. O'Brien RJ, Simone PM. Tuberculosis elimination revisited: obstacles, opportunities and a renewed commitment. Advisory Council for the Elimination of tuberculosis. Centers for Disease Control and Prevention, *MMWR* 1999;48(RR-9).
4. Gasner MR, Maw KL, Feldman GE, et al. The use of legal action in New York City to ensure treatment of tuberculosis. *N Engl J Med* 1999;340:359–366.
5. Wilberschied L. Foreign born tuberculosis cases exceed US-born tuberculosis cases: New York City, 1997. *J Urban Health* 76:143–144.
6. Havlir DV, Barnes PF. Tuberculosis in patients with human immunodeficiency virus infection. *N Engl J Med* 1999;340: 367–373.
7. Pablos-Mendez A, Raviglione MC, Lazlo A, et al. Global surveillance of antituberculosis-drug resistance, 1994–1997. *N Engl J Med* 1998;338:1641–1649.
8. Anonymous. Progress toward the elimination of tuberculosis: United States. *MMWR* 1999;48:732–736.
9. Puttick MPE, Stein HB, Chan RMT, et al. Soft tissue tuberculosis: a series of 11 cases. *J Rheumatol* 1995;22:1321–1325.
10. Alvarez S, McCabe WR. Exptrapulmonary tuberculosis revisited: a review of experience at Boston city and other hospitals. *Medicine* 1984;63:25–55.
11. Division of TB Elimination, CDC Surveillance Reports. *Reported tuberculosis in the US 1996 and 1997.* Atlanta: Centers for Disease Control and Prevention, 1998.
12. Weissler JC. Tuberculosis: immunopathogenesis and therapy. *Am J Med Sci* 1993;305:52–65.
13. Frieden TR, Fujiwara PI, Washko RM, et al. Tuberculosis in New York City: turning the tide. *N Engl J Med* 1995;333: 229–333.
14. Huebner RE, Castro KG. The changing face of tuberculosis. *Annu Rev Med* 1995;46:47–55.
15. Haas DW, Des Prez RM. *Mycobacterium tuberculosis.* In: Mandell GL, Bennett JE, Dolin R, eds. *Principles and practice of infectious diseases,* 4th ed. New York: Churchill Livingstone, 1995:2213–2242.
16. Evanchick CC, Davis DE, Harrington TM. Tuberculosis of peripheral joints: an often missed diagnosis. *J Rheumatol* 1986;13:187–189.
17. Newton P, Sharp J, Barnes KL. Bone and joint tuberculosis in greater Manchester, 1969–79. *Ann Rheum Dis* 1982;41:1–6.
18. Chaisson RE, Schecter GF, Theuer LP, et al. Pulmonary tuberculosis in patients with AIDS. *Am Rev Respir Dis* 1987;136: 570–574.
19. Rieder HL, Snider DE, Cauthen GM. Extrapulmonary TB in the US. *Am Rev Respir Dis* 1990;141:347–351.
20. Garrido G, Gomez-Reino JJ, Fernandez-Dapica P, et al. A review of peripheral tuberculous arthritis. *Semin Arthritis Rheum* 1988;18:142–149.
21. Grosskopf I, Ben David A, Charach G, et al. Bone and joint tuberculosis: a 10-year review. *Israel J Med Sci* 1994;30: 278–283.
22. Ellis ME, El-Ramahi KM, Al-Dalaan AN. Tuberculosis of peripheral joints: a dilemma in diagnosis. *Tubercle Lung Dis* 1993;74:399–404.
23. Kutzbach GA. Tuberculous arthritis. In: Spinoza LR, ed. *Infections in the rheumatic diseases.* Orlando: Grune & Stratton, 1988:131–138.
24. Mitchison DA, Chalmers J. Musculoskeletal tuberculosis. In: Hughes SPF, Fitzgerald RH, eds. *Musculoskeletal infections.* Chicago: Year Book Medical, 1986:186–215.
25. Boachie-Adjei O, Squllante RG. Tuberculosis of the spine. *Orthop Clin North Am* 1996;27:95–103.
26. Vohra R, Kang HS. Tuberculosis of the elbow. *Acta Orthop Scand* 1995;66:57–58.
27. Valdazo JP, Perez-Ruiz F, Albarracin A, et al. Tuberculous arthritis: report of a case with multiple joint involvement and periarticular tuberculous abscesses. *J Rheumatol* 1990;17:399–401.
28. Linares LF, Valcarcel A, Mesa Del Castilla J, et al. Tuberculous arthritis with multiple joint involvement. *J Rheumatol* 1991;18: 635–636.
29. Zahraa J, Johnson D, Lim-Dunham JE, et al. Unusual features of osteoarticular tuberculosis in children. *J Pediatr* 1996;129: 597–602.
30. Ruggieri M, Pavone V, Polizzi A, et al. Tuberculosis of the ankle in childhood: clinical, roentgenographic and computed tomography findings. *Clin Pediatr (Phila)* 1997;36:529–534.
31. Garrido G, Gomez-Reinao J, Fernandez-Dapacia P, et al. A review of peripheral tuberculous arthritis. *Semin Arthritis Rheum* 1988;18:142–149.
32. Valdazo J, Perez-Ruiz F, Albarracin A, et al. Tuberculous arthritis: report of a case with multiple joint involvement and periarticular tuberculous abscesses. *J Rheumatol* 1990;17:399–401.
33. Muradali D, Gold WL, Vellend H, et al. Multifocal osteoarticular tuberculosis: report of four cases and review of management. *Clin Infect Dis* 1993;17:204–209.
34. Fancourt GJ, Ebden P, Garner P, et al. Bone tuberculosis: results and experience in Leicestershire. *Br J Dis Chest* 1986;80: 265–272.
35. Grosskopf I, Ben DA, Charach G, et al. Bone and joint tuberculosis: a 10 year review. *Isr J Med Sci* 1994;30:278–283.
36. Olive A, Gonzalez-Ustes J, Fuiz J. On tuberculosis of the bones and joints. *J Rheumatol* 1998;25:11.
37. King AD, Griffith J, Rushton A, et al. Tuberculosis of the greater trochanter and the trochanteric bursa. *J Rheumatol* 1998;25:391–393.
38. Kulshrestha A, Misra RN, Agarwal P, et al. Magnetic resonance appearance of tuberculosis of the knee joint with ruptured Baker's cyst. *Australas Radiol* 1995;39:80–83.
39. Tsai YH, Ueng SW, Shih CH. Tuberculosis of the ankle: report of four cases. *Chang-Keng I Hsueh Tsa Chih* 1998;21:481–486.
40. Spinner RJ, Sexton DJ, Goldner RD, et al. Periprosthetic infections due to *Mycobacterium tuberculosis* in patients with no prior history of tuberculosis (review). *J Arthroplasty* 1996;11: 217–222.
41. Gravallese EM, Weissman BN, Brodsky G, et al. Loosening of a revision total hip replacement in a 60 year old woman with longstanding rheumatoid arthritis. *Arth Rheumatol* 1995;38: 1315–1327.
42. Berbari EF, Hanssen AD, Duffy MC, et al. Prosthetic joint infection due to *Mycobacterium tuberculosis:* a case series and review of the literature. *Am J Orthoped* 1998;27:219–227.
43. Chen WS, Eng HL. Tuberculous tenosynovitis of the wrist mimicking de Quervain's disease. *J Rheumatol* 1994;21: 763–765.
44. Roverano S, Freyre H, Paira S. Soft tissue tuberculosis in systemic lupus erythematosus presentation of two cases. *J Clin Rheumatol* 1999;5:107–109.
45. Puttick MPE, Stein HB, Chan RMT, et al. Soft tissue tuberculosis: a series of 11 cases. *J Rheumatol* 1995;22:1321–1325.
46. Cramer K, Swiler JG, Milek MA. Tuberculous tenosynovitis of the wrist. Two case reports. *Clin Orthop Rel Res* 1991;262: 137–140.
47. Southwood TR, Hancock EJ, Petty RE, et al. Tuberculous

rheumatism (Poncet's disease) in a child. *Arthritis Rheum* 1988; 31:1311–1313.

48. Dall L, Long L. Stanford Poncet's disease: tuberculous rheumatism. *Rev Infect Dis* 1989;11:105–107.

49. Southwood TR, Gaston JS. The molecular basis of Poncet's disease? *Br J Rheumatol* 1990;29:72–74.

50. DeHart DJ. Poncet's disease. Case report. *Clin Infect Dis* 1992; 15:560.

51. Mankin H. Weekly clinicopathological exercise. *N Engl J Med* 1996;334:784–790.

52. Pertuiset E, Beaudreuil J, Liote, F, et al. Spinal tuberculosis in adults: a study of 103 cases in a developed country, 1980–1994. *Medicine* 1999;78:309–320.

53. Rezai AR, Lee M, Cooper PR, et al. Modern management of spinal tuberculosis. *Neurosurgery* 1995;36:87–97.

54. Pouchot J, Vinceneux P, Barge J, et al. Tuberculosis of the sacroiliac joint: clinical features, outcome and evaluation of closed needle biopsy in 11 consecutive cases. *Am J Med* 1988; 84:622–628.

55. Kim NH, Lee HM, Yoo JD, et al. Sacroiliac joint tuberculosis: classification and treatment. *Clin Orthop Rel Res* 1999;358: 215–222.

56. Felson B, Akers PV, Hall GS, et al. Mycotic tuberculous aneurysm of the thoracic aorta. *JAMA* 1977;237:1104–1108.

57. Friedland JS. Tuberculosis. In: Armstrong D, Cohen J, eds. *Infectious diseases.* London: CV Mosby, 1999 (Sect 2): 30.1–30.16.

58. Centers for Disease Control, Advisory Council for the Elimination of Tuberculosis (ACET). Tuberculosis elimination revisited: obstacles, opportunities, and a renewed commitment. *MMWR* 1999;48(RR-9).

59. Havlir DV, Barnes PF. Tuberculosis in patients with the human immunodeficiency virus infection. *N Engl J Med* 1999; 340:367–373.

60. Witebsky FG, Conville PS. The laboratory diagnosis of mycobacterial diseases. *Infect Dis Clin North Am* 1993;7:359–376.

61. Miller N, Hernandez SG, Cleary TJ. Evaluation of Gen-Probe amplified *Mycobacterium tuberculosis* direct test and PCR for direct detection of *Mycobacterium tuberculosis* in clinical specimens. *J Clin Microbiol* 1994;32:393–397.

62. Agerton TB, Valway SE, Blinkhorn RJ, et al. Spread of strain W, a highly drug-resistant strain of *Mycobacterium tuberculosis* across the United States. *Clin Infect Dis* 1999;29:85–92.

63. Berk RH, Yazici M, Atabgey N, et al. Detection of *Mycobacterium tuberculosis* in formaldeyde solution fixed paraffin-imbedded tissue by polymerase chain reaction in Pott's disease. *Spine* 1996;21:1991–1995.

64. Haygood TM, Williamson SL. Radiographic findings of extremity tuberculosis in childhood: back to the future? *Radiographics* 1994;14:561–570.

65. Buchelt M, Lack W, Kutschera HP, et al. Comparison of tuberculous and pyogenic spondylitis. *Clin Orthop* 1993;296: 192–199.

66. Silverman JF, Larkin EW, Carney M, et al. Fine needle aspiration cytology of tuberculosis of the lumbar vertebrae (Pott's disease). *Acta Cytologica* 1986;30:538–542.

67. Mondal A. Cytological diagnosis of vertebral tuberculosis with fine needle aspiration biopsy. *J Bone Joint Surg* 1994;76: 181–184.

68. Stanley DJ. Tuberculosis of the spine: imaging features. *Am J Roentgenol* 1995;164:659–664.

69. Kim NH, Lee HM, Suh JS. Magnetic resonance imaging for the diagnosis of tuberculous spondylitis. *Spine* 1994;19:2451–2455.

70. National Center for HIV, STD and TB Prevention, Division of Tuberculosis Elimination. Self-Study Modules on Tuberculosis. *www.cdc.govphtntbmodules* April 23, 1999.

71. The Medical Letter. Drugs for tuberculosis. *Med Lett Drugs Ther* 1995;37:67–70.

72. American Thoracic Society. Treatment of tuberculosis and tuberculosis infection in adults and children. *Am J Respir Crit Care Med* 1994;149:1359–1374.

73. Lee AS, Campbell JA, Hoffman EB. Tuberculosis of the knee in children. *J Bone Joint Surg (Br)* 1995;77:313–318.

74. Negusse W. Bone and joint tuberculosis in childhood in a children's hospital. *Ethiop Med J* 1993;31:51–61.

75. Laforgia R, Murphy JCM, Redfern TR. Low friction arthroplasty for old quiescent infection of the hip. *J Bone Joint Surg (Br)* 1988;70:373–376.

76. Martini M, Adjrad A, Boudjemaa A. Tuberculous osteomyelitis: a review of 125 cases. *Int Orthop* 1986;10:201–207.

77. Upadhyay SS, Sahi MJ, Sell P, et al. Longitudinal changes in spinal deformity after anterior spinal surgery for tuberculosis of the spine in adults. *Spine* 1994;19:542–549.

78. Louw JA. Spinal tuberculosis with neurological deficit: treatment with anterior vascularised rib grafts, posterior osteotomies, and fusion. *J Bone Joint Surg (Br)* 1990;72: 686–693.

79. Omari B, Robertson JM, Nelson RJ, et al. Pott's disease: a resurgent challenge to the thoracic surgeon. *Chest* 1989;9;5: 145–150.

80. Colmenero JD, Jimenez-Mejias ME, Sanchez-Lora FJ, et al. Pyogenic, tuberculous, and brucellar vertebral osteomyelitis: a descriptive and comparative study of 219 cases. *Ann Rheum Dis* 1997;56:709–715.

81. Pattisson PRM. Pott's paraplegia: an account of the treatment of 89 consecutive patients. *Paraplegia* 1986;24:77–91.

82. Dankner WM, Waecker NJ, Essey MA, et al. *Mycobacterium bovis* infections in San Diego: a clinicoepidemiologic study of 73 patients and a historical review of a forgotten pathogen. *Medicine* 1993;72:11–37.

83. Wang MN, Chen WM, Lee KS, et al. Tuberculous osteomyelitis in young children. *J Pediatr Orthoped* 1999; 19:151–155.

84. Chazerain P, Desplaces N, Mamoudy P, et al. Prosthetic total knee infection with a *Bacillus Calmette Guérin* strain after BCG therapy for bladder cancer. *J Rheumatol* 1993;20:2171–2172.

85. Guerra CE, Betts RF, O'Keefe RJ, et al. *Mycobacterium bovis* osteomyelitis involving a hip arthroplasty after intravesicular bacille Calmette-Guerin for bladder cancer. *Clin Infect Dis* 1998;27:639–640.

86. Aljada IS, Crane JK, Corriere N, et al. *Mycobacterium bovis* BCG causing vertebral osteomyelitis (Pott's disease) following intravesical BCG therapy. *J Clin Microbiol* 1999;37:2106–2108.

87. Xerri B, Chretien Y, Le Parc JM. Reactive polyarthritis induced by intravesical BCG therapy for carcinoma of the bladder. *Eur J Med* 1993;2:503–505.

88. Belmatoug N, Levy-Djebbour S, Appelbom T, et al. Polyarthritis in four patients treated with intravesical Baccillus of Calmette-Guérin for bladder carcinoma. *Rev Rheumatismo* 1993; 60:130–134.

89. Buchs N, Chevrel G, Miossec Pl. Bacillus Calmette-Guerin induced aseptic arthritis: an experimental model of reactive arthritis (editorial). *J Rheumatol* 1998;25:1662–1665.

90. Lamm DL, Stodgill VD, Stodgdill BJ, et al. Complications of *Bacillus Calmette-Guérin* immunotherapy in 1278 patients with bladder cancer. *J Urol* 1986;135:272–274.

91. Ochsenkuhn T, Weber MM, Caselmann WH. Arthritis after *Mycobacterium bovis* immunotherapy for bladder cancer. *Ann Intern Med* 1990;112:882.

92. Yangco BG, Espinoza CG, Germain BF. Nontuberculous mycobacterial joint infections. In: Espinoza L, Goldenberg D, Arnett F, et al., eds. *Infections in the rheumatic diseases.* Orlando: Grune & Stratton, 1988:139–157.

93. Butt AA, Janney A. Arthritis due to *Mycobacterium fortuitum*. *Scand J Infect Dis* 1998.30:525–527.

94. Woods GL, Washington JA. Mycobacteria other than *Mycobacterium tuberculosis*: review of microbiological and clinical aspects. *Rev Infect Dis* 1987;9:275–294.

95. Travis WD, Travis LB, Robert GD, et al. The histopathologic spectrum in *Mycobacterium marinum* infection. *Arch Pathol Lab Med* 1985;109:1109–1113.

96. Schnadig VJ, Quadri SF, Boyvat F, et al. *Mycobacterium kansasii* osteomyelitis presenting as a solitary lytic lesion of the ulna: fine-needle aspiration finding and morphologic comparison with other mycobacteria. *Diagn Cytopathol* 1998; 19:94–97.

97. Iredell J, Whitby M, Blacklock Z. *Mycobacterium marinum* infection: epidemiology and presentation in Queensland, 1971–1990. *Med J Aust* 1992;157:596–598.

98. Horsburgh CR. *Mycobacterium avium* complex infection in the acquired immunodeficiency syndrome. *N Engl J Med* 1991; 324:1332–1338.

99. Griffith DE. Nontuberculosis mycobacteria. In: Armstrong D, Cohen J, eds. *Infectious diseases*. London: CV Mosby, 1999(Sect 2):31.1–31.10.

100. Ekerot L, Jacobsson L, Forsgren A. *Mycobacterium marinum* wrist arthritis: local and systemic dissemination caused by concomitant immunosuppressive therapy. *Scand J Infect Dis* 1998; 30:84–87.

101. Blumenthal DR, Zucker JR, Hawkins CC. *Mycobacterium avium* complex—induces septic arthritis and osteomyelitis in a patient with the acquired immunodeficiency syndrome [Letters]. *Arthritis Rheum* 1990;33:757–758.

102. Yuen K, Fam AG, Simor A. *Mycobacterium xenopi* arthritis [Review] *J Rheumatol* 1998;25:1016–1018.

103. Hurr H, Sorg T. *Mycobacterium szulgai* osteomyelitis. *J Infect* 1998;37:191–192.

104. Glickstein S, Nashel DJ. *Mycobacterium kansasii* septic arthritis complicating rheumatic disease. *Semin Arthritis Rheum* 1987; 16:231–235.

105. Sherer Rl, Sable R, Sonnenberg M, et al. Disseminated infection with *Mycobacterium kansasii* in the acquired immunodeficiency syndrome. *Ann Intern Med* 1986;105:710–712.

106. Alloway JA, Evangelisti SM, Sartin JS. *Mycobacterium marinum* arthritis. *Semin Arthritis Rheum* 1995;24:382–390.

107. Barton A, Bernstein RM, Struthers JK, et al. *Mycobacterium marinum* infection causing septic arthritis and osteomyelitis. *Br J Rheumatol* 1997,36:1207–1209.

108. Benson CA, Ellner JJ. *Mycobacterium avium* complex infection and AIDS: advances in theory and practice. *Clin Infect Dis* 1993;17:7–20.

109. Sheppard DC, Sullam PM. Primary septic arthritis and osteomyelitis due to *Mycobacterium avium* complex in a patient with AIDS. *Clin Infect Dis* 1997;25:925–926.

110. Mahowald ML, Messner RP. *Chronic infective arthritis*. In: Schlossberg D, ed. *Orthopedic infection*. New York: Springer-Verlag, 1988:76–91.

111. Ip FK, Chow SP. *Mycobacterium fortuitum* infections of the hand. *J Hand Surg (Br)* 1992;17B:675–677.

112. Samuels LE, Sharma S, Morris RJ, et al. *Mycobacterium fortuitum* infection of the sternum: review of the literature and case illustration. *Arch Surg* 1996;131:1344–1346.

113. Hirsch R, Miller SM, Kazi S, et al. Human immunodeficiency virus-associated atypical mycobacterial skeletal infections. *Semin Arthritis Rheum* 1996;25:347–356.

114. Straus WL, Ostroff SM, Hernigan DB, et al. Clinical and epidemiologic characteristics of *Mycobacterium haemophilum*, an emerging pathogen in immunocompromised patients. *Ann Intern Med* 1994;120:118–125.

115. Britton WJ. Leprosy. In *Infectious diseases*. In: Armstrong D, Cohen J, eds. London: CV Mosby, 1999(Sect 6):16.1–16.

116. Barbosa LSG, Scheinberg MA. Articular manifestations of leprosy. In: Espinoza L, Goldenberg D, Arnett F, et al., eds. *Infections in the rheumatic diseases*. Orlando: Grune & Stratton, 1988:159–163.

117. Gelber RH. Leprosy (Hansen's disease). In: Mandell GL, Bennett JE, Dolin R, eds. *Principles and practice of infectious diseases*. New York: Churchill Livingstone, 1995:2243–2250.

118. Gibson T, Ahsan Q, Hussein K. Arthritis of leprosy. *Br J Rheumatol* 1994;33:963–966.

119. Pernambuco JC, Cossermelli-Messina W. Rheumatic manifestations of leprosy: clinical aspects. *J Rheumatol* 1993;20:897–899.

120. Atkin SL, el-Ghobarey A, Kamel M, et al. Clinical and laboratory studies of arthritis in leprosy. *Br Med J* 1989;298: 1423–1425.

121. Carpintero P, Logrono C, Carreto A, et al. Progression of bone lesions in cured leprosy patients. *Acta Leprologica* 1998;11: 21–24.

122. Terreri MTA, Lutti D, Len C, et al. Leprosy: an unusual cause of arthritis in children. *J Trop Pediatr* 1997;24:184–186.

123. Chavez-Legaspi M, Gomez-Vazquez A, Garcia-de la Torre I. Study of rheumatoid manifestations and serologic abnormalities in patients with lepromatous leprosy. *J Rheumatol* 1985;12: 738–741.

124. Garcia-de la Torre I. Autoimmune phenomena in leprosy, particularly antinuclear antibodies and rheumatoid factor. *J Rheumatol* 1993;20:900–903.

125. Mitchell TG. Systemic fungi. In: Armstrong D, Cohen J, eds. *Infectious diseases*. London: CV Mosby, 1999(Sect 8): 27.1–27.18.

126. Cuellar ML, Silveira LH, Citera G, et al. Other fungal arthritides. *Rheum Dis Clin North Am* 1993;19:439–455.

127. Kushwaha VP, Shaw BA, Gerardi JA, et al. Musculoskeletal coccidioidomycosis: a review of 25 cases. *Clin Orthop* 1996;332: 190–199.

128. Bayer AS, Guze LB. Fungal arthritis II. Coccidioidal synovitis: clinical, diagnostic, therapeutic and prognostic considerations. *Semin Arthritis Rheum* 1979;8:200–211.

129. Sarosi GA, Davies SF. Therapy for fungal infections. *Mayo Clin Proc* 1994;69:1111–1117.

130. Perez-Gomez A, Prieto A, Torresano M, et al. Role of the new azoles in the treatment of fungal osteoarticular infections. *Semin Arthritis Rheum* 1998 27:226–244.

131. Bried JM, Galgiani, JN *Coccidioides immitis* infection in bones and joints. *Clin Orthop Rel Res* 1985;211:235–243.

132. Klein BS, Vergeront JM, Week RJ, et al. Isolation of *Blastomyces dermatitidis* in soil associated with a large outbreak of blastomycosis in Wisconsin. *N Engl J Med* 1986;314:529–534.

133. Pappas PG, Threlkeld MG, Bedsole GD, et al. Blastomycosis in immunocompromised patients. *Medicine* 1993;72:311–325.

134. George AL, Hays JT, Graham BS. Blastomycosis presenting as monoarticular arthritis: the role of synovial fluid cytology. *Arthritis Rheum* 1985;28:516–521.

135. Abril A, Campbell MD, Cotton VR Jr, et al. Polyarticular blastomycotic arthritis. *J Rheumatol* 1998;25:1019–1021.

136. Ricciardi DD, Sepkowitz DV, Berkowitz LB, et al. Cryptococcal arthritis in a patient with acquired immune deficiency syndrome: case report and review of the literature. *J Rheumatol* 1986;13:455–458.

137. Stead KJ, Klugman KP, Painter ML, et al. Septic arthritis due to *Cryptococcus neoformans*. *Br J Infect* 1988;17:139–145.

138. Raftopoulos I, Meller JL, Harris V, et al. Cryptococcal rib osteomyelitis in a pediatric patient (review). *J Pediat Surg* 1998; 33:771–773.

139. Hansen K, St. Clair EW. Disseminated histoplasmosis in sys-

temic lupus erythematosus: case report and review of the literature. *Semin Arthritis Rheum* 1998;28:193–199.

140. Como JA, Dismukes WE. Oral azole drugs as systemic antifungal thearpy. *N Engl J Med* 1994;330:263–272.

141. Darouche RO, Cadle RM, Zenon GJ, et al. Articular histoplasmosis. *J Rheumatol* 1992;19:1991–1993.

142. Rex JH. *Sporothrix schenckii.* In: Mandel GL, Bennett JE, Dolin R, eds. *Principles and practice of infectious diseases,* 4th ed. New York: Churchill Livingstone, 1995:2321–2324.

143. Gullberg RM, Quintanilla A, Levin ML, et al. Sporotrichosis: recurrent cutaneous, articular and central nervous system infection in a renal transplant recipient. *Rev Infect Dis* 1987;9: 369–375.

144. Lipstein-Kresch E, Isenberg HD, Singer C, et al. Disseminated *Sporothrix schenckii* infection with arthritis in a patient with acquired immune deficiency syndrome. *J Rheumatol* 1985; 12:805–808.

145. Zachiaris J, Crosby LA. Sporotrichal arthritis of the knee. *Am J Knee Surg* 1997;10:171–174.

146. Lipovsky MM, Hoepelman AIM. Opportunistic fungi. In: Armstrong D, Cohen J, eds. *Infectious diseases.* London: CV Mosby, 1999(Sect 8):26.1–26.16.

147. Luhmann JD, Luhmann SJ. Etiology of septic arthritis in children: an update for the 1990s. *Pediatr Emerg Care* 1999;15: 40–42.

148. Cuende E, Barbadillo C, E-Mazzucchelli R, et al. Candida arthritis in adult patients who are not intravenous drug addicts. *Semin Arthritis Rheum* 1993;22:224–241.

149. Brooks DH, Pupparo F. Successful salvage of a primary total knee arthroplasty infected with *Candida parapsilosis* (review). *J Arthroplasty* 1998;13:707–712.

150. Tunkel AR, Thomas CY, Wispelwey B. Candida prosthetic arthritis. *Am J Med* 1993;94:100–103.

151. Silvera LH, Cuellar ML, Citera G, et al. Candida arthritis. *Rheum Dis Clin North Am* 1993;19:427–437.

152. Weems JJ. *Candida parapsilosis:* epidemiology, pathogenicity, clinical manifestations, and antimicrobial susceptibility. *Clin Infect Dis* 1992;14:756–766.

153. Dupont B, Drouket E. Cutaneous, ocular, and osteoarticular candidiasis in heroin addicts: new clinical and therapeutic aspects in 38 patients. *J Infect Dis* 1985;152:577–591.

154. Murphy O, Gray J, Wagget J, et al. Candida arthritis complicating long term total parenteral nutrition. *Ped Infect Dis J* 1997;16:329.

155. Yousefzadeh DK, Jackson JH. Neonatal and infantile candidal arthritis with or without osteomyelitis: a clinical and radiographic review of 21 cases. *Skeletal Radiol* 1980;5:77–90.

156. Marcus J, Grossman ME, Yunakov MJ, et al. Disseminated candidiasis: *Candida* arthritis and unilateral skin lesions. *J Am Acad Dermatol* 1992;26:295–297.

157. Patel R. Antifungal agents. Part I. Amphotericin B preparations and flucytosine. (review). *Mayo Clin Proc* 1998, 73:1205–1225.

158. Weers-Pothoff G, Havermans JF, Kamphuis J, et al. *Candida tropicalis* arthritis in a patient with acute myeloid leukemia successfully treated with fluconazole: case report and review of the literature. *Infection* 1997;25:109–111.

159. Deleted.

160. Terrell CL. Anti-fungal agents. Part II. The azoles [review]. *Mayo Clinic Proc* 1999;74:78–100.

161. Flanagan PG, Barnes RA. Hazards of inadequate fluconzaole dosage to treat deep-seated or systemic *Candida albicans* infection. *J Infect* 1997;35:295–297.

162. Barson WJ, Marcon MJ. Successful therapy of *Candida albicans* arthritis with a sequential intravenous amphotericin B and oral fluconazole regimen. *Pediatr Infect Dis J* 1996;23: 1179–1180.

163. Ten Broeke R, Walenkamp G. The Madura foot: an "innocent foot mycosis." *Acta Orthopaed Belgica* 1998;64:242–248.

164. McGinnis MR. Mycetoma. *Dermatol Clin* 1996;14:97–104.

165. Hazra B, Bandyopadhyay S, Saha SK, et al. A study of mycetoma in eastern India. *J Commun Dis* 1998;30:7–11.

166. Riviti EA, Aoki V. Deep fungal infections in tropical countries. *Clin Dermatol* 1999;17:171–190.

167. Paugam A, Tourte-Schaefer C, Deita A, et al. Clinical cure of fungal Madura foot with oral itraconazole. *Cutis* 1997;60: 191–193.

168. Richardson MD. Subcutaneous mycoses. In: Armstrong D, Cohen J, eds. *Infectious diseases.* London: CV Mosby, 1999(Sect 8):28.1–28.10.

169. Dinulos JG, Darmstadt GL, Wilson CB, et al. *Nocardia asteroides* septic arthritis in a healthy child. *Pediatr Infect Dis J* 1999;18:308–310.

170. Dellestable F, Kures K, Mainard D, et al. Fungal arthritis due to *Pseudallescheria boydii* (*Scedosporium apiospermum*). *J Rheumatol* 1994;21:766–768.

171. Ostrum RF. Nocardia septic arthritis of the hip with associated avascular necrosis. *Clin Orthop Rel Res* 1993;288:282–286.

172. Bocanegra TS, Vasey FB. Musculoskeletal syndromes in parasitic diseases. *Rheum Dis Clin North Am* 1993;19:505–513.

173. Corman LC. Acute arthritis occurring in association with subcutaneous *Dirofilaria tenuis* infection. *Arthritis Rheum* 1987;30: 1431–1434.

174. Atkin SL, Kamel M, el-Hady AM, et al. Schistosomiasis and inflammatory polyarthritis: a clinical, radiological, and laboratory study of 96 patients infected by *S. mansoni* with particular reference to the diarthrodial joint. *Q J Med* 1986;59: 479–487.

175. Ferrari TC. Spinal cord schistosomiasis: a report of 2 cases and review emphasizing clinical aspects. *Medicine* 1999;78: 176–90.

LYME DISEASE

STEPHANIE ANN CALL

Lyme disease is a vector-borne infectious disorder caused by the spirochete *Borrelia burgdorferi*. Transmitted by the bite of a tick, the infection and resulting inflammation can affect several organ systems and thus has been referred to as the next "great imitator" in medicine. Lyme arthritis is a common presentation of the disease.

EPIDEMIOLOGY

Lyme disease was first recognized as a clinical entity in 1975 when a cluster of children thought to have juvenile rheumatoid arthritis was identified in Lyme, Connecticut (1). Investigation of this geographic cluster led to the identification of the mode of transmission and eventually the implication of ticks of the *Ixodes* genus as the vectors of the disease. The disease is now known to occur in a wide geographic distribution, primarily in temperate climates. Cases have been reported from 48 states in the United States, Europe, Asia, the Soviet Union, and possibly Australia.

Lyme disease is a reportable infection in the United States. A uniform case definition for surveillance was adopted by the Centers for Disease Control and Prevention in 1990. Through surveillance, three endemic regions have been identified in the United States: the Northeast, the Midwest, and the West. The number of cases reported in the United States has progressively increased each year. More than 100,000 cases have been reported since reporting started in 1982. A dramatic increase in incidence was noted in 1996 and was felt to represent "a combination of increased tick density, enhanced health-care provider awareness and reporting, and improved laboratory surveillance" (2). (See Tables 29.1 and 29.2.)

A bimodal age distribution of cases has been described in the United States, with most cases occurring in children under the ages of 15 and middle-aged adults. This distribution is related to the activities that predispose a person to contact with the tick vectors. Most cases are reported between May and November, with typical peaks in incidence rates in June and July. There do not appear to be gender- or race-specific differences in the incidence of Lyme disease.

PATHOPHYSIOLOGY/PATHOGENESIS

Lyme disease develops after inoculation of skin with *Borrelia burgdorferi* from an infected tick of the genus *Ixodes*. After a period of latency (3 to 32 days), the organisms migrate outward in the skin, causing inflammation that results in the herald skin lesion, erythema chronicum migrans (EM) (3,4). Histologically, these lesions show extracellular spirochetes in association with an inflammatory infiltrate consisting of lymphocytes, histiocytes, and plasma cells. The organisms are then thought to disseminate from the primary site to secondary skin sites and other organ systems, which may include the central nervous system, joints, heart, spleen, liver, kidney, bone marrow, and skeletal muscle. Infection appears to trigger both local and systemic immune responses, accounting for the varied presentations. It is unknown whether the chronic manifestations of the disease are associated with live organisms or a parainfectious etiology.

CLINICAL FEATURES

Lyme disease is characterized by three progressive clinical stages. However, this staging system is somewhat arbitrary; patients may be initially asymptomatic and present at a later stage.

Early Disease

The early, localized stage (Stage I) of disease is characterized by the classic erythema chronicum migrans (EM) skin lesion. The thighs, groin, buttocks, and axilla are common sites. The rash begins as a red macule or papule at the site of a previous tick bite, although most individuals are

TABLE 29.1. LYME DISEASE CASES REPORTED TO CENTERS FOR DISEASE CONTROL BY STATE HEALTH DEPARTMENTS, 1990–1999

State	Region	1990	1991	1992	1993	1994	1995	1996	1997	1998	1999	Total	1995 POP	INC 98	INC 99	ANN INC
Alabama	ESC	33	13	10	4	6	12	9	11	24	20	142	4.246	0.57	0.47	0.33
Alaska	PAC	0	0	0	0	0	0	0	2	1	0	3	0.603	0.17	0.00	0.05
Arizona	MT	0	1	0	0	0	1	0	4	1	3	10	4.305	0.02	0.07	0.02
Arkansas	WSC	22	31	20	8	15	11	27	27	8	7	176	2.485	0.32	0.28	0.71
California	PAC	345	265	231	134	68	84	64	154	135	139	1,619	31.565	0.43	0.44	0.51
Colorado	MT	0	1	0	0	1	0	0	0	0	3	5	3.748	0.00	0.08	0.01
Connecticut	NE	704	1,192	1,760	1,350	2,030	1,548	3,104	2,297	3,434	3,215	20,634	3.271	104.99	98.30	63.09
Delaware	SA	54	73	219	143	106	56	173	109	77	167	1,177	0.717	10.74	23.29	16.41
District of Columbia	SA	5	5	3	2	9	3	3	10	8	6	54	0.555	1.44	1.08	0.97
Florida	SA	7	35	24	30	28	17	55	56	71	59	382	14.184	0.50	0.42	0.27
Georgia	SA	161	25	48	44	127	14	1	9	5	0	434	7.209	0.07	0.00	0.60
Hawaii	PAC	2	0	2	1	0	0	1	0	0	0	6	1.179	0.00	0.00	0.05
Idaho	MT	1	2	2	2	3	0	2	4	7	3	26	1.166	0.60	0.26	0.22
Illinois	ENC	30	51	41	19	24	18	10	13	14	17	237	11.790	0.12	0.14	0.20
Indiana	ENC	15	16	22	32	19	19	32	33	39	21	248	5.797	0.67	0.36	0.43
Iowa	WNC	16	22	33	8	17	16	19	8	27	24	190	2.843	0.95	0.84	0.67
Kansas	WNC	14	22	18	54	17	23	36	4	13	16	217	2.564	0.51	0.62	0.85
Kentucky	ESC	18	44	28	16	24	16	26	20	27	19	238	3.857	0.70	0.49	0.62
Louisiana	WSC	3	6	7	3	4	9	9	13	15	9	78	4.338	0.35	0.21	0.18
Maine	NE	9	15	16	18	33	45	63	34	78	41	352	1.239	6.30	3.31	2.84
Maryland	SA	238	282	183	180	341	454	447	494	659	899	4,177	2.039	13.08	17.84	8.29
Massachusetts	NE	117	265	223	148	247	189	321	291	699	787	3,287	6.071	11.51	12.96	5.41
Michigan	ENC	134	46	35	23	33	5	28	27	17	11	359	9.538	0.18	0.12	0.38
Minnesota	WNC	70	84	197	141	208	208	251	256	261	283	1,959	4.615	5.66	6.13	4.25
Mississippi	ESC	7	8	0	0	0	17	24	27	17	4	104	2.696	0.63	0.15	0.39
Missouri	WNC	205	207	150	108	102	53	52	28	12	72	989	5.319	0.23	1.35	1.86
Montana	MT	0	0	0	0	0	0	0	0	0	0	0	0.870	0.00	0.00	0.00
Nebraska	WNC	0	25	22	6	3	6	5	2	4	11	84	1.639	0.24	0.67	0.51
Nevada	MT	2	5	1	5	1	6	2	2	6	2	32	1.533	0.39	0.13	0.21
New Hampshire	NE	4	38	44	15	30	28	47	39	45	27	317	1.148	3.92	2.35	2.76
New Jersey	MA	1,074	915	688	786	1,533	1,703	2,190	2,041	1,911	1,719	14,560	7.950	24.04	21.62	18.32
New Mexico	MT	0	3	2	2	5	1	1	1	4	1	20	1.690	0.24	0.06	0.12
New York	MA	3,244	3,944	3,448	2,818	5,200	4,438	5,301	3,327	4,640	4,402	40,762	18.191	25.51	24.20	22.41
North Carolina	SA	87	73	67	86	77	84	66	34	63	74	711	7.202	0.87	1.03	0.99
North Dakota	WNC	3	2	1	2	0	0	2	0	0	1	11	0.642	0.00	0.16	0.17
Ohio	ENC	36	112	32	30	45	30	32	40	47	47	451	11.134	0.42	0.42	0.41
Oklahoma	WSC	13	29	27	19	99	63	42	45	13	8	358	3.284	0.40	0.24	1.09
Oregon	PAC	11	5	13	8	6	20	19	20	21	15	138	3.149	0.67	0.48	0.44
Pennsylvania	MA	553	718	1,173	1,085	1,438	1,562	2,814	2,188	2,760	2,781	17,072	12.060	22.88	23.06	14.16
Rhode Island	NE	101	142	275	272	471	345	534	442	789	546	3,917	0.992	79.56	55.06	39.50
South Carolina	SA	7	10	2	9	7	17	9	3	8	6	78	3.667	0.22	0.16	0.21
South Dakota	WNC	2	1	1	0	0	0	0	1	0	0	5	0.730	0.00	0.00	0.07
Tennessee	ESC	28	35	31	20	13	28	24	45	47	59	330	5.247	0.90	1.12	0.63
Texas	WSC	44	57	113	48	56	77	97	60	32	72	656	18.801	0.17	0.38	0.35
Utah	MT	1	2	6	2	3	1	1	1	0	2	19	1.958	0.00	0.10	0.10
Vermont	NE	11	7	9	12	16	9	26	8	11	26	135	0.585	1.88	4.45	2.31
Virginia	SA	129	151	123	95	131	55	57	67	73	122	1,003	6.615	1.10	1.84	1.52
Washington	PAC	30	7	14	9	4	10	18	11	7	14	124	5.448	0.13	0.26	0.23
West Virginia	SA	11	43	14	50	29	26	12	10	13	20	228	1.825	0.71	1.10	1.25
Wisconsin	ENC	337	424	525	401	409	369	396	480	657	490	4,488	5.122	12.83	9.57	8.76
Wyoming	MT	5	11	5	9	5	4	3	3	1	3	49	0.479	0.21	0.63	1.02
U.S. TOTAL		**7,943**	**9,470**	**9,908**	**8,257**	**13,043**	**11,700**	**16,455**	**12,801**	**16,801**	**16,273**	**122,651**	**262.889**	**6.39**	**6.19**	**4.67**
NE subtotal	NE	946	1,659	2,327	1,815	2,827	2,164	4,095	3,111	5,056	4,642	28,642	13.305	38.00	34.89	21.53
MA subtotal	MA	4,871	5,577	5,309	4,689	8,171	7,703	10,305	7,556	9,311	8,902	72,394	38.200	24.37	23.30	18.95
ENC subtotal	ENC	552	649	655	505	530	441	498	593	774	586	5,783	43.381	1.78	1.35	1.33
WNC subtotal	WNC	310	363	422	319	347	306	365	299	317	407	3,455	18.351	1.73	2.22	1.88
PAC subtotal	PAC	388	277	260	152	78	114	102	187	164	168	1,890	41.944	0.39	0.40	0.45
SA subtotal	SA	699	697	683	639	855	726	823	792	977	1,353	8,244	47.013	2.08	2.88	1.75
WSC subtotal	WSC	82	123	167	78	174	160	175	145	68	96	1,268	28.899	0.24	0.33	0.44
ESC subtotal	ESC	86	100	69	40	43	73	83	103	115	102	814	16.046	0.72	0.64	0.51
MT subtotal	MT	9	25	16	20	18	13	9	15	19	17	161	15.750	0.12	0.11	0.11

NOTE: Population is in millions. INC, incidence (cases) per 100,000 population; ANN INC, mean annual incidence 1990–99; excludes two cases reported from Guam, one each in 1992 and 1998.
From the Centers for Disease Control and Prevention, Division of Vector-Borne Infectious Diseases, web site (www.cdc.gov).
ENC, east north central; ESC, east south central; MA, mid-Atlantic; MT, mountain; NE, northeast; PAC, Pacific coast; SA, south Atlantic; WNC, west north central, WSC, west south central.

TABLE 29.2. THE TEN STATES IN WHICH 90% OF LYME DISEASE CASES OCCURRED, 1989–1998

State	Total Number Cases Reported, 1989–1998	Annual Incidence per 100,000 Persons
New York	39,370	21.6
Connecticut	17,728	54.2
Pennsylvania	14,870	12.3
New Jersey	13,428	16.9
Wisconsin	4,760	9.3
Rhode Island	3,717	37.5
Maryland	3,410	6.8
Massachusetts	2,712	4.5
Minnesota	1,745	3.8
Delaware	1,003	14.0

Adapted from Questions and answers about Lyme disease from the Centers for Disease Control and Prevention's Web Site (www.cdc.gov).

unaware of the original bite. Over several days to weeks, the erythema expands annularly to a diameter of 15 cm or more and an area of central clearing develops, forming the hallmark "bull's eye" lesion (Fig. 29.1). The lesion was at one time considered pathognomonic for Lyme disease, but similar lesions may be seen in other diseases. Variants of EM include rashes with multiple EM-type lesions, and vesicular or necrotic lesions. The EM site may be asymptomatic, pruritic, or painful and usually resolves spontaneously after several weeks, even without treatment.

Secondary lesions often develop within days of disease onset. These are multiple annular lesions and are felt to represent early dissemination of the spirochete (Fig. 29.1). EM lesions are also often accompanied by systemic symptoms, such as malaise, fatigue, headache, musculoskeletal pain, and stiff neck. Gastrointestinal and respiratory symptoms are extremely rare. Signs and symptoms recorded in a series of 314 patients are presented in Tables 29.3 and 29.4 (3). These early signs and symptoms may be intermittent, may be migratory, and may occur for up to 6 months.

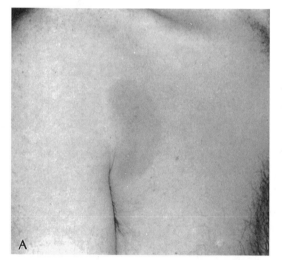

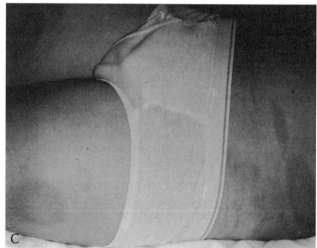

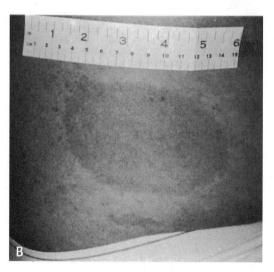

FIGURE 29.1. Dermatologic manifestations of Lyme disease. **A:** Erythema migrans (*EM*). An early lesion is seen 4 days after detection. **B:** In a 10-day lesion of EM, the red outer ring has expanded, and central clearing is beginning. **C:** Eight days after onset of EM, similar secondary lesions have appeared, and several of their borders have merged. (Reproduced with permission from Steere AC, Bartenhagen NH, Craft JE, et al. The early clinical manifestations of Lyme disease. *Ann Intern Med* 1983;99:76–82.)

TABLE 29.3. EARLY SIGNS OF LYME DISEASE

Signs	No. of Patients	
	N = 314	%
Erythema migrans[a]	314	100
Multiple annular lesions	150	48
Lymphadenopathy		
Regional	128	41
Generalized	63	20
Pain on neck flexion	52	17
Malar rash	41	13
Erythematous throat	38	12
Conjunctivitis	35	11
Right upper quadrant tenderness	24	8
Splenomegaly	18	6
Hepatomegaly	16	5
Muscle tenderness	12	4
Periorbital edema	10	3
Evanescent skin lesions	8	3
Abdominal tenderness	6	2
Testicular swelling	2	1

[a]Erythema migrans was required for inclusion in this study.
From Steere AC, Bartenhagen NH, Craft JE, et al. The early clinical manifestations of Lyme disease. *Ann Intern Med* 1983;99:79, with permission.

TABLE 29.4. EARLY SYMPTOMS OF LYME DISEASE

Symptoms	No. of Patients	
	N = 314	%
Malaise, fatigue, and lethargy	251	80
Headache	200	64
Fever and chills	185	59
Stiff neck	151	48
Arthralgias	150	48
Myalgias	135	43
Backache	81	26
Anorexia	73	23
Sore throat	53	17
Nausea	53	17
Dysesthesia	35	11
Vomiting	32	10
Abdominal pain	24	8
Photophobia	19	6
Hand stiffness	16	5
Dizziness	15	5
Cough	15	5
Chest pain	12	4
Ear pain	12	4
Diarrhea	6	2

From Steere AC, Bartenhagen NH, Craft JE, et al. The early clinical manifestations of Lyme disease. *Ann Intern Med* 1983;99:79, with permission.

Early Disseminated and Chronic Disease

Cardiac, neurologic, and rheumatologic manifestations dominate the second and third clinical stages of Lyme disease. The distinction between the two stages is made on a basis of time course and chronicity of symptoms. Early disseminated (Stage II) disease occurs weeks to months after the initial tick bite, whereas chronic (Stage III) signs and symptoms may occur and persist for years after the inciting incident.

Both the central and peripheral nervous system may be affected in Lyme disease. The most common subacute neurologic manifestations include cranial neuropathy, meningitis, and radiculoneuritis. The most common cranial neuropathy is a peripheral 7th nerve palsy that may present as a bilateral palsy. The meningitis associated with Lyme disease is a lymphocytic meningitis in which the cerebrospinal fluid (CSF) shows several to several hundred cells per cubic millimeter, mild protein elevation, and normal glucose. The radiculoneuritis may present with acute onset of severe pain or motor weakness either in a radicular pattern or an asymmetric multifocal pattern. All three of these subacute presentations generally resolve spontaneously within months.

Chronic neurologic manifestations include a chronic peripheral neuropathy, typically paresthesias with an unremarkable sensory and motor examination. Chronic encephalopathy and encephalomyelitis may present years after the onset of disease and is usually subtle as well as difficult to diagnose. These chronic sequelae generally do not remit spontaneously, but progression can halt after treatment with antibiotics.

Atrioventricular block is the most common cardiovascular manifestation of Lyme disease, occurring in approximately 1% to 8% of patients (5). This block may be first degree, Wenckebach, or complete heart block, and typically occurs within weeks to months of onset of disease. These patients present with symptoms typical of heart block: palpitations, lightheadedness, and syncope. Acute myopericarditis is a much rarer but possible cardiac complication.

Lyme arthritis is a common manifestation of infection with *Borrelia burgdorferi.* Occurring from weeks to years after initial infection, 50% to 60% of patients develop frank arthritis that is characterized by intermittent attacks of asymmetric, typically nonpainful joint inflammation (6). The knee is the most commonly involved site, but other large joints may be affected. Frequently noted is the temporomandibular joint. Small joints are rarely involved. Effusions are typical; synovial fluid analysis generally reveals an elevated white blood cell count of 500 to 100,000 (predominantly polymorphonuclear cells), total protein levels of 3 to 8 g/dL, normal or slightly elevated glucose levels, negative rheumatoid factor, and negative antinuclear antibody (7). Joint fluid accumulation may be massive and, in the knee, may lead to the formation of Baker cysts, which can dissect into the calf and rupture. These individual attacks of arthritis usually resolve spontaneously after several weeks but may recur.

Chronic arthritic symptoms may be a result of chronic joint inflammation leading to pannus formation and erosion of cartilage and bone. This is thought to occur most frequently in patients with human leukocyte antigen (HLA) class II antigen DR4 and mimics the histopathology of rheumatoid arthritis (8).

Other

Borrelial lymphocytoma is a skin lesion seen predominantly in European patients with Lyme disease. It presents as a nodule, usually on the pinna of the ear or on the nipple of the breast. Like EM, it usually resolves spontaneously.

Another dermatologic manifestation more commonly seen in European patients is a chronic skin lesion, *acrodermatitis chronica atrophicans*. These lesions begin as violaceous plaques or nodules primarily occurring on the extremities.

Rarer sites of involvement include ophthalmologic involvement such as uveitis, keratitis, and neuritis.

CLINICAL EVALUATION

The diagnosis of Lyme disease is a clinical diagnosis and should be made based on signs and symptoms consistent with the disease. Testing should be used to confirm the diagnosis when suspected. In 1990 the CDC developed a surveillance definition for Lyme disease. Although these criteria were developed for epidemiologic purposes, they have been applied to the clinical setting as well. Table 29.5 outlines these criteria (9). Notably, serologic or culture evidence of disease is not required to make the diagnosis by these criteria.

Culture

A definitive diagnosis of Lyme disease can be made by culture of the organism *Borrelia burgdorferi*. Studies of culture from EM lesions have reported successful culture rates in 30% to 80% of specimens. This is a reasonable initial diagnostic procedure in patients presenting with EM. Culture rates appear to be more successful with 2-mm punch biopsy of the leading edge of the lesion, but sterile saline lavage aspiration has also been shown to be effective. Direct visualization of the organism and newer special staining techniques are low-yield, as are culture attempts from sites other than skin.

TABLE 29.5. CENTERS FOR DISEASE CONTROL AND PREVENTION SURVEILLANCE DEFINITION FOR CONFIRMED CASE OF LYME DISEASE

Clinical description: A systemic, tick-borne disease with protean manifestations, including dermatologic, rheumatologic, neurologic, and cardiac abnormalities. The best clinical marker for the disease is the initial skin lesion, erythema migrans, which occurs in 60% to 80% of patients.

Clinical case definition: Erythema migrans or at least one of late manifestation, as defined below, and laboratory confirmation of infection

Laboratory criteria:
- Isolation of *Borrelia burgdorferi* from clinical specimen or
- Demonstration of diagnostic levels of IgM and IgG antibodies to the spirochete in serum or cerebrospinal fluid or
- Significant change in IgM or IgG antibody response to *Borrelia burgdorferi* in paired acute- and convalescent-phase serum samples

Late manifestations (include any of the following when an alternate explanation is not found):
- *Musculoskeletal:* recurrent, brief attacks (lasting weeks or months) of objective joint swelling in one or a few joints, sometimes followed by chronic arthritis in one or a few joints. Manifestations not considered criteria for diagnosis include chronic progressive arthritis not preceded by brief attacks and chronic symmetric polyarthritis. Arthralgia, myalgia, or fibromyalgia syndromes alone are not criteria for musculoskeletal involvement.
- *Nervous system:* Any of the following, alone or in combination: lymphocytic meningitis; cranial neuritis, particularly facial palsy (may be bilateral); radiculoneuropathy; or, rarely, encephalomyelitis. Encephalomyelitis must be confirmed by showing antibody production against *Borrelia burgdorferi* in the cerebrospinal fluid, demonstrated by a higher titer of antibody in cerebrospinal fluid than in serum. Headaches, fatigue, paresthesias, or mild stiff neck alone are not criteria for neurologic involvement.
- *Cardiovascular:* Acute-onset, high-grade (2 or 3) atrioventricular conduction defects that resolve in days to weeks and are sometimes associated with myocarditis. Palpitations, bradycardia, bundle-branch block, or myocarditis alone are not criteria for cardiovascular involvement.

IgG, immunoglobulin G; IgM, immunoglobulin M.

Enzyme-Linked Immunosorbent Assay and Western Blot

Serology is the most common diagnostic test employed in the evaluation of persons suspected of having Lyme disease. The use of these tests requires an understanding of their role in evaluation as well as an understanding of their limitations. The enzyme-linked immunosorbent assay (ELISA) is the most widely available and utilized test. This is usually performed on serology, but may also be performed on synovial or CSF fluid. One may measure either IgM or IgG antibodies to *Borrelia burgdorferi.* IgM may not be detectable for up to 4 weeks after infection, whereas IgG may not be detectable for up to 8 weeks, thus limiting the role for ELISA testing in patients with EM lesions (acute disease).

Early treatment may also have an effect on the antibody response. Patients who are treated empirically or partially treated may not have reactive ELISA results, although they did have infection at some time. The Lyme ELISA test is fairly nonspecific. False-positive tests have been seen in patients with other infections and other chronic illnesses such as syphilis, HIV, parvovirus, EBV infection, systemic lupus erythematosus, and rheumatoid arthritis. False-positive results have also been documented in normal subjects.

A Western blot assay is available for Lyme disease. The CDC has proposed distinct criteria for the definition of a positive Western blot analysis that includes the bands that have been shown to be most specific for Lyme disease. The current recommendations for the use of the Western blot is as a confirmatory test for ELISA results. Indeterminate and positive results on ELISA should be followed by Western blot testing. A negative Western blot would decrease the probability of Lyme disease. A major criticism of both the ELISA and the Western blot in the evaluation of Lyme disease is the lack of standardization and reproducibility between different laboratories and different assays.

Polymerase chain reaction (PCR) has been used to detect *Borrelia burgdorferi* in both serum and other body fluids; however, it is not yet a standard diagnostic technique. Other tests that may assist in evaluation in the future include an anti–*Borrelia burgdorferi* antibody assay, a urinary antigen assay, and a T-cell proliferation assay; none of which are currently clinically available.

Summary of Diagnostic Evaluation

A recent set of guidelines for the laboratory evaluation in the diagnosis of Lyme disease has been published (10). In a person who presents with an acute EM rash in an endemic area (or with a history of a tick bite), serologic evaluation is not indicated and will most likely be negative. Empiric treatment is reasonable, and cultures from the lesion may be helpful. Table 29.5 outlines the current CDC surveillance definition. Diagnostic testing should be reserved for persons in whom the health care provider has a reasonable clinical suspicion, as false positives are extremely likely and actually more common than true positive results when the clinical suspicion is low. An indeterminate or positive ELISA should be followed by a Western blot for confirmation.

PREVENTION

Lyme disease prevention methods are similar to prevention methods for other vector-borne diseases. Vector control for ticks has not been a major focus in the past, and methods are not as well established as they are for other insect vectors. Insecticides for tick control are now available both to individuals and to professionals. Knowledge of the life cycle of the tick is important in applying and using the insecticides properly in endemic areas.

Control of wildlife hosts of disease is another aspect of prevention of vector-borne diseases. In Lyme disease endemic areas this has primarily been attempted by deer enclosure techniques such as fencing.

On an individual level, education, information, and recognition of signs and symptoms are the key to prevention of disease. Persons in endemic areas must be informed of the mode of transmission of disease and alerted to activities that put them at risk. The use of tick repellents is encouraged in those engaging in high-risk exposures in endemic areas. Recognition of ticks is essential. People are instructed to inspect themselves daily for ticks and to wear light-colored clothing to make tick sighting easier. Prompt removal of a tick with fine forceps will prevent disease, as the transmission of the causative organism does not occur for 24 to 48 hours after the tick has attached. In addition, the early recognition and treatment of EM lesions can prevent the sequelae of Lyme disease.

Vaccine

Recombinant outer-surface protein A vaccine (LYMErix) has recently been licensed by the U.S. Food and Drug Administration for use in the United States. The vaccine uses recombinant *B. burgdorferi* lapidated outer-surface protein A (rOspA) as immunogen. However, in February 2002, the vaccine's manufacturer, SmithKline Beecham, announced that the vaccine would no longer be commercially available (11). The following applies to vaccine currently in supply. The vaccine is administered in three doses: the first two, given 1 month apart, followed by a booster dose the following year. The need for further booster doses beyond the first year is unknown. The decision about whether to vaccinate a patient should take into account individual risk, including geographic risk and likely personal exposure to ticks based on activities and behaviors (Table 29.6) (11).

TABLE 29.6. SUMMARY OF CENTERS FOR DISEASE CONTROL AND PREVENTION ADVISORY COMMITTEE ON IMMUNIZATION PRACTICES (ACIP) RECOMMENDATIONS REGARDING LYMERIX VACCINE

Persons who reside, work, or recreate in areas of high or moderate risk	
Persons aged 15–70 years whose exposure to tick-infested habitat is frequent or prolonged	Vaccine should be considered
Persons aged 15–70 years who have some exposure to tick-infested habitat but whose exposure is neither frequent nor prolonged	Vaccine may be considered
Persons whose exposure to tick-infested habitat is minimal or none	Vaccine not recommended
Persons who reside, work, or recreate in areas of low or no risk	Vaccine not recommended
Travelers to areas of high or moderate risk	
Travelers aged 15–70 years whose exposure to tick-infested habitat is frequent or prolonged	Vaccine should be considered
Children aged <15 years	Vaccine not recommended
Pregnant women	Vaccine not recommended
Persons with history of Lyme disease	
Persons aged 15–70 years with previous uncomplicated Lyme disease who are at continued high risk	Vaccine should be considered
Persons with treatment-resistant Lyme arthritis	Vaccine not recommended
Persons with musculoskeletal disease	Limited data available
Persons with immunodeficiency	No available data

Adapted from *Questions and answers about Lyme disease* from the Centers for Disease Control and Prevention's web site (*www.cdc.gov*).

TABLE 29.7. TREATMENT RECOMMENDATIONS

Early Lyme disease[a]
   Doxycycline, 100 mg twice daily for 21 days
   Amoxicillin, 500 mg three times daily for 21 days[b]
   Cefuroxime axetil, 500 mg twice daily for 21 days
   Azithromycin, 500 mg daily for 7 days[c] (less effective than other regimens)
Neurologic manifestations
   Bell-like palsy (no other neurologic abnormalities)
      Oral regimens for early disease suffice
   Meningitis (with or without radiculoneuropathy or encephalitis)[d]
      Ceftriaxone, 2 g daily for 14–28 days
      Penicillin G, 20 million units daily for 14–28 days
      Doxycycline, 100 mg twice daily (oral or intravenous) for 14–28 days[e]
      Chloramphenicol, 1 g four times daily for 14–28 days
Arthritis[f]
   Doxycycline, 100 mg twice daily for 30 days
   Amoxicillin and probenecid, both at 500 mg three times daily for 30 days[g]
   Ceftriaxone, 2 g daily for 14–28 days
   Penicillin G, 20 million units daily for 14–28 days
Carditis
   Ceftriaxone, 2 g daily for 14 days
   Penicillin G, 20 million units daily for 14 days
   Doxycycline, 100 mg orally twice daily for 21 days[h]
   Amoxicillin, 500 mg three times daily for 21 days[h]
Pregnancy
   Localized early disease
      Amoxicillin, 500 mg three times daily for 21 days
   Any manifestation of disseminated disease
      Penicillin G, 20 million units daily for 14–28 days
   Asymptomatic seropositivity
      No treatment necessary

[a]Without neurologic, cardiac, or joint involvement. For early Lyme disease limited to single erythema migrans lesion, 10 days is sufficient.
[b]Some experts advise addition of probenecid, 500 mg three times daily.
[c]Experience with this agent is limited; optimal duration of therapy is unclear.
[d]Optimal duration of therapy has not been established. There are no controlled trials of therapy longer than 4 weeks for any manifestation of Lyme disease.
[e]No published experience in the United States.
[f]An oral regimen should be selected only if there is no neurologic involvement.
[g]Amoxicillin is generally administered three times daily, but the only trial of this agent for Lyme arthritis used a four-times-daily regimen.
[h]Oral regimens have been reserved for mild carditis limited to first-degree heart block with PR 0.30 seconds and normal ventricular function.
From Malawista SE. Lyme disease. In: Koopman WJ, ed. *Arthritis and allied conditions: a textbook of rheumatology,* 14th edition. Philadelphia: Lippincott Williams & Wilkins, 2001:2629–2648, with permission.

TREATMENT

Similar to syphilis, many of the signs and symptoms of Lyme disease resolve spontaneously, even without treatment. Treatment will, however, prevent chronic disease and sequelae of chronic infection. Treatment recommendations vary, depending on the stage of disease presentation, systems involved, and age of the patient. Antibiotics are the foundation of treatment; several agents have been shown to be efficacious, including doxycycline, tetracycline, amoxicillin, penicillin, and cephalosporins. Oral therapy is effective for early disease, particularly in patients who present with EM lesions and isolated facial palsy. Intravenous antibiotic therapy is indicated in late stages of the disease. Current treatment recommendations are summarized in Table 29.7.

A Jarisch–Herxheimer reaction has been observed in up to 10% of patients during the first 24 hours of treatment (12). The reaction is characterized by fever, rash, and sometimes pain. Currently, the optimal duration of therapy is unclear, but most authorities recommend 2 to 4 weeks of antibiotics. Resolution of symptoms may be slow and may lag behind antibiotic therapy. Recurrence of disease can occur, particularly when a patient receives inadequate or incomplete therapy.

Specific recommendations have been made for the treatment of pregnant patients with suspected Lyme disease, included in Table 29.7. The treatment varies based on the stage of disease and is aimed at preventing maternal–fetal transmission of *Borrelia burgdorferi*.

REFERENCES

1. Steere AC, Malawista SE, Snydman DR, et al. Lyme arthritis: an epidemic of oligoarticular arthritis in children and adults in three Connecticut communities. *Arthritis Rheum* 1977;20:7–17.
2. Anonymous. Lyme disease—United States, 1996. *MMWR* 1997; 46:531–535.
3. Steere AC, Bartenhagen NH, Craft JE, et al. The early clinical manifestations of Lyme disease. *Ann Intern Med* 1983;99:76–82.
4. Steere AC. Diagnosis and treatment of Lyme arthritis. *Med Clin North Am* 1997;81:179–194.
5. Nadelman RB, Wormser GP. Lyme borreliosis. *Lancet* 1998;352: 557–565.
6. Steere AC, Schoen R, Taylor E. The clinical evolution of Lyme arthritis. *Ann Intern Med* 1987;107:725–731.
7. Steere AC, Malawista SE, Hardin JA, et al. Erythema chronicum migrans and Lyme arthritis: the enlarging clinical spectrum. *Ann Intern Med* 1977;86:685–698.
8. Steere AC, Gibofsky A, Pattarroyo ME, et al. Chronic Lyme arthritis: clinical and immunogenetic differentiation from rheumatoid arthritis. *Ann Intern Med* 1979;90:286–291.
9. CDC. Case definitions for infectious conditions under public health surveillance. *MMWR* 1997;46(RR-10):20.
10. Tugwell P, Dennis DT, Weinstein A, et al. Laboratory evaluation in the diagnosis of Lyme disease. *Ann Intern Med* 1997;127: 1109–1123.
11. Centers for Disease Control and Prevention. Recommendations for the use of Lyme disease vaccine. Recommendations of the Advisory Committee on Immunization Practices. *MMWR* 1999; 48:1–17.
12. Steere AC, Hutchinson GJ, Rahn DW, et al. Treatment of the early manifestations of Lyme disease. *Ann Intern Med* 1983;99: 22–26.

30

VIRAL ARTHRITIS

MARTA L. CUELLAR
LUIS R. ESPINOZA

Viruses have long been recognized to play an important role in the pathogenesis of a variety of acute and chronic arthritic disorders. From the original description by Graves of arthritis in the prodromal phase of hepatitis in 1842 (1) to the most recently recognized viral outbreaks, including human immunodeficiency virus (HIV) and Ebola virus infections, a great deal of evidence has emerged in support of an important role of viruses in the triggering of inflammatory articular disease in humans (2).

The intimal pathogenic mechanism(s) involved in viral-induced arthritis remains to be elucidated, but accumulated evidence supports multiple factors, some directly related to the virus itself and others related to its interaction with components of the immune system (3,4) (Table 30.1).

An increasing number of viruses can be associated with the presence of arthritis (Table 30.2), but this section will place emphasis only on those viral disorders that commonly impact and are recognized as etiologic agents of acute and/or chronic arthritis in humans.

HEPATITIS C VIRUS

In the last decade, hepatitis C infection has emerged as a leading cause of liver disease. It is often associated with a

TABLE 30.1. POSSIBLE PATHOGENIC MECHANISMS IN VIRUS-INDUCED ARTHRITIS

Direct effect on endothelial, synovial, and other hematopoietic
  cells, resulting in
    Increased cytopathic activity
    Destruction of CD4+ cells
    Apoptosis
    Shortened telomere
Indirect effect
  Immune complex formation
  Dysregulation of lymphocyte subsets
  Increased expression and production of cytokines:
    Th1 to Th2 switch
  Molecular mimicry
  Superantigen activation of immunocytes
  Infection with arthritogenic microorganisms

TABLE 30.2. VIRUSES ASSOCIATED WITH ARTHRITIS

Hepatitis A, B, and C
Parvovirus B19
Rubella
Retroviruses: HIV, HTLV-1, HRV-5
Herpes virus family: Varicella-Zoster, Herpes simplex, EBV, CMV
Alpha viruses: Chikungunya, O'nyong-nyong, Ross River,
  Mayaro, Sindbis, Barmah Forest
Miscellaneous: adenovirus, cocksackie, mumps, ebola

CMV, cytomegalovirus; EBV, Epstein–Barr virus; HIV, human
immunodeficiency virus; HRV-5, human retrovirus 5; HTLV-1, human
T-cell leukemia virus type I.

wide clinical spectrum of immune and autoimmune abnormalities (5,6) (Table 30.3).

The prevalence of hepatitis C virus (HCV) is 1% to 2% in the general population. Risk factors for HCV include a history of blood transfusion, intravenous drug use, sexual promiscuity, and low socioeconomic status.

Polyarthralgias may occur during the acute stage of HCV infection but generally resolve despite persistence of circulating HCV RNA and anti-HCV antibodies. Polyarthritis following acute posttransfusional HCV infection has also been described, but it appears to be an unusual occurrence.

Chronic HCV infection, however, is often associated with a variety of extrahepatic clinical manifestations. The first well-characterized extrahepatic manifestation associated

TABLE 30.3. CHARACTERISTICS OF HEPATITIS C VIRUS–RELATED RHEUMATIC MANIFESTATIONS

Polyarthralgias during acute stage
Polyarthralgias, myalgias, arthritis during chronic stage
Wide spectrum of immune and autoimmune abnormalities
Classic rheumatoid arthritis–like syndrome may
  occur
Erosive joint involvement does not occur
Sjögren-like syndrome described
Cryoglobulinemia common
Rheumatoid factor and antinuclear antibodies positivity common

with chronic HCV infection was the constellation of symptoms and signs including purpuric rash, arthralgias, renal involvement, and/or neuropathy induced by mixed cryoglobulinemia. Polyarthralgias, polyarthritis, and myalgias frequently occur during chronic HCV infection or may be the presenting complaints. A positive rheumatoid factor and antinuclear antibody (ANA) may be present in up to 50% of affected patients, and may make the differential diagnosis of rheumatoid arthritis from the polyarthritis of HCV extremely difficult, particularly in the presence of normal liver function tests. Erosive arthritis is seldom seen, however. At times, differential diagnoses with other connective-tissue disorders such as Sjögren disease and systemic lupus erythematosus (SLE) may also be difficult to establish (Table 30.3). Diagnosis of HCV infection is usually made by a positive anti-HCV using an enzyme immunoassay (EIA) in the setting of normal or abnormal liver function tests, and confirmed by a recombinant immunoblot assay (RIBA).

Treatment of HCV infection remains to be defined, although interferon-α, 3 million units, three times per week for 24 weeks has been approved by the United States Food and Drug Administration. Other treatment modalities available include once-weekly interferon (pegylated interferon) and interferon combined with ribavarin. The latter combination is the most effective at inducing long-term biochemical and virologic outcomes. All these therapies appear to be effective in the presence of mixed cryoglobulinemia, although it may be accompanied by the development or exacerbation of autoimmune disease.

HEPATITIS B VIRUS

The triad of urticaria, arthritis, and fever characteristically occurs in the prodromal phase of hepatitis B virus (HBV) infection (7).

The frequency of arthralgias in the prodromal phase of hepatitis B varies between 30% and 68%, whereas that for arthritis is much lower, usually less than 5%. The small joints of the hands are most frequently involved, but any joint including knees can be affected. The pattern of involvement is usually symmetric and migratory, and can be either nonadditive or additive. The duration of joint involvement lasts an average of 3 weeks but may persist for several months. In the latter situation, differential diagnosis with RA may prove to be difficult. Polyarteritis nodosa may occur during the course of chronic HBV infection. This subset of patients may require treatment with steroids, immunosuppressive agents with or without antiviral agents.

PARVOVIRUS B19 INFECTION

Human parvovirus B19 consists of single-stranded, small DNA viruses, and was first recognized in 1975. A variety of clinical manifestations including erythema infectiosum, transient aplastic crisis, and bone marrow suppression in immunosuppressed individuals, and arthritis may follow naturally occurring parvovirus infection (8,9).

Arthralgias and arthritis may occur both in children and adults, being more commonly seen in adults. Acute infection in children tends to be asymptomatic or mild, whereas adults have a more severe, flu-like illness. The characteristic facial rash, or "slapped cheeks," is seen mostly in children, although at times patients may exhibit a subtle reticular rash on the torso or extremities.

Joint involvement usually appears 1 to 3 weeks after the initial infection and tends to be self-limited in most patients. The joint pattern is symmetric or RA-like, affecting wrists, small joints of hands, knees, and ankles. A chronic rheumatoid-like arthropathy, most commonly seen in women, may also be seen. Joint symptoms in this group of patients may persist for several months, and in some cases they last for several years. Erosions or joint destruction, however, do not occur in B19-associated arthropathy.

Diagnosis is confirmed by the presence of anti-B19 IgM antibodies, which are usually positive at the time of onset of rash or joint symptoms.

A multitude of autoantibodies, including rheumatoid factor, anti-DNA, antiphospholipid, antilymphocyte, and ANAs, may be present and suggest the diagnosis of RA or SLE. These autoantibodies, however, are only transiently present and, together with an absence of subcutaneous nodules, joint erosions, and lack of association with human leukocyte antigen (HLA)-DR4, allow distinction of B19-related arthropathy from classic RA. Most patients exhibit clinical improvement to nonsteroidal antiinflammatory drugs (NSAIDs).

RUBELLA VIRUS

Sir William Osler in 1906 first described arthritis in association with rubella infection. Both natural infection and rubella vaccination can be accompanied by a similar inflammatory articular involvement and may occur at all ages—from childhood to older age groups—although there is a strong predilection for adolescent and adult women (10).

Joint symptoms characteristically occur within a few days of the onset of rash in natural rubella infection or 2 to 4 weeks after vaccination. The presenting joint manifestations are migratory polyarthralgias and, less frequently, polyarthritis affecting the small joints of hands, wrists, and knees, and much less commonly ankles, elbows, and small joints of feet. Synovial fluid examination reveals inflammatory changes with elevated protein content and leukocyte count, predominantly mononuclear cells. Most acute arthritic episodes last an average of 2 to 3 weeks, although a small proportion of patients may develop chronic or recurrent joint symptoms that may persist for some years.

At times, rubella-associated arthritis may progress to a seropositive disease resembling RA, but the inflammation eventually subsides without permanent damage to the joint. Some patients, in addition to the arthritis, may also develop carpal tunnel syndrome, peripheral neuropathy, and tenosynovitis, which generally tend to run a self-limited course.

Rubella virus has been isolated from peripheral blood and/or synovial fluid mononuclear cells from patients with rheumatoid arthritis (RA) and juvenile RA (JRA), but its role as a causative agent in RA is not well established. Conventional antiinflammatory therapy with NSAIDs provides substantial relief in most patients.

RETROVIRUSES

Various inflammatory musculoskeletal disorders have been described in association with retroviral infection (11–13). Further evidence implicating retroviruses in rheumatologic disorders is the development of RA-like disorder in goats infected with Caprine arthritis–encephalitis virus.

HUMAN IMMUNODEFICIENCY VIRUS INFECTION

Infection with HIV is associated with a broad spectrum of clinical manifestations that ranges from the asymptomatic state to frank acquired immunodeficiency syndrome (AIDS). Musculoskeletal manifestations can occur at any phase of the infection, although in the Western world they tend to occur much more frequently in the last phase. Various manifestations have been described, including distinct rheumatic disorders such as Reiter syndrome or polymyositis to isolated symptoms like arthralgias and myalgias (Table 30.4).

The prevalence of inflammatory musculoskeletal manifestations, particularly that of spondyloarthropathy (SpA) in patients with HIV infection, remains somewhat contro-

TABLE 30.4. HUMAN IMMUNODEFICIENCY VIRUS–ASSOCIATED RHEUMATIC MANIFESTATIONS

Arthralgias
Human immunodeficiency virus–associated arthritis
Reiter syndrome or reactive arthritis
Psoriatic arthritis
Undifferentiated spondyloarthropathy
Sjögren-like syndrome
Polymyositis, dermatomyositis
Vasculitis
Fibromyalgia
Aseptic vascular necrosis

versial. Recently reported data from Central Africa, however, may shed light on and further clarify reported discrepancies in the prevalence of HIV-associated SpA (14,15). Njobvu et al. (14) reported an overall prevalence for SpA of 84%, with a prevalence of 180/100,000 in HIV-positive individuals versus 15/100,000 in the non-HIV patient population. This was a large, prospective study performed in Lusaka, Zambia, during the years 1994 to 1996. Studies of this nature are yet to be performed in Western countries. The incidence and prevalence of rheumatic disorders in HIV infection may vary among populations studied and may depend on the mode of HIV transmission, ethnic background, geographic location, and exposure to different infectious agents.

Arthralgias and/or arthritis appear to be the most common rheumatic complaints, often transient, lasting an average of 3 to 4 weeks, and seen at any stage of HIV infection. At times, arthralgias are extremely painful, requiring the use of narcotic analgesics. Reiter syndrome, usually incomplete, is the most common rheumatic syndrome and may have a prevalence of as much as 11% in some HIV-infected populations. The prevalence of HLA-B27 positivity is lower in HIV-infected populations than in non-HIV-associated Reiter syndrome. In Western countries, Reiter syndrome is predominantly seen in homosexuals, whereas in Central Africa it occurs in heterosexuals. Of interest, the incidence of Reiter's appears to be much lower in whites with intravenous drug use as the risk factor for HIV transmission. Reiter syndrome and other SpA syndromes were extremely unusual in Central Africa before the advent of HIV infection. At times, Reiter syndrome may be the initial manifestation of HIV infection.

Psoriasis and psoriatic arthritis (PsA) occur with increased prevalence in HIV-infected individuals. Both can precede or follow the clinical onset of immunodeficiency. The joint pattern is more frequently polyarticular and asymmetric, accompanied by enthesopathy and dactylitis. Sacroiliac joint and spine involvement may occur. The clinical course is variable, although some patients exhibit a rapidly progressive, deforming, and incapacitating course despite the use of aggressive antiinflammatory therapy (16).

Some HIV patients exhibit an oligoarticular and asymmetric peripheral arthritis, affecting mostly weight-bearing joints—knees and ankles, self-limited course, lasting a few weeks, and not associated with HLA-B27 and/or rheumatoid factor positivity, and occurring in late stages of the disease.

Other rheumatic syndromes (Table 30.4) may also be seen. Most HIV patients presenting with rheumatic manifestations do respond to NSAIDs. Patients refractory to NSAIDs may require the judicious use of steroids and systemic and/or intraarticular, immunosuppressive drugs (e.g., methotrexate). Newer biologic agents, particularly tumor necrosis factor antagonists, can be highly effective, but should be used only in extreme circumstances due to their propensity to precipitate septic complications with multiple microorganisms such as *Staphylococcus aureus, S. pyogenes,* and *Pseudomonas aeruginosa.*

Human T-Cell Leukemia Virus Type I

Human T-cell leukemia virus type I (HTLV-1) is endemic in Japan and Jamaica; it also occurs sporadically in the United States. HTLV-1 infection may induce a chronic, proliferative synovitis, RA-like with erosive arthritis. Elevation of erythrocyte sedimentation rate (ESR), C reactive protein (CRP), and positive rheumatoid factor are present in a large proportion of patients (17). Synovial fluid is characterized by the presence of atypical lymphocytes with nuclear indentations and T-cell infiltration. It may also be associated with other autoimmune disorders, including Sjögren syndrome, thyroiditis, uveitis, and thrombocytopenia.

HUMAN RETROVIRUS 5

Human retrovirus 5 (HRV-5) is a recently identified retrovirus, distinct from HIV or HTLV-I, and not detectable in normal human DNA. A recent report demonstrated its presence in 53% of synovial samples from patients with RA, and in 16% from SLE patients. Others have been unable to confirm these findings, however (18,19).

HERPES VIRUS FAMILY

Several members of the Herpes virus family—including Varicella-Zoster, Herpes simplex, Epstein–Barr virus (EBV), and cytomegalovirus (CMV)—may be associated with arthritis. This is a rare event but can occur with all members. Joint pattern is usually oligoarticular (knees), but polyarticular involvement may also develop. Arthritis when present is transient, lasting days to a few weeks, although occasionally it may last months. A RA-like appearance has been described, and EBV DNA and CMV DNA have been detected by polymerase chain reaction. Although not conclusive, these findings provide some support for a role of these viruses in the etiopathogenesis of RA (20,21).

OTHER VIRUSES

Arthritis is a prominent clinical feature of a multitude of viral infections, some common and some uncommon, some seen in the North American subcontinent, and others seen in other parts of the world, predominantly Africa, Asia, Australia, and the jungles of Central and South America.

Alphaviruses are members of the Togaviridae family, transmitted by percutaneous inoculation of virus from highly infective mosquito saliva. A number of them—including Chikungunya, O'nyong-nyong, Ross River, Mayaro, Sindbis, and Barmah forest virus—are not indigenous to the North American subcontinent, are responsible for well-defined outbreaks of disease, and can induce arthritis (22).

They also share some clinical characteristics, including fever, rash, and rheumatic complaints. They affect both sexes with the same preponderance, with a peak incidence in the second through the fourth decade of life.

Arthralgias and arthritis are the most prominent symptoms of these infections. They occur right after the appearance of fever and involve small and large joints of upper and lower extremities in a symmetric pattern. The axial skeleton is unaffected, although nonspecific back pain is present. At times, as in other viral disorders such as HIV, joint pain is very intense, severe, and incapacitating. Duration of arthritis is usually limited to a few days to a few weeks, although chronic polyarthritis may be seen, especially in Chikungunya and Ross River virus infection. Radiologic evidence of joint destruction is seldom seen, although RA-like presentation with subcutaneous nodules and joint erosions has been occasionally reported. The arthritis of Mayaro infection differs from that of the others because it often is mono- or oligoarticular. Mayaro virus is indigenous to the tropical and subtropical areas of South and Central America. Sindbis is the most widely distributed of the alphaviruses associated with arthritis in humans. It is widely distributed in Europe, Africa, Asia, Australia, and the Philippines. Tenosynovitis and tendonitis are relatively common in patients with Sindbis arthritis. In addition to arthritis, Alphavirus infection often is accompanied by a myriad of symptoms, including malaise, weakness, myalgias, generalized lymphadenopathy, photophobia, conjunctivitis, headaches, retroorbital pain, and gastrointestinal disturbance. Rheumatoid factor and ANA testing are usually negative, but leukopenia with relative lymphocytosis, mild elevation of the ESR, thrombocytopenia (particularly with Chikungunya infection), and transient proteinuria may be seen. The diagnosis is made on clinical grounds, particularly during epidemic outbreaks. A definite diagnosis is made by viral isolation, or serologically in paired sera during the acute and convalescent phases of the infection. Symptomatic treatment with analgesics, bed rest, and hydration are indicated. Hyperplasia of the synovial layer, prominent vascular proliferation and mononuclear cell infiltration, and detection of viral ribonucleic acid have been found in inflamed synovium in Ross River virus infection (23). The use of NSAIDs should be avoided, particularly in Chikungunya infection, because of the propensity to develop hemorrhagic rash. Antimalarial agents have been proposed for use in chronic arthritis.

Other common viral infections such as adenovirus and coxsackie viruses A9, B3, B4, and B6 may also induce recurrent episodes of polyarthritis. Other more uncommon viral infection such as Ebola virus (2) may also be accompanied by myalgias and arthralgias.

REFERENCES

1. Graves RJ. In: Gerhard WW, Barrington ED, Hassell GD, eds. *Clinical lectures.* Philadelphia: 1842:122–123.
2. Baxter AG. Symptomless infection with Ebola virus. *Lancet* 2000;355:2178–2179.
3. Andras P. Mechanisms of viral pathogenesis in rheumatic disease. *Ann Rheum Dis* 1999;58:454–461.
4. Ytterberg SR. Viral arthritis. *Curr Opin Rheumatol* 1999;11:275–277.
5. McMurray RW. Hepatitis C-associated autoimmune disorders. *Rheum Dis Clin North Am* 1998;24:353–374.
6. Rivera J, Garcia-Monforte A, Pineda A, et al. Arthritis in patients with chronic hepatitis C virus infection. *J Rheumatol* 1999;26:420–424.
7. Inman RD. Rheumatic manifestations of hepatitis B infection. *Semin Arthritis Rheum* 1982;11:406–420.
8. White DG, Woolf AD, Mortimer PP, et al. Human parvovirus arthropathy. *Lancet* 1985;1:419–421.
9. Naides SJ. Rheumatic manifestations of parvovirus B19 infection. *Rheum Dis Clin North Am* 1998;24:375–401.
10. Smith CA, Petty RE, Tingle AJ. Rubella virus and arthritis. *Rheum Dis Clin North Am* 1987;13:265–274.
11. Winchester R, Bernstein DH, Fisher HD, et al. The co-occurrence of Reiter's syndrome and acquired immunodeficiency. *Ann Intern Med* 1987;106:19–21.
12. Berman A, Espinoza LR, Diaz JD, et al. Rheumatic manifestations of human immunodeficiency virus infection. *Am J Med* 1988;85:59–63.
13. Cuellar ML. HIV infection-associated inflammatory musculoskeletal disorders. *Rheum Dis Clin North Am* 1998;24:403–421.
14. Njobvu P, McGill P, Kerr H, et al. Spondyloarthropathy and human immunodeficiency virus infection in Zambia. *J Rheumatol* 1998;25:1553–1559.
15. Cuellar ML, Espinoza LR. Human immunodeficiency virus associated spondyloarthropathy: lessons from the third world. *J Rheumatol* 1999;26:2071–2073.
16. Espinoza LR, Berman A, Vasey FB, et al. Psoriatic arthritis and acquired immunodeficiency syndrome. *Arthritis Rheum* 1998;31:1034–1038.
17. Nishioka K, Nakajima T, Hasunuma T, et al. Rheumatic manifestations of human leukemia virus infection. *Rheum Dis Clin North Am* 1993;19:489–496.
18. Griffiths DJ, Cooke SP, Hervé C, et al. Detection of human retrovirus 5 in patients with arthritis and systemic lupus erythematosus. *Arthritis Rheum* 1999;42:448–454.
19. Gaudin P, Moutet F, Tuke PW, et al. Absence of human retrovirus 5 in French patients with rheumatoid arthritis. *Arthritis Rheum* 1999;42:2492–2493.
20. Mousavi-Jazi M, Bostrom L, Lovmark C, et al. Infrequent detection of cytomegalovirus and Epstein-Barr virus DNA in synovial membrane of patients with RA. *J Rheumatol* 1998;25:623–628.
21. Einsele H, Steidle M, Muller CA, et al. Demonstration of cytomegalovirus (CMV) DNA and anti-CMV response in the synovial membrane and serum of patients with rheumatoid arthritis. *J Rheumatol* 1992;19:677–681.
22. Alarcón GS, Castaneda O. Arthritis associated with alphavirus infection. In: Espinoza LR, ed. *Infection in the rheumatic diseases.* Orlando: Grune & Stratton, 1988:109–112.
23. Soden M, Vasudevan H, Roberts B, et al. Detection of viral ribonucleic acid and histologic analysis of inflamed synovium in Ross River virus infection. *Arthritis Rheum* 2000;43:365–369.

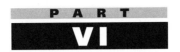

SPECIAL THERAPEUTIC
CONSIDERATIONS

TECHNIQUES OF ARTHROCENTESIS AND INJECTION THERAPY

GERALD F. MOORE

Arthrocentesis, removal of fluid from a joint cavity, has been a routine medical procedure since it was first described in the early 1950s (1). Analysis of joint fluid is required to make a diagnosis in conditions such as gout or to confirm the possibility of a septic joint.

Intraarticular therapy, most commonly performed using a corticosteroid preparation, has been a valuable adjunct to the treatment of many types of arthritis. Early trials with cortisone were disappointing (1). One-third of patients receiving a relatively small dose of hydrocortisone intraarticularly returned to pretreatment status within 1 week of the injection. Other trials with hydrocortisone (2) and later triamcinolone (3) demonstrated more long-lasting effects. Therapeutic injection of a corticosteroid preparation and/or local anesthetic administration have been found to be effective treatments for soft-tissue disease as well as joint pathology.

ARTHROCENTESIS

Joint fluid has been examined since the time of Hippocrates. Rodnan's review of several treatises on joints and joint fluid, and the anatomy and physiology of the synovial membrane found in works by Hippocrates, Celsus, Galen, and Bichat, as well as Jean-Louis Margueron's description on the chemical analysis of synovium, is worth reading (4).

Joint aspiration is easily performed without major complications. One review of more than 100,000 injections in more than 4,000 patients found only 14 infections with coagulase-positive *Staphylococcus*; a rate of one per 286 patients (5). Another study reviewing 3,000 joint injections found no infectious complications (6).

In 1961, McCarty and Hollander (7) were the first to do a systematic analysis of synovial fluid in patients with gout. Uric acid crystals were identified in 15 of 18 (83%) specimens from patients with clinical gout. Incubation with uricase destroyed the crystals in 13 of 15 samples studied. Polarized light increased the rate of positive identification of uric acid crystals from 61% to 83%. The relationship between the crystals and acute gouty attacks was not elucidated.

Indications

Arthrocentesis is required to fully evaluate a patient presenting with monoarticular arthritis. Arthrocentesis also provides a route for the intraarticular injection of corticosteroids, radiopharmaceutical agents used to induce radiation synovectomy, or viscosupplementation with hyaluronan. Arthrocentesis may be used for the diagnosis and treatment of traumatic arthritis or intraarticular fractures. Pain from distention of the joint capsule by fluid accumulation from hemarthrosis or synovitis can be relieved by removal of fluid via arthrocentesis. If more than one or two joints are involved, systemic therapy may be a more appropriate means of treatment.

1. *Evaluation of Monoarticular Arthritis.* Arthrocentesis is the only definitive method to confirm the presence of an infectious agent in septic arthritis or crystals in gout or calcium pyrophosphate deposition disease. All patients with monoarticular arthritis should undergo joint aspiration when the diagnosis is not obvious from the history and physical examination. Examination of fluid can also help differentiate inflammatory from noninflammatory joint disease.

2. *Injection of Therapeutic Agents.* Intraarticular injections of corticosteroids are useful in the treatment of many local and systemic joint disorders. Many conditions (other than trauma and infection) respond at least temporarily with a decrease in swelling and other signs of inflammation. Corticosteroids should not be injected into infected joints in view of the risk of enhanced joint and bone destruction by responsible bacteria.

McCarthy (8) recently listed indications for intraarticular corticosteroid injections: (a) to correct flexion deformities accompanying joint inflammation, (b) to control inflammation in one or more particularly troublesome joints in patients with polyarticular synovitis, (c) to control monoarticular or oligoarticular arthritis, and (d) to provide longer-term control of joint or tendon sheath inflammation, essentially a medical synovectomy.

On occasion, injection of a local anesthetic such as lidocaine benefits the patient by immediately relieving pain.

Relief of pain also indicates to the clinician that a corticosteroid preparation injected into the area might be helpful for long-term control of symptoms. Saline lavage to reduce the inflammatory components of synovial fluid may be helpful in selected patients. Viscosupplementation using hyaluronan preparations has recently been popularized as treatment for severe degenerative joint disease refractory to other measures. (See the following discussion.)

3. *Diagnosis and Treatment of Traumatic Arthritis.* Occasionally, a patient does not remember a minor traumatic event necessitating joint aspiration to rule out septic or crystal-induced disease. The presence of significant amounts of blood in synovial fluid should suggest a traumatic event (either before or during arthrocentesis). Increased intraarticular pressure that decreases range of motion and causes pain in the joint may be reduced by removal of fluid.

4. *Diagnosis of Intraarticular Fracture.* Rarely, an occult fracture can be suggested by finding fat globules mixed with intraarticular blood. This finding should prompt radiographic evaluation and early orthopedic consultation and management as appropriate.

5. *Relief of Pain from Tense Effusion, Hemarthrosis.* Fluid accumulates in response to an inflammatory condition or irritant such as blood. As the volume of fluid increases, the joint capsule becomes stretched, causing pain and discomfort. As fluid accumulates in the knee joint, the semimembranosus–gastrocnemius bursa distends and may develop into a popliteal cyst via a check valve mechanism (9). Injection of corticosteroids into the joint space may help to decrease the production of synovial fluid and the pain associated with capsule distention.

Medical management was found to be superior to surgical treatment in one large review of more than 80 articles comparing needle aspiration to surgical drainage for septic joints (10). Seventy-five percent of the medically managed group responded favorably, compared with 57% of the surgically treated group. Surgical drainage should be used when medical management of the septic joint is unsuccessful or for joints such as the hip that are technically difficult to aspirate.

6. *Obtaining Fluid for Gram Stain and Culture.* One of the most important reasons for doing an arthrocentesis is to rule out infection. Arthrocentesis provides easy access to joint fluid for Gram stain and culture. Repeated, frequent joint aspirations (up to several times per day) may be necessary in septic arthritis to remove cellular debris and speed healing.

RELATIVE CONTRAINDICATIONS TO ARTHROCENTESIS

There are no absolute contraindications to arthrocentesis. If septic arthritis is suspected, the joint should be aspirated to obtain fluid for Gram stain and culture, even when a relative contraindication is present. However, caution should be used in the following situations.

1. *Overlying cellulitis.* Entering the joint space after the needle has passed through an infected area such as a cellulitis theoretically increases the risk of spread of infection into the joint cavity. The use of appropriate technique and avoidance of areas of obvious infection reduces the chance of transmitting infection into the joint space.

2. *Bacteremia.* Likewise, performing an arthrocentesis in a patient with documented bacteremia may spread infection into the joint. However, if the joint is suspected to be infected, it is still necessary to perform a diagnostic arthrocentesis for Gram stain and culture and to facilitate the removal of excessive fluid accumulation.

3. *Bleeding disorders.* Disorders such as hemophilia, thrombocytopenia, or other coagulation disorders may result in intraarticular bleeding after insertion of the needle. Excessive movement of the needle tip while in the joint cavity should be avoided. Bleeding into the joint is infrequently seen and can usually be avoided by using the smallest-gauge needle that allows fluid to be easily aspirated or therapeutic injection performed (e.g., 22 to 25 gauge).

4. *A prosthetic joint.* The presence of a prosthetic joint makes joint aspiration technically more difficult because of scarring from the surgical procedure and resulting change in anatomy. The prosthesis is a foreign body that increases the risk of infectious complications in the joint. Aspiration of the artificial joint should be avoided unless absolutely necessary for diagnosis. If there is any question of loosening of the prosthesis or underlying osteomyelitis, the patient should undergo orthopedic evaluation.

5. *Failure of previous injections.* A single joint should not be injected more than two or three times in 1 year (excluding viscosupplementation; see later). Complications are more likely with more frequent injections. The failure of injections to be effective suggests the need for reevaluation of the treatment regimen and consideration of other intraarticular therapy, systemic therapy, or orthopedic intervention.

6. *Uncooperative patient.* Arthrocentesis should not be performed on a patient who is unable to cooperate. Any unnecessary movement of the joint during aspiration can lead to damage of the cartilage or bleeding that will make interpretation of the joint fluid more difficult.

Technique

Appropriate equipment should be readied (Table 31.1). Knowledge of the anatomy of the joint being aspirated is essential. The aspiration site is carefully chosen (usually on extensor surfaces except for the hip and ankle) to avoid contact with critical structures such as blood vessels and nerves. Appropriate body fluid precautions are observed, including the use of disposable latex gloves. The site is cleansed appro-

TABLE 31.1. EQUIPMENT NEEDED

Disposable gloves (do not need to be sterile)
Povidone–iodine solution (or similar)
Alcohol wipes
Anesthetic: 1 to 2 mL lidocaine (1% without epinephrine)
  or ethyl chloride
Syringes and needles
  One 3-mL syringe with 25-gauge needle for lidocaine
    (if used)
  One 5-mL syringe with 18- to 22-gauge needle for
    administration of corticosteroid/lidocaine preparation (if
    used)
  One (or more) 3- to 50-mL syringes with 18- to 25-gauge
    needles for obtaining fluid (size of syringe depends on
    volume of fluid expected and size of needle depends upon
    size of joint being aspirated)
Plastic bandage
Sterile container for culture and sensitivity
Test tube(s) with liquid anticoagulant for laboratory testing
Polarizing microscope with red filter, slides, and coverslips

From Moore GF. Arthrocentesis technique and intraarticular
therapy. In: Koopman WJ, ed. *Arthritis and allied conditions: a
textbook of rheumatology,* 14th ed. Philadelphia: Lippincott
Williams & Wilkins, 2001:848–859, with permission.

priately with an iodophor (or similar) preparation. A sterile field preparation is unnecessary. In one small study, field preparations using a "swipe" with isopropyl alcohol or an "aseptic" technique using chlorhexidine demonstrated no difference in the incidence of positive cultures from needles used in either group (11). Local anesthesia is obtained with either an ethyl chloride spray or lidocaine injected subcutaneously. The needle is directed into the joint cavity. (See specific joint techniques discussed later.) Fluid should flow easily into the syringe.

If there is no fluid or very sluggish flow, several options should be considered.

1. No fluid is present.
2. Tissue is obstructing the lumen of needle—try rotating the syringe and needle.
3. The needle is not actually in the joint cavity—pull back to the skin surface and reinsert at a slightly different angle.
4. No fluid obtained because the patient has tensed muscles around the joint and obstructed synovial fluid flow. In this situation, keeping the needle still until the patient relaxes may allow synovial fluid to flow into the syringe.

If corticosteroids or other agents are to be injected, the syringe should be removed from the needle while it is still in the joint space. The syringe containing the corticosteroid should be attached to the needle in the joint and an attempt should be made to reaspirate fluid to document that the needle remains in the joint space. If it is still in the joint space, corticosteroid can be safely injected. The injection

should not require much pressure on the plunger. If significant pressure is required, the needle has left the joint space and should be reinserted properly.

A long-acting corticosteroid such as prednisolone or triamcinolone should be used for injection. The amount of corticosteroid administered is determined by the size of the joint injected. Because the knee is a large joint, a volume of 1 to 2 mL is appropriate (usually 40 to 80 mg of triamcinolone). Other joints may accommodate only 0.25 to 0.5 mL of a corticosteroid preparation.

Prolonged joint rest after injection for up to 3 weeks for upper-extremity joints and 6 weeks for lower-extremity joints has been recommended (8). A comparison of ordinary activity versus 24 hours of rest following corticosteroid injections of knees demonstrated that at 3 and 6 months, pain and stiffness assessments favored those patients treated with 24 hours of rest (12). A regimen of decreased activity for a few hours to days after injection is probably adequate.

Complications

Infections

If proper aseptic techniques for arthrocentesis are used, the risk of introducing infection into a joint is negligible. Most reports place the incidence significantly below 1% of all procedures (5,6). A review of the literature identified 443 cases of reported postinjection bacterial arthritis (13). Predisposing factors for infection were diabetes mellitus, rheumatoid arthritis, systemic steroid therapy, immunosuppressive therapy, and infection elsewhere in the body. Slightly less than half of the infections were due to staphylococcal species.

Iatrogenic infection can occur when a needle enters a joint through infected skin or subcutaneous tissue. This complication is estimated to occur in less than one in 10,000 arthrocenteses and may be increased by previous corticosteroid injection (14,15). A case report of *Staphylococcus aureus* infection of the wrist after injection of the carpal tunnel has been reported (16). Another report reviewing more than 3,000 periarticular and intraarticular injections noted no infections (6).

Bleeding

Significant bleeding after arthrocentesis is rare. It is best prevented by pressure over the puncture site after arthrocentesis. Arthrocentesis can safely be performed in patients with a bleeding diathesis or in patients taking anticoagulants if one is careful to avoid vessels and use a small-gauge needle. Bleeding into a joint following arthrocentesis is usually self-limited and usually requires only observation. Treatment may rarely be required to reverse anticoagulation or replace clotting factors.

Cartilage Injury

Injury to the cartilage by the needle is rare. Injury to cartilage can lead to focal degenerative change. This complication can be prevented by utilizing the following techniques.

1. Aspirate as the joint space is entered to avoid going too deep.
2. Do not move the needle from side to side while in the joint.
3. Select a site and needle path that stays away from the cartilage.

Corticosteroid-Related Complications

Table 31.2 lists potential corticosteroid-related complications.

When injected into soft tissues, fluorinated corticosteroids can cause significant atrophy of collagenous tissue and lead to ligament or tendon rupture or subcutaneous calcification. (The atrophy may disappear in 2 to 3 years.) Therefore fluorinated corticosteroids are not recommended for use for extraarticular injections. A crystal-induced arthritis (postinjection flare) sometimes occurs within hours of injection and can last for several days in up to 10% of patients (17).

Isolated reports of tendon rupture following soft-tissue injections with corticosteroids have been documented following excessive administration of a corticosteroid preparation in one area or when the corticosteroid is injected directly into the tendon (18,19).

Three case reports of intraarticular injections illustrate other post–corticosteroid arthrocentesis complications (16). One patient developed rupture of four digital flexor tendons after 29 corticosteroid injections. Another devel-

TABLE 31.2. POTENTIAL SEQUELAE FROM INTRA-ARTICULAR AND PERI-ARTICULAR CORTICOSTEROID INJECTIONS

Elevated serum glucose in diabetic patients
Erythema, warmth, diaphoresis of face and torso
Iatrogenic infection
Nerve damage (injection into nerve)
Pancreatitis
Posterior subcapsular cataracts
Postinjection flare
Radiologic changes
   Charcot arthropathy
   Osteonecrosis
   Steroid arthropathy
Suppression of the hypothalamic/pituitary/adrenal axis
Tendon rupture
Tissue atrophy, fat necrosis, calcification
Uterine bleeding

From Moore GF. Arthrocentesis technique and intraarticular therapy. Koopman WJ. *Arthritis and allied conditions: a textbook of rheumatology,* 14th ed. Philadelphia: Lippincott Williams & Wilkins, 2001:848–859, with permission.

oped a typical bowstring deformity involving the volar aspect of the hand at the metacarpophalangeal joint after 10 injections. The third case described flushing and warmth of the face and neck after intraarticular triamcinolone.

Side effects are not more common in children receiving intraarticular corticosteroid injections (20). Aseptic necrosis was found in one injected hip but could not be shown to be attributable to the corticosteroid injection. Repeated joint injections in children probably do not increase the rate of radiographic deterioration of the joint.

Hormonal changes may be secondary to intraarticular or soft-tissue injections. Up to one-half of women in one series reported either delayed or early menstrual cycles (21). Rarely, patients receiving frequent intraarticular corticosteroid injections may demonstrate suppression of the hypothalamic–pituitary–adrenal axis (22). Plasma cortisol levels may be suppressed within hours of intraarticular injection with the effect lasting for several days (23).

Significant elevation of the blood sugar may follow the intraarticular injection of corticosteroids. Type I diabetic patients should be warned to pay close attention to their blood sugar levels for several days following injection.

Allergic/Local Reactions

Subcutaneous use of local anesthetics should be avoided in patients with known allergies. In these patients, local anesthesia may be obtained by ethyl chloride spray. Ethyl chloride works as a vaporcoolant spray. Second-degree epidermolysis may occur if overzealous freezing of the skin occurs. An erythematous area may develop around the site and last for several days but will usually resolve without any significant long-term effects. Two reports of flushing following intraarticular injections have been described (16,21). The incidence of postinjection flare, probably due to the ingestion of corticosteroid crystals by polymorphonuclear leukocytes, is quite low (2% of 100,000 injections in one series) (5).

Joint Instability

Instability of the joint may be seen with frequent joint injections (more than two per year per joint). Whether this results from a steroid or Charcot-like arthropathy or from progression of the underlying disease is unknown. In one large series of joint injections followed for 10 years, repeatedly injected joints had less than a 1% incidence of joint instability (5). That number is probably close to the incidence of disease-related joint instability. The antiinflammatory effects of the corticosteroid preparation may increase the likelihood of developing joint instability.

Hypodermic Needle Separation

Two cases of hypodermic needle separation from the plastic hub during arthrocentesis have been reported (24).

Removal of the separated needle from the soft tissue may require minor surgical exploration.

Dry Tap

Failure to obtain fluid may result from many factors (25). Most commonly, this is because no fluid is present. It may be difficult to determine whether fluid is present on physical examination, particularly in an obese patient. In the knee, the needle may enter the triangular fat pad on the medial aspect of the patellofemoral compartment. Chronically inflamed synovium may undergo fat replacement (lipoma arborescens), making aspiration difficult. A medial plica in the knee may obstruct the lumen of the needle. Long-standing fluid with reabsorption over time can lead to development of a gelatinous material that is extremely difficult to aspirate.

Technique for Specific Joints

The technique for each individual joint is described later. Video examples of individual joint injections are available (26).

Knee

The patient should be in the supine position with both legs extended as completely as possible. The knee to be aspirated should be completely exposed. A sheet or towel can be arranged around the knee to protect the patient's clothing. If the patient is unable to straighten the knee completely, a pillow should be placed beneath the knee to provide support.

The knee is usually aspirated through either a medial or lateral approach, although some prefer an anterior approach with the knee flexed at 90 degrees. Locate the patella and ask the patient to relax so that the patella is freely movable. Injections are usually made at one of four positions (supe-

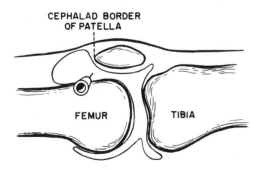

FIGURE 31.1. Arthrocentesis of the right knee, lateral approach to the suprapatellar pouch. (From Moore GF. Arthrocentesis technique and intraarticular therapy. In: Koopman WJ, ed. *Arthritis and allied conditions: a textbook of rheumatology,* 14th ed. Philadelphia: Lippincott Williams & Wilkins, 2001:848–859, with permission.)

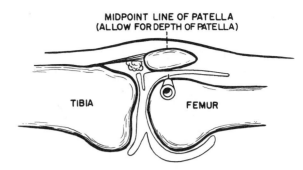

FIGURE 31.2. Arthrocentesis of the right knee, medial approach under the patella. (From Moore GF. Arthrocentesis technique and intraarticular therapy. In: Koopman WJ, ed. *Arthritis and allied conditions: a textbook of rheumatology,* 14th ed. Philadelphia: Lippincott Williams & Wilkins, 2001:848–859, with permission.)

rior or inferior lateral and superior or inferior medial) in the palpable depression between the patella and femur.

Use a 22-gauge or larger needle (some prefer an 18- or 20-gauge needle) attached to a 3- to 5-mL syringe. After appropriate anesthesia is obtained, insert the needle into the space between the patella and femur parallel to the inferior border of the patella. Direct the needle toward the center of the patella. Insertion depth ranges from 2 cm in a normal, thin knee to more than 4 to 5 cm in grossly obese subjects, requiring the use of a 2.5-inch spinal needle. On entry into the synovial cavity, a small "give" may be felt. At that time, fluid should aspirate easily (Figs. 31.1 and 31.2).

Hip

Hip injections are usually performed under fluoroscopic guidance. The hip joint should only be injected by an experienced individual familiar with the anatomy of the joint. The patient is placed supine on a table with the hip extended and slightly internally rotated.

An 18- to 22-gauge spinal needle attached to a 10-mL syringe is typically used. In the anterior approach, a location approximately 2 to 3 cm below the anterior superior iliac spine and 2 to 3 cm lateral to the femoral artery can be used (Fig. 31.3).

After appropriate site preparation and administration of anesthetic, insert the needle under fluoroscopic guidance at a 60-degree angle in a posterior–medial direction. Be careful to avoid the neurovascular bundle that lies medial to the injection site. Advance the needle until bone is encountered and then withdraw it slightly. After radiologic confirmation that the tip of the needle is in the vicinity of the joint capsule, aspiration and/or injection can be performed. Use a long-acting corticosteroid such as prednisolone or triamcinolone. Little pressure on the plunger of the syringe should be required.

Less commonly, a lateral approach is used: insert the needle anterior to the proximal tip of the greater trochanter

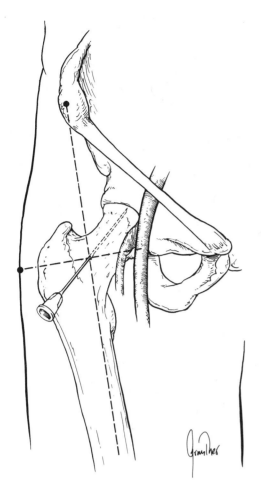

FIGURE 31.3. Right hip. (From Moore GF. Arthrocentesis technique and intraarticular therapy. In: Koopman WJ, ed. *Arthritis and allied conditions: a textbook of rheumatology,* 14th ed. Philadelphia: Lippincott Williams & Wilkins, 2001:848–859, with permission.)

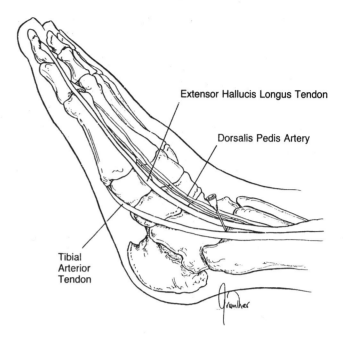

FIGURE 31.4. Right ankle, anteriomedial view. (From Moore GF. Arthrocentesis technique and intraarticular therapy. In: Koopman WJ, ed. *Arthritis and allied conditions: a textbook of rheumatology,* 14th ed. Philadelphia: Lippincott Williams & Wilkins, 2001:848–859, with permission.)

and directed at a point midway between the symphysis pubis and the anterior superior iliac spine.

Ankle Joint

Ankle arthrocentesis is performed with the patient supine in a comfortable position. The foot should be in a neutral position with the heel resting on the table. Use an anterior approach. The area between the extensor hallicus longus and the tibialis anterior tendon should be identified near the medial malleolus (Fig. 31.4). A similar position and technique can be used for a subtalar approach (Fig. 31.5).

Use an 18- to 22-gauge needle attached to a 3- to 5-mL syringe. After preparing the site and administering the anesthetic, insert the needle parallel to the upper surface of the talus in the groove between the talus and tibia. At a depth of approximately 2 cm, the needle will enter the joint space. If present, fluid should easily be aspirated.

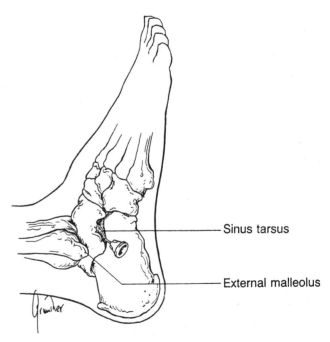

FIGURE 31.5. Right subtalar joint, lateral view. (From Moore GF. Arthrocentesis technique and intraarticular therapy. In: Koopman WJ, ed. *Arthritis and allied conditions: a textbook of rheumatology,* 14th ed. Philadelphia: Lippincott Williams & Wilkins, 2001:848–859, with permission.)

Metatarsophalangeal and Interphalangeal Joints of the Foot

Use a 25-gauge needle attached to a 1-mL syringe. After appropriate site preparation and administration of anesthetic, insert the needle perpendicular to the skin lateral to the extensor tendons, being careful to avoid the neurovascular bundle (Fig. 31.6). Because of the small size of these joints, careful probing of the area may be necessary to ensure that the joint is entered appropriately. Insertion depth will be approximately 0.5 cm. Fluid is not usually easily aspirated.

When aspirating the first metatarsal–phalangeal joint to obtain fluid for crystals, use a medial approach. Because of possible severe discomfort for the patient, it may be appropriate to wait until acute inflammation begins to resolve. Crystals can usually be found between acute attacks of gout.

Shoulder

The patient is seated with the forearm flexed. Palpate the joint to determine the best place to aspirate.

Any of three approaches for arthrocentesis of the shoulder can be used: anterior, lateral, or posterior. Anterior arthrocentesis is done in the groove between the coracoid process and the humerus. Lateral injections are done inferior to the distal end of the acromion process. Posterior injections are done at the posterior tip of the acromion aiming toward the coracoid process.

1. *Anterior approach.* The groove between the coracoid process and the humerus is identified. A 22-gauge or larger needle attached to a 3- to 5-mL syringe should be used. After appropriate site preparation and administration of anesthetic, insert the needle into the area just lateral and slightly inferior to the coracoid process (Fig. 31.7). The needle should be directed posteriorly. A small

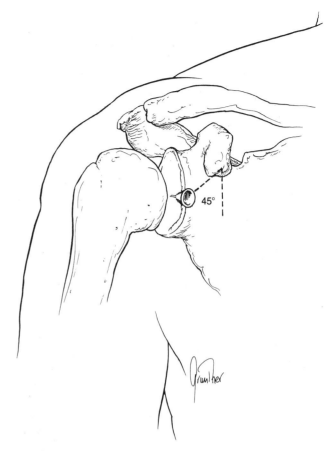

FIGURE 31.7. Right shoulder. (From Moore GF. Arthrocentesis technique and intraarticular therapy. In: Koopman WJ, ed. *Arthritis and allied conditions: a textbook of rheumatology,* 14th ed. Philadelphia: Lippincott Williams & Wilkins, 2001:848–859, with permission.)

"give" may be felt when the joint capsule is entered. Insertion depth is approximately 2 cm in a normal-sized individual. Fluid should be aspirated easily if present.
2. *Lateral approach.* Palpate for the slight indentation just lateral to the distal acromion. Insert the needle horizontally in a medial and slightly posterior direction.
3. *Posterior approach.* Identify the posterior tip of the acromial process. Insert the needle medial to the head of the humerus in the general direction of the coracoid process.

Elbow

Arthrocentesis of the elbow is usually performed in the posterior–lateral area between the lateral epicondyle and the olecranon. The elbow should be partially flexed (approximately 30 to 90 degrees) with the hand placed on the upper leg if sitting or on the abdomen if the patient is supine.

A 22-gauge or larger needle attached to a 3- to 5-mL syringe should be used. After appropriate site preparation and administration of anesthetic, insert the needle perpen-

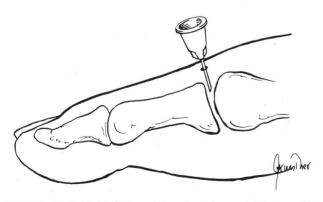

FIGURE 31.6. Right first metatarsal–phalangeal joint, medial view. (From Moore GF. Arthrocentesis technique and intraarticular therapy. In: Koopman WJ, ed. *Arthritis and allied conditions: a textbook of rheumatology,* 14th ed. Philadelphia: Lippincott Williams & Wilkins, 2001:848–859, with permission.)

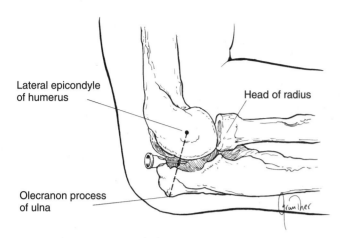

FIGURE 31.8. Right elbow, lateral view. (From Moore GF. Arthrocentesis technique and intraarticular therapy. In: Koopman WJ, ed. *Arthritis and allied conditions: a textbook of rheumatology,* 14th ed. Philadelphia: Lippincott Williams & Wilkins, 2001:848–859, with permission.)

dicular to the skin in the area between the lateral epicondyle and the olecranon. The needle may also be positioned parallel to the radius and directed toward the hand (Fig. 31.8). The needle will need to be inserted approximately 1 cm in a normal-sized individual. Aspirate any fluid present. An alternative approach is to enter the joint posteriorly, inserting the needle superior to the olecranon and just lateral to the triceps tendon.

Wrist

Have the patient place his or her hand on a flat surface with the palm down. Place a small rolled-up towel beneath the wrist to flex the joint slightly. Arthrocentesis of the wrist is best performed on the dorsum of the wrist distal to the tip

of the radius and to the ulnar side of the extensor tendon of the thumb. Alternatively, arthrocentesis may be performed distal to the ulnar styloid at the ulnar–carpal articulation (Fig. 31.9).

After appropriate site preparation and administration of anesthetic, insert the needle perpendicular to the skin directly over the radiocarpal joint between the extensor tendons of the thumb and the fingers (alternatively, the needle can be inserted distal to the ulnar styloid). The needle will need to be inserted approximately 1 cm before entering the joint. Fluid should be easily aspirated if present.

Metacarpophalangeal and Interphalangeal Joints of the Hand

Place the hand palmar side down on a table. The metacarpophalangeal joints of the hand are usually injected through a lateral approach entering the joint space superior to the neurovascular bundle as it runs down the lateral aspect of the finger. The joint line is usually easily identified by moving the finger and palpating the area.

For interphalangeal joint injections, an assistant can put pressure on the joint line opposite the intended insertion point to open up the joint. Enter the joint space superior to the neurovascular bundle on either side of the joint (Fig. 31.10).

A 25-gauge needle attached to a 1-mL syringe should be used. After appropriate site preparation and administration of anesthetic, insert the needle perpendicular to the joint space superior to the neurovascular bundle. Because of the small size of these joints, careful probing of the area may be

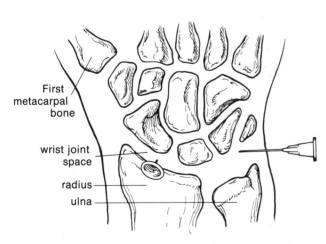

FIGURE 31.9. Right wrist. (From Moore GF. Arthrocentesis technique and intraarticular therapy. In: Koopman WJ, ed. *Arthritis and allied conditions: a textbook of rheumatology,* 14th ed. Philadelphia: Lippincott Williams & Wilkins, 2001:848–859, with permission.)

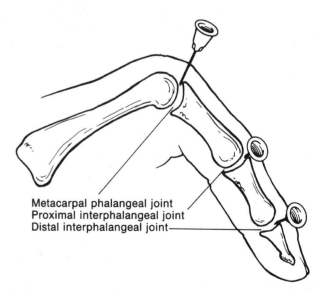

FIGURE 31.10. Small joints of the hand. (From Moore GF. Arthrocentesis technique and intraarticular therapy. In: Koopman WJ, ed. *Arthritis and allied conditions: a textbook of rheumatology,* 14th ed. Philadelphia: Lippincott Williams & Wilkins, 2001:848–859, with permission.)

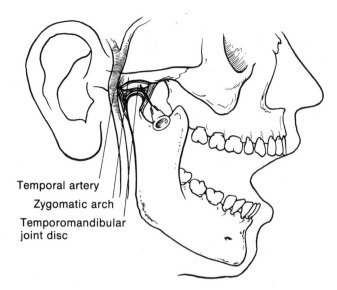

FIGURE 31.11. Right temporomandibular joint. (From Moore GF. Arthrocentesis technique and intraarticular therapy. In: Koopman WJ, ed. *Arthritis and allied conditions: a textbook of rheumatology,* 14th ed. Philadelphia: Lippincott Williams & Wilkins, 2001:848–859, with permission.)

necessary to ensure that the joint is entered appropriately. Insertion depth will be approximately 0.5 cm. Ordinarily, fluid is not easily aspirated.

Temporomandibular Joint

The patient should be asked to open his or her mouth. The temporomandibular joint (TMJ) is best injected at a point approximately 2 cm in front of the tragus just below the zygomatic arch. Care should be taken to avoid the temporal artery as well as the joint disc (Fig. 31.11).

INTRAARTICULAR THERAPY

Corticosteroids

The first information in the literature concerning the use of intraarticular corticosteroids was a personal communication by Thorn in 1950 on the use of 10 mg of hydrocortisone injected intraarticularly into the inflamed knee of a patient with rheumatoid arthritis (2). The knee improved significantly, but because of a generalized improvement thought to be due to a systemic effect, no further experiments were performed. During the next year, Hollander subsequently injected seven knees of patients with rheumatoid arthritis with 25 mg of cortisone and found minimal benefit (2). Comparison of hydrocortisone with cortisone in 129 patients with 700 local injections demonstrated the superiority of hydrocortisone for intraarticular injections (2). The hypothesis was that hydrocortisone, one-seventh less soluble than cortisone, resulted in a significant and durable "reservoir" of antiinflammatory compound in the joint.

Corticosteroids act through intracellular steroid receptors to control the rate of synthesis of mRNA and proteins (27). Corticosteroids have effects on T and B cells and inhibit phospholipase A2 with resultant decrease in the derivatives of arachidonic acid. They also may work by decreasing synthesis of the proteolytic enzyme stromelysin and the pro-inflammatory cytokine interleukin I (IL-1) in addition to reducing expression of the oncogenes *c-fos* and *c-myc,* which are important for the regulation of metalloproteinases and cytokine gene expression (27,28). In biopsy specimens of cartilage from the tibial plateaus of osteoarthritis patients who previously had received intraarticular injections with corticosteroids, metalloprotease activity was found to be normal compared with increased levels in controls not receiving the injections (29).

Neutrophil ingress into the joint is decreased by intravenous injection of 1 g of methylprednisolone, but egress from the joint is not affected (30). Magnetic resonance imaging with gadolinium performed before and after prednisolone sodium succinate injected into the knees of six individuals with rheumatoid arthritis demonstrated reduced thickness of the synovium in two of six knees (31). Five of six patients improved clinically.

Efficacy in Osteoarthritis

Most studies in osteoarthritis have found that intraarticular corticosteroids result in short-term benefit but are usually not any better than placebo after several months. A high placebo response to any injection is usually found in most studies. A review of seven controlled trials involving more than 300 osteoarthritis patients treated with intraarticular steroids found that corticosteroid injections appear to be better than placebo in the first few weeks but no long-term effect was found (27).

An early study of patients with osteoarthritis receiving either placebo, hydrocortisone, saline, novocaine, or lactic acid plus novocaine did not demonstrate any differences between the modalities at a 6-week follow-up (32). Significant improvement in the symptoms of osteoarthritis was found in each group (varying from 78% to 92%). At 6-month follow-up, all groups remained improved.

A controlled trial comparing methylprednisolone to saline given 8 weeks apart in the same joint demonstrated significant short-term benefit of the corticosteroid over the placebo. No clinical predictors of response were found (33). Another study of patients with osteoarthritis of the knee treated with either triamcinolone or placebo demonstrated early benefit for the triamcinolone-treated subjects (78% response in the first week, compared with 49% for the placebo) (34). At 6 weeks, the response rate was equal in the two groups (57% versus 55%). Response to the injection was best predicted by the presence of joint effusion and aspiration of fluid at the time of injection.

Efficacy in Rheumatoid Arthritis

The long-term effectiveness of intraarticular corticosteroids in patients with rheumatoid arthritis is similar to that found in osteoarthritis. In a 2-year follow-up study of patients with rheumatoid arthritis, 63 of 70 patients treated with corticosteroids did not have synovitis, whereas 28 of 59 patients not treated with corticosteroids had synovitis (16).

Most studies have recognized the benefit of using a longer-acting corticosteroid preparation such as triamcinolone. A randomized comparison of triamcinolone versus methylprednisolone in patients with rheumatoid arthritis revealed that at 6 months, three-fourths of those treated with triamcinolone continued to have benefit, compared with 58% of those treated with methylprednisolone (35).

An uncontrolled study of more than 100,000 injections in 4,000 patients over a 10-year period noted a 90% response rate to corticosteroid injection (5). A 7-year follow-up of some of those patients (100 patients with rheumatoid arthritis and 100 patients with osteoarthritis), demonstrated that twice as many of the patients with osteoarthritis still required injections to control their arthritis. (One interesting side note: the authors reported using corticosteroids 142 times in one joint without harm!)

Efficacy in Capsulitis

The use of corticosteroids appears to be more efficient at increasing range of motion in patients with capsulitis than distention of the capsule with both air and a local anesthetic (36).

Viscosupplementation

Viscosupplementation was approved for use in the United States in 1997 as a medical device useful for treating refractory osteoarthritis of the knee. Hyaluronan (hyaluronic acid) is a long-chain polysaccharide made up of repeating disaccharide units of *N*-acetyl-glucosamine and glucuronic acid produced by chondrocytes and synoviocytes (37). It is thought to have chondroprotective properties resulting perhaps from its binding of inflammatory mediators and free radicals (38). Hyaluronan for medical use is extracted from umbilical cords, rooster comb, or bacterial cultures (38). Three to five weekly injections are usually recommended, depending on the preparation used. Before injection, synovial fluid should be removed from the joint so that the hyaluronan is not diluted.

Studies on the use of hyaluronan have not demonstrated a marked benefit of the treatment over conventional forms of therapy. However, in selected individuals with osteoarthritis of the knee, hyaluronan may be appropriate therapy. A large, controlled, randomized double-blind trial compared five weekly intraarticular injections of sodium hyaluronate (Hyalgan) to the nonsteroidal naproxen and to placebo in patients with osteoarthritis of the knee (37). Reduction of pain with a 50-foot walk was found in all groups and persisted for the entire 6 months of the study. The only major complication was injection site discomfort in those receiving sodium hyaluronate. Other controlled studies of osteoarthritis of the knee have not shown any benefit of hyaluronan over placebo (39–41). However, the subset of patients older than 60 years with significant symptoms may be more likely to respond to intraarticular hyaluronan than to placebo.

At present, studies appear to show that hyaluronan may be as effective as nonsteroidal medications in the treatment of osteoarthritis of the knee (38). Patients who have failed conservative therapy and who are not candidates for orthopedic joint replacement may benefit from viscosupplementation. The high cost of the treatment (wholesale cost in 1999 for the injection material alone was between $495 and $600) may limit its usefulness.

REFERENCES

1. Hollander JL. The local effects of Compound F (hydrocortisone) injected into joints. *Bull Rheum Dis* 1951;2:21–22.
2. Hollander JL, Brown EM Jr, Jessar RA, et al. Hydrocortisone and cortisone injected into arthritis joints. *JAMA* 1951;147:1629–1635.
3. McCarty DJ. Treatment of rheumatoid joint inflammation with triamcinolone hexacetonide. *Arthritis Rheum* 1972;15:157–173.
4. Rodnan GP, Benedek TG, Panetta WC. The early history of synovia (joint fluid). *Ann Intern Med* 1966;65:821–842.
5. Hollander JL, Jessar RA, Brown EM Jr. Intra-synovial corticosteroid therapy: a decade of use. *Bull Rheum Dis* 1961;11:239–240.
6. Fitzgerald RH Jr. Intrasynovial injection of steroids. *Mayo Clin Proc* 1976;51:655–659.
7. McCarty DJ, Hollander JL. Identification of urate crystals in gouty synovial fluid. *Ann Intern Med* 1961;54:452–460.
8. McCarthy GM, McCarty DJ. Intrasynovial corticosteroid therapy. *Bull Rheum Dis* 1994;43:2–4.
9. Dixon AstJ, Graber J. *Local injection therapy in rheumatic diseases,* 3rd ed. Basel: Eular, 1989.
10. Broy SB, Schmid FR. A comparison of medical drainage (needle aspiration) and surgical drainage (arthrotomy or arthroscopy) in the initial treatment of infected joints. *Clin Rheum Dis* 1986;12:501–522.
11. Cawley PJ, Morris IM. A study to compare the efficacy of two methods of skin preparation prior to joint injection. *Br J Rheumatol* 1992;31:847–848.
12. Chakravarty K, Pharoah PDP, Scott DGI. Intra-articular steroid therapy for knee synovitis: role of postinjection rest. *Arthritis Rheum* 1992;35:S200.
13. Von Essen R, Savolainen HA. Bacterial infection following intraarticular injection: a brief review. *Scand J Rheum* 1989;18:7–12.
14. Hasselbacher P. Arthrocentesis, synovial fluid analysis, and synovial biopsy. In: Klippel JH, Weyand CM, Wortnab RL, et al., eds. *Primer on rheumatic diseases,* 11th ed. Atlanta: Arthritis Foundation, 1997:98–104.
15. Östensson A, Geborek P. Septic arthritis as a non-surgical complication in rheumatoid arthritis: relation to disease severity and therapy. *Br J Rheumatol* 1991;30:35–38.

16. Gottlieb NL, Riskin WG. Complications of local corticosteroid injections. *JAMA* 1980;243:1547–1548.

17. Kahn CB, Hollander JL, Schumacher HR. Corticosteroid crystals in synovial fluid. *JAMA* 1970;211:807–809.

18. Schaffer TC. Joint and soft-tissue arthrocentesis. *Prim Care* 1993;20:757–770.

19. Morgan J, McCarty DJ. Tendon ruptures in patients with systemic lupus erythematosus treated with corticosteroids. *Arthritis Rheum* 1974;17:1033–1036.

20. Sparling M, Malleson P, Wood B, et al. Radiographic followup of joints injected with triamcinolone hexacetonide for the management of childhood arthritis. *Arthritis Rheum* 1990;33:821–826.

21. Mens JMA, De Wolf AN, Berkhout BJ, et al. Disturbance of the menstrual pattern after local injection with triamcinolone acetonide. *Ann Rheum Dis* 1998;57:700.

22. Reid DM, Eastmond C, Rennie JAN. Hypothalamic-pituitary-adrenal axis suppression after repeated intra-articular steroid injections. *Ann Rheum Dis* 1986;45:87.

23. Bird HA, Ring EFJ, Bacon PA. A thermographic and clinical comparison of three intra-articular steroid preparations in rheumatoid arthritis. *Ann Rheum Dis* 1979;38:36–39.

24. Gottlieb NL. Hypodermic needle separation during arthrocentesis. *Arthritis Rheum* 1981;24:1593–1594.

25. Roberts WN, Hayes CW, Breitbach SA, et al. Dry taps and what to do about them: a pictorial essay on failed arthrocentesis of the knee. *Am J Med* 1996;100:461–464.

26. Moore GF. Arthrocentesis. In: Wigton RS, Tape TG, eds. *Mosby's primary care procedures.* CD-ROM Series. St Louis: CV Mosby, 1999.

27. Creamer P. Intra-articular corticosteroid injections in osteoarthritis: do they work and if so, how? *Ann Rheum Dis* 1997;56:634–636.

28. Anastassiades TP, Dwosh IL, Ford PM. Intra-articular steroid injections: a benefit or a hazard? *CMAJ* 1980;122:389–390.

29. Pelletier JP, Martel-Pelletier J, Cloutier JM, et al. Proteoglycan-degrading acid metalloprotease activity in human osteoarthritic cartilage, and the effect of intraarticular steroid injections. *Arthritis Rheum* 1987;30:541–548.

30. Youssef PP, Cormack J, Evill CA, et al. Neutrophil trafficking into inflamed joints in patients with rheumatoid arthritis, and the effects of methylprednisolone. *Arthritis Rheum* 1996;39:216–225.

31. Leitch R, Walker SE, Hillard AE. The rheumatoid knee before and after arthrocentesis and prednisolone injection: evaluation by Gd-enhanced MRI. *Clin Rheumatol* 1996;15:358–366.

32. Miller JH, White J, Norton TH. The value of intra-articular injections in osteoarthritis of the knee. *J Bone Joint Surg* 1958;40B:636–643.

33. Jones A, Doherty M. Intra-articular corticosteroids are effective in osteoarthritis but there are no clinical predictors of response. *Ann Rheum Dis* 1996;55:829–832.

34. Gaffney K, Ledingham J, Perry JD. Intra-articular triamcinolone hexacetonide in knee osteoarthritis: factors influencing the clinical response. *Ann Rheum Dis* 1995;54:379–381.

35. Jalava S, Saario R. Treatment of finger joints with local steroids. *Scand J Rheumatol* 1983;12:12–14.

36. Jacobs LGH, Barton MAJ, Wallace WA, et al. Intra-articular distension and steroids in the management of capsulitis of the shoulder. *BMJ* 1991;302:1498–1501.

37. Altman RD, Moskowitz R, Hyalgan Study Group. Intraarticular sodium hyaluronate (Hyalgan) in the treatment of patients with osteoarthritis of the knee: a randomized clinical trial. *J Rheumatol* 1998;25:2203–2212.

38. George E. Intra-articular hyaluronan treatment for osteoarthritis. *Ann Rheum Dis* 1998;57:637–640.

39. Dahlberg L, Lohmander LS, Ryd L. Intraarticular injections of hyaluronan in patients with cartilage abnormalities and knee pain. *Arthritis Rheum* 1994;37:521–528.

40. Lohmander LS, Dalén N, Englund G, et al. Intra-articular hyaluronan injections in the treatment of osteoarthritis of the knee: a randomised, double blind, placebo controlled multicentre trial. *Ann Rheum Dis* 1996;55:424–431.

41. Henderson EB, Smith EC, Pegley F, et al. Intra-articular injections of 750 kD hyaluronan in the treatment of osteoarthritis: a randomised single centre double-blind placebo-controlled trial of 91 patients demonstrating lack of efficacy. *Ann Rheum Dis* 1994;53:529–534.

32

MONITORING OF PATIENTS ON ANTIRHEUMATIC THERAPY

W. WINN CHATHAM

The chronicity of the majority of rheumatic diseases often involves the long-term use of antirheumatic therapies. Multiple inflammatory mediators and mechanisms of tissue injury operative in both acute and chronic inflammation frequently require the concurrent use of several agents to adequately suppress disease activity. Moreover, the increased prevalence of rheumatic disease with age dictates that use of antirheumatic therapies must often be prescribed in the context of co-morbidities. It is therefore imperative that clinicians involved in the care of patients with rheumatic disease be mindful of the short-term as well as long-term consequences of antirheumatic therapies, not only upon organ systems affected by therapy but also upon the course or treatment of coexisting disease.

CORTICOSTEROIDS

Glucocorticoids have broad inhibitory effects on specific immune responses mediated by T- and B-cell lymphocytes as well as potent suppressive effects on the effector functions of monocytes and neutrophils. Although these attributes coupled with their rapid onset of action render steroids extremely valuable in suppressing undesired inflammatory processes, corticosteroids have similar broad effects on the function of cells comprising other organ systems. The immunocompromised status and catabolic consequences associated with use of corticosteroids limits their long-term use in high doses and dictate the need for careful surveillance and preventive interventions to avoid undesired complications.

Use of high doses of corticosteroids first and foremost requires vigilance for the development of intercurrent infections. Patients with either rheumatoid arthritis or SLE have an intrinsic susceptibility to infection, and the administration of glucocorticoids enhances the risk of infection. In addition to typical bacterial organisms, infections with mycobacteria, cryptococci, listeria, and nocardia have been associated with corticosteroid therapy. The combination of steroid use with cytotoxic agents such as cyclophosphamide has been associated with higher risk of infection with *Pneumocystis carinii* pneumonia, most notably among patients with lymphopenia. Unless life- or organ-threatening disease complications dictate otherwise, in the setting of serious intercurrent infection doses of corticosteroids should be attenuated to that required to avoid adrenal crisis.

Given the significant catabolic effects of glucocorticoids on muscle, skin, and bone, patients taking moderate or high doses of steroids for prolonged intervals require periodic assessment for the evolution of steroid myopathy or development of steroid-induced osteoporosis. Since steroid myopathy most commonly affects the proximal hip girdle musculature, assessment of hip girdle strength by having the patient squat or arise from a chair unassisted is a simple maneuver that can be employed during clinic visits. Corticosteroid-induced muscle wasting and weakness may be difficult to distinguish from inflammatory muscle diseases for which they are prescribed. Muscle tenderness and elevation in CK favor the presence of active myositis. On muscle biopsy, inflammatory cells in fibrils or perivascular spaces favor inflammatory myopathy but are inconstant findings in myositis. Loss of type 1 and type 2 fibers as well as vacuolar changes may be observed in steroid-induced myopathy or myositis.

Periodic assessment for osteoporosis is becoming a standard of care for patients on chronic corticosteroids. The employment of alternate-day dosing regimens does not appear to confer protection from steroid-induced osteopenia. Exogenous administration of estrogen with calcium and vitamin D may suffice to protect patients from steroid-induced osteopenia. Glucocorticoid-induced suppression of adrenal DHEA production may render women at increased risk for the catabolic effect of steroids on bone, but a role for DHEA administration in the prevention of bone complications has not yet been confirmed. Bisphosphonates, including alendronate and risedronate, are emerging as proven therapies for the prevention and treatment of glucocorticoid-induced osteoporosis (1). Yearly assessment of bone density is recommended to assess the efficacy of these interventions in patients on chronic steroid therapy.

The predictable metabolic consequences of steroids include salt and water retention as well as variable degrees of insulin resistance with hyperglycemia. The mineralocorticoid effects of steroids warrant expectant observation for the development of hypertension or heart failure exacerbations in patients who have or are at risk for these cardiovascular disorders. Long-term metabolic consequences of corticosteroid use in patients with rheumatic disease may include accelerated atherogenesis. Attention to other cardiovascular risk factors, including assessment for and treatment of hypercholesterolemia, may slow the progression of atherogenesis and lower the risk for vascular events in patients who require long-term steroid use for management of rheumatic disease manifestations.

Other complications of corticosteroid therapy are less predictable but nonetheless require vigilance for their occurrence so as to avoid unfavorable outcomes. Corticosteroids may have untoward effects on the central nervous system (CNS), including emotional irritability, difficulty in concentration, depression, confusion, or psychosis. High-dose corticosteroid therapy has been implicated as a possible inducer of pancreatitis. Since pancreatitis may be a manifestation of lupus, the occurrence of pancreatitis in lupus patients receiving glucocorticoid therapy may result in a therapeutic dilemma. Osteonecrosis is a recognized complication of high-dose steroid use. In patients with lupus, other disease-related factors may account for the development of osteonecrosis, but the incidence appears to correlate with the cumulative steroid dose. Since routine radiographs typically fail to reveal the presence of osteonecrosis during its early stages, patients on high doses of steroids who develop otherwise unexplained pain in the shoulders, hips, knees, or ankles should be evaluated with magnetic resonance imaging to rule out the presence of osteonecrosis.

NONSTEROIDAL ANTIINFLAMMATORY DRUGS

Nonsteroidal antiinflammatory drugs (NSAIDs) constitute the most frequently prescribed class of medication used in treatment of patients with rheumatic disorders. A rapid onset of action and their combined analgesic/antiinflammatory attributes render NSAIDs very useful in the management of rheumatic disease. Although a number of cellular effects distinct from those related to prostaglandin production have been described for various NSAIDs, the major therapeutic effect of NSAIDs relates to their ability to inhibit cyclooxygenase (COX)-mediated synthesis of prostaglandins affecting vascular permeability and hyperalgesia. However, prostaglandins generated by cyclooxygenase also play an important role in hemostasis, in maintaining

the integrity of the intestinal mucosa, and in regulating renal blood flow. These physiologic effects of prostaglandins account for the majority of NSAID side effects and toxicity, most notably bleeding, intestinal ulceration, azotemia, and retention of salt and water.

Certain toxic effects of a given NSAID may be governed by its specificity for the respective isoforms of COX: COX-1 and COX-2. COX-1 is expressed constitutively in most organ systems and is the isoform primarily responsible for synthesis of prostaglandins maintaining the integrity of the GI mucosa and the hemostatic function of platelets. COX-2 is primarily induced and expressed in response to cytokines at sites of tissue injury and inflammation and is not expressed in platelets. Traditional nonselective NSAIDs inhibit both COX-1 and COX-2, whereas more recently developed NSAIDs (celecoxib, rofecoxib, and valdecoxib) selectively inhibit COX-2, substantially sparing activity of COX-1.

Monitoring of patients taking NSAIDs, particularly those not selective for COX-2, entails careful attention to symptoms referable to the GI tract and the possibility of bleeding complications. As the majority of NSAID-induced ulcerations are silent, periodic assessment of the hematocrit and red cell indices is prudent in patients taking NSAIDs for extended durations. Although there are no published studies to provide guidelines for how frequently such monitoring should occur, risk factors for NSAID-induced gastrointestinal bleeding and perforation are now well recognized (Table 32.1) (2,3), and the presence of these risk factors in a given patient should guide the frequency of blood count or hemoccult monitoring.

Both COX-1 and COX-2 are constitutively expressed in the kidney and generate prostaglandins (PGE$_2$ and PGI$_2$) that regulate renal blood flow under conditions of volume contraction and/or decreased effective arterial blood volume. PGE$_2$ and PGI$_2$ furthermore stimulate secretion of renin with attendant release of aldosterone and potassium secre-

TABLE 32.1. RISK FACTORS FOR NONSTEROIDAL ANTIINFLAMMATORY DRUG (NSAID)-INDUCED GASTROINTESTINAL BLEEDING AND PERFORATION

Previous peptic ulcer disease
Previous gastrointestinal bleed
Previous hospitalization for gastrointestinal disease
History of NSAID-induced gastritis or dyspepsia
Use of H$_2$-blocker or antacid for dyspepsia
Concurrent corticosteroid use
Older age
Higher dose of NSAID
History of cardiovascular disease
Higher arthritis-related disability score
Concurrent anticoagulant use
Smoking
Alcoholism

Compiled from the ARAMIS database and outcomes in the MUCOSA trial (2,3).

tion. Accordingly, diminution in glomerular filtration rate (GFR) with salt and water retention and/or hyperkalemia may occur as a consequence of treatment with either nonselective or COX-2 selective NSAIDs. Patients with preexisting renal disease or diminished effective arterial blood volume (congestive heart failure, cirrhosis, renal vascular disease) are at particular risk for effects of NSAIDs on glomerular perfusion. Effects of NSAIDs on GFR may cause significant complications in diabetic patients with type IV renal tubular acidosis (hyporeninemic hypoaldosteronism), as the attendant inhibition of renin release accompanied by diminution of salt load to distal nephrons may precipitate significant hyperkalemia. Careful monitoring for fluid retention and elevations of creatinine or potassium should be undertaken in these at-risk patient populations within several days of instituting treatment with a NSAID.

In addition to their potential effects on glomerular perfusion and renin secretion, NSAIDs may induce idiosyncratic, drug-specific complications of interstitial nephritis. While this complication may occur with any NSAID, interstitial nephritis has been reported most commonly in patients receiving fenoprofen. Although an appropriate frequency of monitoring renal function in patients taking NSAIDs has not been established by relevant outcome studies, at least semiannual assessment of creatinine and urinalysis is prudent for patients on long-term NSAID therapy to minimize the risk of permanent kidney damage from drug-induced interstitial nephritis.

Colchicine

Colchicine is most commonly used in the treatment of acute gout or pseudogout; the drug may be used for extended periods of time to prevent repeated flares of acute crystalline-induced arthritis. The antiinflammatory effects of colchicine are attributed to the drug's interference with the function of tubular microfilaments required for chemotaxis, migration, and release of granule constituents by neutrophils. The toxicity of colchicine when used acutely is primarily related to effects on the intestinal mucosa when administered excessively. Inappropriate use of intravenous colchicine in the setting of renal insufficiency may result in serious bone marrow toxicity. When used in the appropriate setting of an acute attack of crystalline-induced arthritis of less than 24 hours' duration, it is seldom necessary to administer oral dosing of colchicine that induces diarrhea. Three to four oral doses of 0.6 mg administered over the course of a day usually suffice in this setting. Provided renal function is normal and there has been no immediate antecedent use of oral colchicine, a single 2.0-mg intravenous dose of colchicine can be administered safely in this setting without toxicity. Attacks of crystalline-induced arthritis of greater than 24 hours' duration are less likely to resolve with administration of colchicine, and alternative therapies such as NSAIDs or corticosteroids should be considered in this setting.

A vacuolar myopathy may evolve in the setting of chronic colchicine use, particularly among patients with renal insufficiency. For patients treated with colchicine over extended periods, monitoring for the development of myopathy with periodic assessment for serum elevations in creatine kinase is prudent. Patients with renal insufficiency may also be at greater risk for marrow toxicity and should also be monitored periodically for evidence of cytopenias when taking colchicine over extended periods.

DISEASE-MODIFYING ANTIRHEUMATIC DRUGS

Use of one or more disease-modifying antirheumatic drugs (DMARDs) is now the standard of care for patients with active rheumatoid arthritis. Many DMARDs—including methotrexate, hydroxychloroquine, and azathioprine—are used to manage manifestations of diseases other than rheumatoid arthritis, including lupus and polymyositis. Use of DMARDs entails titration of the dose to achieve the desired clinical benefit without inducing toxicity. Selection and successful use of a DMARD or DMARD combination for a given patient rests upon multiple clinical considerations, including stage and activity of the disease, patient comorbidities, concurrent medication use, and known side effect profiles of the respective DMARDs. Monitoring for DMARD toxicity and side effects is therefore critical to the appropriate use of these drugs.

Methotrexate

An analog of folic acid, methotrexate inhibits folic acid–dependent pathways through numerous mechanisms. At high doses, methotrexate is an effective chemotherapeutic agent for the treatment of lymphoid neoplasms and some solid tumors. At lower doses methotrexate has immunosuppressive and significant antiinflammatory effects, most likely mediated by effects of its polyglutamated metabolites on aminoimidazole carboxamide ribonucleotide (AICAR)–transformylase. Inhibition of AICAR-transformylase by polyglutamated methotrexate results in impaired synthesis of purines and pyrimidines as well as accumulation of AICAR, a potent inducer of adenosine release. The latter may account for methotrexate's antiinflammatory effects, as engagement of adenosine receptors on leukocytes attenuates their adherence to endothelial cells.

Although uncommon in the doses usually employed for management of rheumatoid arthritis, mucositis, bone marrow suppression, and hepatocellular injury constitute the primary toxicities associated with use of methotrexate. Less common complications include acute interstitial pneumonitis, interstitial nephritis, and transient postdose syndromes that may include fever, neurocognitive impairment, arthralgia, and/or myalgia. The occurrence of mucositis or cytopenias may depend in part on folate stores, as these complications can be prevented or significantly reduced with folic acid supplementation (4). Folic acid does not impair the formation of polyglutamated methotrexate metabolites, and use of folic acid supplements has been shown not to alter the antirheumatic efficacy of methotrexate.

Effects of methotrexate on hematopoiesis are typically dose-dependent, but there is considerable individual variability in the dose threshold for development of methotrexate-induced cytopenias. Rare, severe idiosyncratic cytopenias may develop even in the setting of low weekly doses and adequate folate stores. Renal insufficiency greatly enhances the likelihood of marrow toxicity, due in large part to the prominent role of renal excretion in elimination of the drug. Use of methotrexate in patients with end-stage renal disease, even while on regular hemodialysis, may have deleterious and irreversible consequences. Although serum levels of methotrexate can be efficiently lowered by hemodialysis using high-flux dialyzers, peritoneal dialysis is ineffective at lowering serum levels of methotrexate, and dialysis of any type likely has little effect on removal of the active polyglutamated metabolites within cells.

Guidelines for monitoring of patients with rheumatoid arthritis receiving methotrexate have been established (Table 32.2) (5). Before starting methotrexate, a complete blood count with serum levels of liver transaminases (ALT, AST), albumin, and creatinine should be checked. Screening for hepatitis B and hepatitis C infection should also be done. Transaminase levels and complete blood cell counts should be checked within 4 weeks of instituting therapy, and within 4 weeks of any dose increment. More frequent assessment of blood counts may be indicated for patients with renal insufficiency. Alternatively, the interval between assessment of blood counts and liver function tests may be extended to 8 weeks for patients who have been on a stable dose of methotrexate in excess of 6 months. Creatinine levels should be checked at least every 6 months.

For patients who develop cytopenias [white blood cell count (WBC) <3,000/mm³; hematocrit <30%; platelets <130,000/mm³)], methotrexate should be withheld until the cause of the cytopenia is elucidated or the level of the depressed blood element recovers. A similar strategy should be employed for patients who develop elevation in liver transaminases in excess of twice the upper limit of normal. In either case, if it is deemed the abnormality was due to methotrexate, treatment with methotrexate at a lower dose can often be employed with success. Elevations of creatinine while on methotrexate warrant exclusion of interstitial nephritis and attention to the need for dose adjustment to avoid marrow toxicity. The occurrence of cough, dyspnea, and fever should prompt withholding of methotrexate until it can be established that the syndrome is not likely attributable to methotrexate pneumonitis.

The reported occurrence of cirrhosis among patients with psoriasis treated with long-term weekly methotrexate initially prompted recommendations for routine liver biopsy in patients with rheumatoid arthritis treated with methotrexate once the cumulative dose approached 2.0 g. However, given the infrequent occurrence of serious liver disease observed among patients with rheumatoid arthritis treated with methotrexate (estimated risk at 5 years < 1 in 1,000), current guidelines do not advocate routine liver biopsy for patients treated with long-term methotrexate who have normal liver function. Liver biopsy is advocated pretreatment for patients with known history of previous heavy alcohol use, active hepatitis B, or hepatitis C infection, and for patients on methotrexate who develop persistent elevation in liver transaminases or a fall in serum albumin despite well-controlled rheumatoid arthritis.

TABLE 32.2. GUIDELINES FOR MONITORING PATIENTS RECEIVING METHOTREXATE

Baseline evaluation:
 Complete blood count
 Liver function tests—AST, ALT, bilirubin, alkaline
  phosphatase, albumin
 Hepatitis B surface antigen, hepatitis C antibody
Pretreatment liver biopsy for patients with
 Prior history of excessive alcohol consumption
 Persistent abnormal elevations in transaminases (AST, ALT)
  levels
 Evidence of persistent infection with hepatitis B or C
Monitor CBC, AST, ALT, and albumin at 4- to 8-week intervals
Monitor creatinine at 3- to 6-month intervals
In setting of cytopenia or elevation in AST, ALT twice upper
 range of normal:
  Hold methotrexate, resume at lower dose once lab
   abnormality resolves
Perform liver biopsy before continuing treatment if
 5 of 9 or 6 of 12 AST determinations in a 1-year time frame
  are abnormal, or
 Albumin decreases below normal range despite adequate
  control of synovitis

ALT, alanine transaminase; AST, aspartate transaminase; CBC, complete blood count.

Antimalarials: Hydroxychloroquine and Chloroquine

Most commonly employed in the management of lupus or rheumatoid arthritis, antimalarials have multiple effects on immunologic function and have a very favorable toxicity/benefit profile. Hydroxychloroquine and chloroquine do not suppress bone marrow function, and liver toxicity is uncommon. Side effects consist primarily of cutaneous reactions, gastrointestinal intolerance, and mild CNS symptoms. With the exception of severe skin eruptions, many of the gastrointestinal and neurologic side effects may abate with reduction in the dose of antimalarials. Although rare, cardiac conduction abnormalities, cardiomyopathy, and neuromyopathy have been reported as more serious complications. As is recommended following initiation of therapy with most antirheumatic drugs, assessment of liver transaminases should be performed within the first 2 or 3 months of treatment to ensure the absence of idiosyncratic liver toxicity.

Although uncommon in the doses employed (200 to 400 mg/d), ocular toxicity may occur with use of antimalarials. Corneal deposits associated with perception of halos around lights may occur, but often remit spontaneously even with continued antimalarial use. CNS effects of hydroxychloroquine or chloroquine following initiation of either drug may result in transient defects in accommodation or convergence. Retinopathy is a more serious complication that may result in permanent visual impairment. Although opinion varies with regard to the appropriate frequency of monitoring, patients on hydroxychloroquine should undergo at least yearly ocular evaluation for evidence of hydroxychloroquine retinopathy (6,7). Antimalarial-induced retina toxicity is often, although not uniformly, identifiable before any perceived alterations in visual acuity. With regular ocular assessment for pigmentary abnormalities in the retina, alterations in visual field, and changes in acuity or color perception, permanent visual impairment from antimalarial use can usually be avoided.

Sulfasalazine

Sulfasalazine consists of a salicylate (5-aminosalicyclic acid) and a sulfapyridine molecule adjoined by an azo bond that is cleaved by bacterial organisms in the gut. In addition to the antiinflammatory effects afforded by the liberated salicylate, sulfapyridine and/or its metabolites appear to have immunomodulatory effects that are of benefit in the management of patients with rheumatoid arthritis, ankylosing spondylitis, or one of the other spondyloarthropathies. Gastrointestinal symptoms are usually the most common side effects reported with use of sulfasalazine, but these often resolve with dose attenuation. The less common but potentially more serious hematologic consequences of sulfasalazine use include aplastic anemia, agranulocytosis, or hemolytic anemia, with the latter occurring predominantly in patients with glucose-6-phosphate dehydrogenase deficiency. Leukopenia most often occurs during the first several months of treatment but may occur at any time. In decreasing order of frequency, cutaneous, hepatic, pulmonary, and renal hypersensitivity reactions may also occur.

When initiating therapy with sulfasalazine, it is advisable to check baseline blood counts, perform liver function tests, and screen for glucose-6-phosphate dehydrogenase deficiency. The drug is best introduced incrementally, starting with a 500 mg/d dose and then increasing by 500 mg weekly until the therapeutic target dose of 1 to 2 g twice daily is reached. Blood counts and liver function tests should be assessed at 2-week intervals until the patient has been on the target maintenance dose for at least 1 month. Blood counts and liver transaminase levels can then be monitored less frequently, but should be assessed at least every 3 months. As leukopenia may occur precipitously, patients should be instructed to promptly report the occurrence of fever, malaise, mouth ulcers, or sore throat.

Leflunomide

Leflunomide is an inhibitor of dihydroorotate dehydrogenase, an enzyme mediating synthesis of pyrimidines. Leflunomide has significant inhibitory effects on proliferation of lymphocytes and has demonstrated efficacy in the management of rheumatoid arthritis. Adverse effects of leflunomide are relatively mild and infrequent, and include reversible alopecia, skin rash, diarrhea, and elevation in liver enzymes. Leflunomide is teratogenic in animals and is contraindicated in women who are or wish to become pregnant.

Liver function tests should be assessed at baseline and at monthly intervals following initiation of therapy. Frequency of testing can be extended to every 3 months for patients who have been on therapy for more than 6 months without signs of liver toxicity. Leflunomide should be promptly discontinued if significant elevations in liver transaminases occur. The serum half-life of the major active metabolite of leflunomide (referred to as M1) exceeds 2 weeks, but because of significant enterohepatic circulation the serum levels of M1 can be rapidly decreased with administration of cholestyramine. In the setting of significant liver toxicity or the occurrence of pregnancy, a 10- to 14-day course of 8.0 g cholestyramine taken three times daily should be administered to enhance rapid elimination of the drug and bring the serum levels of M1 below 0.02 μg/mL. It is recommended that sequential determinations of M1 be performed at 2-week intervals until elimination is complete.

Gold Salts: Aurothioglucose and Auranofin

Gold salts have a variety of effects on cells and enzymes that regulate immune responses and inflammatory reactions relevant to the pathogenesis and expression of rheumatoid arthritis. The most common preparations currently in use are aurothioglucose, administered parenterally, and auranofin, administered orally. Another parenteral gold preparation, gold sodium thiomalate (aurothiomalate) is no longer in common use. Although parenteral gold salts such as aurothioglucose are very effective disease-modifying drugs, the frequency of side effects patients experience has traditionally limited their use.

The most common adverse events limiting use of gold compounds are mucocutaneous reactions, including stomatitis, pruritus, and any number of various forms of dermatitis. Although rarely reported with use of auranofin, proteinuria is a less common complication of parenteral gold salt therapy that may require either attenuation or cessation of therapy. Leukopenia, thrombocytopenia, or aplastic anemia are rare but potentially fatal consequences that may occur at any time during the course of gold therapy. Other rare complications of gold therapy include pneumonitis, enterocolitis, cholestasis, pancreatitis, and cranial or peripheral neuropathy. Corneal or lens deposits (chrysiasis) commonly occur with use of parenteral gold but are usually of little consequence and do not require discontinuation of therapy.

Nitritoid reactions are vasomotor responses to injection of gold sodium thiomalate that induce symptoms of flushing, nausea, vomiting, sweating, or dizziness. Such reactions are rarely seen following administration of aurothioglucose but have been reported with use of auranofin. The peripheral vasodilatation associated with nitritoid reactions is usually well tolerated but in elderly patients with arteriosclerotic vascular disease may result in stroke or myocardial infarction.

Monitoring of patients on gold therapy requires attention to the occurrence of skin rash, pruritus, or mouth ulcers. Before each injection of parenteral gold, patients should be questioned as to the occurrence of mucocutaneous symptoms. Patients on oral gold should be advised to report the occurrence of skin rash or symptoms of stomatitis that may arise between monthly blood checks. Most mucocutaneous side effects are best managed by interruption of therapy, then resuming treatment at a lower dose once the dermatitis or stomatitis has resolved. Topical steroid preparations may be of benefit in hastening the resolution of mouth ulcers or severe skin reactions. Gold compounds should not be reinstituted in patients who develop bullous eruptions, exfoliative dermatitis, or lichen planus.

For patients on parenteral gold therapy, blood counts and a urinalysis should be checked before each injection during the first year of treatment. Once a patient is on a stable regimen beyond the initial year, the monitoring interval for proteinuria and cytopenias can be extended to every other injection. The development of significant leukopenia (<3,500/mm^3), thrombocytopenia (<100,000/mm^3), or a persistent downward trend in the platelet count or hematocrit should prompt cessation of chrysotherapy. In the absence of other identifiable causes for observed cytopenia(s), treatment with gold compounds should not be reinstituted.

Proteinuria during treatment with gold compounds is often transient, responding to temporary withholding of gold; most patients can resume treatment at lower doses without recurrence of the proteinuria. Gold should not be reinstituted in patients who develop significant proteinuria (>1 g protein excreted every 24 hours). Although many patients with this degree of proteinuria improve spontaneously over several months following cessation of therapy, treatment with corticosteroids may be required to effect res-

olution of the proteinuria. The prognosis for recovery of patients developing gold-induced nephrotic syndrome is good, with more than 70% of patients recovering fully. Progression or persistence of proteinuria following withdrawal of gold should prompt evaluation to rule out other factors such as amyloidosis, glomerular toxicity induced by other drugs, or nephrosclerosis from poorly controlled hypertension.

D-Penicillamine

Derived from biochemical modification of penicillin or synthesized de novo, penicillamine is a sulfhydryl amino acid with demonstrated efficacy in the treatment of rheumatoid arthritis. Penicillamine does not have direct antiinflammatory effects, nor is it immunosuppressive, but the highly reactive sulfhydryl moiety appears to impart a distinct immunomodulatory effect on the function of T- and B-cell lymphocytes. Now used infrequently as a disease-modifying drug, penicillamine may be most useful in selected patients with rheumatoid arthritis (RA) unresponsive to other therapies or who have extraarticular manifestations such as vasculitis, severe nodulosis, or rheumatoid lung disease. Although penicillamine has been used in the management of scleroderma, its efficacy in this disorder remains controversial.

Adverse effects of penicillamine are similar to those observed with gold compounds, with mucocutaneous reactions, cytopenias, and proteinuria being the most common. Erythematous rashes or pruritus occurring during the first few weeks or months of treatment are usually transient and can be managed with antihistamines without altering the administered dose. Rashes occurring later in the course of treatment may respond to attenuation followed by slow reescalation of the administered dose. Stomatitis or rashes that occur after 6 months of treatment warrant exclusion of evolving autoimmune complications such as pemphigoid, pemphigus, or lupus that may be associated with use of penicillamine.

In addition to attention to cutaneous reactions, surveillance for leukopenia and thrombocytopenia is mandatory in the monitoring of patients taking penicillamine. Blood counts should be determined at baseline and every 2 weeks following the initiation of therapy or after any increment in the administered dose. Once the target dose has been achieved for several months, blood counts can be monitored at monthly intervals. Treatment should be withheld in the presence of leukopenia (WBC < 3,000 cells/mm^3) or thrombocytopenia (platelets < 100,000/mm^3). Thrombocytopenia may be dose related and responsive to lowering the administered dose. For patients who develop leukopenia, penicillamine should not be reinstituted unless appropriate investigations reveal an alternative cause.

Since penicillamine may induce a membranous nephropathy or rapidly progressive glomerulonephritis, monthly surveillance for proteinuria is recommended.

Microscopic hematuria occurs not uncommonly in the setting of penicillamine therapy, but in the absence of associated proteinuria or elevation in the serum creatinine does not require cessation of therapy. Gross hematuria requires exclusion of infection, coagulopathy, overt nephritis, or anatomic lesions. In the absence of other identifiable causes of urinary tract bleeding penicillamine should be stopped.

Tetracyclines: Minocycline and Doxycycline

In addition to their well-established antimicrobial effects, tetracyclines have a variety of effects on leukocytes and enzymes involved in immune responses that likely account for their moderate efficacy in the management of rheumatoid arthritis. Tetracyclines inhibit the activity of matrix metalloproteases and have demonstrated efficacy in preventing bone resorption in patients with periodontal disease. The inhibitory effect of tetracyclines on metalloprotease activity in articular cartilage has provided a rationale for assessing their efficacy in the prevention of cartilage loss in osteoarthritis.

In controlled trials examining the efficacy of minocycline in the treatment of RA, very few side effects were experienced that required discontinuation of the drug. Side effects most commonly experienced among patients using tetracyclines over extended periods of time include nausea and anorexia. Photosensitivity is not uncommon and is particularly associated with use of doxycycline. Vertigo and the development of slate-gray skin pigmentation are most often associated with use of minocycline. Rare complications other than hypersensitivity reactions include hepatitis, interstitial nephritis, pronounced eosinophilia, leukemoid reactions, and drug-induced lupus syndromes.

Given the adverse effects of tetracyclines on skeletal development in the fetus as well as pigmentation of unerupted teeth, tetracyclines should not be given to pregnant women or to young children. Although there are no published guidelines for adult patients taking tetracyclines over extended time periods, surveillance at 3-month intervals for possible hematologic, liver, or renal abnormalities with routine blood counts, serum creatinine, and liver transaminases is advisable. Flare of joint symptoms while on minocycline requires consideration of the possibility of an evolving drug-induced lupus syndrome. The syndrome is often associated with hepatitis and is usually associated with a positive antinuclear antibody test and prompt resolution of joint symptoms upon withdrawal of the drug.

CYTOTOXIC DRUGS

Cyclophosphamide

The effects of cyclophosphamide are mediated through its active metabolites, hydroxycyclophosphamide and phosphoramide mustard, which alkylate DNA, resulting in breaks in DNA, decreased DNA synthesis, and cell apoptosis. Although the relationship between the drug's cytotoxic effects and its immunoregulatory effects remains unclear, T-cell proliferation as well as the proliferation and function of B-cell lymphocytes are significantly affected by cyclophosphamide. Daily oral cyclophosphamide is frequently the drug of choice for the management of patients with systemic necrotizing vasculitis and for patients with active lung inflammation associated with autoimmune disease. Intermittent intravenous "pulse" cyclophosphamide is commonly employed in patients with certain manifestations of lupus. The toxicities of cyclophosphamide include reversible myelosuppression, bladder toxicity, ovarian failure, and irreversible oligospermia.

The adverse effects of cyclophosphamide are dependent in part upon the administered dose and whether the drug is given as a daily oral dose or as a periodic intravenous pulse. Effects of intravenous pulse dosing on peripheral leukocyte counts are fairly predictable, with a nadir in the leukocyte count occurring within 8 to 14 days following a single intravenous dose and full recovery 21 days following the dose. To achieve the desired clinical effects in lupus patients without inducing severe leukopenia and the attendant risk of infection, subsequent doses of intravenous cyclophosphamide are usually adjusted based upon the WBC nadir 10 to 14 days after administering the dose, attenuating the dose if the WBC nadir is <1,500/mm^3 or increasing the dose if the WBC nadir is >4,000/mm^3. It is also prudent to assess the WBC immediately before each intravenous dose. In the doses employed for management of rheumatologic disorders, pulse intravenous doses of cyclophosphamide generally have minimal, if any, impact on platelet counts.

The hematologic effects of daily oral cyclophosphamide are much less predictable. Drug-induced leukopenia as well as thrombocytopenia may occur at any time during the course of treatment. Blood counts should be monitored a minimum of every 2 weeks following initiation of therapy. For management of vasculitides such as Wegener granulomatosis, clinical efficacy does not require induction of cytopenia. Once a stable target dose (usually 2 mg/kg/day) has been established and blood counts have been stable for a minimum of 6 to 8 weeks, the interval between blood count determinations can be extended to every 4 weeks; longer intervals between blood count determinations are not recommended.

Toxic effects of cyclophosphamide on the bladder are also related to the route of administration as well as the duration of therapy. With attention to hydration at the time of administration, pulse intravenous cyclophosphamide in doses employed for management of lupus generally does not result in bladder toxicity. Bladder toxicity occurs primarily in the setting of long-term daily oral cyclophosphamide and is due to exposure of vesicular epithelium to acrolein, a cyclophosphamide metabolite. Microscopic or gross hematuria is the common presenting feature of acrolein toxicity. In the setting of either oral or intravenous cyclophosphamide therapy, urinalysis should be performed monthly, with prompt urologic evaluation of nonglomerular hematuria. The risk of bladder cancer is significantly increased in patients who receive cyclophosphamide. Major risk factors are daily oral dosing, a history of cyclophosphamide-induced cystitis, smoking, duration of therapy of more than 2 years, and a cumulative dose in excess of 100 g (8). For patients who have experienced an episode of cyclophosphamide-induced cystitis, life-long surveillance for bladder cancer is recommended, with yearly urinalysis and urine cytologic evaluation.

Regardless of the route of administration there is a 45% to 71% risk of ovarian failure following treatment with cyclophosphamide, with highest rates observed among women who are older and who have received a higher cumulative dose. Similar rates of azospermia are reported for males receiving alkylating agents such as cyclophosphamide. To preserve future fertility, sperm or ova can be banked before treatment with cyclophosphamide. There is no evidence that prior treatment of either parent with cyclophosphamide is associated with genetic abnormalities in subsequent offspring.

Treatment with oral cyclophosphamide is associated with a two- to fourfold increased risk of malignancy. Bladder, skin, myeloproliferative, and oropharyngeal cancers have been reported more commonly among patients with RA treated with daily cyclophosphamide than among RA patients not treated with cyclophosphamide. Although there is insufficient data to render a quantifiable risk for malignancy following treatment with pulse intravenous cyclophosphamide, few malignancies have been reported in this setting.

Chlorambucil

Chlroambucil and its primary metabolite, phenyl acetic acid mustard, are potent alkylating agents. The clinical effects are comparable to cyclophosphamide, although slower in onset. Chlorambucil does not induce bladder toxicity and is most often used as an alternative to cyclophosphamide when cytotoxic therapy is indicated. It is often the drug of choice to suppress clones of immunoglobulin light chain secreting cells in patients with primary (AL) amyloidosis. The primary toxicity of chlorambucil is that of myelosuppression, which may occur abruptly at anytime during the course of treatment. Although reversible, chlorambucil-induced leukopenia may persist for months following discontinuation of the drug.

Because of the occurrence of precipitous leukopenia in patients taking chlorambucil, frequent surveillance for cytopenia is imperative. Following the initiation of treatment, complete blood counts should be assessed a minimum of every 2 weeks. Once the dose and leukocyte count

are stable, the monitoring interval can be extended to every 4 weeks. The risk of myeloid leukemias as well as lymphomas is increased among patients who have been treated with chlorambucil, an association to be considered should chlorambucil-treated patients develop persistent cytopenia, adenopathy, or otherwise unexplained constitutional symptoms.

Azathioprine and 6-Mercaptopurine

Azathioprine is a purine analog antimetabolite that is converted following ingestion by glutathione-S-transferase and sulfhydryl groups to 6-mercaptopurine. Thiopurine metabolites of 6-mercaptopurine decrease the synthesis of purine nucleotides, resulting in antiproliferative effects, whereas incorporation of thiopurine nucleotides into DNA and RNA results in cytotoxicity. The net immunosuppressive effects of azathioprine and 6-mercaptopurine are comparable, but azathioprine is better tolerated, favoring its use. Although efficacious as a disease-modifying drug in the treatment of rheumatoid arthritis, azathioprine is used most commonly as a steroid-sparing agent in the management of lupus and inflammatory myositis.

The myelosuppressive effects of azathioprine are dose related and vary considerably among individuals. Severe myelosuppression is most often associated with a genetic polymorphism in the activity of thiopurine methyltransferase (TPMT), one of the two enzymes (xanthine oxidase being the other) that convert 6-mercaptopurine to inactive metabolites. TPMT activity has a trimodal distribution, with 90% of the population having normal activity, just under 10% having intermediate activity, and about one in 300 individuals homozygous for poorly functioning TPMT. Median TPMT activity is reported to be lower among blacks than among whites (9). Myelosuppression associated with impaired TPMT appears anywhere from 1 to 3 months following initiation of treatment with azathioprine. While screening for TPMT activity is now available, prudent approaches at present to avoid severe myelosuppression are to carefully follow blood counts in all patients at 2-week intervals following initiation of treatment with azathioprine. Once the target dose has been achieved with stable blood counts, the interval for blood count surveillance can be extended to monthly.

Inhibitors of xanthine oxidase such as allopurinol must be used with extreme caution in patients taking azathioprine. Concomitant use of these two drugs should be avoided if possible by employing alternative immunosuppresants (e.g., mycophenolate, cyclosporine) or alternative urate-lowering drugs (uricosurics). If no effective alternative options exist, the dose of azathioprine should be attenuated 75% to 80% and blood counts should be monitored weekly.

Gastrointestinal symptoms are the most common side effects associated with use of azathioprine. Nausea, vomiting, or diarrhea often responds to dose attenuation followed by more gradual dose increases (25 mg/week) as clinically indicated. It is important to recognize that relative leukopenia is not required to achieve therapeutic immunosuppression with azathioprine. Although severe hepatitis and cholestasis are rare complications of azathioprine use, mild increases in liver enzymes occur in up to 10% of patients. Liver function tests should be checked within the first month of initiating treatment and every 3 to 4 months thereafter. A reasonable approach to patients who develop serum levels of liver transaminases in excess of twice the upper limit of normal is to withhold therapy and reinitiate treatment at a lower dose.

Other rare complications of azathioprine use include acute hypersensitivity syndromes, eosinophilia, drug fever, and drug-induced pancreatitis. The data with regard to any increased risk of malignancy associated with azathioprine use are conflicting. Although not approved for use during pregnancy, favorable outcomes have been reported when azathioprine has been used to manage and suppress the emergence of severe lupus complications through the course of pregnancy.

OTHER IMMUNOMODULATING DRUGS

Cyclosporine

Originally developed and employed to suppress graft rejection in recipients of organ transplants, cyclosporine is also used as a disease-modifying drug in the management of rheumatoid arthritis and other autoimmune disorders, including chronic recurrent anterior uveitis, psoriatic arthritis, and Behçet syndrome. Cyclosporine inhibits the activation of T cells and secretion of interleukin (IL)-2 (a major T-cell growth factor) by forming a cytoplasmic complex with cyclophilin. The resulting complex inactivates a phosphatase (calcineurin) required for the translocation of a factor to the nucleus that activates transcription of IL-2 and other genes associated with activation of T cells.

Although cyclosporine is generally well tolerated, measurable but reversible decreases in renal function occur in most patients treated. A small rise in serum creatinine within the first 3 months of treatment is fairly predictable but often remains stable thereafter. However, an increase in serum creatinine that exceeds 30% of the baseline value portends possible irreversible nephrotoxicity. In such instances the administered dose should be attenuated by 1 mg/kg/day and temporarily discontinued if the serum creatinine remains elevated. Provided the serum creatinine level returns to within 15% of the established baseline level, cyclosporine can be safely restarted at the attenuated dose (10). Hypertension is reported to occur in approximately 20% of patients but can be managed with either attenuation in the dose of cyclosporine or addition of antihypertensive drug therapy.

Other common side effects of cyclosporine include tremor, paresthesia, hypertrichosis, hyperkalemia, hypo-magnesemia, and hyperuricemia. Liver enzyme abnormalities, particularly a rise in serum alkaline phosphatase, occur not uncommonly but are seldom of clinical significance. Although cyclosporine use in recipients of organ transplants has been associated with an increased risk of skin cancer and lymphoma, this association has not been confirmed among smaller cohorts of RA patients treated with cyclosporine.

Mycophenolate Mofetil

Similar to cyclosporine, mycophenolate mofetil is an established therapy for the suppression of graft rejection in organ transplant recipients that is acquiring an expanded role as an immunosuppressant in the management of patients with autoimmune disease. Following ingestion, the drug is hydrolyzed to its active metabolite, mycophenolic acid, an inhibitor of inosine monophosphate dehydrogenase. As lymphocytes are particularly dependent upon this enzyme for de novo synthesis of purines, mycophenolate selectively targets proliferation of T- and B-cell lymphocytes without attendant myelotoxicity.

Although data with regard to tolerability and adverse events in patients with autoimmune disease are presently limited, mycophenolate is generally well tolerated. Most adverse events relate to gastrointestinal intolerance, including nausea, vomiting, diarrhea, and abdominal pain. Because liver enzyme abnormalities may occur, patients taking mycophenolate should have a liver function test performed at baseline, 1 month following initiation of therapy, and every 3 to 4 months thereafter.

Dapsone

Originally employed in the treatment of leprosy, dapsone is a sulfone with significant inhibitory effects on the function of neutrophils. Although there are few controlled trials examining its efficacy, dapsone is most commonly used in the management of cutaneous leukocytoclastic vasculitis, urticarial vasculitis, bullous or ulcerative cutaneous lupus, and orogenital ulcers associated with Behçet syndrome.

Use of dapsone requires attention to dose-dependent effects of the drug on erythrocytes and the potential for drug-induced agranulocytosis. Reversible agranulocytosis affecting as many as one of every 250 individuals may occur during the first 2 months of treatment. Some degree of methemoglobinemia and hemolysis is seen in almost all patients receiving doses of 100 mg daily or higher. Although individual variation exists, the adverse effects of dapsone on red cell membranes are usually well tolerated and often stabilize or resolve after 6 weeks. However, patients deficient in glucose-6-phosphate dehydrogenase are particularly susceptible to hemolysis that may be severe and life-threatening, and it is advisable to prescreen patients for evidence of this deficiency before instituting treatment with dapsone.

TABLE 32.3. SUGGESTED TESTS AND MONITORING INTERVALS FOR PATIENTS TAKING ANTIRHEUMATIC DRUGS

Drug	CBC	AST, ALT	Albumin	Creatinine	Urinalysis	Other
NSAIDs	q 6 mos	First month q 6 mos		First month q 6 mos	q 6 mos	
Hydroxychloroquine		First month q 6 mos				Ocular exam q 6–12 mos
Methotrexate	q 4 wks[a] q 4–8 wks	q 4–8 wks	q 8 wks	q 3–6 mos		Pre-Rx screen for Hepatitis B & C
Sulfasalazine	q 2 wks[a] q 3 mos	First month q 3 mos		q 6 mos	q 6 mos	Pre-Rx screen G-6-PD
Leflunomide		q month				
Aurothioglucose	Each Rx				q mo	
Auranofin	q mo				q mo	
Minocycline and other tetracyclines	q 3 mos	First month q 3 mos		q 3 mos	q 6 mos	
Cyclosporine				q 2 wks[b] q mo		BP q 2 wks[b] BP q mo
Penicillamine	q 2 wks[a] q mo				q mo	
Azathioprine	q 2 wks[a] q mo	First month q 3 mos				
Cyclophosphamide	q 2 wks[a] q mo				q mo	WBC 2 wks p i.v. dose
Mycophenolate	q 3 mos	First month q 3 mos				
Dapsone	q 2 wks[a] q mo	First month q 3 mos				Pre-Rx G-6-PD screen

[a]Until target dose reached and continued for 1 month.
[b]Until target dose reached and continued for 3 months.
ALT, alanine transaminase; AST, aspartate transaminase; BP, blood pressure; CBC, complete blood count; PD, Glucose-6-phosphate dehydrogenase; WBC, white blood cell.

The drug is best tolerated starting with a daily dose of 25 mg and advancing to the target therapeutic dose of 100 mg daily over the course of several weeks. Blood counts should be monitored weekly until the target dose has been achieved for a month, then monthly thereafter. Should a significant fall in hematocrit and hemoglobin levels occur, the drug should be withheld and reintroduced at a lower dose. Liver function tests should be assessed within the first several weeks of treatment, following any dose increments, and periodically every 3 months thereafter. A rare hypersensitivity syndrome characterized by fever, exfoliative rash, jaundice, and hemolysis may occur with dapsone use; patients with this complication should not be retreated.

See Table 32.3 for a list of suggested tests and monitoring intervals for patients taking antirheumatic drugs.

Thalidomide

Following its withdrawal in 1961 due to its well-publicized and dramatic teratogenic effects, thalidomide was reintroduced specifically for the management of erythema nodosum leprosum, presently its only approved indication. Thalidomide has inhibitory effects on the production of tumor necrosis factor-α and has been reported to be efficacious in the treatment of severe mucocutaneous ulcers asso-ciated with Behçet syndrome as well as severe cutaneous lesions associated with lupus, sarcoidosis, and pyoderma gangrenosum. It has also been reported to be of benefit in the management of graft-versus-host disease.

In addition to the known teratogenic effects, peripheral neuropathy is a frequent complication of thalidomide use and, aside from the teratogenic effects, is the major limiting factor in its long-term use. Nerve damage from thalidomide is usually manifest by symmetric, painful paresthesias that often persist despite discontinuation of the drug. Since nerve conduction abnormalities may be noted before the onset of neuropathy symptoms, periodic electrophysiologic testing of peripheral nerves has been advocated for patients receiving thalidomide over extended time intervals, with discontinuation of the drug if neuropathy occurs.

BIOLOGIC TUMOR NECROSIS FACTOR-α ANTAGONISTS

Etanercept

Etanercept is a genetically engineered chimeric molecule comprising two of the human p75-soluble receptors for tumor necrosis factor-α (TNF) adjoined to the Fc portion of a human immunoglobulin G. By binding TNF, etanercept precludes ligation of TNF receptors on effector cells participating in immune and inflammatory responses promoted by this cytokine. Administered as a subcutaneous injection twice weekly, etanercept is predominantly used for the management of rheumatoid arthritis. An expanded role for etanercept is evolving for the management of other rheumatic diseases, including psoriatic arthritis, ankylosing spondylitis, and Behçet syndrome.

Since etanercept is a fully humanized molecule, its overall tolerance is excellent and its use does not require routine laboratory monitoring. Injection site reactions consisting of mild erythema and swelling lasting 1 to 3 days occur in more than one-third of patients but are well tolerated and do not preclude continuation of therapy. Since TNF-α likely plays a role in host defense, patients who are taking etanercept should be cautioned about the occurrence of infection. It is generally advisable to withhold etanercept in the setting of acute bacterial infection, resuming treatment once the infection has resolved with appropriate antibiotic therapy. Postmarketing studies and clinical trials of other anti-TNF agents have documented reactivation of *Mycobacterium tuberculosis* in the setting of anti-TNF therapy. Patients with known previous infection of *M. tuberculosis* who are treated with etanercept should accordingly be monitored closely for signs of reactivation.

Up to 15% of patients taking etanercept are reported to develop new positive antinuclear antibodies, antibodies to double-stranded DNA, or both. Although no patients in premarket controlled clinical trials who developed such antibodies developed clinical manifestations of systemic lupus erythematosus, a number of postmarket case reports have documented the occurrence of demyelinating syndromes following initiation of treatment with etanercept. Although laboratory monitoring for emergence of autoantibodies is unnecessary, etanercept should be discontinued should autoimmune disease manifestations not normally associated with rheumatoid arthritis emerge. These considerations render use of etanercept (or other anti-TNF therapies) inadvisable in patients with systemic lupus erythematosus.

Infliximab and Anti-Tumor Necrosis Factor-α Monoclonal Antibodies

Infliximab is a chimeric monoclonal antibody consisting of a murine domain in the variable region with binding specificity for human TNF-α; the remainder of the antibody is of human origin. Administered by intravenous infusion, infliximab binds and neutralizes secreted TNF-α. Binding of infliximab to cells expressing surface TNF-α may also result in antibody-mediated cytotoxicity. Originally approved for use in patients with severe complications of Crohn disease, infliximab is approved for and most commonly used in the management of rheumatoid arthritis. Fully humanized antibodies to TNF-α have been developed and are anticipated to be of benefit in the management of rheumatoid arthritis. An expanded role for monoclonal anti-TNF reagents in the treatment of other inflammatory diseases is evolving.

Infliximab is well tolerated and routine laboratory monitoring for toxicity is not required. Human antichimeric antibody responses to murine components of the antibody develop in up to 40% of patients given infliximab. Infusion reactions with pruritis, urticaria, and/or chills occur in a very small minority of patients and respond favorably to halting of the infusion and administration of antihistamines. Retreatment of patients who have experienced a serious infusion reaction is not recommended. Although not required for initial efficacy, co-treatment with low-dose weekly methotrexate has been shown to decrease (but not abrogate) human antichimeric antibody responses and extend the duration of infliximab efficacy.

Anti-TNF-α antibodies such as infliximab should not be administered to patients with evidence of active bacterial infection and should be used with caution in patients predisposed to serious bacterial infections. Reported reactivation of tuberculosis in patients given anti-TNF-α reagents emphasizes the need for caution and careful surveillance when administering infliximab or other TNF-α neutralizing antibodies to patients with known prior history of tuberculosis. As occurs with other TNF-α antagonists, administration of anti-TNF-α monoclonal reagents is associated with the development of antinuclear antibodies in a minority of patients. Clinical manifestations of lupus have been reported to occur following administration of infliximab, and anti-TNF-α antibodies are not recommended for use in patients with systemic lupus erythematosus.

REFERENCES

1. Saag KG, Emkey R, Schnitzer TJ, et al. Alendronate for the prevention and treatment of glucocorticoid-induced osteoporosis. *N Engl J Med* 1998;339:292–299.
2. Fries JF. The epidemiology of NSAID gastropathy: the ARAMIS experience. *J Clin Rheumatol* 1998;4(Suppl):S11.
3. Silverstein FE, Graham DY, Senior JR, et al. Misoprostol reduces serious gastrointestinal complications in patients with rheumatoid arthritis receiving nonsteroidal anti-inflammatory drugs. *Ann Intern Med* 1995;123:241.
4. Morgan SL, Baggott JE, Vaughn WH, et al. The effect of folic acid supplementation on the toxicity of low-dose methotrexate in patients with rheumatoid arthritis. *Arthritis Rheum* 1990;33:9.
5. Kremer JM, Alarcon GS, Lightfoot RW Jr, et al. Methotrexate for rheumatoid arthritis: suggested guidelines for monitoring liver toxicity. *Arthritis Rheum* 1994;37:316.
6. Easterbrook M. Detection and prevention of maculopathy associated with antimalarial agents. *Int Ophthalmol Clin* 1999;39:49–57.
7. Blyth C, Lane C. Hydroxychloroquine retinopathy: is screening necessary? *BMJ* 1998;316:716–717.
8. Talar-Williams C, Hijazi YM, Walther MM, et al. Cyclophosphamide-induced cystitis and bladder cancer in patients with Wegener's granulomatosis. *Ann Intern Med* 1996;124:477.
9. McLeod HL, Lin JS, Scott EP, et al. Thiopurine methyltransferase activity in American white subjects and black subjects. *Clin Pharmacol Ther* 1994;55:15.
10. Panayi GS, Tugwell P. The use of cyclosporine A microemulsion in rheumatoid arthritis: conclusions of an international review. *Br J Rheumatol* 1997;36:808.

SUBJECT INDEX

Page numbers followed by "f" indicate figures. Page numbers followed by "t" indicate tables.